Decriminalizing Mental Illness

Decriminalizing Mental Illness

Edited by

Katherine Warburton
Medical Director, California Department of State Hospitals, and Associate Clinical Professor at University of California, Davis, California

Stephen M. Stahl
Professor of Psychiatry, University of California at Riverside and at San Diego, Riverside and San Diego, California

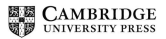

CAMBRIDGE
UNIVERSITY PRESS

University Printing House, Cambridge CB2 8BS, United Kingdom

One Liberty Plaza, 20th Floor, New York, NY 10006, USA

477 Williamstown Road, Port Melbourne, VIC 3207, Australia

314–321, 3rd Floor, Plot 3, Splendor Forum, Jasola District Centre, New Delhi – 110025, India

79 Anson Road, #06–04/06, Singapore 079906

Cambridge University Press is part of the University of Cambridge.

It furthers the University's mission by disseminating knowledge in the pursuit of education, learning, and research at the highest international levels of excellence.

www.cambridge.org
Information on this title: www.cambridge.org/9781108826952
DOI: 10.1017/9781108920698

© Katherine Warburton and Stephen M. Stahl 2021

First published 2021

Printed in the United Kingdom by TJ Books Limited, Padstow Cornwall

A catalogue record for this publication is available from the British Library.

Library of Congress Cataloging-in-Publication Data
Names: Warburton, Katherine D., editor. | Stahl, Stephen M., 1951– editor.
Title: Decriminalizing mental illness / edited by Katherine Warburton, Stephen M. Stahl.
Description: Cambridge ; New York, NY : Cambridge University Press, 2021. | Includes bibliographical references and index.
Identifiers: LCCN 2020031748 (print) | LCCN 2020031749 (ebook) | ISBN 9781108826952 (paperback) | ISBN 9781108920698 (ebook)
Subjects: MESH: Forensic Psychiatry – methods | Commitment of Mentally Ill – legislation & jurisprudence | Criminal Law – methods | Institutionalization | Psychotic Disorders – therapy | Insanity Defense
Classification: LCC RA1148 (print) | LCC RA1148 (ebook) | NLM W 740 | DDC 614/.15–dc23
LC record available at https://lccn.loc.gov/2020031748
LC ebook record available at https://lccn.loc.gov/2020031749

ISBN 978-1-108-82695-2 Paperback

Cambridge University Press has no responsibility for the persistence or accuracy of URLs for external or third-party internet websites referred to in this publication and does not guarantee that any content on such websites is, or will remain, accurate or appropriate.

Every effort has been made in preparing this book to provide accurate and up-to-date information that is in accord with accepted standards and practice at the time of publication. Although case histories are drawn from actual cases, every effort has been made to disguise the identities of the individuals involved. Nevertheless, the authors, editors, and publishers can make no warranties that the information contained herein is totally free from error, not least because clinical standards are constantly changing through research and regulation. The authors, editors, and publishers therefore disclaim all liability for direct or consequential damages resulting from the use of material contained in this book. Readers are strongly advised to pay careful attention to information provided by the manufacturer of any drugs or equipment that they plan to use.

The findings and conclusions in this book are those of the authors and do not necessarily represent the views or opinions of the California Department of State Hospitals or the California Health and Human Services Agency.

Contents

Contributors

Oona Appel
Office of Diversion and Reentry, Los Angeles County Department of Health Services, Los Angeles, CA, USA
and
Department of Psychiatry and Biobehavioral Sciences, David Geffen School of Medicine at UCLA, Los Angeles, CA, USA

Juan Carlos Arguello
Assistant Deputy Director Chief, Office of Medical and Psychiatric Services, Clinical Operations, California Department of State Hospitals, CA, USA

Tyler M. Argüello
California State University, Sacramento, CA, USA

Ai-Li W. Arias
Department of Psychiatry, University of California, Irvine, Patton, CA, USA

Chloe Auletta-Young
Department of Psychiatry University of California, Davis, Sacramento, CA, USA

Allen Azizian
California Department of State Hospitals, Sacramento, CA, USA
and
California State University, Department of Criminology, Fresno, CA, USA

Shannon M. Bader
New Hampshire Department of Corrections, Office of the Forensic Examiner, Centurion Managed Care, Concord, NH, USA

Justin Barry-Walsh
Fixated Threat Assessment Centre New Zealand (FTACNZ) Capital and Coast District Health Board

Andrea Bauchowitz
California Department of State Hospitals, CA, USA

Amanda Beltrani
Department of Psychology, Fairleigh Dickinson University, Teaneck, NJ, USA

Nigel Blackwood
Institute of Psychiatry, Psychology and Neuroscience, King's College London, London, UK

Ashley M. Breth
California Department of State Hospitals, Sacramento, CA, USA

Charles Broderick
California Department of State Hospitals, Sacramento, CA, USA

Clarissa Bush
Zuckerberg San Francisco General Hospital, University of California San Francisco School of Nursing, San Francisco, CA, USA

Alberto Carrara
Pontifical Academy for Life, Rome, Italy
and
Neurobioethics Research Group (GdN), Pontifical Athenaeum Regina Apostolorum, Rome, Italy
and
UNESCO Chair in Bioethics and Human Rights, Rome, Italy
and
Faculty of Psychology, European University of Rome (UER), Rome, Italy

Tim Coffey
Eleventh Judicial Circuit Criminal Mental Health Project, Miami-Dade County, Miami, FL, USA

Michael A. Cummings
Department of Psychiatry, University of California, Riverside, CA, USA
and
Department of Psychiatry, University of California, Irvine, Patton, CA, USA

Brendan Daugherty
University of New South Wales, Sydney, Australia

Kimberlie Dean
School of Psychiatry, University of New South Wales, Australia
and
Justice Health and Forensic Mental Health Network, New South Wales, Australia

Elizabeth Deckler
University of Miami, Miller School of Medicine, Miami, FL, USA

Darci Delgado
California Department of State Hospitals, Sacramento, CA, USA

Charles Dempsey
Crisis Response Support Section, Mental Evaluation Unit, Administration-Training Detail, Los Angeles Police Department, Los Angeles, CA, USA

Sarah L. Desmarais
North Carolina State University, Raleigh, NC, USA

Joel A. Dvoskin
Department of Psychiatry, University of Arizona College of Medicine, Tucson, AZ, USA

Andrew Ellis
School of Psychiatry, Faculty of Medicine, University of New South Wales, Sydney, New South Wales, Australia

Matthew W. Epperson
School of Social Service Administration, University of Chicago, Chicago, IL, USA

Sean E. Evans
California Department of State Hospitals, Clinical Operations, Office of Clinical Research and Program Implementation, Sacramento, CA, USA

Seena Fazel
Department of Psychiatry, University of Oxford, Oxford, UK

William H. Fisher
Senior Consultant, National Association of State Mental Health Program Directors Research Institute, Falls Church, Virginia, USA
and
Adjunct Professor of Psychiatry and Community Health, University of Massachusetts Medical School, Worcester, MA, USA

Mary Gable
Department of Psychiatry, Division of Psychiatry and the Law, University of California, Davis, Sacramento, CA, USA

Anthony Gale
University of California Davis, Davis, CA, USA

W. Neil Gowensmith
The Denver Forensic Institute for Research, Service, and Training (Denver FIRST), Graduate School of Professional Psychology, University of Denver, Denver, CO, USA

Philip D. Harvey
Department of Psychiatry, University of Miami, Miami, FL, USA
and
Bruce W. Carter VA Medical Center, Miami, FL, USA

Shelley Hill
California Department of State Hospitals, Sacramento, CA, USA
and
University of California, Davis, CA, USA

Vera Hollen
Senior Director of Research and Consulting, National Association of State Mental Health Program Directors Research Institute, Falls Church, Virginia, USA

David V. James
Fixated Threat Assessment Centre New Zealand (FTACNZ) Capital and Coast District Health Board

Mackenzie T. Jones
Department of Psychiatry and Behavioral Sciences, University of Miami, Miller School of Medicine, Miami, FL, USA

Elizabeth Kim
Office of Diversion and Reentry, Los Angeles County Department of Health Services, Los Angeles, CA, USA

Scott E. Kirkorsky
Department of Psychiatry, Division of Psychiatry and the Law, University of California, Davis, Sacramento, CA, USA

James L. Knoll
Department of Psychiatry, SUNY Upstate Medical University, Syracuse, NY, USA and Central New York Psychiatric Center, Marcy, NY, USA

Rebecca Kornbluh
California Department of State Hospitals, Sacramento, CA, USA

Kelly Kruger
San Francisco Police Department, San Francisco, CA, USA

H. Richard Lamb
Professor Emeritus of Psychiatry and the Behavioral Sciences, Keck School of Medicine of USC, Los Angeles, CA, USA

Richard Latham
South London and Maudsley NHS Foundation Trust, London, UK

Judge Steven Leifman
Miami-Dade County Court, Eleventh Judicial Circuit of Florida, Miami-Dade County, Miami, FL, USA

Evan M. Lowder
George Mason University, Fairfax, VA, USA

Katherine E. McCallum
The Denver Forensic Institute for Research, Service, and Training (Denver FIRST), Graduate School of Professional Psychology, University of Denver, Denver, CO, USA

Barbara E. McDermott
University of California Davis, Davis, CA, USA

Jonathan M. Meyer
California Department of State Hospitals, Patton, CA, USA

Sean M. Mitchell
Department of Psychiatry, University of Rochester Medical Center, Rochester, New York, USA
and
Department of Psychological Sciences, Texas Tech University, Lubbock, TX, USA

Robert D. Morgan
Department of Psychological Sciences, Texas Tech University, Lubbock, TX, USA

Paul E. Mullen
Fixated Threat Assessment Centre New Zealand (FTACNZ) Capital and Coast District Health Board

Vanessa Nascimento
University of Miami, Miller School of Medicine, Miami, FL, USA

Viet Nguyen
Office of Diversion and Reentry, Los Angeles County Department of Health Services, Los Angeles, CA, USA
and
Department of Psychiatry and Biobehavioral Sciences, David Geffen School of Medicine at UCLA, Los Angeles, CA, USA

Kristen Ochoa
Office of Diversion and Reentry, Los Angeles County Department of Health Services, Los Angeles, CA, USA
and
Department of Psychiatry and Biobehavioral Sciences, David Geffen School of Medicine at UCLA, Los Angeles, CA, USA

Jennifer O'Day
California Department of State Hospitals, Norwalk, CA, USA

Megan Pollock
California Department of State Hospitals, Sacramento, CA, USA

George J. Proctor
Department of Psychiatry, Loma Linda University School of Medicine, Patton, CA, USA

David Pyo
California Department of State Hospitals, CA, USA

Cameron Quanbeck
Cordilleras Mental Health Rehabilitation Center,
San Mateo County Health, San Mateo, CA, USA

Tiffany Rector
California Department of State Hospitals,
Sacramento, CA, USA

Benjamin Rose
California Department of State Hospitals,
Sacramento, CA, USA

Leon Sawh
School of Social Service Administration,
University of Chicago, Chicago, IL, USA

Sophia P. Sarantakos
School of Social Service Administration,
University of Chicago, Chicago, IL, USA

Faith Scanlon
Department of Psychological Sciences,
Texas Tech University, Lubbock, TX, USA

Eric Schwartz
California Department of State Hospitals, Napa, CA,
USA

Charles L. Scott
Department of Psychiatry and Behavioral Sciences,
University of California, Davis, Sacramento, CA,
USA

Mollie Silva
Offices of Joel A. Dvoskin, Ph.D., Tucson, AZ, USA

Sara Singh
School of Psychiatry, University of New South Wales,
New South Wales, Australia

Yin-Lan Soon
Justice Health and Forensic Mental Health Network,
New South Wales, Australia

Stephen M. Stahl
Professor of Psychiatry, University of California at
San Diego, San Diego, CA, USA

and
University of Cambridge, UK

Martin T. Strassnig
Department of Psychiatry, University of Miami,
Miami, FL, USA

Helga Thordarson
California Department of State Hospitals,
Sacramento, CA, USA

Stephanie A. Van Horn
Department of Psychological Sciences,
Texas Tech University, Lubbock, TX, USA

Susan Velasquez
California Department of State Hospitals, CA,
USA

Katherine Warburton
Medical Director, California Department of State
Hospitals and University of California, Davis, CA,
USA

Linda E. Weinberger
Professor Emerita of Clinical Psychiatry and the
Behavioral Sciences, Keck School of Medicine of USC
and
Chief Psychologist, USC Institute of Psychiatry, Law
and Behavioral Sciences, Los Angeles, CA, USA

Amanda Wik
Research Associate, National Association of State
Mental Health Program, Directors Research
Institute, Falls Church, VA, USA

Hannah Kate Williams
Forensic Psychotherapy, South West London and
St. George's Mental Health NHS Trust, London, UK

Denis Yukhnenko
Department of Psychiatry, University of Oxford,
Oxford, UK

Patricia A. Zapf
Division of Continuing and Professional Studies,
Palo Alto University, Palo Alto, CA, USA

Balancing the Pendulum: Rethinking the Role of Institutionalization in the Treatment of Serious Mental Illness

Katherine Warburton and Stephen M. Stahl

The history of serious mental illness (SMI) is grim, from a cultural as well as a treatment perspective. The conditions of individuals with psychotic disorders have swung, like a pendulum, from institutional neglect to community neglect and back again over the past several hundred years.[1-4] At the core of treatment failure is a failure in mental health policy and funding, with the result usually framed as the degree of human institutionalization in jails, prisons, and asylums.[5-7] In the middle of the nineteenth century, institutions designed to deliver moral treatment were considered the humane answer to care properly for the SMI population. By the mid-twentieth century, those same, now overcrowded, institutions were blamed for the horrible conditions of mistreatment of individuals with SMI. Now, as we approach the middle of the twenty-first century, deinstitutionalization (the answer to the cruel asylums) is purportedly at fault for homelessness, lack of treatment, and criminalization. As the pendulum swings, we are hearing cries to "bring back" the asylums.[8]

Care providers currently working in the trenches delivering public mental health services to people with SMI know that society has failed to care adequately for this group. Individuals living with mental illness are now often living on the open streets or incarcerated, and on average die 20 years sooner than the rest of us.[9-12] An examination of the history of the approach to people with SMI across time and geography indicates that we are just one data point on a cyclical pattern of treatment and policy failure through time.[1-4]

Figure 1.1 is an oversimplification but illustrates the issue if you consider the current state of homelessness, criminalization, forensic institutionalization, and incarceration of people living with SMI in the wake of deinstitutionalization. The criminalization crisis is currently reaching the tipping point where it will begin to drive changes in policy. And so, we are at

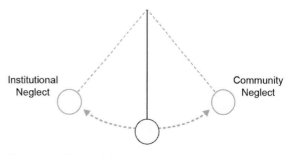

Figure 1.1: The pendulum.

risk of watching the familiar pendulum swing in the same pattern: lock them up, let them out, lock them up. When a society fails to take care of humans with SMI in either setting, the pendulum will continue to swing between these two extremes. The social choices have historically been to either neglect them in state hospitals and prisons or let them fall apart in the community (until such time as they are incarcerated, or dead).

It is a fact, and we must accept it, that 1–2% of the population will develop a SMI. A significant fraction of that population will require high levels of publicly funded care, including medications, housing, and programs to find meaning through human contact. This care will be expensive, and it will be long-term. But it is cheaper than the alternatives.[13]

As leaders in the field of mental health, how do we make provision of that care a priority? In other words, how do we prevent the policy pendulum from continuing to swing between extremes of neglect within institutions and neglect outside of institutions? The institutionalization debate thus far has been whether we should lock up human beings with brain disease. Perhaps we need to broaden our understanding of what institutionalization means.

The term institutionalization has more than one definition. In addition to (1) *the state of being placed or*

Institutional Neglect

Figure 1.2: History of mental health policy.

Community Neglect

Table 1.1 Are we institutionalizing the wrong things?

Deinstitutionalize	Institutionalize
Human beings	Compassion
Clinical certitude	Humility
Treatment ideology	Flexibility
Polarized policymaking	Data collection, simple outcomes
Funding disparities	Responsibility

kept in a residential institution (www.lexico.com), the word also refers to (2) *the act of establishing a new norm in a society* (https://sociologydictionary.org). Using the second definition, let's consider what has been institutionalized by human society vis-à-vis the approach to individuals with psychotic disorders. Medical treatment and psychological interventions have been routinely institutionalized. Whether it be insulin shock therapy, psychoanalysis, lobotomies, or indiscriminate polypharmacy, the mental health field has taken vague conceptual models for approaching this complex and poorly understood condition and institutionalized them to a point where they lack adequate flexibility. To that end, clinical certitude about these treatments is also cyclically institutionalized, only to be later exposed as hubris.

From a social perspective, funding sources, and a lack thereof, have also been institutionalized. Examples include the prohibition against federal reimbursement for inpatient psychiatric treatment, the enduring lack of mental health parity, and the fractured funding streams from local, state, and federal resources, none of which fully address the full continuum of needs required to care for psychotic illnesses. The very process of policymaking has also been institutionalized into an incoherent cacophony of diametrically opposed stakeholders forcing their ideology and certitude into the process, rather than a nuanced approach to balancing paternalism and autonomy, or medicine and recovery, in a way that works in the best interest of this population. The result has been extremes such as unrealistic thresholds for involuntary treatment, the exclusion of individuals with criminal justice involvement from community resources, inadequate prioritization of psychotic disorders by systems at all levels, the overvaluation of privacy over family involvement

and the subsequent unchecked explosion in forensic commitments, and incarceration as a result of all of these factors.[14–16]

And most important, even though this illness impacts 1–2% of the population and virtually everyone knows someone who has fallen victim to a psychotic illness, human society has institutionalized a lack of responsibility for, moral judgement for, and a lack of compassion for people whose brains develop in such a way that they misperceive stimuli and reality. The deinstitutionalization debate needs to include a discussion of letting go of these rigid societal approaches to the 77 million people currently living in the world with SMI. We need to search for ways to institutionalize an ethic of responsibility and compassion for this 1% of our population who, in addition to losing their individual sense of reality as a function of disease, also lose their humanity and dignity as a function of social approaches to the treatment of this disease.

Is it possible to institutionalize compassion? Is it possible to institutionalize clinical flexibility, where mental health clinicians are open to the idea that biopsychosocial interventions of all types (including stable housing) are needed? Is it possible to institutionalize a practice of data collection and analysis, so that if systems are failing (for example a 74% increase in forensic patients in state hospitals) it doesn't take decades to identify and respond?[17] Can we focus on real outcomes, such as lack of engagement with treatment, homelessness, incarceration, arrest, and death; outcomes we know are pervasive?

Can we institutionalize humility? Psychotic syndromes are complex and poorly understood, and no one really knows from one patient to the next what caused or what will improve the symptoms. Yes, we have seen promising advances in neurobiology and psychopharmacology in the last few decades, but this knowledge is useless if the field of medicine fails to recognize our limitations without proper psychosocial support, and if society fails to deliver balanced treatment due to a lack of coherent mental health funding and policy.

But mostly, as a profession and moreover a society, can we institutionalize a sense of responsibility to care for these patients, who are our parents, children, neighbors, and friends? Psychotic disorders are not going away, increasing forensic mental health budgets are not going away, the homelessness issue is not going away, just because we are ignoring it. The knowledge that SMI is characterized by a departure from reality, combined with a lack of insight, means that these individuals need our help. The good news is, there are things that work. With compassion, a sense of responsibility, and a coherent approach, individuals living with SMI can live meaningful lives, for less money than the current state of criminalization.

Once we institutionalize an ethic of compassion and responsibility for the least fortunate members of our society, we will be able to manifest the obvious, logical, economical, and evidence-based continuum of care necessary to balance the pendulum. Once we recognize the limitations of rigid clinical ideology and polarized policymaking, we can create an adequate, balanced, and properly funded system of care. This will prevent fractured mental health systems from continuing to collapse under the weight of the need.

The vision for a continuum is simple: it must address all stages of this relapsing and remitting illness, in the same way that medical care is delivered for other chronic conditions. This is achieved with adequate supplies of acute community hospital beds, crisis services, assertive community treatment, housing, vocational support, peer support, early intervention, therapy, socialization, case management, informed psychopharmacology, and a few straightforward metrics to monitor the need and maintain effectiveness.

In other words, a modern health delivery system that focuses on prevention, takes responsibility for all patients, and has adequate resources when there is a crisis or exacerbation. We have the science and the collective intelligence, we just need the will. As the reader takes in the following material on decriminalizing mental illness, we encourage you to widen the lens beyond this moment in time and consider a new approach to the deinstitutionalization debate. Let's make room in our medical, psychological, advocacy, and academic environments to talk about

changing the ethics of our approach to this disease. Let's also have this conversation in our dining rooms, courtrooms, churches, treatment spaces, and board rooms. We can stop the pendulum, for the first time in history, by creating a responsible and sustained approach to caring for SMI.

References

1. Dvoskin JA, Knoll JL, Silva M. A brief history of the criminalization of mental illness. *CNS Spectr*. 2020; **Mar 20**: 1–13.

2. Scull A. *Madness in Civilization*. London: Thames and Hudson Ltd; 2015.

3. Shorter E. *A History of Psychiatry*. New York: John Wiley & Sons, Inc; 1997.

4. Doughty B, Warburton K, Stahl SM. A social history of psychotic illness. *CNS Spectr*. 2020; **May 12**: 1–9.

5. Penrose IS. Mental disease and crime: outline of a comparative study of European statistics. *Med Psych*. **XVIII**: 1–15.

6. Torrey EF, Kennard AD, Eslinger D, Lamb R, Pavle J. More mentally ill persons are in jails and prisons than hospitals: a survey of the states. Treatment Advocacy Center and National Sheriff's Association; 2010. www.treatmentadvocacycenter.org/storage/documents/final_jails_v_hospitals_study.pdf (accessed June 2020).

7. Lamb HR, Weinberger LE. Persons with severe mental illness in jails and prisons: a review. *Psychiatr Serv*. 1998; **49**(4): 483–492.

8. Sisti DA, Segal AG, Emanuel EJ. Improving long-term psychiatric care: bring back the asylum. *J Am Med Assoc*. 2015; **313**(3): 243–244.

9. Fazel S, Seewald K. Severe mental illness in 33,588 prisoners worldwide: systematic review and meta-regression analysis. *Br J Psychiatry*. 2012; **200**: 364–373.

10. Parks J, Svendsen D, Singer P, Foti ME. Morbidity and mortality in people with serious mental illness. National Association of State Mental Health Program Directors; October 2006. www.nasmhpd.org (accessed June 2020).

11. Druss BG, Zhao L, Von Esenwein S, et al. Understanding excess mortality in persons with mental illness: 17-year follow up of a nationally representative US survey. *Med Care*. 2011; **49**(6): 599–604.

12. Colton CW, Manderscheid RW. Congruencies in increased mortality rates, years of potential life lost, and causes of death among public mental health clients in eight states. *Prev Chronic Dis*. 2006; **3**(2): 1–14.

13. Delgado D, Breth A, Warburton K, Stahl SM. Economics of decriminalizing mental illness: when doing the right thing costs less. *CNS Spectr.* 2020; **Jan 8**: 1–5.

14. Torrey, EF. *American Psychosis: How the Federal Government Destroyed the Mental Illness Treatment System.* New York: Oxford University Press; 2013.

15. Jaffe, DJ. *Insane Consequences.* Amhurst, NY: Prometheus Books; 2017.

16. Powers, R. *No One Cares About Crazy People.* New York: Hachette Books; 2018.

17. Wik A, Hollen V, Fisher W. Forensic patients in state psychiatric hospitals: 1999–2016. *CNS Spectr,* 2020; **25**(2): 196–206.

Deinstitutionalization and Other Factors in the Criminalization of Persons with Serious Mental Illness and How it is Being Addressed

H. Richard Lamb and Linda E. Weinberger

The United States prison population, including both federal and state prisons and county and city jails, was 2,162,400 inmates as of December 31, 2016.[1] The percentage of jail and prison inmates assumed to be seriously mentally ill (as defined in various studies as schizophrenia, schizophrenia spectrum disorder, schizoaffective disorder, bipolar disorder, brief psychotic disorder, delusional disorder, and psychotic disorder, not otherwise specified) has generally been estimated at about 16%.[2] Using these numbers (2,162,400 × 16%) yields an estimate of 345,984 incarcerated persons with serious mental illness (SMI) in jails, and state and federal prisons. The actual number may be somewhat higher or lower, depending on the accuracy of the percentage.

The figures noted above represent a substantial number of persons with SMI in correctional facilities. In a previous era, many more persons with SMI who came to the attention of law enforcement would have been hospitalized rather than arrested and incarcerated.[3] The extent to which persons with SMI have been arrested has significantly impacted both the mental health and criminal justice systems. This phenomenon has been referred to as the "criminalization of the mentally ill."

One of the major concerns in present-day psychiatry is that placement in the criminal justice system poses a number of important problems for and obstacles to the treatment and rehabilitation of persons with SMI.[4,5] Even when quality psychiatric care is provided in jails and prisons, the inmate/patient still has been doubly stigmatized as both a person with mental illness and a criminal. Furthermore, correctional facilities have been established to mete out punishment and to protect society; their primary mission and goals are not to provide treatment. The correctional institution's over-riding need to maintain order and security, as well as its mandate to implement society's priorities of punishment and social control, greatly restricts the facility's ability to establish a therapeutic milieu and provide all the necessary interventions to treat mental illness successfully.[6]

How can we explain these large numbers of people with SMI being arrested and falling under the jurisdiction of the criminal justice system? They come to the attention of law enforcement because they appear to have engaged in illegal behavior. It may well be that they have done so because their mental illness is not being treated adequately in the community. Some of the reasons for this are given in the following sections.

Psychiatric Hospitalization and Deinstitutionalization

Beginning in the late 1950s, the number of hospital beds declined precipitously. For example, in 1955, when the number of patients in state hospitals in the United States reached its highest point, 559,000 persons were institutionalized in state mental hospitals out of a total national population of 165 million (339 beds per 100,000 population). However, by 2016 (as a result of hospital closures and bed eliminations), the number of persons in state mental hospitals dropped to 37,679 for a total population of approximately 324,000,000, or 11.7 beds per 100,000 population. This rate is similar to that found in 1850 when persons with SMI received little care and concern.[7]

What were some of the reasons for the reduction of the number of involuntary psychiatric beds? It was the confluence of the following factors: the introduction of chlorpromazine (Thorazine) and other powerful antipsychotic medications; the development of more efficacious community treatment interventions, such as assertive community treatment (ACT); the creation of federal programs (e.g. SSI, SSDI, Medicaid, and Medicare), which fund community treatment and housing for persons with mental illness; the influence of the civil rights movement; and the high cost of institutionalizing persons with mental illness.[8]

Deinstitutionalization is one of the leading causes that has been viewed as increasing the number of persons with mental illness entering the criminal justice system. The community mental health system was developed in the 1960s and 1970s as a more appropriate setting than psychiatric hospitals to provide treatment for persons with mental illness who had moderate needs and could be maintained in the community. Consequently, the number of public psychiatric hospital beds was reduced with the belief that current and future psychiatric patients could be treated adequately in the community mental health system. Although deinstitutionalization held the promise of persons with SMI being able to live successfully in the community, that outcome did not occur for a sizeable number of people. Part of the reason for the failure was attributed to a lack of planning before or during deinstitutionalization, as well as a lack of adequate funding for the community mental health systems. As a result, many of the important components of a community care system were not sufficiently provided (i.e. housing, medical and psychiatric care, social services, and social and vocational rehabilitation) for the formerly hospitalized patients.

Despite this, the majority of deinstitutionalized patients were able to adapt successfully in the community; however, this was not the case for a substantial minority. Some of these individuals presented challenges in treatment – such as not seeing themselves as mentally ill, not taking their medications, abusing substances, and in many cases, becoming violent when stressed. Many of these persons needed highly structured care to replace that which had been provided to them, albeit imperfectly, in psychiatric hospitals. The flawed implementation of deinstitutionalization would thus appear to be a significant factor accounting for many persons with SMI migrating to jails and prisons as well as to homelessness (between one-fourth and one-third of homeless persons have a SMI).[9]

Initially, concerns about deinstitutionalization tended to focus on those persons with SMI who were discharged into the community after many years of living in state hospitals. However, treating the new generation that has appeared since the implementation of deinstitutionalization policies has proven to be even more difficult.[10] These individuals are different from those who were hospitalized for long periods and who tended to become institutionalized and not experienced in living outside a highly structured setting. When they are placed in a community living situation that has sufficient support and structure to meet their needs, most tend to remain there and to accept treatment. However, this has not been the case for the new generation of persons with SMI; they have not been institutionalized, they have not lived for long periods of time in hospitals and have developed considerable dependence on others, and for the most part they have spent only brief periods in acute care facilities. The lack of community resources capable of adequately treating this challenging new generation of persons with SMI, who often pose difficult clinical problems in treatment and rehabilitation, and may also suffer from homelessness, has contributed to their inappropriate incarceration.

Civil Commitment Criteria

In 1969, California enacted new legislation regarding civil commitment law, known as the Lanterman–Petris–Short Act (LPS). One of the intents of LPS was to "end the inappropriate indefinite and involuntary commitment of mentally disordered persons" (Section 5001 Welfare and Institutions Code). Under LPS, the commitment procedures and criteria were better defined than before; consequently, fewer people were involuntarily committed. Within a decade, every state made similar changes to their civil commitment codes. Such universal and significant changes are virtually unprecedented.

The new civil commitment laws tended to incorporate three major changes. The first change referred to the criteria for involuntary psychiatric hospitalization. The criteria changed from being general in their focus on mental illness and the need for treatment to becoming more specific in addressing how the individual's mental illness contributed to the person's danger to self or others, or the person's ability to care for themselves. The second change impacted the duration of commitment; that is, the length of involuntary psychiatric hospitalization went from an indeterminate period to one with a specific time duration that was often brief. The third change addressed the patient's civil liberty and due process rights to have prompt access to independent hearings and trials, as well as the assistance and representation of patient advocates and attorneys at the various hearings/trials.

These revised civil commitment laws resulted in fewer, as well as shorter, commitments. In fact, many patients who were discharged from the psychiatric hospitals because they no longer met the strict criteria for involuntary hospitalization were released into the community, often without the resources to help them adjust. They may have had difficulties maintaining psychiatric stability, controlling their impulses, living in unstructured community settings, and adapting to the demands of community living. Thus, some of these individuals might have decompensated to the point where they committed criminal acts and entered the criminal justice system.

Community Support Systems Tend to Be Inadequate

Another factor that both leads to and perpetuates the criminalization of persons with SMI is the lack of adequate support systems in the community. This includes mental health treatment, case management, housing, and rehabilitation resources. The inadequacy of these support systems has three important aspects.

First, given the very large numbers of persons with SMI in the community, there may not be sufficient resources to serve them. For instance, case management has come to be viewed as one of the essential components of an adequate mental health program.[11] However, the mental health system is ill prepared to provide quality case management services to all persons with SMI who require it, including those leaving jails and prisons.

Second, the community treatment services that are available may be inappropriate for some of the population to be served. For example, there may be an expectation that persons with SMI go to the clinic when in fact a large proportion of them need outreach services.

Third, persons with SMI who have been released from correctional facilities may not be accepted into community treatment or housing, even when it is available. Clinicians may not want to treat this population because they are thought to be resistant to treatment, dangerous, and serious substance abusers.

These individuals can be intimidating because of previous violent and fear-inspiring behavior. Working with this group is very different from helping passive, formerly institutionalized patients adapt quietly to life in the community. Thus, these are individuals who generally may not be considered desirable by most community agencies and staff. Moreover, some of these agencies may not have the capability to provide the structure and limit setting necessary to enhance safety for staff who work with these persons.

A Difficult Population

A large proportion of persons with SMI who commit criminal offenses are found to be highly resistant to psychiatric treatment. They may refuse referral, may not keep appointments, may not be adherent with psychiatric medications, may not abstain from substance abuse, and may refuse appropriate housing placements. There is evidence that many of these persons suffer from a disorder called anosognosia (a biologically based inability to recognize that one has a mental illness, and thus a biologically based lack of insight).[12] Consequently, such individuals are less likely to believe they need treatment and seek it when needed.

It should also be mentioned that some researchers suggest that criminogenic factors are a stronger predictor for criminal recidivism than mental illness.[13] On the other hand, active psychosis has been found to be a risk factor for violent behavior, independent of criminogenic factors such as antisocial personality characteristics or substance abuse.[14]

The Plight of Family Members

Generally, family members can be an important source of support for persons with SMI. However, they will have to overcome a number of hurdles. These include coping with the symptoms of their relative's mental illness, dealing with their own emotions (e.g. frustration, denial, anxiety, guilt, feeling inadequate), and ambivalence about involving the police when the relative is violent.[15] Given the many obstacles in dealing with their relatives with SMI, as well as obtaining treatment for them, family members may feel overwhelmed and discouraged in their attempt to help their loved ones. As mentioned earlier, these challenges include not being able to obtain adequate involuntary treatment because of the insufficient number of inpatient psychiatric beds, as well as the increasingly restrictive civil commitment criteria. In addition, community treatment services may not be sufficient in addressing the needs of the mentally impaired relative. Moreover, the nature of the individual's mental illness, which may also include substance abuse disorders, may pose additional problems for both the family and their relative with SMI. Finally, resistance to obtaining treatment is a common phenomenon among those with SMI and thus can contribute to the family's frustration, which results from their inability to resolve their relative's problems.

Police and Criminalization

Police play an important role in the criminalization of persons with SMI. Often, instead of directing the individual with mental illness to treatment, the person may be arrested and placed in jail.[16] There are several reasons for this.

When urgent situations arise in the community involving persons with mental illness, the police are typically the first responders.[17] Consequently, they play a major role as a mental health resource in determining what to do with the individuals they encounter. The police have dual roles. They are responsible for recognizing the need for the treatment of an individual with mental illness and connecting the person with the proper treatment resources, as well as making the determination whether the individual has committed a type of illegal act for which the person should be arrested. These responsibilities thrust them into the position of primary gatekeepers who determine if the individual will enter the mental health or the criminal justice system.

For many years, police have had the legal authority to transport persons with SMI whom they believe are a danger to self, others, or gravely disabled to psychiatric institutions for involuntary treatment. This authority forces police to make decisions about the individual's mental condition and welfare. Police also have the discretion to use informal tactics, such as attempting to calm the individual by talking to them or taking them home instead of transporting them to a psychiatric hospital.

Generally, the police have a great deal of discretion in determining what to do when they encounter a person with acute mental illness in the community. In some cases, however, public policy limits the police officer's discretionary power. For instance, if the person with mental illness is alleged to have committed

a major crime, the disposition is clear – that person is taken to jail because of the seriousness of the offense. However, in cases where persons with SMI are believed to have committed a minor offense, the officer may use discretion; that is the officer may arrest the individual, transport the individual to an inpatient psychiatric facility for treatment, or refer the individual to an outpatient clinic for mental health treatment. A major issue is that law enforcement officers do not have the training and experience that mental health professionals have in recognizing symptoms of mental illness in their determination of dispositions.[18] Mental illness may appear to the police as simply alcohol or drug intoxication, especially if the person with mental illness has been using these substances at the time of the interaction with the police. Moreover, in the heat and confusion of an encounter with the police and other citizens, which may include forcibly subduing the person with mental illness, signs of a psychiatric disorder may go unnoticed.

Another major issue contributing to the criminalization of persons with SMI is that even if the police recognize the individual's need for treatment, treatment services are not always available. For example, there are often very few accessible hospital beds for psychiatric inpatients; however, the police are well aware that if they arrest a person with mental illness, that person will be dealt with in a more systematic and predictable way under the criminal justice system.

Efforts to Address the Criminalization of Persons with SMI

Diversion from the Criminal Justice System

There have been extensive efforts to divert persons with SMI from the criminal justice system to the mental health system. Diversion before the person is actually booked into jail, or pre-booking diversion, has gained recent attention and is exemplified by large-scale efforts to create community mobile crisis teams of police officers and/or mental health professionals.

A number of jurisdictions use sworn police officers who have special and extensive mental health training to provide crisis intervention services as part of crisis intervention teams (CIT programs) and to act as liaisons to the mental health system.[19] This approach is often referred to as the "Memphis model" because it was developed in

Memphis, Tennessee. These specially trained officers may deal with mental health emergency situations on-site or act as consultants to the officers at the scene. This model places a heavy reliance on psychiatric emergency services that have agreed to a "no refusal policy" for persons brought to them by the police. Although this strategy has a close liaison with mental health, it does not require the actual participation of mental health professionals in the field.

In addition, mental health training for all law enforcement officers, and not only those who are on mobile crisis teams, may help them gain a better understanding of mental illness and result in their seeking treatment for such individuals rather than arresting them. The interventions of mobile crisis teams and law enforcement education of mental illness can reduce the number of people who previously may have been arrested and entered the criminal justice system.[20]

However, not all people with mental illness are diverted by law enforcement officers prior to booking. For those who are arrested and taken to jail, post-booking diversion occurs through a variety of other forms. These include specialized mental health courts that handle exclusively offenders with mental illness. Mental health consultation to other courts may also assist the judge by offering recommendations for treatment in lieu of incarceration.

Mental Health Courts

Post-booking diversion strategies are being used increasingly by special courts called mental health courts.[21] The first widely known mental health court was established in Broward County, Florida, in 1997. Since then, the number of mental health courts in the United States has increased greatly. Initially, these courts were set up to hear cases of persons with mental illness who were typically charged with misdemeanors, but now also include those charged with felonies. In mental health courts, all the courtroom personnel (i.e. judge, prosecutor, defense counsel, and other relevant professionals) have experience and training in mental health issues and available community resources. These mental health courts have a particular set of characteristics: they hear specialized cases involving defendants with mental illness; they use a nonadversarial team of professionals (e.g. judge, attorneys, and mental health clinician); they are linked to the mental health system that will

provide treatment; and they use some form of adherence monitoring that may involve sanctions by the court.

Underlying the concept of mental health courts is the principle of therapeutic jurisprudence, which emphasizes that the law should be used, whenever possible, to promote the mental and physical well-being of the people it affects. The concept of therapeutic jurisprudence operates on the belief that the application of the law can have therapeutic consequences.[22] It should be emphasized that therapeutic jurisprudence does not diminish the importance of public safety, which is fully taken into account by the court.

Under the tenets of therapeutic jurisprudence, people with SMI charged with crimes may be diverted into programs designed to address their treatment and service needs rather than simply being incarcerated, with their treatment needs either being neglected or not fully addressed. Even individuals with SMI convicted of serious crimes can be provided with humane and appropriate treatment while incarcerated. Generally, mental health courts facilitate linking offenders with SMI to appropriate needed services and supports on discharge from jail in order to enable them to successfully re-enter their communities.

Mental health courts were developed as a strategy to divert persons with mental illness from the criminal justice system into the mental health system. When offenders with mental illness are arrested, their case may be handled by mental health courts in lieu of traditional courts. Mental health courts work in a collaborative effort among the personnel in the criminal justice and mental health systems to devise, coordinate, and implement a treatment plan that includes medications, therapy, housing, and social and vocational rehabilitation, all in an effort to address the individual's mental illness and reduce the risk of recidivism.

Mental Health Consultation to the Court

In non-mental-health courts, the use of mental health consultation for persons with SMI who are being tried for criminal offenses may be helpful in influencing the court's disposition. By providing mental health evaluation, it may become clear to the court what factors may have played a role in the defendant's criminal behavior. If these appear to be more likely the result of inadequate treatment regarding the individual's mental illness rather than the person's criminal tendencies, the court may be inclined to place the individual in a mental health treatment program instead of jail or prison.

Clearly, the quality of services plays an influential role in the success of mental health courts. However, as seen in the past, community psychiatric treatment, rehabilitation, and housing capabilities have been historically insufficient to accommodate all persons with SMI. Will the necessary resources be provided for those who are diverted? Can the mental health system expand adequately to what is needed to serve this particular population? Another question is whether those in the mental health system would be willing to work with those who are diverted from the criminal justice system, given their denial of illness and tendency for many to be violent.

Outpatient Treatment to Reverse or Prevent Criminalization

In order to decriminalize persons with SMI, it is necessary to find ways to help them become stabilized outside of jails and prisons and, to the extent possible, not enter the criminal justice system at all. Thus, the community treatment of persons with SMI who are or may become offenders has developed into an increasingly important and urgent issue. Many criminalized persons with SMI can be treated at mainstream mental health clinics on their release from jails and prisons, especially those who were arrested for non-dangerous and minor crimes.

Moreover, it must be acknowledged that there are a number who are discharged from correctional institutions who have multiple problems that cannot be adequately treated in traditional community-based facilities. This would include persons with SMI who have a history of violence. Rather, these individuals need special, highly structured and adequately secured (metal detectors, alarm buttons, security personnel) clinics staffed by professionals who understand dangerous offenders with mental illness and are willing to provide treatment to them. Usually, these clinics are an actual part of the criminal justice system (e.g. run by parole departments).

Finally, it should not be assumed that persons with SMI engage in criminal behavior solely as a result of their mental illness; there may be other influencing factors such as antisocial characteristics or situational circumstances (e.g. poverty, homelessness). If so, the following treatment interventions may not be very effective in reducing their criminal recidivism, unless concerted efforts are made to modify those particular risk factors, if possible.

Treatment of Co-occurring Disorders

It is estimated by professionals and other personnel in the criminal justice system who are knowledgeable about incarcerated persons with SMI that many of them also meet criteria for substance use disorders.[23] Clearly, if treatment after release is to be successful, both the mental illness and the substance abuse must be addressed. These services should be integrated in the community for the released offender. Treatment of co-occurring disorders very frequently needs to be a long-term process.

Assisted Outpatient Treatment

An important treatment modality that is available in almost all of the states is assisted outpatient treatment (AOT). AOT is an outpatient court-ordered civil commitment initiated by the mental health system and not the criminal justice system. The purpose of AOT is to ensure that persons with mental illness and a history of hospitalizations or violence participate in services in the community that are appropriate to their needs.[24] AOT is for persons with mental illness who are capable of living in the community with the help of family, friends, and mental health professionals, but have a history of and are presently resistant to psychiatric treatment, including medications. Without such treatment, they may continue to relapse and become violent and/or dangerous to themselves and require involuntary hospitalization. Because of these characteristics, this population is also prone to be arrested, incarcerated, and criminalized. To prevent recurrent decompensation, these persons with SMI can be ordered to participate in outpatient psychiatric treatment, with their progress closely monitored by the court.

For AOT to be successful, intensive and evidence-based practices of treatment should be used. These include assertive community treatment (ACT) and forensic assertive community treatment (FACT). ACT is a community-based program with mobile mental health treatment teams that provide an array of treatment, rehabilitation, and housing services that are available 24 hours a day. Although similar to ACT, FACT is for individuals who have been convicted of crimes and includes legal leverage from the criminal justice agencies (e.g. adding probation officers to the treatment team, use of court sanctions to encourage participation) in an effort to reduce recidivism.[25] The goal of ACT and FACT is to help persons with SMI stay out of the hospital and avoid incarceration, as well as develop skills for living in the community.

Working in Collaborative Efforts

Not all persons with SMI who have a history of incarceration are obtaining treatment in the community with ACT or FACT. There are many who are being released from jail or prison on probation or parole and are required to attend outpatient treatment in community mental health clinics. Given these requirements, agents of the criminal justice system, including probation and parole officers, as well as judges, are vested in knowing the mental health status of the client. Consequently, the treating mental health clinicians may be asked to communicate directly with these justice personnel regarding the client's psychiatric condition and progress, as well as the client's potential threat of harm. Similarly, clinicians may want to obtain information about their clients' criminal history in order to better understand the extent of their clients' problems. Therefore, clinicians should feel comfortable maintaining a liaison with the criminal justice personnel.

The Importance of Structure

The need for structure is an essential concept for persons with SMI. Often, they lack internal controls and have difficulty coping with stressful life demands. Structure provides external controls and organization which is needed by these individuals. Generally, mental health professionals who treat this population believe that their patients' days should be structured through meaningful, therapeutic activities such as work, day treatment, and various forms of social therapy.

Another form of structure that is essential for most of this population is that treatment be mandatory, and compliance be reviewed by the court or other criminal justice agent. Knowing that their community status may be revoked can be an influential factor in motivating these clients to adhere to treatment.

Management of Violence

Not all persons with SMI who are incarcerated have been convicted of violent offenses or have a history of violence. However, for those who do, the need for them to control their impulses and inappropriate expressions of anger should be a priority in treatment. Persons whose violence is rooted in a major mental illness often experience their violence as a frightening loss of control. A clinician who is not aware of their destructive potential may be perceived as unable to protect them. They tend to establish that knowledge by testing the clinician for limits. Therefore, the clinician must not only be aware of their potential for violence, but must also be continuously alert and firm in order not to risk being perceived as uncaring and unable to protect their patient from their destructiveness.

Persons with SMI, especially those with histories of violent behavior, generally need continuous rather than episodic care, as well as adherence to psychiatric medications. Thus, regular monitoring is needed, especially when symptoms are absent or at a low ebb, in order to deal with individual and situational factors that may arise and result in violence. In addition, behavioral, cognitive, and psychoeducational techniques emphasizing anger management have been widely used and have been successful in the treatment and management of violence.

Therapeutic Living Arrangements

An important factor in determining community survival for the majority of persons with SMI appears to depend on an appropriately supportive and structured living arrangement.[26] Often, this can be provided by family members. In many cases, however, the kind and degree of structure the client needs can be found only in a living arrangement outside of the family home with a high staff–patient ratio, dispensing of medication by staff, enforcement of curfews, and therapeutic activities that structure most of the client's day.

Working with the Family

The role of family members or significant others can be critical in the treatment of offenders with mental illness. However, their involvement may not always be possible. The treatment team should determine whether these individuals were the victims of the client's aggression, whether they have maintained contact with the client, and whether they are able and interested in continuing such contact.

Clinicians should help family members in understanding the client's mental condition, teach them to recognize symptoms of decompensation, emphasize the importance of self-protection, and explain the client's current legal situation.

24-Hour Structured Inpatient Care

Community treatment is not necessarily the most efficacious or benign intervention at all times for all people with SMI.[10] There is a substantial minority who need the structure and support of acute, intermediate, or long-term care in a hospital setting or a highly structured, locked 24-hour care community facility. Providing access to care in psychiatric facilities when needed and for as long as required is absolutely essential if deinstitutionalization and the reduction of criminalization are to be successful.

A Final Word

In this time of extreme overcrowding in our jails and prisons, decarceration has become a necessity. Inmates with SMI have been included in those released from correctional facilities. Acknowledging that sufficient treatment resources did not exist following deinstitutionalization and that this contributed to the criminalization of persons with SMI, we are now at a place where we can aim to prevent the recurrence of this event. Mental health professionals are poised to provide persons with SMI the mental health treatment and supportive social services that were lacking for so many, and thus leading to their decompensation and criminal behavior. If the goals of reducing the criminalization of persons with SMI are to be accomplished, the mental health and criminal justice systems must be provided with all the necessary resources and funding, as mentioned in this chapter, to identify and treat these individuals in the most appropriate setting. It cannot be emphasized enough that the criminal justice system should not be used as a substitute for the mental health system in the treatment of persons with SMI.

Disclosures

Regarding disclosures of financial or other potential conflicts of interest, there are none for H. Richard Lamb or Linda E. Weinberger.

References

1. Kaeble D, Cowhig M. Correctional populations in the United States, 2016. US Department of Justice, Office of Justice Programs, Bureau of Justice Statistics; 2018. www.bjs.gov/content/pub/pdf/cpus16.pdf (accessed June 2020).

2. Torrey EF, Kennard AD, Eslinger D, Lamb R, Pavle J. More mentally ill persons are in jails and prisons than hospitals: a survey of the states. Treatment Advocacy Center; 2010. www.treatmentadvocacycenter.org/storage/documents/final_jails_v_hospitals_study.pdf (accessed June 2020).

3. Lamb HR, Weinberger LE. Decarceration of our jails and prisons: where will persons with serious mental illness go? *J Am Acad Psychiatry Law*. 2014; **42**(4): 489–494.

4. Olley MC, Nichols TL, Brink, J. Mentally ill individuals in limbo: obstacles and opportunities for providing psychiatric services to corrections inmates with mental illness. *Behav Sci Law*. 2009; **27**(5): 811–831.

5. Blevens, KR, Soderstrom, IR. The mental health crisis grows on: a descriptive analysis of DOC systems in America. *J Offender Rehabil*. 2015; **54**(2): 142–160.

6. Adams, K. Ferrandino, J. Managing mentally ill inmates in prisons. *Crim Justice Behav*. 2008; **35**(8): 913–927.

7. Torrey EF, Fuller DA, Geller J, Jacobs C, Ragosta K. No room at the inn: trends and consequences of closing public psychiatric hospitals 2005–2010. Treatment Advocacy Center; 2012. www.treatmentadvocacycenter.org/storage/documents/no_room_at_the_inn-2012.pdf (accessed June 2020).

8. Harcourt BE. Mass incarceration: causes, consequences, and exit strategies. Reducing mass incarceration: lessons from the deinstitutionalization of mental hospitals in the 1960s. *Ohio St J Crim L*. 2011; **9**: 53–88.

9. Folsom DP, Hawthorne W, Lindamer L, et al. Prevalence and risk factors for homelessness and utilization of mental health services among 10,340 patients with serious mental illness in a large public mental health system. *Am J Psychiatry*. 2005; **162**(2): 370–376.

10. Lamb HR, Bachrach LL. Some perspectives on deinstitutionalization. *Psychiatr Serv*. 2001; **52**(8): 1039–1045.

11. Anthony WA, Cohen M, Farkas M, Cohen B. Clinical care update: the chronically mentally ill – case management – more than a response to a dysfunctional system. *Community Ment Health J*. 2000; **36**(1): 97–106.

12. Lehrer DS, Lorenz J. Anosognosia in schizophrenia: hidden in plain sight. *Innov Clin Neurosci.* 2014; **11** (5–6): 10–17.

13. Andrews DA, Bonta J, Wormith SJ. The recent past and near future of risk and/or need assessment. *Crime Delinq.* 2006; **52**(1): 7–27.

14. Lamberti, JS. Understanding and predicting criminal recidivism among adults with psychotic disorders. *Psychiatr Serv.* 2007; **58**(6): 773–781.

15. Rowaert S, Vandevelde S, Lemmens G, et al. The role and experiences of family members during the rehabilitation of mentally ill offenders. *Int J Rehabil Res.* 2016; **39**: 11–19.

16. Lamb HR, Weinberger LE, DeCuir WJ. The police and mental health. *Psychiatr Serv.* 2002; **53**(10): 1266–1271.

17. Patch PC, Arrigo BA. Police officer attitudes and use of discretion in situations involving the mentally ill: the need to narrow the focus. *Int J Law Psychiatry.* 1999; **22**(1): 23–35.

18. Lurigio AJ, Smith A, Harris A. The challenge of responding to people with mental illness: police officer training and special programmes. *Police J.* 2008; **81**(4): 295–322.

19. Compton MT, Bahora M, Watson AC, Oliva JR. A comprehensive review of extant research on crisis intervention team (CIT) programs. *J Am Acad Psychiatry Law.* 2008; **36**(1): 47–55.

20. Ritter C, Teller JLS, Marcussen K, Munetz MR, Teasdale B. Crisis intervention team officer dispatch, assessment, and disposition: interactions with individuals with severe mental illness. *Int J Law Psychiatry.* 2011; **34**(1): 30–38.

21. Redlich AD. The past, present, and future of mental health courts. In: Wiener RL, Brank EM, eds. *Problem Solving Courts: Social Science and Legal Perspectives.* New York: Springer; 2013: 147–163.

22. Wexler DB, Winnick BJ. Therapeutic jurisprudence as a new approach to mental health law policy analysis and research. *Univ Miami Law Rev.* 1991; **45**(5): 979–1004.

23. Peters HP, Wexler KW, Lurigio AJ. Co-occurring substance use and mental disorders in the criminal justice system: a new frontier of clinical practice and research. *Psychiatr Rehabil J.* 2015; **38**(1): 1–6.

24. Swartz MS, Wilder CM, Swanson JW, et al. Assessing outcomes for consumers in New York's assisted outpatient treatment program. *Psychiatr Serv.* 2010; **61**(10): 976–981.

25. Lamberti SJ, Deem A, Weisman RL, LaDuke C. The role of probation in forensic assertive community treatment. *Psychiatr Serv.* 2011; **62**(4): 418–421.

26. Slate RN, Buffington-Vollum JK, Johnson WW. *Criminalization of Mental Illness, 2nd edn.* Durham, NC: Carolina Academic Press; 2013.

A Brief History of the Criminalization of Mental Illness

Joel A. Dvoskin, James L. Knoll, and Mollie Silva

Introduction

For a very long time, mental illness was viewed not as a disease, but as a manifestation of evil spirits.[1] Confusion and apprehension have been the legacy view of mental illness, even as far back as ancient Greece. In 380 B.C., Socrates wrote in *The Republic* that "The offspring of the inferior...will be put away in some mysterious, unknown place, as they should be." During the middle ages, an obsession with evil in the form of witches became prominent. The official practice guidelines for detecting evil and witches, the *Malleus Maleficarum* (1486), assisted inquisitors in finding evil lurking amidst women, the socially disenfranchised, and those suffering from mental illness.[2] In 1494, theologian Sebastian Brant wrote *The Ship of Fools,* which detailed the phenomenon of sending away persons with mental illness aboard cargo ships through the canals of Europe and overseas. During the Renaissance (fourteenth to seventeenth centuries) families were expected to care for relatives with mental illness, which often involved confinement in the home.[3] Lay concepts of evil often fuse with professional ethics of mental illness, and threaten to confound each other's ideologies.[4] Even today, there remains a deeply ingrained societal prejudice that persons with mental illness are "ticking time bombs, ready to explode into violence."[5] Thus, the primitive association between mental disorder and moral depravity has yet to be completely dissolved. The age-old concept that depravity is somehow involved in the origin of mental disease lingers in the shadows and waits to be resurrected.[6,7]

In 1656, the first Hôpital-Général was opened in Paris. These institutions were for the "insane" (sic), as well as those deemed to pose a threat to normality and progress. Within three years, the Hôpital-Général in Paris became home to more than 6000 people – approximately 1% of the French population. In London, the famous Bethlem Hospital began showing its patients off for a price in 1815. The hospital earned an annual revenue from this weekly event of almost 400 pounds from 96,000 visitors who came (the equivalent today of a little more than US $44,000).

Early in the nineteenth century, the idea of "moral treatment" came to the United States. According to Patricia D'Antonio of the University of Pennsylvania, "The moral treatment of the insane was built on the assumption that those suffering from mental illness could find a way to recovery and an eventual cure if treated kindly and in ways that appealed to the parts of their minds that remained rational. It repudiated the use of harsh restraints and long periods of isolation that had been used to manage the most destructive behaviors of mentally ill individuals. It depended instead on specially constructed hospitals that provided quiet, secluded, and peaceful country settings; opportunities for meaningful work and recreation; a system of privileges and rewards for rational behaviors; and gentler kinds of restraints used for shorter periods."[8]

Moral treatment led to the asylum movement, which was based on a belief that separation from the community, coupled with long periods of rest, would allow the person to regain their senses and faculties.[9] It was not uncommon that a stay in an asylum lasted a lifetime, resulting in a severely restricted existence and limited exposure to life beyond the walls of the institution.[10]

Initially, the moral treatment philosophy and the asylums that practiced it were reserved for those who could afford this kind of care. In 1841, Dorothea Dix, while teaching in a Massachusetts jail, observed that a high number of inmates were not criminals, but people with mental illnesses. During the 1850s and 1860s, she travelled the country urging states to create public asylums, practicing moral treatment, that would be available to people who could not afford private care. By the end of the nineteenth century, every state had such a public institution.[11] Unfortunately, those facilities quickly became incredibly large and over-crowded, resulting in conditions that were nothing like those envisioned by Dorothea Dix and other advocates.[12]

Clearly, the problem of criminalization of mental illness is not a new one. The reality that initially motivated Dorothea Dix to action (i.e. the large numbers of people with mental illness in jails) is remarkably similar to the situation in which we find ourselves today, where the prevalence of mental illness in jails is significantly higher than for the population in general.[13,14]

From the mid to late 1800s, public advocacy drew national attention to the plight of persons confined in institutions. *Isaac Ray,* a founder of forensic psychiatry in the U.S., advocated for clarification of civil commitment laws. Despite this, civil commitment laws were commonly misused, as in the 1860 case of *Elizabeth Packard* who was committed to an institution for the insane based on an Illinois statute which allowed husbands to commit their wives for reasons other than mental illness. Many of the long-term civilly committed patients may not have been mentally ill at all. Most importantly, the effects of trauma were poorly understood. Women were especially vulnerable to psychiatric commitment when they rebelled against their husbands, including cases where the husband was physically abusive.[15]

From about the 1870s to 1920s, eugenics and biological theories of crime regarded habitual criminality as a form of intellectual disability.[16] Eugenic "segregation" in public institutions for "defectives" and "the feebleminded" was pervasive.

In the decades following the Civil War there was a gradual return to more relaxed procedural standards and physician decision-making in terms of commitment. Psychiatric hospitalization was available only on an involuntary basis until 1881 when Massachusetts enacted the first state law that allowed persons to admit themselves voluntarily. However, the standards for admission were lax and subsequently began to receive greater scrutiny. In 1917, the Minnesota's Children's Code was enacted as a package of laws that affirmed the state's role as protector of disadvantaged children who were defined as "defectives," and thus a "public menace." The Code empowered probate judges to commit "defectives" (defined as feebleminded, inebriate, and/or insane) to state guardianship, regardless of the wishes of parents or family. As wards of the state, committees could not vote, own property, or make their own medical decisions. By 1923, nearly 43,000 individuals were confined in custodial institutions for "the feebleminded." It was not until 1942 that the U.S. Supreme Court ruled that punitive sterilization was unconstitutional in *Skinner v. Oklahoma*, yet the decision left "eugenic" sterilization laws intact. By 1946, President Truman signed the National Mental Health Act – which created the NIMH and allocated Government funds toward research into the causes of and treatments for mental illness.

In 1952 the antipsychotic effects of chlorpromazine (Thorazine) were discovered, and led to a much more optimistic view about the ability of doctors to treat the symptoms of psychosis. For a variety of reasons beyond the scope of this article, the promise of Thorazine exceeded its performance. The presence of severe and disfiguring side effects (especially tardive dyskinesia) led many people to resist taking this medication, and for those who did take it, the results were not always satisfactory. Nevertheless, the promise of this drug and its progeny ushered in an era of optimism that would help to fuel a movement to move people out of institutions and into the community.

That same year, the U.S. Government's Draft Act Governing Hospitalization of the Mentally Ill was published. The Draft Act proposed two criteria for involuntary commitment: (1) a risk of harm to self or others, and (2) the need for care or treatment when mental illness rendered someone lacking in insight or capacity and therefore unable to seek voluntary hospitalization.

At about the same time, the treatment of people with mental retardation (now called developmental and intellectual disabilities) was decried as inhumane warehousing of people who posed little or no risk to public safety. The Willowbrook State School in Staten Island, NY, became a national symbol of disgrace. Among the many horrors uncovered at Willowbrook were physical violence, use of persons with intellectual disabilities for medical research without consent, understaffing, overcrowding, and a virtually complete lack of education and habilitative programs. Once these atrocities came to light, the residents of Staten Island filed a 1972 class action that was finally resolved by a consent decree in 1975. Not coincidentally, federal policy was changed by Willowbrook as well. For example, the Protection and Advocacy System for Persons with Disabilities was created in 1975, and in 1980, Congress passed the Civil Rights of Institutionalized Persons Act, which continues to hold various mental hygiene and correctional institutions accountable to this day.[17]

As the inhumane institutional conditions became clear to the public, public sentiment and eventual involvement of the Federal Courts made it clear that the conditions of confinement for committed psychiatric patients were going to become much more expensive. As a result, there were two powerful tides at work moving toward deinstitutionalization: human rights and money.

In 1960, attorney-physician Morton Birnbaum published a seminal article, "The Right to Treatment,"[18] advancing the "revolutionary thesis" that each mental patient had a legal right to such treatment as would give him "a realistic opportunity to be cured or to improve his mental condition." Failing that, Birnbaum argued, the patient should be able "to obtain his release at will in spite of the existence or severity of his mental illness." Birnbaum saw right to treatment as a way to impel improved hospital treatment.[19] He advocated for a standard of care for state hospitals, which involved improvements such as better staffing ratios and ending overcrowding. He believed such standards could be enforced (given) adequate federal funding.[20]

Change and intended reformation was the theme of this period, with Thomas Szasz publishing *The Myth of Mental Illness*,[21] and Erving Goffman publishing *Asylums: Essays on the Social Situation of Mental Patients and Other Inmates*.[22] The 1960s–1970s was a period of substantial sociocultural change in which civil rights took center stage. On an even grander scale, the attention to human rights occurred in the context of radical changes in regard to the civil rights of African Americans (and later other marginalized and disenfranchised groups). The Civil Rights Act of 1964 emphasized ideals of equal rights, freedom from government intrusions, the right to procedural protections when individual liberty was at stake, and outlawed discrimination on the basis of race, color, religion, sex, or national origin.[23]

Deinstitutionalization and the Decline of Civil Commitment

Thus began the process of deinstitutionalization in Western countries – the process of replacing long-stay psychiatric hospitals with less isolated community mental health services. Deinstitutionalization was driven by many factors, including:

- Socio-political movement for community mental health services
- The advent of psychotropic medications
- Class action lawsuits on behalf of institutionalized patients
- The rising cost of constitutionally adequate inpatient care
- Financial imperatives to shift costs from state to federal budgets
- Civil rights movements that asserted constitutional rights for certain classes of people

Civil commitment has dramatically decreased over the past 40 to 50 years. A 40-year review of case law in Oregon found that Oregon Court of Appeals rulings significantly contributed to a dramatic reduction in civil commitment.[24] Beginning in 1955, the state hospital population in the U.S. peaked at 550,000.[25] By 1980, it had fallen to 137,000 and to approximately 45,000 by the turn of the twenty-first century. Unfortunately, outpatient care did not replace inpatient care, and state mental hospitals were not successfully replaced by community-based facilities. In the 1950s to 1960s, the process of replacing long-stay psychiatric hospitals with less isolated community mental health services began. In 1963 the Community Mental Health Act was passed to provide federal funding for community mental health centers in the United States and furthered deinstitutionalization. During this period, the pendulum of change swung away from a need for treatment (*parens patriae*) justification, and towards a dangerousness standard. Washington, DC was the first to adopt a "dangerousness standard" in 1964, marking the shift from medical model of "in need of treatment" to a legal model of danger to self and/or others. Medicare and Medicaid were introduced in 1965, and provided federal funds to states for treatment of persons with mental illness, but only if they lived in the community. This created an incentive to discharge patients to defer the cost of treatment to federal government. Three years later, in 1969, the Lanterman–Petris–Short Act (LPS Act) was passed in California. The LPS Act endorsed voluntary treatment and repealed indefinite commitment, while including provisions for procedural protection in the case of involuntary interventions. It set a tone of reform that influenced commitment statutes across the U.S.

Civil commitment saw its high-water mark set in 1972, and began its decline with two important cases, both of which took place in the early 1970s. In *Lessard v. Schmidt*,[26] the court drew strong comparisons between civil and criminal commitment. The standard of proof for civil commitment was held to be "beyond a reasonable doubt," and procedural safeguards similar to criminal commitment were mandated for Wisconsin. The U. S. Supreme Court then set the constitutional minimum standard of proof required for civil commitment at "clear and convincing" evidence. The net effect of all these changes was to reduce psychiatric hospitalization, as well as make it more difficult to involuntarily commit patients.[27]

The Role of Federal Courts

In the early 1970s, the federal courts became increasingly concerned about the unacceptable state of institutional care in some facilities. In *Wyatt v. Stickney*, Federal Court Judge Frank Johnson ruled that the conditions at Bryce (Alabama) State Hospital were so bad that they violated the due process clause of the constitution.[28] For example, at the time there was one psychiatrist at Bryce, serving approximately 5,000 patients. Ironically, while Morton Birnbaum's goal was to drastically improve the conditions in state hospitals, other attorneys (e.g. Bruce Ennis) working on the case had a very different goal: to make involuntary hospitalization prohibitively expensive. *Wyatt* was soon followed by similar suits in Louisiana, Minnesota, and Ohio.[19,29]

As Ennis and others hoped, the cost of involuntarily committing psychiatric patients skyrocketed, and the number of people housed in state hospitals began to decrease. As Birnbaum feared, however, there were not nearly enough facilities and services in the community to care for the people who were released.[30] As a result of these many forces, between 1955 and 1968, the residential psychiatric population in the United States dropped by 30%.[31] But the bright new reality promised by the Community Mental Health Centers (CMHC) Act never materialized. Of the 1,500 community mental health centers that were envisioned in the CMHC Act, only half were ever constructed, and most were not fully funded.[32]

The Theory of Trans-Institutionlization

Trans-institutionalization is a term used to describe the proposed link between deinstitutionalization and increased rates of serious mental illness (SMI) in jails and prisons. It is based in part on the *Penrose Hypothesis* which posits an inverse relationship between prison and mental hospital populations. If one of these forms of confinement is reduced, the other will increase. Penrose's hypothesis remains unresolved.[33] There are methodological problems with its study, including time points, politics, and legal reforms. Nevertheless, there is broad consensus that people with SMI are over-represented in correctional settings.[34] There is less agreement about what policy trends may have created this situation.[35]

The Penrose Hypothesis continues to be the subject of contentious debate.[36,37] Some 80 years after its formulation, the Penrose Hypothesis has neither been rejected nor confirmed.[38] Nevertheless, it appears to remain a credible hypothesis, not just in the U.S. but in other countries as well.[39]

Investigation is ongoing, with different elements being studied to confirm or refute trans-institutionalization. For example, the term "compensation imprisonment" is used to describe a convicted person who is unable or unwilling to pay the requisite fine for a crime, resulting in a mandatory jail sentence. Compensation prisoners suffer disproportionately from SMIs, leading to trans-institutionalization and further criminalization.[40] Similarly, many people are detained in jail while awaiting trial simply because they cannot pay the required cash bail,[41,42] drawing a nearly straight line from poverty to incarceration. Whether trans-institutionalization or the Penrose Hypothesis are confirmed or not, there is general agreement that the correctional system was never intended to care for persons with SMI, and has had largely negative effects on this vulnerable population.

To be sure, for many of the folks who would previously have been hospitalized for life, their life in the community was better. Many were able to get psychiatric and psychological assistance from CMHCs, many were able to live with families, and many were able to maintain steady employment.[43] But for many others, life in the community resulted in a barrage of bad outcomes, including unemployment, homelessness, and victimization. More importantly for the purposes of this chapter, many of the people who would have formerly remained in psychiatric hospitals were now vulnerable to the vagaries of the criminal justice system.[44]

Fisher et al. found that "individuals with mental illness had significantly higher odds of having at least one arrest across all charge categories, often for misdemeanors."[45]

The Growth of Incarceration

It is impossible to discuss the increase in incarceration rates for people with SMI without discussing the massive increase in incarceration rates in general throughout the U.S. From 1970 until the present, there has been a sea change in the manner in which the United States has responded to fear of crime, especially crimes involving interpersonal violence and illegal drugs. The growth of American corrections has been astronomical, from about 200,000 in 1970 to 1.6 million today, this despite any significant change in the levels of violent crime during the same period. The reasons for this dramatic increase include: (1) political strategies to gain power by claiming to be "tough on crime";[46] (2) a handful of high profile murders committed by recently released prisoners, especially Willie Horton;[47] (3) a misguided "war on drugs" that unsuccessfully sought to alleviate a perceived epidemic of addiction by incarcerating addicts;[48] and (4) a shift in criminal justice policies that removed discretion from judges, who exercised discretion in the light of day, to prosecutors who made charging decisions behind closed doors.[49]

The growth of corrections populations especially affected people with SMIs, many of whom had co-occurring substance abuse problems, and a high percentage of whom were living in communities of poverty.[50–52] Communities of poverty that have higher levels of violent crime place people with mental illness in jeopardy of being victimized, and there has been substantial co-variation between victimization and violent offending that can land a person in jail.[53]

In 1986, Willie Horton, a convicted murderer serving a life sentence without parole, was allowed a weekend furlough from his Massachusetts prison. Instead of returning from his furlough, Horton committed a number of serious crimes, including armed robbery and rape, before being arrested in Maryland. It is widely believed that this incident effectively scuttled the 1988 presidential campaign of Michael Dukakis, who was the Governor of Massachusetts during this episode. "Tough on crime" (or more accurately, "Tough on criminals") had moved from a political slogan to an essential stance for anyone seeking elective office.

It is important to understand that all crimes are not equal. The relationship between SMI and crime is complicated and grossly misunderstood.[54,55] For example, use of the phrase "violent crime" is so vague as to be misleading. In some studies, it is considered a violent crime to push or shove a family member, just as it is considered a violent crime to take someone's life. What we now know is that the majority of crimes committed by people with SMI is of the former type, pushing and shoving family and friends.[56]

It is a matter of wide consensus that the reduction in long-term psychiatric hospital beds dramatically increased the number of people with SMI who live in the community. It is equally clear that as the number of people incarcerated in America has risen, so has the number of inmates and detainees with SMI. What is less clear is the extent to which mental illness itself has become criminalized. Peterson, Skeem, Hart, Vidal, and Keith tested the criminalization hypothesis in a study of 220 parolees with and without SMI. Interestingly, they found that "a small minority (7%) of parolees fit the criminalization hypothesis," in that their crimes were the result of either psychosis or minor, "survival crimes" related to poverty. For both groups, crime was chiefly driven by "hostility, disinhibition, and emotional reactivity." They concluded, "Offenders with serious mental illness manifested heterogeneous patterns of offending that may stem from a variety of sources. Although psychiatric service linkage may reduce recidivism for a visible minority, treatment that targets impulsivity and other common criminal needs may be needed to prevent recidivism for the larger group."[57]

Jeffery Draine came to a similar conclusion: "Conceptualizing mental illness too generally as a cause of criminal involvement is not useful for policy or service implications. Such a strategy decontextualizes the experience of people with mental illness from broader incarceration patterns in the U.S. When the reasons people go to jail or return to jail are examined, it becomes clear that the key issues are social difficulties complicated by mental illness – but not caused by mental illness."[58]

Despite a great deal of rhetoric associating SMIs with violent crime, this alleged association is consistently belied by research data. That being said, there are other, predictable consequences of undertreated psychosis, including homelessness, living in distressed and often violent neighborhoods, unemployment, hunger, and victimization; all of which are well-known criminogenic factors.[59-61]

It is important to distinguish between at least three types of crimes when discussing people with SMI. A small number of seriously violent crimes that truly endanger the public are committed by people with SMI.[62-64] Further, the characteristics, situations, and stressors that lead to those crimes are in most cases similar for people with or without SMI. For non-dangerous acts, even those that are technically counted as violent (e.g. pushing or shoving), the necessity of confinement, especially long-term confinement, is dubious, and there is little evidence that it is effective. Long stays in hospital or jail tend to disrupt those parts of a person's life that are working, so that they might lose a job or an apartment, making things worse instead of better.

Crimes of survival are especially vexing when managed by the criminal justice system. For example, a homeless person who has no address may be unable to get disability checks; when such a person steals food, not a single ostensible purpose of criminal justice is served by sending them to jail. There will be no deterrence; hungry people will beg or steal food if they have no other option. It would be kinder and infinitely cheaper to give them a box lunch every day than to lock them up in jail.

On the other hand, some people with SMIs do commit serious crimes of violence. For the relatively small number of people with SMI who pose a serious threat to public safety, at least some type of involuntary confinement – whether in psychiatric or correctional institutions – will continue to be necessary. Prior to deinstitutionalization, that would have likely meant a long stay in a psychiatric hospital.

But humane psychiatric hospitals are expensive, costing hundreds of thousands of dollars per bed to build and almost as much annually to operate. As local, state, and federal budget crises have exploded, governments are increasingly seeking ways to save money, and the threshold for hospital care has risen. Those who cannot gain access to inpatient hospital beds are now housed in large numbers in local jails and state prisons across the United States.

The solution does not mean a return to the vast expense of massive long-term hospitalization. A host of examples have proven that most people with SMI

can live safely in the community if they have access to housing, necessities, as well as varying levels of support, structure, scrutiny, supervision, and services, but only to the degree that they are actually necessary. For example, the best community mental health care costs much less than a state hospital bed or a jail or prison bed for a person with a mental disability. One good example is Forensic Assertive Care Teams (FACT), which provide high intensity treatment and case management for people with SMI who have been involved in the criminal justice system.[65]

Corrections as the New Asylums

In 1974 and 1975 Robert Martinson published findings suggesting that treatment programs in New York State prisons had failed to reduce recidivism.[66] The Martinson Report helped set off a national debate over the report's implication that "nothing works." Ironically, "Martinson's intention was to improve prison rehabilitative programs, not to give up on them. He thought that his well-publicized skepticism about rehabilitation would empty most prisons."[67] Instead, it was asserted that inmates must necessarily have the proper internal motivation and commitment to be able to benefit from programming which should not be mandatory. Finally, their release from prison should be based on an objective schedule, and not on an arbitrary, subjective determination, as seen in indeterminant sentencing. Society turned to embrace new, more punitive correctional philosophies, which reflected public demands and concerns about safety. The Martinson report sparked the end of the "medical model" of corrections, and ushered in an era of explicitly punitive and retributive criminal justice policies.[68]

Diminishing liberal attitudes and increasingly conservative politics in the 1980s helped usher in a renewed societal desire for punishing offenders and "getting tough" on crime. Society had lost faith and interest in promoting correctional rehabilitation. Rather, the "certainty" of a punitive model became attractive in as much as it appeared to ensure that offenders received their "just desserts." Indeterminate sentences were replaced by fixed determinate sentences, with the ultimate outcome being that incarceration rates increased significantly. Correctional facilities began to fill beyond their capacities and America's move toward mass incarceration had begun.[67]

It was during the era of the Retributive Model that the number of mentally ill persons in jails and prisons began dramatically increasing. Correctional facilities began to house mentally ill persons in record numbers, and became "the new asylums." Research conducted over the last two to three decades clearly shows that the rates of severe mental illness, such as schizophrenia and mood disorders, are three to six times greater in the prison population than in the community at large.[69] The present-day dilemma is that jails and prisons were not prepared to provide services to the large numbers of mentally ill inmates in their facilities. The incarceration of large numbers of mentally ill persons has led to the challenge of providing quality psychiatric care within facilities that are oriented primarily toward security and custodial care. Caring for people with serious and disabling mental illnesses in corrections places a significant financial burden upon state governments, and is a poor long-term financial strategy.[70] Nevertheless, until adequate community resources and innovative alternatives (e.g. jail diversion, mental health courts) are established in much greater numbers, mental health services in corrections will remain a pressing and obligatory duty. This duty is commonly ensured via litigation and class action lawsuits because correctional facilities tend to be reactive to deficiencies. As a result, change comes mainly through legal action. Individual cases may be litigated, or they may be settled with settlement agreements or consent decrees.[71]

Why Correctional Institutions Are Harmful to People with Mental Illnesses

The mental health system has been "recreated" inside U.S. jails and prisons at considerable cost and effort, to treat the rising numbers of inmates with SMI. Patients with SMI require competent, well-coordinated mental health treatment. Treatment in a correctional environment presents many unusual challenges and stresses. Unfortunately, if patients are to fare well in this new corrections-based mental health system, they must adapt to it. They must make its ways their own, and many of these customs are contrary to what most in free society would consider psychologically healthy. Patients with SMI, along with all inmates, must undergo a process of "prisonization," the success of which can be measured by how closely they can come to resemble other inmates in their attitudes and behaviors. As can be imagined, many of these new behaviors would be maladaptive upon re-entry into the

community. Some of the effects of prisonization on inmates with SMI include:

- Over-reaction to perceived "disrespect"[72]
- Reluctance to discuss problems
- Preference for isolation (impaired ability to trust)
- Reliance on verbal threats or intimidation
- Medication noncompliance
- Manipulation to achieve goals
- Increased disciplinary infractions[73]
- Increased likelihood of restrictive housing[74]
- Increased likelihood of recruitment into gangs

During society's renewed interest in punishment and retribution over the past several decades, the lay public may sometimes have the misimpression that prison life is too comfortable and affords too many privileges to inmates. To the contrary, "Life, in even the kindest of prisons is truly punishing."[75] While the barbarous practices condemned by John Howard may no longer exist, life in today's prisons is neither privileged nor comfortable. At the very core of the experience of incarceration is the inescapable deprivation which is most punishing.[76] It is difficult for many in free society to conceptualize life in a "total institution," cut off from loved ones, friends, and other supports most may take for granted. In a total institution, one is removed from society, and utterly subject to an "administered" form of living.[77] Thus, it is not necessarily the deprivation of material possessions that produces the greatest suffering. Rather, it is the isolation from society and the lack of control over one's basic life circumstances which is most punishing.

Through prisonization, inmates adapt to an institutional way of life that requires less independent thinking, fewer complicated decisions, and less healthy interpersonal emotional connections. Due to the relentless structure and repetition, it is not uncommon for seemingly trivial circumstances to take on critical importance in the eyes of inmates. Clinicians must remain sensitive to this fact. The new generation of correctional mental health professionals must be fully cognizant of the fact that unwritten rules govern inmates' code of conduct. They must adapt not only to official prison rules, but also to the rules of the inmate subculture, the effects of which may have a direct impact upon the success of their treatment plans. For example, the phrase, "Do your own time" could almost be considered a sacred mantra among inmates. It refers to keeping one's affairs to oneself, and not interfering in the affairs of others.

In doing so, inmates hope to spend their prison time with the least amount of interpersonal conflict, avoid disciplinary infractions, and steer clear of intra-prison retribution. Other unwritten codes of inmate conduct involve avoiding displays of emotional "weakness," which ultimately encourages emotional isolation, even from fellow inmates. The code also demands that the inmate shows primary allegiance to other inmates, and general distrust of correctional officers. "Ratting out" a fellow inmate to correctional staff may cost an inmate his or her life, or at the very least cause them to live an anxious, paranoid existence.

All of these learned behaviors are antithetical to living in treatment settings, or even one's family in the community, leaving offenders with more problems than they had before their incarceration.

Theories of Punishment

The basis of punishment may be generalized into four different underlying principles: Rehabilitation, Restraint, Retribution, and Deterrence.[78] Of note is the fact that only one of the four is ostensibly related to "bettering" the state of the offender.

Particularly after the fall of the medical model, the notion of "rehabilitation" lost its appeal to many. Thus, the primary objection to rehabilitation is the assertion, perhaps premature, that it simply does not work. Supporters of this argument point to a wealth of data on the high degree of recidivism among offenders to bolster their claims. In addition, it can be persuasively argued that the very nature of the prison system runs counter to the goal of rehabilitation. For example, locking a criminal up with other criminals can be compared to requiring an individual who has engaged in terrorist attacks to associate only with other terrorists. The conclusion of this line of logic is clear: prisons increase rather than decrease the criminal propensities of inmates. Finally, some argue that it is unjust to use scarce public resources to rehabilitate individuals who have demonstrated their disregard for lawful behavior with recidivism.

Restraint refers to the act of removing offenders from society to prevent them from committing further crimes. The length of restraint will depend upon the danger that offenders appear to present to society, and whether they are amenable to some lesser form of restraint. Whether restraint should be coupled with rehabilitation and to what degree is a perpetual source of debate. Specifically, those arguing in favor of rehabilitation point out that confinement without meaningful rehabilitation merely defers criminal conduct until the inevitable release from restraint.

Retribution aims to literally "pay back" the harm to the offender who caused it. The obvious objection to retribution is that it is barbarous and not compatible with enlightened civilization due to the fact that it often involves doing some harm to the offender, either mentally or physically. Those in favor of retribution often argue from a moralistic standpoint, and/or a belief that institutionalized retribution is necessary to prevent private or personal retribution. Yet philosophical arguments aside, society has made itself abundantly clear in this matter – it demands some form of retribution.

Legal theorists generally speak of two types of deterrence – individual and general deterrence. Individual deterrence has as its goal precluding further criminal activity by that particular defendant who is before the court. The theory behind general deterrence is that punitive sanctions imposed on a single criminal will dissuade others with similar propensities. It is not uncommon for judges (who may be up for re-election) to proclaim they are handing down a particularly harsh sentence to "make an example" of one offender, and thereby serve as a "general deterrent" to others who might commit the crime at issue. Critics of general deterrence argue that most prospective criminals are more or less unaware of sentences that the courts are imposing. Further, even those who are aware do not tend towards thoughtful, cautious reflection on the risk/benefit ratios of their actions. The counterpoint is simply the reverse; that the certainty of harsh punishment does in fact influence their thinking to some degree, an argument frequently used in support of the death penalty.

In summary, decisions regarding punishment are extremely complex. Yet punishment alone as resolution to society's "crime problem" seems lacking. Indeed, this may be because in reality, it is inaccurate to say that America has a "crime problem"; rather, we have a number of very different people who engage in antisocial conduct for a number of different reasons, and to achieve a number of different outcomes.

The job of corrections is made more difficult by the fact that society appears to have abandoned the concept of formal rehabilitation, and is likely to express outrage when prisons subjectively appear to be too pleasant or comfortable. Conversely, society reacts with horror when riots, suicides, and prisoner abuse confirm appalling prison conditions. These sentiments constitute the essence of the conflicting message that society gives corrections: transform, but do not rehabilitate; cure, but do not treat; salvage, but do not restore.

Jails

Jails, sometimes referred to as County Houses of Correction, confine persons who are awaiting trial (pre-trial detainees) or offenders (in most states) serving a sentence of (typically) one year or less.[79] Federal jails are often referred to as Metropolitan Correctional Centers, and house inmates who are serving short sentences or awaiting trial on federal crimes. In reality, there is no one standard type of jail due to the fact that they vary in size and function across the country.[80] They range from massive facilities in urban areas to small "lockups" or "drunk tanks" in sheriff's stations. Functions range from the initial stop for police after arrest to the last resort for people who are homeless or mentally ill. Since jail inmates are often "fresh off the street," intoxication and/or mental illness may be in the acute stages. The initial booking and admission to jail is frequently a stressful and traumatic experience for a new inmate. These factors are thought to contribute to the high rate of suicide seen in jails.

Jail populations are complex and varied, consisting of both sentenced and unsentenced offenders. Pre-trial detainees and offenders serving a year or less make up the majority of jail inmates. Other jail inmates include: probation/parole violators, convicted but pre-sentencing offenders, and offenders waiting for transfer to prison. The jail population is rather transient due to a high turnover among the population. The typical jail population turns over 20 to 25 times per year, versus the prison population which turns over once every two years.[81] The high turnover presents a challenge to mental health staff who may have little time to develop a rapport, treatment plan, or even discharge plans for the jail inmate.

Jails across the country have been sued over a variety of unconstitutional conditions, especially in regard to their inadequate mental health services. In a similar way, the U.S. Department of Justice Civil Rights Division has conducted many investigations of local jails, the vast majority of which result in settlement agreements.[82]

Prisons

Prisons are correctional facilities that confine offenders who are serving sentences in excess of one year. They are operated at both the state and federal levels. State prisons typically confine offenders who are found guilty of violating state criminal statutes. Federal prisons generally hold offenders found guilty of federal offenses such as tax fraud, international drug trafficking, or crimes involving federal property. Federal prisons are operated by the Federal Bureau of Prisons. Compared to jails, prisons generally house larger numbers of inmates. There are far fewer prisons in the country than jails. Prisons range from large high security complexes to smaller rural facilities or camps. By the time offenders arrive in prison, most have either spent time in jail, or have had some prior confinement.

Prisons across the country have been sued for a variety of unconstitutional conditions, frequently regarding inadequate mental health services.[83] State prisons now have a great deal more forced idleness, and far too many inmates with SMI still find their way into segregated housing, despite federal court cases in CA, NY, WI, MS, and many other states.

Prison Overcrowding

Beginning in the 1970s, state and federal prison populations began a steady increase with no reprieve. By 2005, 24 state prison systems were operating at or above their highest capacity, and the federal system was 40% over capacity.[84] The conditions caused by overcrowding resulted in a steady wave of litigation and consent decrees aimed at resolving the problem. However, the prison population has continued to soar, and has reached approximately 2.1 million in prisons and jails, with another 5 million in probation and parole programs.[85]

Prisons may struggle with overcrowding in different ways. For example, some prisons may attempt to double and triple bunk the usually small, 8 ft. by 10 ft. cells intended to house single inmates. When limited cell space has been exhausted, it is common for inmates to be assigned to mattresses lining the hallways outside of cells. Some prisons are able to assemble pre-fabricated trailers or tents on the prison grounds for housing the population overflow. Those prisons unable to afford such amenities may have to resort to using gym, education, or dayroom space for housing, which results in these services becoming nonoperational.

In addition, the close-quarter living conditions that overcrowding produces facilitates the spread of communicable diseases such as tuberculosis and hepatitis.[80] Viral respiratory and gastrointestinal illnesses spread easily in poorly ventilated, crowded prison housing areas. Huey and McNulty have theorized that overcrowded conditions may increase the risk of prison suicides.[86] Thus, the adverse effects of prison overcrowding are manifold, ranging from basic health to basic institutional functioning.

In *Brown v. Plata* (2011),[87] the U.S. Supreme Court issued a five to four decision that is the court's most important decision impacting correctional health care at least since *Farmer v. Brennan*[88] in 1994. The Court upheld the lower courts' decision to require a total prison population not to exceed 137.5% of rated capacity within a five-year period of time. This involved a reduction of some 46,000 prisoners, but California was allowed to transfer some inmates to local jails, provide for enhanced good time credits leading to a somewhat earlier release, or even build new facilities. In sum, the doors to California's prisons were not suddenly opened.

The overcrowding was linked to the cause of inadequate health care, including mental health care. Its relief, then, simply cleared the path to hiring adequate numbers of treatment staff, creating an adequate number of beds that were varied as to the conditions treated, and assuring reasonable access by eligible inmates to staff and bed space.

California's prison reduction, which decreased its census by 15,493 persons from 2010 to 2011, constituted the most significant prisoner reduction in the nation in that period. A "Realignment" plan, effective October 1, 2011, now promises to be the most ambitious correctional reform in the nation, and with a significant impact on health care. Realignment transfers significant numbers of convicted felons from the state prison and parole systems to the state's 58 counties. This includes nearly all drug and property crimes.[89] Jails accustomed to providing pre-trial detention or relatively short-term incarceration now house offenders serving as many as 10 years, which means chronic health and mental health care is on the agenda, and despite some state funding, the jails

seem remarkably unprepared as to physical plant, staffing, training, and culture. In short, jails and prisons are counter-therapeutic for people with SMIs.

As evidenced by overcrowding, the lack of programming, inadequate education and mental health services, it is easy to see why it is frequently alleged that mass and long-term incarceration has been an ineffective way to change criminal behavior. Indeed, it has been argued that current criminal justice policies make offenders worse instead of better.[90] Dvoskin et al. wrote:

> An objective look at today's criminal and juvenile justice programs reveals the sad truth: If this were a boxing match, there would be an investigation, because it looks like we are trying to lose. In the United States, billions of dollars are spent annually on a punitive system that consistently fails to increase public safety. Given our policy of mass incarceration, generations of minority children are growing up without a father in their home. Money that could be spent on community development and the creation of jobs is being poured into the construction and operation of prisons.[94 (p. 299)]

What Do We Do Now?

Whatever its etiology, there is little debate that America incarcerates a very large number of people with SMI, people whose mental health needs would be better served in mental health settings.[91] It is equally clear that there seems to be little about the experience of incarceration that reduces their likelihood of future crime. If America is to successfully reduce its reliance on jails and prisons as the locus of treatment for people with SMI, a number of changes will be needed.

First, the sheer number of incarcerations and detentions, especially for offenders who pose no significant threat to public safety, needs to be reduced. Reducing the number of inmates could free up more money for correctional programs that are aimed at criminogenic factors.

Second, for those inmates with SMI who truly need to be incarcerated, there must be an investment in adequate mental health care for the duration of their confinement. Even if mental illness was not the cause of the person's criminal behavior, untreated mental illness in jails and prisons will prevent inmates and detainees from participating in correctional and educational programs aimed at criminogenic factors. Substantial numbers of inmates with and without SMIs have experienced significant trauma. Evidenced-based therapies to address inmates' psychological and emotional problems should become a priority in corrections.[92]

Third, it is essential that law enforcement and mental health agencies be given more and better options for dealing with people in crisis. Unreasonably low rates of Social Security Disability payments mean that many people with SMI will remain homeless. People in crisis need a place to go that is safe, such as drop-in centers and crisis residences. When police officers have options other than jail or emergency rooms, they use them.[93-96]

Fourth, the all-or-nothing rhetoric about reopening vast, long-stay institutions is a waste of energy. Even if such institutions were a good idea, they would be prohibitively expensive. But that does not mean that we have enough inpatient beds to adequately respond to short-stay crises. The dearth of acute inpatient beds has nothing to do with the horrors of psychiatric "warehouses" of the past.

Fifth, the vast majority of incarcerated people will eventually be released. When prisons are overcrowded and lack adequate mental health care, the criminal justice system has arguably made them worse instead of better.

Sixth, the current system of prosecutorial discretion provides no incentives for prosecutors to drop charges in cases of incompetent misdemeanor or minor felony defendants. One of the authors (JD) served as an independent expert in a class action involving incompetent defendants who remained in jail waiting for a bed in a psychiatric center. In a shocking number of cases, the underlying crime was extremely minor (e.g. driving without a license, stealing a sandwich), yet the person had been in jail for months waiting for an inpatient restoration bed, then spent months in an inpatient bed, before being returned to court to stand trial, whereupon they were released with "time served." The person who stole a sandwich because he was hungry lost his freedom for as long as a year, at a cost of more than $100,000 taxpayer dollars, all for the want of a $3 sandwich.

Finally, Lamb and Weinberger have suggested it is important to remember that the vast majority of incarcerated people, including those with SMI, will eventually be released into the community:

The long term consequences of society's choice to use the criminal justice system and corrections as the new asylums have undeniably arrived, and require a thoughtful, evidenced based approach by multiple stakeholders. The present-day reality is that large numbers of persons with SMI are being released in the community, and it is critical that they receive the public sector mental health care they need. Important options to consider for this population upon re-entry include: diversion and mental health courts; the expectation that the mental health system will not avoid such patients; the capabilities, limitations, and realistic treatment goals of community outpatient psychiatric treatment; the use of involuntary commitment (both inpatient and outpatient), appropriately structured, monitored, and supportive housing; and implementation of workable violence prevention plans.[97-100]

Conclusion

The role of SMIs (especially psychoses) in violent crime has been exaggerated in the media. Research has demonstrated that mental illness itself accounts for a small percentage of violent crime in America, and that people with mental illnesses often commit crimes for the same criminogenic reasons as people without SMI. That being said, the combination of deinstitutionalization and inadequate community mental health and housing resources has clearly placed huge numbers of people with SMI in jeopardy of coming into contact with the criminal justice system. Homelessness is especially pernicious, and contributes to poor clinical outcomes and increased likelihood of crime. As a result, we have hundreds of thousands of people with SMI in jails and prisons that are ill-suited to meet their mental health needs.

At least some solutions to this problem are clear:[101]

1. Jails and prisons should be reserved for those offenders who truly pose a serious risk to public safety.
2. Community mental health centers should be adequately funded, so that anyone who needs treatment for their serious mental illness can have access to timely and competent care.
3. Communities must invest in short-, intermediate-, and long-term housing for people with serious mental illnesses.
4. Police officers and other first responders must be trained (e.g. crisis intervention team, Mental Health First Aid) in how to identify and respond

to symptoms of mental illness and emotional crisis; more importantly, communities must create user-friendly options for people in emotional crisis.

5. While there are excellent reasons to avoid a return to long-term hospitalization of large numbers of Americans, there must be an adequate number of beds (in a variety of more or less restrictive settings) to provide short-term and crisis stabilization of people with SMIs during periods of extreme exacerbation that might otherwise be likely to land them in jail or prison.

6. For those people with SMI who truly pose a serious risk, and whose crimes were not the direct result of their illness, jails and prisons must provide adequate mental health services.

7. For offenders who are diverted or returned to the community, treatment programs must attend to both mental health and criminogenic factors.[102]

Disclosures

Joel A. Dvoskin, James L. Knoll, IV, and Mollie Silva declare no conflicts of interest.

Further Reading

Bernstein R, Seltzer T. Criminalization for people with mental illnesses: the role of mental health courts in system reform. *UDC L Rev.* 2003; **7**(1): 143–162.

Chaimowitz G. The criminalization of people with mental illness. *Can J Psychiatry.* 2012; **57**(2).

Draine J, Salzer MS, Culhane DP, Hadley TR. Role of social disadvantage in crime, joblessness, and homelessness among persons with serious mental illness. *Psychiatr Serv.* 2002; **53**(5): 565–573.

Engel RS, Silver E. Policing mentally disordered suspects: a reexamination of the criminalization hypothesis. *Criminology.* 2001; **39**(2): 225–252.

Fisher WH, Silver E, Wolff N. Beyond criminalization: toward a criminologically informed framework for mental health policy and services research. *Adm Policy Ment Health.* 2006; **33**(5): 544–557.

Junginger J, Claypoole K, Laygo R, Crisanti A. Effects of serious mental illness and substance abuse on criminal offenses. *Psychiatr Serv.* 2006; **57**(6): 879–882.

Lamb HR, Weinberger LE. Persons with severe mental illness in jails and prisons: a review. *Psychiatr Serv.* 1998; **49**(4): 483–492.

Powell TA, Holt JC, Fondacaro KM. The prevalence of mental illness among inmates in a rural state. *Law Hum Behav.* 1997; **21**(4): 427–438.

Ringhoff D, Rapp L, Robst J. The criminalization hypothesis: practice and policy implications for persons with serious mental illness in the criminal justice system. *Best Pract Ment Health.* 2012; **8**(2): 1–19.

Skeem JL, Manchak S, Peterson JK. Correctional policy for offenders with mental illness: creating a new paradigm for recidivism reduction. *Law Hum Behav.* 2011; **35**(2): 110–126.

References

1. Høyersten JG. [Possessed! Some historical, psychiatric and current moments of demonic possession]. *Tidsskr Nor Laegeforen.* 1996; **116**(30): 3602–3606.

2. Kramer H, Sprenger J. *The Malleus Maleficarum.* Translated by M. Summers. New York: Dover Publications; 1971.

3. Teague S, Robinson P. The History of Unreason: Social Construction of Mental Illness. In: Martin JM, ed. *Mental Health Policy, Practice, and Service Accessibility in Contemporary Society.* Hershey, PA: IGI Global; 2019: 1–19.

4. Billig M, Condor S, Edwards D, et al. *Ideological Dilemmas: A Social Psychology of Everyday Thinking.* London: Sage; 1988.

5. Appelbaum PS. Law & Psychiatry: "One madman keeping loaded guns": misconceptions of mental illness and their legal consequences. *Psychiatr Serv.* 2004; **55**(10): 1105–1106.

6. Knoll J. The recurrence of an illusion: the concept of "evil" in forensic psychiatry. *J Am Acad Psychiatry Law.* 2008; **36**(1): 105–116.

7. Chiu SN. Historical, religious, and medical perspectives of possession phenomenon. *Hong Kong J Psychiatry.* 2000; **10**(1).

8. D'Antonio P. History of Psychiatric Hospitals. Nursing, History, and Health Care. Penn Nursing. www.nursing.upenn.edu/nhhc/nurses-institutions-caring/history-of-psychiatric-hospitals/ (accessed June 2020).

9. Luchins AS. The rise and decline of the American asylum movement in the 19th century. *J Psychol.* 1988; **122**(5): 471–486.

10. Kiesler CA, Sibulkin AE. *Mental Hospitalization: Myths and Facts about a National Crisis.* Newbury Park: Sage Publications; 1987.

11. Diseases of the Mind: Highlights of American Psychiatry through 1900 – Early Psychiatric Hospitals

and Asylums. U.S. National Library of Medicine. www.nlm.nih.gov/hmd/diseases/early.html (accessed June 2020).

12. Grob GN. *Mental Institutions in America: Social Policy to 1875*. London: Routledge; 2017.

13. Confronting California's Continuing Prison Crisis: The Prevalence And Severity Of Mental Illness Among California Prisoners On The Rise. Stanford Justice Advocacy Project; 2017. https://law .stanford.edu/wp-content/uploads/2017/05/Stanfor d-Report-FINAL.pdf (accessed June 2020).

14. Bronson J, Berzofsky M. Indicators of Mental Health Problems Reported by Prisoners and Jail Inmates, 2011–12; 2017. www.bjs.gov/content/pub/pdf/imhpr pji1112.pdf (accessed June 2020).

15. Stefan S. The protection racket: rape trauma syndrome, psychiatric labeling, and law. *NW Univ Law Rev*. 1994; **88**(4).

16. Ladd-Taylor M. "Ravished by Some Moron": the eugenic origins of the Minnesota Psychopathic Personality Act of 1939. *J Policy Hist*. 2019; **31**(2): 192–216.

17. Goode D. *A History and Sociology of the Willowbrook State School*. Washington, DC: American Association on Intellectual and Developmental Disabilities; 2013.

18. Birnbaum M. The right to treatment. *Am Bar Assoc J*. 1960; **46**(5): 499–505.

19. Right to Treatment: Wyatt v. Stickney – Case Summary. Mental Illness Policy Org. https://menta lillnesspolicy.org/legal/wyatt-stickney-right-treatment.html (accessed June 2020).

20. Birnbaum, R. Remembering the "right to treatment". *Am J Psychiatry*, 2012; **169**(4): 358–359.

21. Szasz TS. The myth of mental illness. *Am Psychol*. 1960; **15**(2): 113–118.

22. Goffman E. *Asylums: Essays on the Social Situation of Mental Patients and Other Inmates*. New York: Doubleday Anchor; 1961.

23. Civil Rights Act of 1964. U.S. Equal Employment Opportunity Commission. www.eeoc.gov/eeoc/his tory/50th/thelaw/civil_rights_act.cfm (accessed June 2020).

24. Bloom JD, Britton J, Berry, W. The Oregon Court of Appeals and the State Civil Commitment Statute. *J Am Acad Psychiatry Law*. 2017; **45**(1): 52–61.

25. Goldman HH, Adams NH, Taube CA. Deinstitutionalization: the data demythologized. *Psychiatr Serv*. 1983; **34**(2): 129–134.

26. *Schmidt v. Lessard*, 414 U.S. 473. 1973.

27. Developments in the Law: Civil Commitment of the Mentally Ill. *Harv L Rev*. 1974; **87**(6): 1190–1406.

28. *Wyatt v. Stickney* 325 F. Supp. 781(M.D.Ala.1971), 334 F. Supp. 1341 (M.D. Ala 1971), 344 F. Supp. 373 (M.D. Ala. 1972), sub nom *Wyatt v. Aderholt*, 503 F. 2d 1305 (5th Cir. 1974).

29. Perez A, Leifman S, Estrada A. Reversing the criminalization of mental illness. *Crime Delinq*. 2003; **49**(1): 62–78.

30. Unfortunately, in 1981 the Omnibus Budget Reconciliation Act consolidated federal funding, and shifted treatment costs back to states. As a result, the funding of community-based mental health services was significantly curtailed.

31. Goldman HH, Adams NH, Taube CA. Deinstitutionalization: the data demythologized. *Psychiatr Serv*. 1983; **34**(2): 129–134.

32. Teich J. Better data for better mental health services. *Issues Sci Technol*. 2016; **XXXII**(2).

33. Mundt AP, Konrad N. Institutionalization, Deinstitutionalization, and the Penrose Hypothesis. *Adv Psychiatry*. 2018; 187–196.

34. Teplin LA. Criminalizing mental disorder: the comparative arrest rate of the mentally ill. *Am Psychol*. 1984; **39**(7): 794–803.

35. Prins SJ. Does transinstitutionalization explain the overrepresentation of people with serious mental illnesses in the criminal justice system? *Community Ment Health J*. 2011; **47**(6): 716–722.

36. Lamb HR. Does deinstitutionalization cause criminalization? *JAMA Psychiatry*. 2015; **72**(2): 105.

37. Kalapos MP. Penrose's Law: methodological challenges and call for data. *Int J Law Psychiatry*. 2016; **49**: 1–9.

38. Schildbach S, Schildbach C. Criminalization through transinstitutionalization: a critical review of the penrose hypothesis in the context of compensation imprisonment. *Front Psychiatry*. 2018; **9**: 534.

39. O'Neill CJ, Kelly BD, Kennedy HG. A 25-year dynamic ecological analysis of psychiatric hospital admissions and prison committals: Penrose's Hypothesis updated. *Ir J Psychol Med*. 2018; 1–4.

40. O'Neill CJ, Kelly BD, Kennedy HG. A 25-year dynamic ecological analysis of psychiatric hospital admissions and prison committals: Penrose's Hypothesis updated. *Ir J Psychol Med*. 2018; 1–4.

41. www.law360.com/access-to-justice/articles/1180373/ risk-assessment-tools-are-not-a-failed-minority-report- (accessed June 2020).

42. Robuy B, Kopf D. Detaining the poor: how money bail perpetuates an endless cycle of poverty and jail time. 2016. www.prisonpolicy.org/reports/income jails.html (accessed June 2020).

43. Drake RE, Latimer E. Lessons learned in developing community mental health care in North America. *World Psychiatry*. 2012; **11**(1): 47–51.

44. Feldman S. Community mental health centers: a decade later. *Int J Ment Health*. 1974; **3**(2–3): 19–34.

45. Fisher WH, Roy-Bujnowski KM, Grudzinskas AJ, et al. Patterns and prevalence of arrest in a statewide cohort of mental health care consumers. *Psychiatr Serv*. 2006; **57**(11): 1623–1628.

46. Smith KB. The politics of punishment: evaluating political explanations of incarceration rates. *J Politics*. 2004; **66**(3): 925–938.

47. Anderson DC, Enberg C. Crime and the politics of hysteria: how the Willie Horton story changed American justice. *J Contemp Crim Justice*. 1995; **11**(4): 298–300.

48. National Research Council. *The Growth of Incarceration in the United States: Exploring Causes and Consequences*. Washington, DC: The National Academies Press; 2014.

49. Cullen, James. The History of Mass Incarceration. Brennan Center for Justice; 2018. www .brennancenter.org/our-work/analysis-opinion/his tory-mass-incarceration (accessed June 2020).

50. Silver E, Mulvey EP, Swanson JW. Neighborhood structural characteristics and mental disorder: Faris and Dunham revisited. *Soc Sci Med*. 2002; **55**(8): 1457–1470.

51. Silver E. Extending social disorganization theory: a multilevel approach to the study of violence among persons with mental illnesses. *Criminology*. 2000; **38** (4): 1043–1074.

52. Silver E. Race, neighborhood disadvantage, and violence among persons with mental disorders: the importance of contextual measurement. *Law Hum Behav*. 2000; **24**(4): 449–456.

53. Silver E, Piquero AR, Jennings WG, Piquero NL, Leiber M. Assessing the violent offending and violent victimization overlap among discharged psychiatric patients. *Law Hum Behav*. 2011; **35**(1): 49–59.

54. Harvard Health Publishing. Mental illness and violence. Harvard Medical School; 2011. www .health.harvard.edu/newsletter_article/mental-illness-and-violence (accessed June 2020).

55. Monahan J, Steadman HJ. *Violence and Mental Disorder: Developments in Risk Assesment*. Chicago, IL: University of Chicago Press; 1994.

56. Steadman HJ, Mulvey EP, Monahan J, et al. Violence by people discharged from acute psychiatric inpatient facilities and by others in the same neighborhoods. *Arch Gen Psychiatry*. 1998; **55**(5): 393–401.

57. Peterson J, Skeem JL, Hart E, Vidal S, Keith F. Analyzing offense patterns as a function of mental illness to test the criminalization hypothesis. *Psychiatr Serv*. 2010; 61(12): 1217–1222.

58. Draine J. Where is the 'illness' in the criminalization of mental illness? In: *Research in Community and Mental Health. Community-Based Interventions for Criminal Offenders with Severe Mental Illness*. Bingley: Emerald Group Publishing Limited; 2002: **12**: 9–21.

59. Teplin LA. Criminalizing mental disorder: the comparative arrest rate of the mentally ill. *Am Psychol*. 1984; **39**(7): 794–803.

60. Silver E. Race, neighborhood disadvantage, and violence among persons with mental disorders: the importance of contextual measurement. *Law Hum Behav*. 2000; **24**(4): 449–456.

61. Andrews DA. The Risk-Need-Responsivity (RNR) model of correctional assessment and treatment. In Dvoskin JA, Skeem JL, Novaco RW, Douglas K, eds. *Using Social Science to Reduce Violent Offending*. New York: Oxford University Press; 2011: 127–156.

62. Appelbaum PS. Public safety, mental disorders, and guns. *JAMA Psychiatry*. 2013; **70**(6): 565.

63. Angermeyer MC. Schizophrenia and violence. *Acta Psychiatr Scand*. 2000; **102**(s407): 63–67.

64. Fazel S, Gulati G, Linsell L, Geddes JR, Grann M. Schizophrenia and violence: systematic review and meta-analysis. *PLoS Med*. 2009; **6**(8): e1000120.

65. Forensic Assertive Community Treatment (FACT). A Service Delivery Model for Individuals With Serious Mental Illness Involved With the Criminal Justice System. Substance Abuse and Mental Health Services Administration. https://store.samhsa.gov/sy stem/files/508_compliant_factactionbrief_0.pdf (accessed June 2020).

66. Empey LT, Lipton D, Martinson R, Wilks J. The effectiveness of correctional treatment: a survey of treatment evaluation studies. *Contemp Sociol*. 1976; **5** (5): 582.

67. Miller JG. The debate on rehabilitating criminals: is it true that nothing works? Washington Post; 1989. www.prisonpolicy.org/scans/rehab.html (accessed June 2020).

68. Macnamara DE. The medical model in corrections: requiescat in pace. *Criminology*. 1977; **14**(4): 439–448.

69. Robins LN, Regier DA. Psychiatric disorders in America The Epidemiologic Catchment Area Study. *Psychiatr Serv*. 1991; **43**(3): 289.

70. Kupers TA. *Prison Madness: the Mental Health Crisis behind Bars and What We Must Do about It*. San Francisco: Jossey-Bass; 1999.

71. Metzner J. Class action litigation in correctional psychiatry. *J Am Acad Psychiatry Law*. 2002; **30**: 19–29.

72. Carr WA, Rotter M, Steinbacher M, et al. Structured Assessment of Correctional Adaptation (SACA). *Int J Offender Ther Comp Criminol*. 2006; **50**(5): 570–581.

73. Toch H, Adams K. Pathology and disruptiveness among prison inmates. *J Res Crime Delinq*. 1986; **23**(1): 7–21.

74. Lovell D, Cloyes K, Allen D, Rhodes L. Who lives in super maximum custody? A Washington State study. *Fed Probat*. 2000; **64**: 33–43.

75. Roberts JW. *Reform and Retribution: an Illustrated History of American Prisons*. Lanham, MD: American Correctional Association; 1997.

76. Stinchcomb JB. *Corrections: Past, Present, and Future*. New York: Routledge; 2011.

77. Goffman E. *Asylums: Essays on the Social Situation of Mental Patients and Other Inmates*. London: Routledge, Taylor & Francis Group; 2017.

78. Loewy AH. *Criminal Law in a Nutshell*, 2nd Edn. St. Paul, MN: West Publishing Co; 1987.

79. American Psychiatric Association. *Psychiatric Services in Jails and Prisons*. Washington DC: American Psychiatric Association; 2000.

80. Stinchcomb JB. *Corrections: Past, Present, and Future*. New York: Routledge; 2005.

81. Weedon J. The role of jails is growing in the community. *Corrections Today*. April 2003.

82. www.justice.gov/crt/rights-persons-confined-jails-and-prisons (accessed June 2020).

83. *Coleman v. Brown*, 938 F. Supp.2d 955, 974, n.35 (E.D. Cal). 2013.

84. Harrison PM, Beck AJ. Prisoners in 2005. U.S. Department of Justice; 2006. www.bjs.gov/content/pub/pdf/p05.pdf (accessed June 2020).

85. Beck A. Testimony on Prison Demographics. Commission on Safety and Abuse in America's Prisons. Newark, NJ. July 19, 2005.

86. Huey MP, McNulty TL. Institutional conditions and prison suicide: conditional effects of deprivation and overcrowding. *Prison J*. 2005; **85**(4): 490–514.

87. *Brown v. Plata* 131 S. Ct. 1910 (2011).

88. *Farmer* v. *Brennan* (92–7247), 511 US 825 (1994) www.law.cornell.edu/supct/html/92-7247.ZS.html

89. Petersilia J, Cullen FT. Liberal but Not Stupid: Meeting the Promise of Downsizing Prisons. *SSRN Electronic Journal*. 2014.

90. Dvoskin JA, Skeem JL, Novaco RW, Douglas KS. What if psychology redesigned the criminal justice system? In: *Using Social Science to Reduce Violent Offending*. New York: Oxford University Press; 2011: 291–302.

91. Slate RN, Buffington-Vollum JK, Johnson WW. *The Criminalization of Mental Illness: Crisis and Opportunity for the Justice System*. Durham, NC: Carolina Academic Press; 2013.

92. Knoll J. Individual psychotherapy. In: Trestman RL, Appelbaum KL, Metzner JL, eds. *Oxford Textbook of Correctional Psychiatry*. New York: Oxford University Press; 2015: 223–228.

93. Beckett K Ph.D. Seattle's Law Enforcement Assisted Diversion Program: Lessons Learned from the First Two Years; 2014. www.fordfoundation.org/media/2543/2014-lead-process-evaluation.pdf (accessed June 2020).

94. Varano SP, Kelley P, Makhlouta N. The city of Brockton's "champion plan": the role of police departments in facilitating access to treatment. *Int J Offender Ther Comp Criminol*. 2019; **63**(15–16): 2630–2653.

95. Crisis Intervention Team (CIT) Programs. National Alliance on Mental Illness. www.nami.org/get-involved/law-enforcement-and-mental-health (accessed June 2020).

96. Teller JLS, Munetz MR, Gil KM, Ritter C. Crisis intervention team training for police officers responding to mental disturbance calls. *Psychiatr Serv*. 2006; **57**(2): 232–237.

97. Lamb HR, Weinberger LE. Understanding and treating offenders with serious mental illness in public sector mental health. *Behav Sci Law*. 2017; **35**(4): 303–318.

98. Baillargeon J, Hoge SK, Penn JV. Addressing the challenge of community reentry among released inmates with serious mental illness. *Am J Community Psychol*. 2010; **46**(3–4): 361–375.

99. Lurigio AJ. Effective services for parolees with mental illnesses. *Crime Delinq*. 2001; **47**(3): 446–461.

100. Dlugacz HA. *Reentry Planning for Offenders with Mental Disorders: Policy and Practice*. Kingston: Civic Research Institute; 2015.

101. Perez A, Leifman S, Estrada A. Reversing the criminalization of mental illness. *Crime Delinq*. 2003; **49**(1): 62–78.

102. Wilson AB, Farkas K, Bonfine N, Duda-Banwar J. Interventions that target criminogenic needs for justice-involved persons with serious mental illnesses: a targeted service delivery approach. *Int J Offender Ther Comp Criminol*. 2017; **62**(7): 1838–1853. *This research describes the development of a targeted service delivery approach that tailors the delivery of interventions that target criminogenic needs to the specific learning and treatment needs of justice-involved people with serious mental illnesses (SMI).*

A Social History of Psychotic Illness

Brendan Daugherty, Katherine Warburton, and Stephen M. Stahl

Have you ever walked down the street andseen someone with mental illness, agitated and yelling, or lying on the sidewalk, and wondered why? Have you ever wondered why, despite myriad reforms from bold thinkers and progressive governments over centuries, does this still occur? Why, despite miraculous technology, comfort, and opportunity for the majority of the Western population, do people living with serious mental illness continue to miss out on a good life? Or even a humane one?

Take the case of a recently arrested man later admitted to a state hospital. In a condition of homelessness and untreated symptoms, he was standing in a fast-food restaurant in an agitated state, yelling at what he perceived to be a manifestation of the devil. The police were called, and when they arrived, they noted that this individual was missing an eye, which he reported to them he'd removed himself as he provided an unintelligible explanation related to a conflict with the devil. The police, understandably, felt the individual was in need of mental health care, and put hands on him to take him into custody, at which point the terrified man took out an imaginary phone to call the "police," and reported into this delusional device that he was being attacked by an agent of the devil. He proceeded to fight for his life, and in the process lashed out physically leading the officers to charge him with two felonies and book him into custody. He was found incompetent to stand trial (did not have the cognitive capacity to participate in the court process), sent to a hospital for restoration to competency and in the process received mental health services. The devil disappeared after a month on antipsychotic medication, the patient was sent back to court, sentenced to a short term in prison, and then discharged back into homelessness. Treatment soon ceased. He returned to the very conditions that led to his arrest. Only now he had one additional burden; as a convicted felon he was denied the already scant social and mental health services in the community.

The historian Grob stated about the failed state of institutional care, "to attribute bad results to evil people or to condemn an entire society may prove psychologically and intellectually satisfying."[1] It would be easy to blame the failure of institutionalization on immoral superintendents, for instance. Or the failure of deinstitutionalization on disorganized governance. It is not so simple. Why then does "good" policy repeatedly fail those with psychotic illness? Why, despite well-intentioned reforms, policies, and treatments, does care for the seriously mentally unwell have a recurrent tendency towards maltreatment?

Societal Treatment of Psychotic Disorders is a Sisyphean Task

In this paper, we suggest that society's treatment of people with psychotic illness is a Sisyphean task – constantly regressing to a baseline of maltreatment. We define maltreatment as neglect, abuse, or other forms of harm. We suggest that, even when treatment is appropriate for some with psychotic disorders, society struggles to maintain this. Many will deal with absent or improper treatment. For some, conditions today are no better than they were centuries or millennia ago.

The criminalization of individuals living with serious mental illness in the United States is a current example of this type of regression to inhumane treatment, but the pattern is global. Institutional care in the nineteenth century is but one example where good intention in mental health policy went awry. Deinstitutionalization in the twentieth century is another. While it is possible to identify isolated examples of positive reform and therefore dispute the degree to which maltreatment exists, we demonstrate the pattern of regression to maltreatment and its ongoing existence.

When the people of the twenty-second century gaze back to now, will they consider psychiatry as a benevolent institution capable of advocating for the vulnerable insane? Or perhaps a misguided tool of social control, unable to correct the neglect and mistreatment that has recurrently haunted the profession? We suggest that

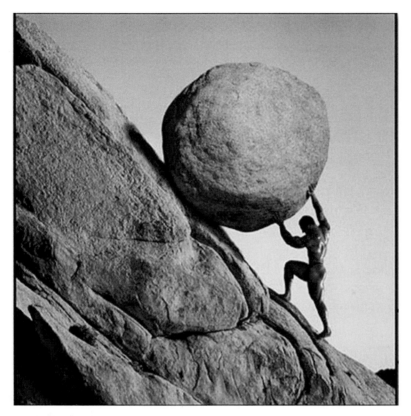

Sisyphus was a deceitful King. He was eternally punished by Zeus, requiring him to push a boulder to the top of a hill, only for the boulder to roll down every time he neared the top.

Credit: Gerard Van der Leun

deeper consideration of history will help guide us toward the former.

A Sampler of Psychiatric (Mis)treatments

To detail the history of treatment, mistreatment, and reforms in the domain of mental illness is beyond the ability of most books, no less a single scientific paper. Herein lies a tour of notable occurrences across time and geography, mostly in chronological order, demonstrating a tendency to maltreatment.

Early Treatment Was Idiosyncratic, but Usually Harmful

In ancient civilization, there was little recognition that mental illness was a disease, and therefore it was not treated as one.[2,3] Conceptualization of madness centered on demonic or other types of supernatural influence. Families, communities, religious healers, and leaders dealt with insanity in idiosyncratic ways to protect themselves and society, and to promote their

institutions. If not able to be contained within a home environment, either humanely or inhumanely, families would seek the help of others, often resulting in ceremony, admonishment, containment, exorcism, or whatever the community and religious sentiment of the time dictated. Treatment was regularly harsh. The insane may have ended up beaten, chained, banished, or dead.[2–4]

This is not to say that examples of humane treatment did not exist. In some ancient indigenous and Eastern cultures in particular, there is evidence of humane treatment and integration into society.[3] But in almost every case, there are certain to be examples of the exact opposite. The tendency to harm was rife.

A Small and Temporary Reform from Spiritual to Corporeal Treatment

Though ancient Chinese society pre-dated a Western shift to physical understandings of disease,[5] ancient Greek society was the first Western society to treat mental afflictions as a medical illness.[3,6] The separation of church from state allowed free thinking individuals, such as Hippocrates, to explore wholly naturalistic causes of disease. It was in the asclepeion, or "healing sanctuary," where those with mental illness were first cared for outside the home, albeit in a temple.[2,6] These sanctuaries were not hospitals, but they provided retreat for the afflicted, a revolutionary idea for the times. A mixture of somatic and mystical treatments including bathing, purging, and dieting, followed by prayer, were common.[6,7] Porter notes that "around the temples religious and secular healing rubbed shoulders."[6]

The religious understanding of mental illness was too intoxicating for most societies, however, and with the decline of Greek civilization, the physical understanding of "madness" again lay dormant in most Western societies.[3]

Here, the Sisyphean pattern is evident. Recognition of corporeal understanding of disease led to more progressive treatment, only for the understanding to be cast aside in many places. For centuries after, beatings and various eclectic exorcisms far outnumbered any semblance of care.

The Beginnings of Institutional "Care"

The first societies to have hospitals in which those with mental illness could be cared for were the ancient Islamic cultures approximately half a millennium later (starting in the eighth century AC).[8] The "bimaristans" (in Persian, "bimar" meaning "ill person" and "stan" denoting "place"), or hospitals, in Baghdad, Damascus, and Cairo were indeed revolutionary, and founded on the ideal in Islamic culture that no individual needing care should be turned away.[8,9] This being the perfect policy for those who had lost their senses, most of the bimaristans had special areas of their hospitals reserved for those with serious mental disorders.[3,9] Though they would be judged as harsh by today's standards, often using chains to contain behavior, they were provided in good will and were a valiant early attempt to help a neglected population.

Roy Porter, the late patient-focused medical historian, clarified that the bimaristans should not be overglorified in their ideals, which were just that.[6] These ideals were symbolic in nature, and though bringing the medical profession together, cared for a "drop in the ocean" of those with mental afflictions. The progress, also, was arguably symbolic. Most with serious mental illness remained neglected. Further, Islamic policy has not always served the mentally ill. Many countries based on Shariah law have previously relied on cautery, exorcism, and physical violence to manage the "mad."[10,11]

The "Progress" of Asylums

Bethlehem Hospital is thought to be the seat of institutional care in the Western World. It opened its doors in 1247 and began to care for the insane sometime between 1377 and 1403.[12] As is well documented, conditions were appalling. This was not so much a regression as a *progression* of maltreatment – the maltreatment now legitimised through institutionalization. Dark and dank rooms (exacerbating the prevailing English climate), minimal or adverse treatment, beatings, and shackling were all prevalent. Despite its prominence, Bedlam (as it became known) held only a handful of patients, with the familial home remaining the dominant place of care until the seventeenth and eighteenth century.[4,12]

Private alms houses and asylums began to proliferate in seventeenth- and eighteenth-century Britain. In this so-called "trade in lunacy," entrepreneurs charged a fee for containing the unwanted within their makeshift and converted "mad-houses."[2,3,13] The demand for such facilities is likely to have justified their existence. The early asylums and alms houses proffered humane alternatives for desperate families, though their marketing pitch was rarely matched by the product.[3] From the beginning, a conflict of interest predestined poor treatment. In other words, the better the care, the lower the profit.

William Parry-Jones, a professor of psychiatry and historian of the Trade in Lunacy, warned against the generalization of horror-stories in the private asylums with the exception of the "pauper" lunatics – who, in fact, were the majority of inpatients until the mid-nineteenth century, when public asylums proliferated.[14] He writes, of "crowded, ill-ventilated cells in converted stables and outbuildings where pallid, half-naked lunatics were housed on filthy straw."[14] Thus, the façade of progression hid the reality of maltreatment for many.

The Spread and Reform of Asylumdom

Regardless of institutional abuses, there was widespread adoption of the asylum as a place of containment throughout the Western World and colonies. Several distinct but connected reforms and reformers in the eighteenth and nineteenth century are mentioned. Though they signified progress, they were unable to stop a regression to the maltreatment so well reported in many asylums, particularly in the United States.[15-17]

The first reform was public oversight of asylums, best documented in England and Wales. The mental illness of King George III and a number of high-profile false imprisonments, especially of women, drove reform.[18] A series of laws led first to licensing requirements for private asylums. From 1845, asylums were mandated in each county, the same year official oversight was required in all asylums by the "Lunacy Commissioners."[18] Other countries enacted protective laws such as the requirement for two doctors to certify insanity (for example, Australia's first "lunacy law" in 1843),[19] or the use of the courts to help determine lunacy (for example, statutes in mid-nineteenth-century USA).[20]

The second reform was "moral treatment," simultaneously enacted by Phillipe Pinel and Jean-Baptiste Pussin at the Bicetre in Paris, William Tuke in England, and Vincenzo Chiarugi in Italy. At its heart, moral treatment reconceptualized the madman as a human, with similar needs of self-esteem, purpose, and interaction, rather than the animalistic "treatments" and containments of the past (such as shackling, seclusion, beatings, verbal degradation, and ostracism).[21] Patients were encouraged to re-exercise their powers of self-control through positive reinforcement of good behavior in a welcoming environment. Increased access to grounds and nicer accommodation might be the rewards for self-control. The small early institutions could give close attention to the individual patient, with a high degree of success to match.[21]

Third, perhaps aided by the former movements, several humanitarian campaigners promoted appropriate asylum-based care. Here we mention but two. Dorothea Dix, an American hero, was a tireless advocate for the expansion of asylums in mid-nineteenth-century America. As a woman, she was unable to attend the Massachusetts legislature at the time, though her written submissions resonated. In her first Memorial to the legislature, she wrote, "I proceed, Gentlemen, briefly to call your attention to the present state of insane persons confined within this Commonwealth, in cages, closets, stalls, pens! Chained, naked, beaten with rods, and lashed into obedience!" To not have asylums, she said, was "aggravated culpability."[3] Dix is credited with establishing 32 new asylums and championed moral treatment within them.[22]

Another campaigner, Sir John Charles Bucknill, an English psychiatrist and reformist, was a determined campaigner for the removal of physical restraints and move toward humane asylum care.[23] Though Robert Gardner Hill, a provincial surgeon, was the first to implement a system of care without restraint in the 1830s,[24] Bucknill's ongoing efforts contributed to the relative absence of restraints in Britain asylums. He was the founder of the *Asylum Journal,* within three years called the *Journal of Mental Science,* ultimately becoming the *British Journal of Psychiatry.*[25] In 1875 he engaged in a tour of the eastern United States and Canada and then published criticism of American psychiatry's widespread use of restraints – the use of which is still ongoing today.[26]

Taken together, these improvements were significant advances for the treatment of those with serious mental illness. Asylum care, when enacted under certain moral terms, provided a humane and specialized service for those with psychotic illness.

Though it is tempting to idealize the asylum model in retrospect in comparison to the failures of today's deinstitutionalized care, a significant proportion of institutions did not adequately protect those within them. From custodial style, untherapeutic care, to downright dangerous and unregulated treatments, overcrowding, disenfranchisement, overmedication, sexual violence, and shackling, the reality for many in asylums was truly treacherous. This is explored in the following sections.

The Reality of Asylum Care for Most Was Custodial and Untherapeutic

In England, the shining light of moral treatment was the Quaker William Tuke's Retreat at York. Just up the road from The Retreat, the York Lunatic Asylum claimed to espouse moral principles before and after The Retreat's opening in 1796, though failed miserably in their enactment.[27]

In a summary of well-documented cases, the historian Anne Digby notes,

> …the York Asylum had many of the characteristics of a "total institution" where patients faced loss of determination and identity. Whippings, rape, and contamination from a filthy environment, threatened physical integrity. Accommodation was overcrowded, damp, gloomy, and ill-ventilated. Violent or incontinent patients were housed indiscriminately with the clean, quiet, or convalescent. Clothing was often conspicuous by its absence, and food was wretched even by the standards of contemporary

workhouses. Lack of attention to patients meant that they were often dirty and could suffer from untreated illnesses.[27]

Mortality was so high that the number of deaths were concealed by the Apothecary and the official record fraudulently altered.[27] An extraordinary level of abuse despite the outward declaration of a moral institution.

Though care for those at the York Asylum (eventually Bootham Park Hospital) undoubtedly improved from this nadir, what of the effects of institutionalization, overcrowding, and then deinstitutionalization, including the recent failed attempt to improve the safety of the 240-year-old building, followed by a sudden requirement to move its vulnerable inpatients and outpatients to distant institutions within five days?[28] The prioritization of patient welfare was lost multiple times.

England, of course, was not the only country where institutional care was less than ideal, despite a number of reforms. Custodial and overcrowded institutions proliferated in many countries.

In early nineteenth-century Australia, unsurprisingly, the priority was the containment of criminals, and as such those recognized as insane and dangerous were typically kept in jails.[19,29,30] The Female Factory in Sydney housed "a motley collection of fallen women and prostitutes, indigents, the elderly and the insane, initially in a loft above a gaol."[19] Political imperative helped find a new space for the mentally ill, with the "less than comfortable converted barracks building" in Castle Hill, Sydney used until 1825. As many as a third of convicts in jail had mental illness, and as asylums were oversubscribed, "many lunatics were being held in both metropolitan and provincial gaols and susceptible to 'the moral injury now too often inflicted on them, by compulsory association with all classes of criminals.'"[19] Unsurprisingly, "commissions of inquiry into shortcomings of the various asylums were commonplace from their inception."[19]

In Africa, asylum care proliferated in the early twentieth century. Parts of jails were transformed into asylums, such as the asylum in Zanzibar "situated physically inside the walls of the prison, overseen by prison guards, run administratively by the Prison Department and operated essentially as an additional cell block in close proximity to the gallows."[31] Or, in the case of Hoima Gaol in Uganda, simply re-established as Hoima Lunatic Asylum in 1923 as it had become, "without any official

designation," a "dumping ground for a variety of inmates whose presence was deemed undesirable or disruptive among the general prison population."[31]

Hospitals in West Africa were "all-purpose institutions," with most superintendents not of a medical background.[32] "Dark, congested cells, poor bathing facilities, lack of basic supplies and the use of chains" were prevalent.[32,33] A 1936 survey noted most asylums "were run down and poorly serviced and were no more than prisons."[32]

Femi Oyebode, a psychiatrist and author, writes "that the asylums were developed, at least partly, in response to a perceived need to assist the mentally ill."[32] Good intention, perhaps. Though, he goes on, "as in other parts of the world, the actual facilities were poorly resourced and maintained." Asylum care was promoted in Africa, but the custodial nature of the institutions undoubtedly caused additional harm to many.

In nineteenth-century India, asylums "were greatly influenced by British psychiatry and catered mostly to European soldiers posted in India at that time. Their function was more custodial and less curative."[34] The law dictating care for the mentally ill in the early twentieth century was "purely custodial, did not understand the medical view, and the need for proper care and cure, but instead viewed these with suspicion."[35] "Financial rather than therapeutic reasoning" guided care, a common theme in the custodial care of those with psychotic illness over time.[35] Here, too, the care needs of the insane were likely forgotten, and harm ensued.

In the USA, despite several, mostly private, asylums based on moral treatment, state asylums became so overcrowded humane care was not possible. One asylum in Georgia contained 14,000 individuals. Repetitive inhumanity and scandal were a notable feature of its history.[36]

Here the pattern of regression to maltreatment was evident across multiple countries and multiple centuries, a Sisyphean task indeed. Morally based institutional care had prima facie merit. Dorothea Dix and others had previously argued this case.[3] Scholars continue to make the case today.[37] If this model of care were to dominate psychiatry again, what would be different this time around? What would stop us regressing to the maltreatment that harmed thousands, if not millions, of vulnerable people? Alas, institutionalization was not the first method of care to harm those with serious mental illness (among others), nor would it be the last.

Twentieth-Century Abusive Treatments

With increasing medicalization of mental illness, the tendency towards harm continued in the twentieth century.

Notwithstanding individual treatments, the guise of "treating" or helping *society,* such as the eugenics movement, caused extensive harm the world over. In total, hundreds of thousands of people considered, at the time, to be "mental defectives" were sterilized in the USA, Scandinavia, Western and Eastern Europe, and Latin America to advance the human race.[38-41] Sobering, was the general acceptance by the academic world and that involuntary sterilization was practiced well into the 1970s in places such as Sweden and the United States.[39,41]

Direct "treatments" of mental illness, however, also irreparably harmed (and sometimes killed) many with mental illness. The extent of harm is documented by authors such as Scull.[3,42,43] Outlined below are some prominent examples.

One of two psychiatrists to be awarded the Nobel Prize in Medicine, Julius Wagner-Jauregg noticed that patients with general paralysis of the insane (GPI; later discovered to be syphilis) sometimes improved when they had a fever. He settled on malaria as the best agent to induce "pyrotherapy" in 1917, injecting the blood of GPI patients with infected blood.[44] Even though this procedure killed 3–20% of patients (records were poorly kept), the desperation and inevitable death of end-stage syphilis justified the treatment at the time.[45] Notwithstanding, the lack of controlled trials of the procedure and uncertain prognosis of GPI clouds the certainty of success.[42] It was not necessarily the harm caused by pyrotherapy in GPI itself that is the lesson. Rather, it was the fervor with which some somatic treatments, including pyrotherapy, were thereafter trialled on the mentally ill in the quest for further success. From unorthodox uses of pyrotherapy (such as injecting blood directly into the brain of those with GPI),[46] to "surgical bacteriology" (the removal of teeth and other organs to rid the body of occult infections leading to insanity),[3] to deep-sleep therapy (prolonged sedation as therapy),[47] and metrazol therapy (inducing intense convulsions),[3] the benefits were few and the harm immense.

Another somatic therapy, "insulin-coma therapy," was developed by the Viennese doctor Manfred Sakel, while working in Berlin in 1927. Schizophrenia cure rates of up to 80% were reported. It was widely adopted by the scientific community and was the standard of care from approximately the 1930s to the 1950s, prior to the advent of chlorpromazine.[48] "The Insulin Myth" was published in 1953 in *The Lancet,* reporting a lack of evidence for the treatment.[49] A subsequent controlled trial found no statistical difference to placebo.[50] But the damage was done. Approximately 1 in 100 patients died during the procedure. Many others suffered brain damage from the resulting hypoglycemic coma or were rendered obese from the effects of insulin. A widely accepted treatment by professionals and academics, later found to have no evidence of beneficial effect whilst damaging many.

In the mid-twentieth century, Egas Moniz, the Portuguese neurologist and to-be Nobel prizewinner, pioneered the frontal lobotomy (earlier called leukotomy). The Americans Walter Freeman and James Watts developed a transorbital method, completed in just 20 minutes with the use of an ice-pick and a mallet.[3,4] Beyond the 0.85% to 2.5% mortality rate (though reported as high as 18% in some centers),[51] the effects on personality and cognition were obvious. Its recipients traded one form of madness for an iatrogenic mental deficiency, often left "soulless," bland, and without emotional capacity.[4] The sister of President John F. Kennedy, Rosemary Kennedy, was a notable case of someone left incapacitated from surgery.[52,53]

The above treatments occurred largely in a time before randomized controlled trials, so they must be viewed in that light. But were these times also absent of regulatory measures? What forces were at play? What checks and balances were lost? For there were certainly detractors in all cases. But this did not stop the inexorable rise of damaging treatments. Is it possible that current treatments will be viewed in retrospect as failed experiments on vulnerable people?

Deinstitutionalization in the USA

In the 1950s USA, institutional abuse was particularly rife. Overcrowded "snake pits" and lack of evidence-based treatment and care led to abhorrent conditions within America's asylums.[3,16,17] At its peak, 560,000 people were institutionalized in 1950s America. Undoubtedly, there were examples of good care. But with this degree of overcrowding it was simply not possible to provide this to most. Preceding the civil rights movement, a number of damning exposes demonstrated the plight of the institutionalized mentally ill, altering the social climate.[15,16]

The reasons for deinstitutionalization are discussed in depth elsewhere. Notable is the certainty of those that promoted deinstitutionalization, similar to the certainty of those that promoted institutionalization centuries before. Nevertheless, the reform's noble intention was to create a community mental health plan that focused on prevention and would negate the need for state hospitals.[53] This plan simultaneously failed in its preventative intent whilst disregarding patients that flooded out of state hospitals.[53] Whereas the relative contribution of deinstitutionalization to the increase in homelessness and incarceration of those with serious mental illness is debated,[54,55] it is well recognized that the clumsy handling of deinstitutionalization contributed to both.[53,54] Thus, the regression to maltreatment continued for many.

The Regression of Indonesia's Promising System

In the wake of the country's independence from Holland and deinstitutionalization in the Western World, Indonesia's mental health system was reformed under the leadership of Professor R. Kusumanto Setyonegoro in the 1960s and 1970s. The commencement of a new mental health law, separate from the general health laws, occurred in 1966. The law emphasized the principles of prevention, treatment, and rehabilitation, which had been enthusiastically agreed upon at a meeting of psychiatrists organized by the Ministry of Health earlier in the same year.[56,57]

Kusumanto, appointed in 1971 as the Director of the Directorate of Mental Health within the Department of Mental Health, opened 22 new mental health hospitals, resulting in a psychiatric hospital in 26 of Indonesia's 31 provinces. The hospitals were integrated with the community mental health program, providing in- and outpatient care, public health education, and consultation to general hospitals. The period from 1970 to 1985 was designated the "golden age" in Indonesian psychiatry by some authors.[56,57]

This peak in Indonesian mental health care was gradually eroded by reductions in funding and a decentralization of mental health provision (almost certainly a move to reduce the burden on the government). The once central place of the community mental health system was threatened. As the mental hospitals were under-resourced, they were no longer able to integrate with the general health programs. As the integration reduced, so did the quality of care.

Indonesia is the fourth most populous country in the world. The current state of care for those with mental illness is, in many places, tragic. Whilst exceptional care can be found in some wealthy private institutions, other private facilities – borne out of declining public facilities – have "deplorable conditions, [where patients] receive inadequate nutrition, suffer from a variety of ailments, and are often restrained."[57] *Pasung,* or chaining, was outlawed in the 1970s, but exists to this day in many places, as demonstrated by the photojournalist Andrea Star Reese in 2012.[58] Some of the treatment facilities are cages with no sanitation facilities.

Criminalization, Homelessness, and Neglect: The Current (Troubling) Picture in the United States

Of the approximately 10 million people with serious mental illness (as a proxy for psychotic illness) in the United States, at least 300,000 people are incarcerated,[59] at least 60,000 people are homeless,[60] and at least 5 million do not receive stable treatment at last reliable measurement.[61] Further, it is estimated that more than two million arrests each year involve people with serious mental illnesses, many of whom are homeless at the time of arrest.[62,63] Perhaps unsurprisingly, this results in at least three times more seriously mentally ill people in jails and prisons than in mental health hospitals.[64] Jails and prisons, therefore, are the principal care facility for those with serious mental illness. Interestingly, in an odd reversal of the nineteenth-century pattern of jails converted to asylums (for example, Africa and Australia – as described above), some state hospitals converted to jails.[65-67] Additionally, there are approximately 4,000 prisoners with mental illness kept in solitary confinement in US prisons.[68]

What Does History Tell Us?

The task of Sisyphus was to push a boulder up a hill. He was able to do this, but invariably it rolled down again and he would start over. We hope to demonstrate the repetition of maltreatment of those with serious mental illness – despite the efforts of many to reform and progress – and whilst doing so, to inspire deeper reflection.

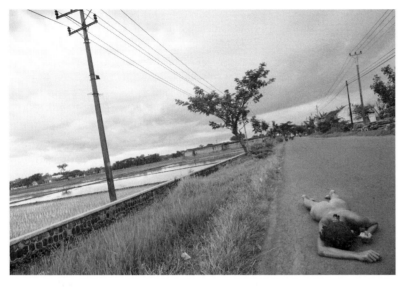

Indonesia
Credit: Andrea Star Reese

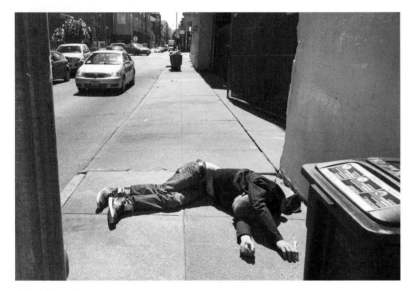

San Francisco
Credit: Associated Press, Ben Margo

We do not suggest that outcomes for those with psychotic illness are universally poor. The authors have seen many inspiring stories of recovery and good policy. In fact, one can choose to see a series of reforms leading to overall improved care. No longer are there witch hunts and exorcisms for souls gone mad. Hospitals of today are, for the most part, better than asylums of yesteryear, with an increasingly professional workforce. Advances in psychopharmacology and evidence-based psychological therapies have improved the lives of those with psychotic illness, but people are often not accessing the treatment.

Because of a lack of access or utilization of care, many people with psychotic disorders are locked up in prisons. Others are homeless and untreated. Those with psychotic illness die, on average, 10–17 years earlier than those without.[69-71]

People with cancer and heart disease are rarely locked up within jails or found lying in the streets for reasons to do with their illness. Why then those with psychotic disorders? Intelligent and passionate policymakers, clinicians, and advocates debate and attempt to implement the best forms of care and treatment. Yet, something is amiss.

We conclude that scientific advancements and policy reform does not seem to be enough to ensure humane treatment for the 1–2% of the population with psychotic illness. We hope this provides a basis for deeper reflection on the context of reform failure and maltreatment through which more resilient policy can be created.

Acknowledgments

We acknowledge Paris Beauregard, Charles Daugherty, Andrew Scull, William Taft, and Sunny Wade for their help in the preparation of this manuscript.

References

1. Grob GN. *Mental Institutions in America*. Piscataway, NJ: Transaction Publishers; 1973.

2. Porter R. *Madness: A Brief History*. New York: Oxford University Press; 2002.

3. Scull A. *Madness in Civilization: A Cultural History of Insanity from the Bible to Freud from the Madhouse to Modern Medicine*. New Jersey, USA: Princeton University Press; 2015.

4. Shorter E, Healy D. A history of psychiatry: from the era of the asylum to the age of prozac. *J Psychopharmacol*. 1997; **11**(3): 287.

5. Tseng W-S. The development of psychiatric concepts in traditional Chinese medicine. *Arch Gen Psychiatry*. 1973; **29**(4): 569–575.

6. Porter R. *The Greatest Benefit to Mankind: A Medical History of Humanity (The Norton History of Science)*. New York: WW Norton & Company; 1999.

7. Risse GB. *Mending Bodies, Saving Souls: A History of Hospitals*. Oxford: Oxford University Press; 1999.

8. Miller AC. Jundi-Shapur, bimaristans, and the rise of academic medical centres. *J R Soc Med*. 2006; **99**(12): 615–617.

9. Youssef HA, Youssef FA, Dening TR. Evidence for the existence of schizophrenia in medieval Islamic society. *Hist Psychiatry*. 1996; **7**(25): 55–62.

10. Dubovsky SL. Psychiatry in Saudi Arabia. *Am J Psychiatry*. 1983; **140**(11): 1455–1459.

11. Pridmore S, Pasha MI. Psychiatry and Islam. *Australas Psychiatry*. 2004; **12**(4): 380–385.

12. Andrews J, Briggs A, Porter R, Tucker P, Waddington K. *The History of Bethlem*. London and New York: Routledge; 2013.

13. Parry-Jones WL. *The Trade in Lunacy: A Study of Private Madhouses in England in the Eighteenth and Nineteenth Centuries*. London: Routledge; 1972.

14. Parry-Jones WL. English private madhouses in the eighteenth and nineteenth centuries. *Proc R Soc Med*. 1973; **66**(7): 659.

15. Maisel AQ. Bedlam 1946: most US mental hospitals are a shame and a disgrace. *Life Mag*. 1946; **20**(18): 102–118.

16. Gorman M. *Oklahoma Attacks Its Snake Pits*. USA: National Mental Health Foundation; 1948.

17. Deutsch A. *The Shame of the States*. California, USA: Harcourt, Brace; 1948.

18. Scull A. *The Most Solitary of Afflictions: Madness and Society in Britain, 1700–1900*. New Haven and London: Yale University Press; 1993.

19. Kirkby KC. History of psychiatry in Australia, pre-1960. *Hist Psychiatry*. 1999; **10**(38): 191–204.

20. Appelbaum PS, Kemp KN. The evolution of commitment law in the nineteenth century: a reinterpretation. *Law Hum Behav*. 1982; **6**(3–4): 343.

21. Scull AT. Moral treatment reconsidered: some sociological comments on an episode in the history of British psychiatry. *Psychol Med*. 1979; **9**(3): 421–428.

22. Dorothea Dix. Encyclopaedia Britannica; 2019. www.britannica.com/biography/Dorothea-Dix (accessed June 2020).

23. Scull A, MacKenzie C, Hervey N. *Masters of Bedlam: The Transformation of the Mad-Doctoring Trade*. New Jersey, USA and Chichester, UK: Princeton University Press; 2014.

24. Topp L. Single rooms, seclusion and the non-restraint movement in British asylums, 1838–1844. *Soc Hist Med*. 2018; **31**(4): 754–773.

25. Langley GE. Sir John Charles Bucknill 1817–1897: our founder. Based on a lecture given at the annual meeting of the Royal College of Psychiatrists in Exeter on 9th July, 1979. *Br J Psychiatry*. 1980; **137**(2): 105–110.

26. Bucknill JC. Notes on asylums for the insane in America. *Am J Psychiatry*. 1876; **33**(2): 137–160.

27. Digby A. Changes in the asylum: the case of York, 1777–1815. *Econ Hist Rev*. 1983; **36**(2): 218–239.

28. Kirby D. Vulnerable patients moved 50 miles after closure of York Psychiatric Hospital. *The Independent*; 2015. www.independent.co.uk/life-style/health-and-families/health-news/vulnerable-patients-moved-50-miles-after-closure-of-york-psychiatric-hospital-a6787061.html (accessed June 2020).

29. Coleborne C, MacKinnon D. Psychiatry and its institutions in Australia and New Zealand: an overview. *Int Rev Psychiatry*. 2006; **18**(4): 371–380.

30. Dax EC. The first 200 years of Australian psychiatry. *Aust N Z J Psychiatry*. 1989; **23**(1): 103–110.

31. Mahone S. Psychiatry in the East African colonies: a background to confinement. *Int Rev Psychiatry*. 2006; **18**(4): 327–332.

32. Oyebode F. History of psychiatry in West Africa. *Int Rev Psychiatry*. 2006; **18**(4): 319–325.

33. Sadowsky J. *Imperial Bedlam: Institutions of Madness in Colonial Southwest Nigeria*. **10**. Berkeley, CA: University of California Press; 1999.

34. Nizamie H, Goyal N. History of psychiatry in India. *Indian J Psychiatry*. 2010; **52**(7): 7.

35. Jain S, Murthy P. Madmen and specialists: the clientele and the staff of the Lunatic Asylum, Bangalore. *Int Rev Psychiatry*. 2006; **18**(4): 345–354.

36. Judd A. America's dark past relived as cycle ends. *Atlanta Journal & Constitution*; 2013. www.ajc.com/news/state-regional/asylum-dark-past-relived-cycle-ends/uq2OK0dgHCeynhFUGba36O/ (accessed June 2020).

37. Sisti DA, Segal AG, Emanuel EJ. Improving long-term psychiatric care: bring back the asylum. *J Am Med Assoc*. 2015; **313**(3): 243–244.

38. Kevles DJ. Eugenics and human rights. *Br Med J*. 1999; **319**(7207): 435–438.

39. Bashford A, Levine P. *The Oxford Handbook of the History of Eugenics*. New York: Oxford University Press; 2010.

40. Adams MB. *The Wellborn Science: Eugenics in Germany, France, Brazil, and Russia*. New York: Oxford University Press; 1990.

41. Broberg G, Roll-Hansen N. *Eugenics and the Welfare State: Sterilization Policy in Denmark, Sweden Norway and Finland*. Michigan: Michigan State University Press; 2005.

42. Scull A. *Psychiatry and Its Discontents*. Oakland, CL: University of California Press; 2019.

43. Scull A. *Madhouse: A Tragic Tale of Megalomania and Modern Medicine*. New Haven and London: Yale University Press; 2007.

44. Wagner-Jauregg J. The history of the malaria treatment of general paralysis. *Am J Psychiatry*. 1946; **102**(5): 577–582.

45. Ouwens IMD, Lens CE, Fiolet ATL, et al. Malaria fever therapy for general paralysis of the insane: a historical cohort study. *Eur Neurol*. 2017; **78**(1–2): 56–62.

46. Lieberman JA. *Shrinks: The Untold Story of Psychiatry*. London: Weidenfeld and Nicholson; 2015.

47. Walton M. Deep sleep therapy and Chelmsford Private Hospital: have we learnt anything? *Australas Psychiatry*. 2013; **21**(3): 206–212.

48. Jones K. Insulin coma therapy in schizophrenia. *J R Soc Med*. 2000; **93**(3): 147–149.

49. Bourne H. The insulin myth. *Lancet*. 1953; **262**(6793): 964–968.

50. Ackner B, Harris A, Oldham AJ. Insulin treatment of schizophrenia: a controlled study. *Lancet*. 1957; **269** (6969): 607–611.

51. Swayze VW. Frontal leukotomy and related psychosurgical procedures in the era before antipsychotics (1935–1954): a historical overview. *Am J Psychiatry*. 1995; **152**(4): 505–515.

52. Larson KC. *Rosemary: The Hidden Kennedy Daughter*. New York: Houghton Mifflin Harcourt; 2015.

53. Torrey EF. *American Psychosis: How the Federal Government Destroyed the Mental Illness Treatment System*. New York: Oxford University Press; 2014.

54. Lamb HR. Deinstitutionalization and the homeless mentally ill. *Psychiatr Serv*. 1984; **35**(9): 899–907.

55. Lamb HR. Does deinstitutionalization cause criminalization?: the Penrose hypothesis. *JAMA Psychiatry*. 2015; **72**(2): 105–106.

56. Pols H. The development of psychiatry in Indonesia: from colonial to modern times. *Int Rev Psychiatry*. 2006; **18**(4): 363–370.

57. Pols H, Wibisono S. Psychiatry and mental health care in Indonesia from colonial to modern times. In: Minas H, Lewis M, eds. *Mental Health in Asia and the Pacific*. New York: Springer; 2017: 205–221.

58. Reese AS. Disorder; 2011–2016. www.andreastarreese.com/disorder (accessed June 2020).

59. Lamb HR, Weinberger LE. The shift of psychiatric inpatient care from hospitals to jails and prisons. *J Am Acad Psychiatry Law*. 2005; **33**(4): 529–534.

60. Fazel S, Khosla V, Doll H, Geddes J. The prevalence of mental disorders among the homeless in western countries: systematic review and meta-regression analysis. *PLoS Med*. 2008; **5**(12): e225.

61. Kessler RC, Berglund PA, Bruce ML, et al. The prevalence and correlates of untreated serious mental illness. *Health Serv Res*. 2001; **36**(6 Pt 1): 987.

62. Iglehart JK. Decriminalizing mental illness—the Miami model. *N Engl J Med*. 2016; **374**(18): 1701–1703.

63. McNiel DE, Binder RL, Robinson JC. Incarceration associated with homelessness, mental disorder, and co-occurring substance abuse. *Psychiatr Serv*. 2005; **56** (7): 840–846.

64. Torrey EF, Kennard AD, Eslinger D, Lamb R, Pavle J. More mentally ill persons are in jails and prisons than

hospitals: a survey of the states. Treatment Advocacy Centre, Arlington, VA and National Sheriffs' Association; 2010. www.treatmentadvocacycenter.org/storage/documents/final_jails_v_hospitals_study.pdf (accessed June 2020).

65. Lima State Hospital.

66. Matteawan State Hospital.

67. St. Joseph State Asylum.

68. The Association of State Correctional Administrators, The Liman Center for Public Interest Law at Yale Law School. Reforming restrictive housing: the 2018 ASCA-Liman nationwide survey of time-in-cell. 2018.

69. Walker ER, McGee RE, Druss BG. Mortality in mental disorders and global disease burden implications: a systematic review and meta-analysis. *JAMA Psychiatry*. 2015; **72**(4): 334–341.

70. Hjorthøj C, Stürup AE, McGrath JJ, Nordentoft M. Years of potential life lost and life expectancy in schizophrenia: a systematic review and meta-analysis. *Lancet Psychiatry*. 2017; **4**(4): 295–301.

71. Chang C-K, Hayes RD, Perera G, et al. Life expectancy at birth for people with serious mental illness and other major disorders from a secondary mental health care case register in London. *PLoS One*. 2011; **6**(5): e19590.

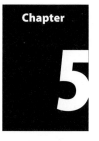

Forensic Patients in State Psychiatric Hospitals: 1999–2016

Amanda Wik, Vera Hollen, and William H. Fisher

Introduction

Recently, mental health officials have expressed concern regarding population shifts occurring in public psychiatric hospitals. Specifically, they have seen an increase in the number of "forensically involved" patients in these facilities. This trend is seen, in part, as an increase in the number of persons who have been brought to court on a criminal charge and subsequently court-ordered to receive inpatient services at state psychiatric hospitals.[1-5] These "forensic patients" are referred to the state psychiatric hospitals to be evaluated (e.g. to determine their mental status at the time of the crime and their ability to comprehend court proceedings and/or assist their attorney with their case because of an apparent mental illness) or to be restored (e.g. to receive treatment services and/or educational interventions aimed at helping defendants regain their ability to understand the court process) prior to adjudication.[1-8] Forensic patients can also consist of patients who have been court-ordered to receive inpatient services after a verdict has been reached on their case (e.g. individuals found to be not guilty but mentally ill, inmates who were transferred from a correctional facility for inpatient services, or individuals involved in the criminal justice system who were involuntarily civilly committed[I] to a state psychiatric hospital for continued treatment).[2,7-9] As can be seen, there are a variety of different types of forensic patients. This descriptive presentation is based on the major findings from a national study.[II] For the purposes of this study, this paper focuses solely on: (1) the overall forensic population, (2) patients who had been court-ordered to receive

pre-trial evaluations at a state psychiatric hospital, and (3) defendants who were found incompetent to stand trial (IST) and court-ordered to receive competency restoration services at a state psychiatric hospital. The term "forensic patients" is used in this paper to refer to all persons found "not guilty by reason of insanity," persons found "guilty but mentally ill," individuals transferred from correctional facilities seeking treatment services that are not available in the correctional setting, and, in some states, individuals involved in the criminal justice system who have been civilly committed to a state psychiatric hospital.

A large portion of forensic patients receiving services at state psychiatric hospitals consist of defendants who have been deemed IST[III] and court-ordered to receive competency restoration services.[2,3,7,10] These services typically involve treatment and/or educational interventions aimed at helping defendants regain their ability to understand the court process and/or assist their attorneys in their defense.[2,6] The apparent growth of this forensic population, in particular, has sparked the concerns of state officials. Many state officials have queried the National Association of State Mental Health Program Directors Research Institute (NRI) as to whether the rising forensic population in state psychiatric hospitals in their state, particularly IST patients, is a phenomenon that is unique to their state, or if this is a national trend.

Despite the growing concern centered around this trend, there are few national studies that have examined this "forensification"[IV] of state hospitals.[7] This is indeed a valid concern. Forensic patients differ from civil patients[V] and patients who are involuntarily civilly

---

[I] Patients who are involuntarily committed because they are a danger to themselves or others but are not involved in the criminal justice system.

[II] For information on the results of other forensic statuses, please email the author, or view the full report at: 1318/tac-paper-9-forensic-patients-in-state-hospitals-final-09-05-2017.pdf.

[III] In some states the term "incompetent to proceed" is used to refer to these patients.

[IV] A term used to refer to the proportional increase in forensic patients present within state psychiatric hospitals.

[V] This term refers to patients who are not involved in the criminal justice system and are being treated at a state psychiatric hospital.

committed.[2,7-9] In cases where a patient is being civilly admitted to a hospital, the hospital has the authority to determine who is to be admitted or discharged. Conversely, the admission and discharge of forensic patients is primarily controlled by the courts. Very few state psychiatric hospitals have the authority to discharge patients who have been court-ordered to receive inpatient services.[2] Even though the admission and discharge process for forensic patients diverges from that of civil patients, the funding for these hospitalizations and their effect on bed supply are the concerns of the mental health system.[9]

Data from a national study are needed for policy-makers to be able to address whether or not: the perceived "forensification" process is "real" and the rise in forensic patients is not a result of a declining civil population (e.g. the trend among forensic patients has remained steady, but the decline in civil patients has made it to appear as if the forensic population is growing).

Due to a lack of information on the scope of the issue and the potential factors that may be contributing to this apparent shift, this national study was developed to examine these factors. In doing so we address three questions regarding the perceived increase in the number of forensic patients: (1) Has there been an increase in the rate of state hospital admissions and census for *all* forensic statuses? (2) Are forensic patients becoming an increasing proportion of these hospitals' census? (3) Has the *absolute number* of patients receiving pre-trial evaluations and the number of IST patients who have been court-ordered to receive competency restoration services in state psychiatric hospitals services increased?

Methodology

State-Level Data on Forensic Patients

The NRI has worked with the Substance Abuse and Mental Health Services Administration (SAMHSA) since 1996 to maintain the State Profiling System (SPS). The SPS collects and maintains qualitative and quantitative data on public behavioral health services, including all state psychiatric hospitals. For the purposes of this report, the NRI used the data collected by the SPS, which captured the number of forensic patients present within state psychiatric hospitals in each state and the amount that these hospitals were spending on those patients.

This study draws on state-level aggregate information from the SPS on the number of forensic patients present within all state psychiatric hospitals on a given "census day."[VI] To assess the trends on forensic utilization, data were collected from each state for the years 1996, 1999, 2002, 2004, 2005, 2006, 2009, 2011, and 2014. Data were also obtained from the SPS regarding the state behavioral health agency's inpatient budget spending on forensic patients versus civil patients for each fiscal year from 2004 to 2015.

Data Collection from States

In addition to the data obtained from the SPS, we also queried state forensic directors. A series of Excel tables was sent to these officials as data collection instruments. The first table collected information for 2016. For each forensic status as well as for the total adult forensic population, the forensic directors were asked to indicate: the number of forensic patients present on the first census day of the state's 2016 fiscal year (FY);[VII] the number of forensic patients admitted to the state psychiatric hospitals in FY 2016;[VIII] the average and median length of stay for forensic patients in FY 2016. A second table contained data on each forensic status from 1996 to 2014. Finally, a third table contained information collected between 2004 and 2015 on the number of patient-days and state psychiatric hospital budget spending on forensic and civil patients. Each forensic director was asked to review the information to verify its accuracy. If inconsistencies were found, the states were allowed to submit updated information.

To gain a better understanding of the challenges faced by each state and the perspectives of each state's forensic director on changes occurring among the forensic population, a questionnaire including 36 items taken from the National Association of State Mental Health Program Directors (NASMHPD) 2014 forensic mental health services report[2] was sent (along with the tables described above) to the forensic

---

VI A state's given census day for 1996 through 2011 was the last day of its fiscal year. In 2014 SAMHSA modified the data collection period, changing census day to the first day of the fiscal year. Since the data used for this study are based on SAMHSA's SPS, the given census day used for this study was changed.

VII It should be noted that the "fiscal year" varies between states. The states were told to code the fiscal year based on their state's definition.

VIII States were asked to code this based on the 2016 FY. However, some states may have used the calendar year.

director within each state and the District of Columbia. The questions were intended to collect information on: the percentage of competency-to-stand-trial (CST) evaluations that were being conducted on an outpatient basis, the percentage of patients who were receiving competency restoration services on an outpatient basis, whether or not there was a limit on how long defendants could be committed to the state psychiatric hospitals for competency restoration services, if the state maintains a waitlist for different types of forensic admissions, the length of time that defendants typically are on the waitlist (if applicable), and whether the state psychiatric hospital has ever been threatened with or held in contempt for not admitting IST defendants court-ordered to receive competency restoration services in a timely manner.[2] To assess the viewpoints of forensic directors and to understand what programs (if any) were being developed to provide mental health treatment to the defendants in a less intensive setting, new questions were developed. A total of 37 states returned completed surveys to the NRI.

Analysis

Data from the questionnaire were analyzed using version 24 of the Statistical Package for the Social Sciences (SPSS). Data collected from the tables were analyzed using Microsoft Excel.

Data on forensic statuses were analyzed in several ways. For each forensic status, as well as the total number of adult forensic patients, the national average and median were calculated for each year. Since responses across states can be impacted by different factors, percent change was used to examine individual state trends in regard to the state psychiatric hospital's forensic population. Percent change calculations were performed for three time periods: 1999–2005, 2005–2014, 1999–2014. To understand if changes were occurring across the nation, an "overall percent change" was computed. Finally, information on the number of patients admitted in 2016 was used to calculate admission rates. The 2016 admission rates were computed by dividing the number of forensic patients admitted to the state psychiatric hospitals in 2016 by the state's adult civilian population[IX] and multiplying the result by 100,000.

The final analysis examined the percentage of adult forensic patients among the state psychiatric hospital populations. In order to conduct this analysis, the NRI needed information on the number of adults (age >18) present within each state psychiatric hospital on a given census day. The NRI collected this information from SAMHSA's Uniform Reporting System (URS). The URS database includes information on the number of patients over the age of 18 present in a state psychiatric hospital on a given census day for every year, which was used to determine the change in forensic population for each state between 2002 and 2014.

Missing Data

Some states were unable to provide the requested information in the stipulated time, and others were only able to provide partial data.

States with missing information could not be represented in the graphs depicting longitudinal trends. Throughout this paper, the trends of states with complete data for the time periods examined are only shown.

It should be noted that our presentation is entirely descriptive. We did not test hypotheses regarding between-state differences or change from year to year. Doing so would have been difficult given the use of aggregate data and the small number of states and data points in this work.

Results

Total Adult Forensic Census

The "total adult forensic" patient census includes all adult forensic inpatients (*regardless of their forensic status/category*) within a state psychiatric hospital on the designated census day. The national average of adult forensic inpatients between 1999 and 2014 has shown an increase during this period. While the average is helpful, it can be influenced by extremely high or extremely low values. However, the national median, which is unaffected by outlying values, shows the population trend to be fairly stable between 1999 and 2014. In essence, the differences between the national average and national median indicate that the outlying numbers impacted the trend line (Figure 5.1).

The results for the states that had complete data for 1999, 2002, 2004, 2005, 2006, 2010, 2011, and 2014 suggest that many of these states were experiencing a rise in state psychiatric hospitals' forensic

---

[IX] This refers to anyone who is >18 years of age living in the state and not a member of the military.

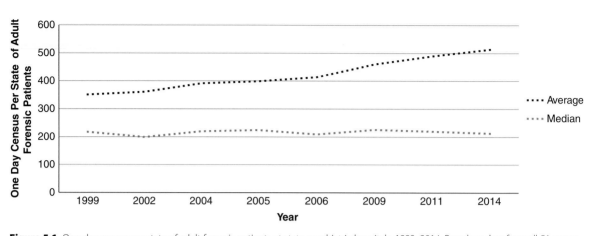

Figure 5.1 One-day census per state of adult forensic patients at state psychiatric hospitals, 1999–2014. Based on data from all 51 states. Sources: 2017 NRI Inpatient Forensic Services Study; 1995–2015 State Mental Health Agency Profiling System.

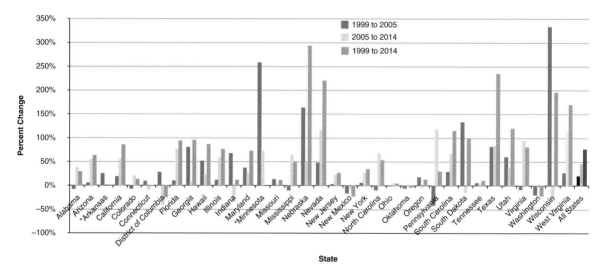

Figure 5.2 Percent change in inpatient forensic population. Based on data from 35 states for 1999, 2005, and 2014.

Notes: Thirty-seven states had numerical data for these years. NH was removed since it reported having 0 forensic patient for *1999, 2005,* and *2014.* MA was removed. Their data are included in the data table for this graph, and was used to conduct the percent change for "All States." AR had a percent change of 1960% for *2005–2014* and a percent change of 2475% for *1999–2014.* MN had a percent change of 517% for *1999–2014.* Sources: 2017 NRI Inpatient Forensic Services Study; 1995–2015 State Mental Health Agency Profiling System.

population. While for the most part the rise in the total adult forensic population was gradual, many of the states experienced a spike in state psychiatric hospitals' total adult forensic population in 2011.

Each state is unique. Therefore, percent change calculations were performed for the 35 states that provided information on the total number of forensic patients present in their state psychiatric hospitals in 1999, 2005, and 2014 (Figure 5.2). Across all the 35 states, there was a 76% increase in the number of adult forensic patients present in their state psychiatric

hospitals between 1999 and 2014. Across all the 35 states, the largest increase occurred between 2005 and 2014 (46% increase across all the 35 states versus a 20% increase between 1999 and 2005). These results suggest that many of the states that had complete data for 1999, 2005, and 2014 experienced an increase in the number of adult forensic patients present in their state psychiatric hospitals between 1999 and 2014.

The SPS does not capture data on the number of admissions to each state psychiatric hospital per year. While the "census day" data can be

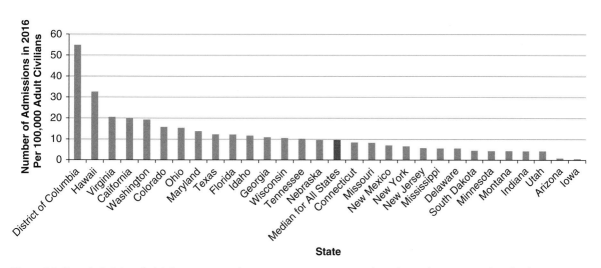

Figure 5.3 Rate of admission of adult forensic patients for inpatient services at state psychiatric hospitals in 2016. Based on data from 29 responding states.

Notes: Thirty-two states reported admission data. NC, NH, and SC had admission rates of 0 per 100,000, so they were not included in the graph. IL, MA, MI, NV, and PA did not report, or did not have data available for 2016.
Source: 2017 NRI Inpatient Forensic Services Study.

informative, it is limited by the fact that it only shows the number of individuals present on one day in a year. Admission rates were calculated using the 2016 data reported by the responding states. Of the 37 responding states, the number of adult forensic admissions in 2016 was reported by 32 states, of which 27 states had an admission rate of over 4 per 100,000 adult civilians (Figure 5.3). Overall, the median admission rate was 9.65 adult forensic patients per 100,000 adult civilians.

Census day information and admission rates are helpful for state comparisons. In addition, this information can be used to compare bed availability and allocation between forensic and civil patients in state hospitals. The number of beds available within state psychiatric hospitals obviously impacts admission rates, which, in turn, impact waitlists for beds. Information on the types of patients occupying these beds is important. This is especially true with regard to forensic patients, since some forensic patients may remain in state psychiatric hospitals for a long period of time.[1–4]

In order to calculate the utilization of beds, the analysis had to be restricted to examining data from 2002 through 2014 since the URS does not contain information prior to 2002. Twenty-five states had complete data for this time period. Changes in each state hospital's forensic composition are shown in Figure 5.4. Accordingly, only one state experienced

a decrease in forensic population between 2002 and 2014. The remaining states experienced a rise in the number of forensic patients within their facilities.

Each analysis of the various adult forensic statuses indicates that there has been an increase in the number of adult forensic patients receiving inpatient services between 1999 and 2014. This rise appears to have resulted in a larger proportion of population in state psychiatric hospitals being forensic patients.

The results lead to further questions. Specifically, is a particular specific forensic status responsible for this increase? Or, is the rise in adult forensic population due to an increase in multiple forensic statuses receiving inpatient services? To answer these questions, a series of analyses were developed and are discussed below.

Pre-Trial Evaluations

The national average for the number of patients present for inpatient pre-trial evaluations on annual census days between 1999 and 2014 is higher than the national median for this population (Figure 5.5). As with the total adult forensic status, the national average for this population is impacted by states with outlying data.

When changes within each state were examined, the percent change calculations suggest that among the 26 states with data for 1999, 2005, and 2014

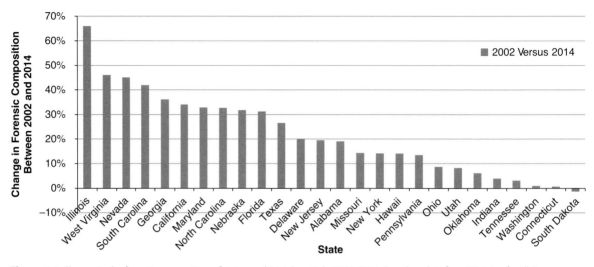

Figure 5.4 Change in the forensic composition of state psychiatric hospitals, 2002–2014. Based on data from 27 states for all 7 years.

Notes: Twenty-eight states had data for 2002 and 2014. NH was removed from graph since it reported 0 forensic patient for either year. MA was removed from the graph due to a not-divisible-by-zero error. IL reported having 1213 forensic patients in 2014, yet 513 patients were 18 or older. Data from 2013 was used for 2014. This made the number of adult state hospital residents 1232 for 2014. This caused a percent change of 66.0%.

Sources: 2017 NRI Inpatient Forensic Services Study; Uniform Reporting System; 1995–2015 State Mental Health Agency Profiling System.

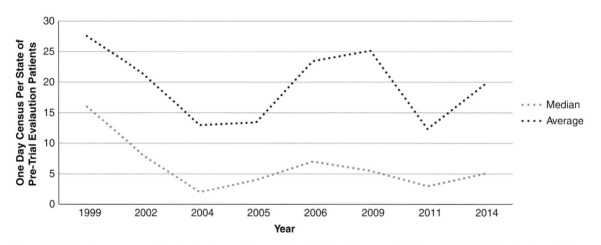

Figure 5.5 One-day census per state of patients present for pre-trial evaluation at state psychiatric hospitals, 1999–2014. Based on data from all 51 states.

Notes: For Arkansas the number of patients present for pre-trial evaluation on the 2014 census day was removed from the average and median calculations for 2014.

Sources: 2017 NRI Inpatient Forensic Services Study; 1995–2015 State Mental Health Agency Profiling System.

(nine of which reported 0 forensic patients under pre-trial status), the rise in the number of patients present for pre-trial evaluation was a relatively new phenomenon. Between 2005 and 2014 these 17 states collectively saw an 84% rise in the number of forensic patients present on a given census day

for pre-trial evaluation at state psychiatric hospitals (Figure 5.6).

Data from 15 of the reporting states included information on the number of patients admitted for pre-trial evaluations in 2016. Each of the 15 states had an admission rate >1 per 100,000 adult

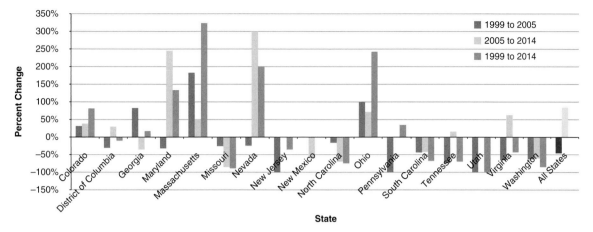

Figure 5.6 Percent change in inpatient population present for pre-trial evaluation, 1999–2014. Based on data from 17 states for 1999, 2005, and 2014.

Notes: Twenty-six states had data for these years. Several states (CA, CT, FL, IN, NE, NH, NY, SD, and TX) were removed since they did not report having any patients present for pre-trial evaluation in 1999, 2005, and 2014. UT reported having 0 patient for pre-trial evaluation on the census days examined in 2005 and 2014.

Sources: 2017 NRI Inpatient Forensic Services Study; 1995–2015 State Mental Health Agency Profiling System.

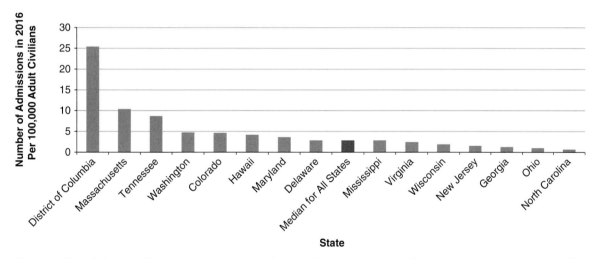

Figure 5.7 Rate of admission of patients to inpatient services for pre-trial evaluation at state psychiatric hospitals in 2016. Based on data from 15 responding states.

Notes: Thirty-four states reported admissions data for 2016. AZ, CA, CT, FL, ID, IL, IN, MN, MT, NE, NH, NY, SD, TX, and UT were removed from the graph since they had admission rates of 0 per 100,000. IA, MO, NM, and SC had admission rates of 0.2 per 100,000. MI, NV, and PA did not report or did not have data available for 2016. Therefore, the data for these states are missing.

Source: 2017 NRI Inpatient Forensic Services Study.

civilians. Eleven had an admission rate between 1 and 5 per 100,000 adult civilians. Three states had admission rates that were relatively high (Figure 5.7).

IST restoration services

The data obtained for this study suggest that there has been a rise in the number of IST patients receiving competency restoration services during our observation period. The national average and median both showed an increase between 2005 and 2014 (Figure 5.8).

The 27 states with complete data for 1999, 2005, and 2014 collectively show a 72% increase in IST patients present on the census day (Figure 5.9).

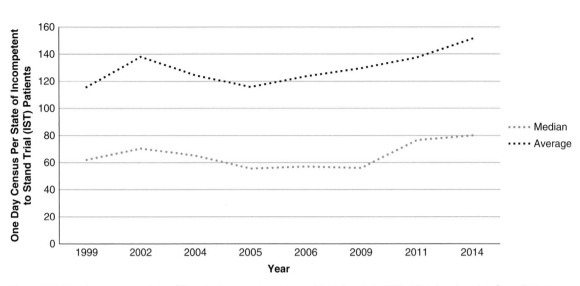

Figure 5.8 One-day census per state of IST patients present at state psychiatric hospitals, 1999–2014. Based on data from all 51 states.
Sources: 2017 NRI Inpatient Forensic Services Study; 1995–2015 State Mental Health Agency Profiling System.

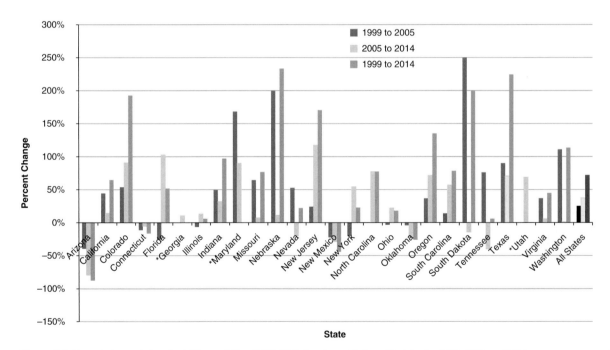

Figure 5.9 Percent change in inpatient IST population, 1999–2014. Based on data from 26 states for 1999, 2005, and 2014.
Notes: Twenty-seven states had data. NH was removed since it had 0 IST patients for 1999, 2005, and 2014. GA had a percent change of 302% for 1999–2005 and 344% for 1999–2014. MD had a percent change of 409% for 1999–2014. UT had a percent change of 629% for 1999–2005 and 1129% for 1999–2014.
Sources: 2017 NRI Inpatient Forensic Services Study; 1995–2015 State Mental Health Agency Profiling System.

Based on the IST admission data for 32 states, the rates of patient admission for IST restoration were higher than that for pre-trial evaluations. The admission rate of IST patients in 32 states (out of the 34 states that responded with complete data) was >3 per 100,000 adult civilians (See Figure 5.10).

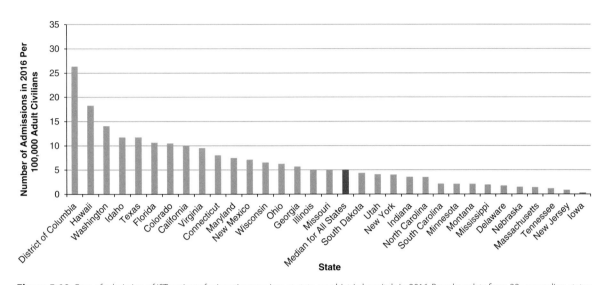

Figure 5.10 Rate of admission of IST patients for inpatient services at state psychiatric hospitals in 2016. Based on data from 32 responding states. Notes: Thirty-four states had admission data for 2016. Two states (NH and AZ) were not included in the graph since NH had an admission rate of 0 per 100,000 and AZ, 0.2 per 100,000. MI, NV, and PA did not report or did not have data available for 2016. These states were not included in the graph. Sources: 2017 NRI Inpatient Forensic Services Study.

Discussion

The results presented here show a rise in the number of adult forensic patients present in state psychiatric hospitals on a given census day between 1999 and 2014. Additionally, based on the data obtained from the SPS, this rise was apparent in a majority of states. Furthermore, when each of the forensic statuses was examined, the data appear to suggest that IST patients – those who might spend a longer period of time in hospitals in an attempt to restore competency – were primarily responsible for the rise in the adult forensic population. Since many of the state psychiatric hospitals are facing pressure to admit civil as well as forensic patients, such information is important. This was occurring at a time when the number of inpatient beds in all sectors had greatly reduced, leading many states to develop waitlists.[1-5,8,9] With regard to competency restoration, IST defendants may be waitlisted anywhere from several days to a year or more.[1-5] Many state psychiatric hospitals have faced legal action as a result of their lengthy wait times;[1-5] indeed, 20 of the 37 responding states (54%) indicated that they had been (or were currently being) threatened with or actually held in contempt of court for failing to reduce wait times. Many of these states reported implementing a variety of strategies to reduce wait times for competency restoration services to IST patients. The commonly reported strategies include,

but are not limited to, implementing outpatient competency restoration programs, creating and/or implementing jail-based competency restoration programs, creating additional state psychiatric hospital beds, hiring more forensic state psychiatric hospital workers, improving their admission processes (e.g. making it centralized and/or developing new prioritization standards), and increasing collaboration between mental health and criminal justice agencies.

Forensic patients are an important but often overlooked population within state psychiatric hospitals, yet state psychiatric hospitals spend approximately one-third of their budgets on forensic patients. As the number of forensic patients has increased over the years, the amount being spent on them has similarly increased.[9] Meanwhile, the proportion of inpatient budget spent on civil patients has decreased (Figure 5.11). It should be noted that while the amount being allocated to forensic patients may be impacted by how much of the inpatient budget can be spent on civil patients (and vice versa), it can also be impacted by additional factors. Specifically, the inpatient budget spent on civil patients is affected by the fact that more civil patients are being served in outpatient and other community-based settings.[9] This, in turn, means that fewer civil patients are being admitted to inpatient settings. In essence, the increasing preponderance of forensic patients in state psychiatric hospitals suggests a shift in the functioning of such facilities as these become an adjunct to the criminal justice system – a direction that was never envisioned as part of the mission of state mental health agencies.

Limitations

Our study has several limitations. As noted in the Methodology section, some states were unable to respond to the survey and so the data pulled from existing data sources could not be verified. The fact that such data were used in the analyses could have impacted the results.

A second limitation is that the data collection methods that state psychiatric hospitals were required to follow may have changed over time. This could lead to significant differences within and between states, which makes comparisons more complicated. A third limitation of the dataset is that it was difficult to determine if the states may have duplicated cases with more than one status (e.g. IST and sex offender). Consequently, the data used for this study might contain duplicated cases, depending on whether each state psychiatric hospital coded forensic patients as belonging to multiple forensic statuses. This limitation can impact the interpretations of state data.

States that did not duplicate information may have prioritized a particular forensic status over others for forensic patients with multiple statuses. Without knowing how each state coded patients with multiple

statuses, comparisons between states need to be done with caution.

Another limitation is that only criminal defendants are "at risk" for forensic admissions, and a better denominator for adjusting these data would be the number of adult criminal court arraignments in each state. However, obtaining such information at the level required would have been difficult and well beyond this study's scope and available resources.

Lastly, one-day census data were used as a proxy for the number of adult beds to compute the total adult forensic composition of state psychiatric hospitals. The reader should keep these limitations in mind when interpreting the results of this study.

Conclusion

The findings of this study support the perceptions of many state officials who are concerned that the forensic population is, indeed, increasing[1–5] and that the phenomenon is not unique to just a couple of states. The results presented here demonstrate that there was a rise in the number of adult forensic patients nationally, specifically IST patients, in state psychiatric hospitals between 1999 and 2014. This trend was not experienced by every state, since each state varies with respect to how it manages competency evaluation and restoration process.

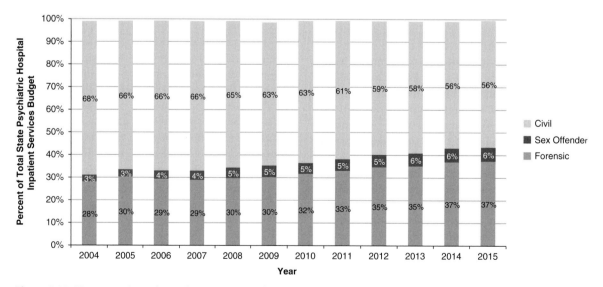

Figure 5.11 US state psychiatric hospital inpatient services budget spending, 2004–2015. Based on data from all 51 states. Source: State Revenues and Expenditure Study.

This study described the trends in the number of defendants being admitted to state psychiatric hospitals. Future studies need to do a more in-depth examination of the types and effectiveness of strategies undertaken by various states to reduce forensic admissions. Such information could help states determine what methods might be most applicable to the management of forensic population, thereby avoiding negative consequences (e.g. held in contempt for lengthy wait times). These data could provide a useful baseline for future analyses.

The study raises several questions. *Why is this increase occurring now? Who are these forensic patients? Are they new to the mental health system, or have they previously received services as "civil patients" and have newly encountered the criminal justice system? Have community-based services had an effect? In an era when many jurisdictions are developing diversion programs, how is it that so many persons displaying symptoms of mental health issues are still appearing in criminal courts? Keeping in mind that these referrals might have an effect on the judiciary, what are judges' views on this increase? Are forensic referrals really about the capacity to stand trial, or are these, in reality, a coping strategy used by judges to ensure access to mental health services for defendants who appear to need them?* Indeed, ordering a CST evaluation may be a simple, temporary – albeit inappropriate – solution to such problems.

Mental health services researchers have paid relatively little attention to this segment of public mental health systems and their clientele. Given an increasing presence of forensic patients and its growing burden on restoration resources across multiple states, the subject deserves a greater focus of attention.

Acknowledgments

The authors gratefully acknowledge the expertise and technical review provided by the following national experts on forensic mental health services: Debra A. Pinals, M.D., W. Lawrence Fitch, J.D., and Katherine Warburton, D.O. Without their guidance, a study of this magnitude could not have been completed. We also extend our appreciation to the State Forensic Directors and other staff collaborators who spent many hours compiling and reviewing data for this study. The authors assume all responsibility for the scientific content of the paper.

Funding

This work was developed under Task 2.2 of NASMHPD's Technical Assistance Coalition contract/task order, HHSS283201200021I/HHS28342003T, and funded by the Center for Mental Health Services/SAMHSA of the Department of Health and Human Services through the NASMHPD.

Disclosures

The authors (Amanda Wik and Vera Hollen) are employees of the NRI, and William Fisher is an NRI paid consultant. The authors maintained full independent control over study design, data collection and analysis, and the contents of written reports.

Ethical Considerations

The authors report no ethical considerations to disclose in regard to this study.

References

1. Colorado Department of Human Services. Needs analysis: current status, strategic positioning, and future planning. Office of Behavioral Health; 2015. www.nri-inc.org/media/1109/2015-colorado-department-of-human-service-behavioral-health-needs-analysis-nri.pdf (accessed June 2020).

2. Fitch LW. Assessment #3: Forensic mental health services in the United States. National Association of State Mental Health Program Directors; 2014. www.nasmhpd.org/sites/default/files/Assessment%203%20-%20Updated%20Forensic%20Mental%20Health%20Services.pdf (accessed June 2020).

3. Nobles J, Randall J. Evaluation report: mental health services in county jails. Office of the Legislative Auditor (OLA), State Of Minnesota; 2016. www.auditor.leg.state.mn.us/ped/pedrep/mhjails.pdf (accessed June 2020)

4. PCG. Initial findings report: Washington mental health system assessment. Public Consulting Group; 2016. www.ofm.wa.gov/reports/MentalHealthSystemAssessmentInitialFindings.pdf (accessed June 2020).

5. Washington State Department of Social and Health Services. Cassie Cordell Trueblood, et al., v. Washington State Department of Social and Health Services, et al. Case No. C14-1178 MJP monthly report to the court appointed monitor - July 15, 2017. www.dshs.wa.gov/sites/default/files/BHSIA/FMHS/Trueblood/2017Trueblood/Trueblood-Report-2017-07.pdf (accessed June 2020).

6. Miller RD. Hospitalization of criminal defendants for evaluation of competence to stand trial or for restoration of competence: clinical and legal issues. *Behav Sci Law*. 2003; **21**: 369–391.

7. Fisher WH, Geller JL, Pandiani JA. The changing role of the state psychiatric hospital. *Health Affairs*. 2009; **28**(3): 676–684.

8. Parks J, Radke AQ. The vital role of state psychiatric hospitals. National Association of State Mental Health Program Directors; 2014. https://nasmhpd .org/content/vital-role-state-psychiatric-hospitals-july-2014-0 (accessed June 2020).

9. Lutterman T, Shaw R, Fisher W, Manderscheid R. Trend in psychiatric inpatient capacity, United States and each state, 1970 to 2014. National Association of State Mental Health Program Directors; August 2017. www.nri-inc.org/media/1319/tac-paper-10-psychiatric-inpatient-capacity-final-09-05-2017.pdf (accessed June 2020).

10. The State of Texas Legislative Budget Board. Texas state government effectiveness and efficiency report: selected issues and recommendations. January 2013. https://www.lbb.state.tx.us/Documents/Publications/ GEER/Government%20Effectiveness%20and%20Effi ciency%20Report%202012.pdf (accessed June 2020).

A Survey of National Trends in Psychiatric Patients Found Incompetent to Stand Trial: Reasons for the Reinstitutionalization of People with Serious Mental Illness in the United States

Katherine Warburton, Barbara E. McDermott, Anthony Gale, and Stephen M. Stahl

Introduction

Recent information indicates that the number of forensic patients in state hospitals has been increasing, largely driven by an increase in patients referred as incompetent to stand trial (IST).[1,2] The surge in referrals for the evaluation and restoration of patients found IST is taxing state hospital systems, as well as the jails that must care for these patients when state hospitals are unable to accommodate the increased referrals.[3,4] Many state mental health authorities are facing litigation pressure to admit IST patients more quickly, raising concerns about overcrowding and reinstitutionalization. Little is known about these national trends of increasing IST populations, and even less is known about what is driving them. This survey was intended to broaden the understanding of IST population trends on a national level.

In 1960, the United States Supreme Court articulated the standard for competence to stand trial, requiring that individuals facing criminal prosecution possess the ability to rationally consult with their attorney and possess a rational and factual understanding of the legal proceedings.[5] Research after this landmark ruling has shown that the majority of defendants deemed IST are suffering from a psychotic disorder.[6–10]

During the same time period, the United States instituted what has been termed "one of the most well-meaning but poorly planned social changes ever carried out in the United States":[11] the closing of long-term psychiatric hospitals. Since that time, numerous scholars have forecasted that these closures would ultimately lead to the seriously mentally ill receiving services in the criminal justice system.[12,13] Recent reports suggest these predictions were accurate: many individuals with serious mental disorders are now receiving mental health treatment via the criminal justice system, not in the community as originally intended.[11,12,14] A poignant example of this is the commonly cited statistic that Cook County, Los Angeles County, and New York City jails are the largest mental health treatment facilities in the United States.[15] This is supported by recent research that documents that an individual with a serious mental disorder is three times more likely to receive psychiatric treatment in the criminal justice system than the mental health system.[11]

More recent data suggest that individuals receiving mental health treatment via forensic hospital systems have been increasing nationally. A 2014 survey of officials responsible for forensic services revealed that 90% of responding states experienced an increased demand for these beds.[1] In 78% of respondents, the increased demand resulted in waitlists to admit patients. Half reported a threat or finding of contempt of court for inability to admit patients in a timely manner. Although this 2014 survey confirmed anecdotal reports and indirect data about increasing forensic admissions, it did not specifically address increases in IST patients within the larger forensic population. Recently, national data have emerged confirming that the number of forensic patients in state hospitals from 1999 to 2016 has increased by 76%, and IST patients are largely responsible for this trend.[2]

Numerous reports have shown that states are struggling to manage the ever-increasing numbers of referrals for competency evaluations and subsequent commitments for restoration. For example, the state of Washington experienced an 82% increase in referrals for competency evaluations between the years 2000 and 2011, and faced litigation because of the increased demand.[16] In Colorado, requests for competency evaluations increased 524% from 2000 to 2017; corresponding requests for restoration increased 931% in the same time frame.[17] In California, defendants judicially determined to be IST have been increasing at an alarming rate. In Los Angeles alone, the County Health Services Agency reported a 350% increase from 2010 to 2015 in IST cases referred by the criminal courts.[18,19]

The decades-long trend of increasing forensic hospitalization and/or incarceration of individuals with serious mental illness has been well studied, and while often attributed to the unintended impacts of deinstitutionalization,[14,20,21] the more recent surge in referrals has not been fully explained. There are many potential explanations for the observed increases such as decreasing access to treatment for mental illness and substance use in the community[11,20,22] and decreasing access to inpatient psychiatric beds.[11,23] Others have postulated that the increased popularity of specialty courts, such as mental health and drug courts, contributes to an increase in competence referrals for defendants who are unable to comply with the guidelines ordered by these courts due to their serious mental illness.[24] Finally, the Director of Community Health and Integrated Programs at the Los Angeles County Department of Health Services suggested that multiple issues have led to increased competency referrals such as increasing awareness of mental illness in the criminal justice system and the complex relationship between homelessness, methamphetamine use, and psychotic symptoms.[18]

Beyond hypotheses, there is little in the way of consensus or data about the proximal causes of the new IST crisis. Without fully understanding the potential reasons for this increase, the criminalization of individuals with serious mental illness will continue. Although multiple suggestions have been discussed for improving the competency evaluation and restoration system (see for example, Gowensmith's review[19]), the fact remains that in order to address this problem and craft a solution, the underlying cause or causes must be clarified and identified. This survey was designed to achieve two goals. First, we sought to confirm anecdotal reports of recent nationwide increases in competency evaluations and commitments. Second, and more importantly, this survey was designed to gather opinions as to the potential causes of the increases and to ascertain if there were commonalties between jurisdictions. Effective interventions to reverse the criminalization of mental illness depend on a full understanding of the forces that drive this trend.

Methods

The authors developed a survey to gather specific information on the processes for IST commitments in each state and the District of Columbia. We first reviewed the statutes for each jurisdiction. From this review, we determined that offenders found IST for misdemeanor offenses were frequently handled differently than those arrested for felony offenses. For this reason, the survey was designed to gather information about each process separately. Additionally, we found from this review that the processes by which individuals are determined to be IST vary between jurisdictions. For example, in some states, defendants are hospitalized to conduct the competence evaluations, whereas in others, community evaluators conduct the assessments while the defendant is in jail. Because of these differences, separate questions were asked about referrals for initial evaluations and referrals for

Table 6.1 Opinions on change in referral rates

	Referrals for evaluations			Referrals for restoration		
	Increasing n (%)	Decreasing n (%)	No change n (%)	Increasing n (%)	Decreasing n (%)	No change n (%)
Misdemeanor	34 (70.8)	1 (2.1)	13 (27.1)	33 (68.8)	1 (2.1)	14 (29.2)
Felony	35 (70.0)	–	15 (30.0)	32 (65.3)	–	17 (34.7)
Combined	41 (82.0)	1 (2.0)	8 (16.0)	39 (78.0)	1 (2.0)	10 (20.0)

restoration. A 30-question survey was developed to focus on trends in referrals, length of stay, and opinions as to the causes of the IST increases, if applicable. The survey was administered via Survey Monkey to all 50 states and the District of Columbia via email.

In order to obtain the most accurate information possible, potential sources were identified by reviewing rosters available on the National Association of State Mental Health Program Directors website. Individual emails were sent to these individuals. In most cases, the initial contact either agreed to take the survey or provided an alternative contact who they determined would be more appropriate and provide more accurate information. Occasionally, either the email address was invalid or the individual did not respond. In those instances, either the state hospitals or largest correctional institutions in those jurisdictions were contacted directly to determine who would be most appropriate to complete the survey. Each individual identified was sent a link to the survey. Non-responders were sent repeat requests via email. When this was not successful, identified individuals were contacted by phone and asked to complete the survey.

Results

Characteristics of Respondents

A total of 50 out of the 51 jurisdictions contacted completed the survey. In most jurisdictions, the survey was completed by an individual in an administrative role. Forty-eight percent (24/50) of individuals identified themselves as a Central Office Administrator (state office position) and 30% (15/50) identified themselves as a State Hospital Administrator (e.g. Executive Director, Medical Director). The remaining 22% (11/50) identified themselves as "Other." Specific roles included: Chief Psychologist, Chief of Forensic Psychology Department, County Behavioral Health Director, State-Wide Forensic Mental Health Program Director, Director of Forensic Services, Psychological Services Director, Area Forensic Director for the Department of Mental Health, Assistant Attorney General, Program Director for Competency Restoration, Chief Forensic Psychologist, and State Forensic Service Director.

IST Rates and Processes

As is shown in Table 6.1, approximately 70% of the respondents indicated referrals for competency evaluations for both misdemeanor and felony offenses were increasing. Only 2% of respondents felt misdemeanor competency evaluation requests were decreasing; no respondent indicated felony requests were decreasing. When combined, fully 82% of states indicated that referrals for competency evaluations for either misdemeanor or felony offenses were increasing. Not surprisingly, states reported that referrals for restoration were increasing as well; 68.8% for offenders with misdemeanor charges and 65.3% for offenders with felony charges. When combined, 78% of respondents thought referrals for restoration of offenders with either felony or misdemeanor offenses were increasing.

In addition to ascertaining if rates of referrals for evaluation and restoration services were changing, we also requested information about the processes for restoration services. When asked where restoration services occur in their jurisdiction, the majority indicated that state hospitals were the primary location for both misdemeanor (n = 30, 61.2%) and felony offenders (n = 41, 82%). Four states (8.2%) reported that misdemeanant offenders were not restored and charges were dropped, whereas only one state (2%) indicated felony offenders were not restored. Some states used both in- and outpatient restoration; more for misdemeanant offenders (n = 7, 14.3%) than for felony offenders (n = 5, 10%). One state restores both misdemeanant and felony offenders in jail. Of those jurisdictions that reported state hospital as the primary site for restoration of misdemeanants, the average length of stay was 93.58 days (SD 39.9), with a range from 33 days to 180 days. In contrast, felony offenders' length of stay ranged from 33 days to 281 days, with an average of 120.7 days (SD 52.2). Fully 70.8% of jurisdictions reported having a waitlist to admit IST patients and 38.8% reported having faced litigation due to length of time on the waitlist.

Table 6.2 provides the descriptive statistics for the factors respondents considered to be the most important cause of increases in IST referrals. Respondents were asked to rank nine factors (including one where they could provide a response other than the eight contained in the survey). Rankings ranged from a 1 (most important) to a 9 (least important). The factors are presented in order from the smallest mean score (suggesting it was ranked as more important by many respondents) to the largest (ranked as less important by many respondents). The modal and median scores also are included in the table to provide a comparison

Table 6.2 Ranking of factors leading to increase in IST referrals

Factor	Number of respondents	Average rank	Modal rank	Median rank	SD
Inadequate general mental health services in the community	38	3.45	1	2.5	2.46
Inadequate crisis services in the community	38	3.71	3	3.0	1.80
Inadequate number of inpatient psychiatric beds in the community	36	3.78	1	3.0	2.50
Inadequate ACT services in the community	37	4.22	4	4.0	1.92
Other	17	4.24	1	3.0	3.35
More awareness of mental illness by the courts/officers of the court	38	4.58	2, 6	5.0	2.45
Homelessness	36	4.92	6	5.0	1.98
Bar for involuntary medication is too high	32	5.56	6	6.0	1.92
Bar for involuntary hospitalization is too high	28	5.75	7	5.5	2.20

between factors. Thirty-eight participants ranked these nine factors, although not all 38 ranked all nine.

The highest ranked response was inadequate general mental health services with an average score of 3.45 (lower numbers indicate a higher ranking). Inadequate crisis services in the community was ranked second, inadequate number of inpatient psychiatric beds in the community was the third highest, with inadequate Assertive Community Treatment (ACT) services in the community ranked fourth. Fifth highest was respondent's opinions on factors not mentioned. Those factors included: the bar for finding defendants incompetent was too low, inadequate jail mental health, increasing rate of substance abuse, inefficiency of the court with involuntary medication orders, and lack of compliance with outpatient treatment. As seen in Table 6.2, homelessness and the bar being too high for involuntary medication or hospitalization were ranked lowest, with each having a modal ranking of 6 or 7, suggesting states believed lack of mental health services in the community were more important to the competency problem. Interestingly, rankings on increased awareness by the courts regarding mental illness were bimodal; with some states believing this was highly relevant, with others thinking it was less relevant than other factors.

Respondents were asked to provide what, if any, methods they have used to address the problem of increased demand for services to restore offenders. The most cited method was implementing diversion programs with 54% of respondents indicating they were developing or had already implemented diversion programs. Forty-two percent tried either increasing the numbers of beds or decreasing length of stay. Ten states (20%) indicated that they have used double-bedding to address the problem. When asked to provide other methods used, some states indicated they were providing restoration services in the community, contracting with private hospitals for restoration, and implementing jail-based restoration services. States were evenly split on whether these methods improved the problem, with 10 (35.7%) saying yes and the same number saying no. Six (21.4%) said it was too soon to tell if their methods addressed the problem, with only two (7.1%) indicating the efficacy was equivocal.

Discussion

The results of our survey indicate that requests for competency evaluations and restoration services are indeed rising. Many of the respondents ranked a lack of community mental health services as a primary reason for the rising numbers of IST commitments, be it community hospital beds, crisis services, ACT teams, or general mental health services. One potential explanation for the perceived lack of services is the economic downturn in 2008. Advocacy groups at that time warned that "massive" cuts to mental health spending in the wake of the great recession would "simply shift financial responsibility to emergency rooms, community hospitals, law enforcement agencies, correctional facilities, and homeless shelters."[25]

Moreover, IST defendants charged with violent offenses have been shown to have a higher degree of marginalization from society, particularly manifested as homelessness and unemployment.[26–28] Cuts in services following the recession could account for the recent sustained increase in IST referrals via a mechanism of patient decompensation, downward drift, and subsequent criminal justice contact.

The opinion that the IST crisis is driven by a lack of community mental health beds is intriguing. Much has been written about what an appropriate number of hospital beds per capita is, and the appropriate location for those beds.[11,29,30] The Treatment Advocacy Center expert consensus guidelines recommend 50 inpatient psychiatric beds per 100,000 population. Recent literature points out that the average in the United States is 22 beds per 100,000, and in California that number is 17 per 100,000.[29–31] There is a suggestion that increasing suicide rates also are related to the decline in beds over time.[29] As such, it is feasible that arrest, incarceration, and forensic hospitalization are also negative outcomes of the decline in community inpatient beds. A compelling explanation is the decision an officer makes about whether to bring a psychiatric patient to a hospital or charge them with a crime and book them into jail. Research suggests that this decision depends on whether the arresting officer thinks the patient will be admitted to a hospital bed.[32] Therefore, a lack of community hospital and/or crisis beds could be a strong driver of an increase in arrests of individuals living with serious mental illness. The combination of these factors may drive both the IST crisis and increasing numbers of psychiatric patients in jails and prisons.

The possibility that a lack of community psychiatric hospital beds is indeed behind the recent surge sheds an ironic cast on the controversy over a call to bring back asylums.[33] The data confirm that people with serious mental illness are growing populations in forensic institutions and the problem of over-representation of persons with serious mental illness in prisons is well documented.[34–36] California alone has added over 400 state hospital beds and approximately 300 treatment beds in local jails in response to the crisis in the last five years. The effort to avoid the stigma of psychiatric hospitalization may in fact be exacerbating the trend of long-term institutionalization.

Understanding the causes behind the recent surge in referrals for IST evaluations and restoration services will benefit states vulnerable to increased

scrutiny and federal lawsuits. For example, in the state of Washington, the outcome of a recent lawsuit resulted in mandates for admission of defendants found IST within a very narrow time range.[16] Fines in that case have topped 80 million dollars as the state struggles to comply in the face of increasing referrals.[37] Failure to comply with mandatory timelines is likely related to the fact that many state mental health authorities have limited or no influence over forensic referrals from the community. Because the entity being sued (State Mental Health Authority) has limited influence on the source of the crisis (increasing referrals from the community), the consequence of judicially mandated admission timelines is increased pressure on an already taxed system in the form of overcrowding and reinstitutionalization of individuals living with serious mental illness. A more logical solution is to find ways of reversing the increased referral trends by addressing the root causes driving them.

Our survey supports the notion that timeline to admission mandates have the potential to dramatically increase state hospital populations, creating a dangerous precedent for overcrowding. That 20% of states responded that they are "double-bedding" to comply with the increased demand indicates a potentially counterintuitive result of legal actions intended to preserve civil liberties.

In addition to creating a situation of reinstitutionalization and overcrowding, the current response to the IST crisis does nothing to address the complex long-term biopsychosocial needs of individuals living with serious mental illness. Once a patient admitted for competency restoration demonstrates the abilities to understand the criminal proceedings and assist counsel, the law mandates a return to court. Once the proceedings have concluded, the patient is released to the same circumstances that precipitated the arrest, institutionalized, or incarcerated, no better off for the state hospital stay.

The opinion data indicate that expanding state hospital capacity is not a remedy to the problem. What then, is? Jail diversion, based on sequential intercept mapping, is a well-studied systemic intervention that provides short-, medium-, and long-term alternatives. As our survey reflected, 54% of states are implementing diversion programs in an effort to reduce the influx of IST commitments. Funding may also provide an answer. In many states, local jurisdictions fund many community mental health programs, while the state authority tends to pay for the state hospital and prison mental health services. This provides a perverse fiscal incentive that supports downward drift to the point of arrest. In short, policy related to services for the serious mental illness population needs to shift funding incentives away from costly state hospital beds and prison mental health services. Instead, these public mental health dollars should focus on robust long-term continuums in the community that include adequate wrap around services, housing, crisis services, and community hospital beds. Finally, to ensure that communities have adequate services to deal with most mentally ill patients, consistent measuring of outcomes is needed. Arrest, incarceration, and institutionalization rates need to be considered metrics by which to measure service delivery.

Conclusion

Whatever the cause, increased demand for competency services is overwhelming state hospital capacity, resulting in a backlog of patients into local jails. Although some states are compelled via litigation to comply with challenging timelines for admitting IST patients, this approach does little to solve the problem of the increasing demand. The data from our survey support a disturbing trend of forensically driven reinstitutionalization of patients living with serious mental illness. Jail diversion and funding incentives are two potential solutions.

Disclaimer

The findings and conclusions in this article are those of the authors and do not necessarily represent the views or opinions of the California Department of State Hospitals or the California Health and Human Services Agency.

Disclosures

Katherine Warburton, Barbara E. McDermott, and Anthony Gale declare no conflicts of interest. Stephen M. Stahl, M.D., Ph.D., over the past 12 months (January–December of 2016), has served as a consultant to Acadia, Alkermes, Allergan, Arbor Pharmaceuticals, AstraZeneca, Axovant, Biogen, Biopharma, Celgene, Forest, Forum, Genomind, Innovative Science Solutions, Intra-Cellular Therapies, Jazz, Lundbeck, Merck, Otsuka, Pam Labs, Servier, Shire, Sunovion, Takeda, and Teva. He is a board member of Genomind and he has served on speakers bureaus for Forum,

Lundbeck, Otsuka, Perrigo, Servier, Sunovion, and Takeda. He has also received research and/or grant support from Acadia, Avanir, Braeburn Pharmaceuticals, Eli Lilly, Intra-Cellular Therapies, Ironshore, ISSWSH, Neurocrine, Otsuka, Shire, Sunovion, and TMS NeuroHealth Centers.

Supplementary Materials

To view supplementary material for this article, please visit http://dx.doi.org/10.1017/S1092852919001585.

References

1. Fitch WL. Forensic mental health services in the United States. National Association of State Mental Health Program Directors Policy Paper; 2014.

2. Wik A, Hollen V, Fisher WH. Forensic patients in state psychiatric hospitals: 1999–2016. National Association of State Mental Health Program Directors Policy Paper; 2017.

3. Grissom B. With state hospitals packed, mentally ill inmates wait in county jails that aren't equipped for them. *Dallas Morning News*; 2016. www.dallasnews.com/news/politics/2016/04/21/with-state-hospitals-packed-mentally-ill-inmates-wait-in-county-jails-that-aren-t-equipped-for-them/ (accessed June 2020).

4. Jail wait times are inhumane for the mentally ill. *The Delaware County Daily Times*; 2016. www.delcotimes.com/opinion/ editorial-jail-wait-times-are-inhumane-for-the-mentally-ill/article_ cb4244 a5-7113-5f8f-96a4-ab1bb0228cc2.html (accessed June 2020).

5. *Dusky v. United States*, 362, 402 (1960).

6. Pirelli G, Gottdiener WH, Zapf PA. A meta-analytic review of competency to stand trial research. *Psychol Public Policy Law*. 2011; **17**(1): 1–53.

7. Warren JI, Murrie DC, Stejskal W, et al. Opinion formation in evaluating the adjudicative competence and restorability of criminal defendants: a review of 8,000 evaluations. *Behav Sci Law*. 2006; **24**(2): 113–132.

8. Bartos BJ, Renner M, Newark C, McCleary R, Scurich N. Characteristics of forensic patients in California with dementia/Alzheimer's disease. *J Forensic Nurs*. 2017; **13**(2): 77–80.

9. Cooper VG, Zapf PA. Predictor variables in competency to stand trial decisions. *Law Hum Behav*. 2003; **27**(4): 423–436.

10. Cochrane RE, Grisso T, Frederick RI. The relationship between criminal charges, diagnoses, and psychelegal opinions among federal pretrial defendants. *Behav Sci Law*. 2001; **19**(4): 565–582.

11. Torrey EF, Kennard AD, Eslinger D, Lamb R, Pavle J. More mentally ill persons are in jails and prisons than hospitals: a survey of the states. Treatment Advocacy Center Policy Paper; 2010.

12. Abramson MF. The criminalization of mentally disordered behavior. *Psychiatr Serv.* 1972; **23**(4): 101–105.

13. Arvanites TM. The impact of state mental hospital deinstitutionalization on commitments for incompetency to stand trial. *Criminology.* 1988; **26**(2): 307–320.

14. Torrey EF. Jails and prisons – America's new mental hospitals. *Am J Public Health.* 1995; **85**(12): 1611–1613.

15. Fields G, Phillips EE. The new asylums: jails swell with mentally ill. *The Wall Street Journal*; September 25, 2013.

16. *Trueblood v. Washington State Department of Social and Health Services* (United States Court of Appeals, Ninth Circuit); 2016.

17. Phillips N. Lawyers take Colorado DHS back to court over mental competency exam backlog. *The Denver Post*; June 14, 2018.

18. Katz MH. Examination of increase in mental competency cases. Report to LA County Supervisors; 2016.

19. Gowensmith WN. Resolution or resignation: the role of forensic mental health professionals amidst the competency services crisis. *Psychol Public Policy Law.* 2019; **25**(1): 1–14.

20. Lamb HR, Weinberger LE. The shift of psychiatric inpatient care from hospitals to jails and prisons. *J Am Acad Psychiatry Law.* 2005; **33**(4): 529–534.

21. Lamb HR, Weinberger LE, Marsh JS, Gross BH. Treatment prospects for persons with severe mental illness in an urban county jail. *Psychiatr Serv.* 2007; **58** (6): 782–786.

22. Bondurant SR, Lindo JM, Swensen ID, National Bureau of Economic Research. Substance abuse treatment centers and local crime; 2016.

23. Toynbee M. The Penrose hypothesis in the 21st century: revisiting the asylum. *Evid Based Mental Health.* 2015; **18**(3): 76.

24. Stafford K, Sellbom M. Assessment of competence to stand trial. In: Weiner I, Otto R, eds. *Handbook of Psychology, Vol 11 Forensic Psychology.* Hoboken, NJ: John Wiley & Sons, Inc.; 2012: 412–439.

25. Honberg R, Diehl S, Kimball A, Gruttadaro D, Fitzpatrick M. *State mental health cuts: a national crisis.* National Alliance on Mental Illness; 2011.

26. Martell DA, Rosner R, Harmon RB. Base-rate estimates of criminal behavior by homeless mentally ill persons in New York City. *Psychiatr Serv.* 1995; **46** (6): 596–601.

27. Martell DA, Rosner R, Harmon RB. Homeless mentally disordered defendants: competency to stand trial and mental status findings. *Bull Am Acad Psychiatry Law.* 1994; **22**(2): 289–295.

28. Schreiber J, Green D, Kunz M, Belfi B, Pequeno G. Offense characteristics of incompetent to stand trial defendants charged with violent offenses. *Behav Sci Law.* 2015; **33**(2–3): 257–278.

29. Bastiampillai T, Sharfstein SS, Allison S. Increase in US suicide rates and the critical decline in psychiatric beds. *J Am Med Assoc.* 2016; **316**(24): 2591–2592.

30. Sisti DA, Sinclair EA, Sharfstein SS. Bedless psychiatry-rebuilding behavioral health service capacity. *JAMA Psychiatry.* 2018; **75**(5): 417–418.

31. California Hospital Association. California's acute psychiatric bed loss. 2019.

32. Green TM. Police as frontline mental health workers: the decision to arrest or refer to mental health agencies. *Int J Law Psychiatry.* 1997; **20**(4): 469–486.

33. Sisti DA, Segal AG, Emanuel EJ. Improving long-term psychiatric care: bring back the asylum. *J Am Med Assoc.* 2015; **313**(3): 243–244.

34. Steadman HJ, Osher FC, Robbins PC, Case B, Samuels S. Prevalence of serious mental illness among jail inmates. *Psychiatr Serv.* 2009; **60**(6): 761–765.

35. Trestman RL, Ford J, Zhang W, Wiesbrock V. Current and lifetime psychiatric illness among inmates not identified as acutely mentally ill at intake in Connecticut's jails. *J Am Acad Psychiatry Law.* 2007; **35** (4): 490–500.

36. Wilper AP, Woolhandler S, Boyd JW, *et al.* The health and health care of US prisoners: results of a nationwide survey. *Am J Public Health.* 2009; **99**(4): 666–672.

37. Bellisle M. After paying $83 million in fines, Washington settles jail mental-health lawsuit. *The Seattle Times.* 2018.

Forensic Psychiatry and Mental Health in Australia: An Overview

Andrew Ellis

Introduction

The indigenous inhabitants of the Australian continent arrived approximately 65,000 years ago. Issues of mental illness and criminal responsibility prior to European arrival are not well known by current professionals. The continent is now home to the Commonwealth of Australia, a parliamentary democracy, established in 1901 following land claims by Britain that began in 1788. The Commonwealth is a federation of six states and two territories that were originally colonies of Britain. The first British colony in Sydney, New South Wales was a penal settlement, which perhaps set the tone for development of forensic mental health services across the country as developing as an offshoot from prison services. Forensic mental health services have been reviewed before,[1,2] and more recent developments are covered.

Forensic Psychiatry in Australia

Australia is now home to 25 million people, approximately one-quarter of whom are immigrants.[3] Each state or territory government is responsible for provision of health services and criminal justice systems. Therefore the legislation covering and service provision to forensic patients varies across each jurisdiction (Table 7.1). There are some crimes that fall under the federal Commonwealth legislation, which has its own provisions for mental health defenses and diversion. Australia is a signatory to international treaties on human rights that impact on forensic mental health care, including the International Covenant on Civil and Political Rights and the Convention on the Rights of Persons with Disabilities. The Australian Constitution does not have a specific bill of rights for citizens; however, some rights (such as to vote or trial by jury) are implied in the constitution, and state governments may pass human rights acts.

The original colonies followed British common law practices and established courts, prisons, and psychiatric hospitals. Civil commitment in public psychiatric hospitals (originally called lunatic asylums) or prisons was possible for mentally ill persons who were deemed to be a danger to themselves or others, be at risk of vagrancy, or in the process of committing a crime. The concepts of fitness to be tried (known as competence to stand trial in the United States), the insanity defense, and the transfer of mentally ill prisoners from prison to hospital were introduced in early legislation. The release of "criminally insane" persons was at the discretion of the State Governor, a practice that continued well into the twentieth and twenty-first centuries in some states. This practice no longer continues, and release decisions are now made by legal and not political bodies. Some state legislation allowed the detention of unfit or insane in prisons as well as hospitals, which is a practice that continues in some states. In 2006, the Australian Health Ministers' Advisory Council published a statement of principles for forensic mental health,[4] which included a principle of equivalent individualized care to nonoffenders, comprehensive forensic mental health services, judicial determination of detention and release, transparency and accountability, and legal reform. It noted that forensic services had been neglected. Arguably, states' compliance with these principles has been inconsistent.[5]

Modern mental health acts are present in all states and territories. These allow for civil commitment in a hospital or in community settings. The least restrictive principle is applied. Some states base commitment on risk, and some on a combination of risk and capacity to make decisions about care. External checks such as legal and administrative review occur. Fitness to be tried for serious offences is based on caselaw, with the lead case being *Presser*.[6] Some states have codified the criteria set out in this case. The insanity defense exists under different names for serious offences, and follows M'Naghten's case. The concept

Table 7.1 Characteristics of state and territory forensic mental health services

	New South Wales	Victoria	Queensland	South Australia	Western Australia	Tasmania	Northern Territory	Australian Capital Territory
Population (millions)	8.0	6.4	5.0	1.7	2.6	0.5	0.2	0.4
Incarceration rate (per 100,000)	215.6	145.4	221.8	223.7	340	146.3	878.4	141.2
Forensic hospitals (beds)	197	116	192	30	38	17	0	25
Mental Health Service in Custody	Yes	Yes	Yes	Yes	Yes	Yes	Yes	Yes
Involuntary medication in custody	Yes (one unit only)	No	No	Yes	No	No	No	No
Court diversion service	Yes	Yes	Yes	Yes	Yes	Yes	No	Yes
Community service	Consultation only	Yes	Yes	Yes	Yes	Yes	No	Yes
Specialist forensic disability provision	No	Yes	Yes	No	No	Yes	No	No

of knowledge of wrongfulness is broader following the case of *Porter* where an element of being able to reflect with a moderate degree and sense of composure on decisions about moral wrongfulness is incorporated.[7] Transfer of mentally ill prisoners to hospital for involuntary care can occur; however, it is often limited by resource availability. Diversion of mentally ill or disordered offenders for lower order offences into clinical care is possible by legislation, and is applied variably across the states.

Forensic hospitals, which specialize in the care of mentally disordered offenders, are present in all but one Australian jurisdictions. The Northern Territory still relies on prison for the detention of adjudicated mentally ill and disordered persons with serious offences. These facilities are generally modern with multidisciplinary mental health care, which also focuses on substance use disorders and offending behaviors. This reflects the multiple psychiatric problems of the patient populations.[8,9] Some hospitals have specialized units for female forensic patients. The number of beds for the population varies state by state and is generally less than other Western nations. Significant waits in prison to enter one of these facilities after legal disposition occurs is the norm. Once released from forensic hospital settings to conditional community care, patients show very low rates of reoffending.[10,11]

Each jurisdiction provides prison in-reach mental health services. Some of these are well developed, as the majority of forensic patients were originally housed in prison environments and forensic services have tended to develop out of prison services. Some jurisdictions have special areas of the prison devoted to care of mentally ill prisoners.[12] Surveys show very high rates of major psychotic and mood disorders, as well as high prevalence of mental disorders in Australian prison settings.[13] This is comparable with international findings on the rates of mental illness in custody. There are very high rates of indigenous persons in custody, and considerable concern about rates of suicide and mental disorder in this group.[14] A Royal Commission into Aboriginal Deaths in Custody established practice changes in order to reduce this. Most jurisdictions are experiencing increasing rates of incarceration, the contributions to which are complex.

Community forensic mental health services are a relatively new development. With repeal of governor's pleasure laws, more forensic patients were released to community settings, based on assessed risk reduction with rehabilitation.[15] Some states adopt a specialist team approach to care of forensic patients in the community, while others provide consultation to generalist mental health services. Services for those forensic patients with intellectual disability are provided in some states. It remains difficult to transfer care of forensic patients across state boundaries.[16] Novel specialist services have been developed, particularly in Victoria with the Problem Behaviour Clinic in their Community Forensic Mental Health Service. Specific assessment and multidisciplinary treatment for stalkers, arsonists, threateners, and sex offenders that deals with both behavior and contributing diagnosis is provided. With the advent of extremist violence and the potential association with mental disorder, some states have teams linked with police fixated threat units and negotiator units.

Court diversion services are provided in all states. These utilize local legislation to link defendants before the courts with treatment services as an alternative to custody or parole. Most diversion involves supervised treatment with review, and disposal of the charges if treatment is successful and sustained. Evaluation of these services shows both positive clinical and justice outcomes, and overall cost savings to the system by reduction in the need for incarceration and re-offending with diverted groups.[17,18]

Hospital, detention, community, and court services are specifically targeted at juvenile offender populations in most states. These services tend to mirror services for adults and serve smaller, but arguably more complex populations. Rates of over-representation of indigenous populations in juvenile services are higher than in adult services.

The development of academic departments and training in forensic psychiatry and mental health is also relatively new. There are three universities that offer postgraduate degrees in forensic mental health and have small academic departments. The Faculty of Forensic Psychiatry has been a part of the Royal Australian and New Zealand College of Psychiatrists since 1968; however, a formal subspecialty training of two years (in additional to general psychiatric training) has only been available since 2004.[19] The training program is shared with New Zealand and 10–12 new forensic psychiatrists complete this each year. Forensic psychiatry training also includes practice in civil law areas such as insurance claims, family law, and guardianship. The training is paired with one of the three academic departments. The Australian Psychological Society College of Forensic Psychology has accredited training for subspecialist psychologists. Mental health nursing, social work, and other allied health disciplines have no specific forensic training pathways, though individual practitioners work in the area.

Conclusion

Whilst there have been significant additional resources and modernization of forensic services the legacy of colonial practices, particularly housing forensic patients in prison environments, continues in some parts of Australia. This is likely at odds with Australia's commitment to human rights instruments and adherence to the least restrictive principle in mental health acts. It is crucial that the growing body of professionals working in the area advocate for continual improvement of services and demonstrate through formal research the opportunities this rights-based practice is likely to have on improved criminal justice outcomes and community safety, as well as clinical care for individuals. The development of forensic specific training for all allied health disciplines, including mangers of forensic mental health services would likely assist with these goals.

Disclosure

Dr. Ellis has nothing to disclose.

References

1. Mullen PE, Briggs S, Dalton T, et al. Forensic mental health services in Australia. *Int J Law Psychiatry*. 2000; **23**: 433–452.

2. Every-Palmer S, Brink J, Chern TP, et al. Review of psychiatric services to mentally disordered offenders around the Pacific Rim. *Asia-Pac Psychiatry*. 2014; **6** (1): 1–7.

3. Australian Bureau of Statistics. www.abs.gov.au/Popu lation (accessed June 2020).

4. Australian Institute of Health and Welfare. www .aihw.gov.au/getmedia/e615a500-d412-4b0b-84f7-fe0 b7fb00f5f/National-Forensic-Mental-Health-Principles.pdf.aspx. Accessed March 30, 2019.

5. Hanley N, Ross S. Forensic mental health in Australia: charting the gaps. *Curr Issues Crim Justice*. 2013; **24**(3): 341–356.

6. Kasinathan J, Le J, Barker A, Sharp G. Presser – the forgotten story. *Australas Psychiatry*. 2016; **24**(5): 478–482.

7. Allnutt S, Samuels A, O'Driscoll C. The insanity defence: from wild beasts to M'Naghten. *Australas Psychiatry*. 2007; **15**(4): 292–298.

8. Ogloff JR, Talevski D, Lemphers A, et al. Co-occurring mental illness, substance use disorders, and antisocial personality disorder among clients of forensic mental health services. *Psych Rehab J*. 2015; **38**(1): 16.

9. Adams J, Thomas SD, Mackinnon T, et al. The risks, needs and stages of recovery of a complete forensic patient cohort in an Australian state. *BMC Psychiatry*. 2018; **18**(1): 35.

10. Hayes H, Kemp RI, Large MM, et al. A 21-year retrospective outcome study of New South Wales forensic patients granted conditional and unconditional release. *Aust N Z J Psychiatry*. 2014; **48**(3): 259–282.

11. Ong K, Carroll A, Reid S, et al. Community outcomes of mentally disordered homicide offenders in Victoria. *Aust N Z J Psychiatry*. 2009; **43**(8): 775–780.

12. Adams J, Ellis A, Brown A, et al. A prison mental health screening unit: a first for New South Wales. *Australas Psychiatry*. 2009; **17**(2): 90–96.

13. Butler T, Andrews G, Allnutt S, et al. Mental disorders in Australian prisoners: a comparison with a community sample. *Aust N Z J Psychiatry*. 2006; **40** (3): 272–276.

14. Butler T, Allnutt S, Kariminia A, et al. Mental health status of Aboriginal and non-Aboriginal Australian prisoners. *Aust N Z J Psychiatry*. 2007; **41**(5): 429–435.

15. Ellis A, Kumar V, Rodriguez M, et al. A survey of the conditionally released forensic patient population in New South Wales. *Australas Psychiatry*. 2010; **18**(6): 542–546.

16. Carroll A, Scott R, Green B, et al. Forensic mental health orders: orders without borders. *Australas Psychiatry*. 2009; **17**(1): 34–37.

17. Soon YL, Rae N, Korobanova D, et al. Mentally ill offenders eligible for diversion at local court in New South Wales (NSW), Australia: factors associated with initially successful diversion. *J Forens Psychiatry Psychol*. 2018; **29**(5): 705–716.

18. Albalawi O, Chowdhury NZ, Wand H, et al. Court diversion for those with psychosis and its impact on re-offending rates: results from a longitudinal data-linkage study. *B J Psych Open*. 2019; **5**(1): e9.

19. Royal Australian and New Zealand College of Psychiatrists. www.ranzcp.org/pre-fellowship/about-the-training-program/certificates-of-advanced-training/forensic-psychiatry (accessed June 2020).

Community Forensic Psychiatric Services in England and Wales

Richard Latham and Hannah Kate Williams

Introduction

This paper is intended to provide a summary and commentary on the extent of community services for mentally disordered offenders in England and Wales. Our focus on England and Wales is because the different countries of the United Kingdom have devolved legislative and administrative powers so that this paper would – by necessity if a United Kingdom paper – be three times as long so as to include Scottish and Northern Irish law, practice, and policy; Wales is considered alongside England as the two countries are sufficiently similar. We have interpreted "community services" broadly and have included descriptions of court liaison and diversion services, and multiagency risk management services. In other words, we have described, in some form, all of the services that are in place to manage mentally disordered offenders after they have been released from prison, discharged from hospital, or diverted from either form of custody to the community.

As in all jurisdictions, the issue of mentally disordered offenders is on the agenda of "justice" and "health," both in political terms and for professionals providing services. Where we refer to forensic community mental health teams, we are describing health services; almost exclusively NHS services. Court and probation services are part of the justice system. The more recent direction of travel has been towards jointly funded services – broadly speaking by the NHS and the National Offender Management Service (NOMS) – and the sharing of responsibility. This is particularly the case with children and young people and with adults with personality disorder.

Multidisciplinary community mental health teams are the backbone of general community psychiatry in England and Wales. Community psychiatry had its origins as early as the 1920s, but the large institutions dominated until much later in the century. More specialized community mental health teams[1] have fallen in and out of fashion over the last 20 years,

sometimes driven by research evidence.[2] Assertive outreach teams have all but disappeared whilst early intervention in psychosis and crisis teams have shown more longevity. Specialist community forensic mental health teams are relatively young and underevaluated but are at the center of the services we have described below.

History of Forensic Psychiatric Services

Arguably, the first forensic psychiatric inpatient facility anywhere in the world was formed by the criminal wings at the Bethlem Hospital in London in 1815. These wings were developed in response to, amongst others, the case of James Hadfield[3] who had, in a deluded state, fired a gun at George III. He missed but was found to be insane. At the time (1800), the legal provisions for his safe confinement were considered to be inadequate and the government swiftly passed the Criminal Lunatics Act.[4] "Criminal lunatics" needed a place to go and specific inpatient services for mentally disordered offenders grew from the nineteenth century with the development of what later became known as the "special hospitals." The first was Broadmoor Hospital, which opened in 1863, and the three hospitals which were developed exist today as "high secure" services. For most of the twentieth century they constituted the full extent of clinical, forensic mental health services.

The Committee of Mentally Abnormal Offenders (the Butler Committee)[5] was set up jointly by two branches of government to consider: (i) law as it applied to people with mental disorder and (ii) services for offenders with mental disorder. They reported in 1975 and recommended (albeit they were not the first to do so) that each region set up secure psychiatric units. This recommendation coincided with the closure of the Victorian asylums. There was perceived contradiction in these policies: on the one hand there was a policy of deinstitutionalization[6] but simultaneously Butler recommended a new kind of institution, the regional secure unit. Initial development was hesitant but "medium secure units" were built, with development accelerating throughout the late 1980s and 1990s. Subsequently, low secure units were developed with each stage of forensic mental health provision arising out of a recognition that people needed somewhere to go next. The Butler Report also recommended forensic community services be developed, although this has been the last of the recommendations to be adopted.

Forensic psychiatry, as a medical specialty in the United Kingdom, has grown over the last 40 years, in tandem with the secure hospital development. What began as a handful of self-identified forensic psychiatrists, is now a faculty within the Royal College of Psychiatrists with a specific training scheme and recognition as a distinct specialty by the General Medical Council, the regulatory body for doctors. Forensic psychiatry grew along traditional medical, ethical lines, by focusing on beneficence and nonmaleficence. With the accelerating growth of the secure hospital system, there was a strong emphasis on removing mentally disordered people from the prison system to places which would provide therapeutic benefit and to a lesser extent reduction of risk.

Through the 1980s and 1990s there was more emphasis on the risk reduction role of psychiatry,[7] driven partly by media publicity of cases where mentally disordered people had committed serious offences. Christopher Clunis killed a stranger, Jonathan Zito, in an underground station. The subsequent media coverage was accompanied by consistent statements from Mr Zito's widow highlighting the absence of adequate care for Christopher Clunis. The influence of these cases and their coverage may have led to policies increasing restrictive care.[8]

The global financial crash in 2008 and subsequent policy of austerity in funding public services has contributed to the deceleration of the expansion of secure hospital services, but the profession continues to grow. The last workforce census indicated that there were approximately 350 forensic psychiatrist posts in England and Wales.[9] Community forensic psychiatry services developed significantly at the start of the twenty-first century, largely in response to the increase – over the preceding two decades – of these new inpatient forensic services; perhaps an obvious and necessary next step. Forensic community services represent the evolving compromise between concern about overzealous control of those with mental disorder (in the deinstitutionalization movement)[10] against the opposing concern about those

discharged from secure hospitals receiving inadequate supervision of their risk to others from community psychiatric teams without forensic expertise.

In 1993, a review of forensic services made scant reference to community forensic services.[11] By 1996, there was a call for a "forensic psychiatry team in each district to own responsibility for mentally disordered offenders."[12] Today, there are both community forensic mental health teams and partnership arrangements with justice agencies. These new services provide an exit route for people detained in the secure hospital system as well as – more inconsistently – people released from prison. The initial pathway for patients discharged from forensic hospitals when they were first developed was to general psychiatric services, which brought some difficulties about "ownership" of people with mental disorders who were considered to have high risks of offending. The tension between forensic and general services persists with no real resolution to the question, "What makes someone a forensic patient?" Essentially, there is now a parallel forensic psychiatric system which exists alongside general psychiatric services albeit under the same umbrella organizations: NHS Trusts (there are 60 mental health trusts in England). The entire forensic psychiatry system is expensive, costing over one billion pounds a year.[13] The vast majority of this is associated with the cost of the secure hospital system.[14] Over 15% of spending on all mental health services is spent on forensic psychiatric services.

The last decade of forensic mental health service development began with The "Bradley Report,"[15] which has driven many of the most recent changes in forensic mental health provision and continues to do so. This report was commissioned by the Government to examine the extent to which offenders with mental health problems or learning disabilities could be diverted from prison to other services. This ambitious remit led to extensive recommendations, published in 2009, including, in relation to the scope of this paper:

- All police custody suites should have access to liaison and diversion services.
- Further research on mental health treatment requirements (community orders).
- Improved continuity of care for prisoners released from custody.
- Development of Criminal Justice Mental Health Teams (in part to facilitate diversion). These teams

were to bridge the gap between the justice and mental health systems in the community.

Forensic Psychiatry Today

The secure hospital system is constructed around three tiers of security: high, medium, and low. There are between 7,000 and 8,000 people in secure mental health services although there is some difficulty in collecting wholly reliable statistics because of the rather vague nature of what constitutes a low secure service.

- High secure hospital beds are all provided by the NHS in three hospitals: Broadmoor, Rampton, and Ashworth.
- Medium secure hospital beds are split between the NHS and private sector with approximately 65% in the NHS. The private sector beds are all funded by the NHS. Half of secure hospital beds are medium secure beds.
- Low secure hospital beds are more diverse with some representing the upper end of security for general psychiatric services and others the lower end of forensic services.

Community forensic services cost very little by comparison to the hospital system and there is little in the way of nationally collected data on their cost.

The increase in the prison population in England and Wales has been mirrored by an increase in the number of people detained in secure hospitals. From 2000 to 2010 the numbers of people sentenced to hospital under Sections 37 and 41 (see below) rose from fewer than 1,000 to over 1,500. Since 2010, as with the prison population, there has been a more gradual but continuing increase in overall numbers of detained forensic patients.

There has, however, been increasing emphasis on reducing the length of stay in secure hospitals and there is some observational (unpublished) data to suggest that where intensive community forensic teams exist there can be a substantial reduction in length of stay. This is providing the impetus for the development of new services.

Core Community Forensic Psychiatry Services

Structure of Community Forensic Services

Community forensic mental health teams in England and Wales are heterogeneous in their design. They are funded according to borough catchment areas.[16] A

patient's borough is determined by the geographical location of the general practitioner (GP) they are registered with. Twenty-eight NHS Trusts provide community forensic psychiatry care (47 provide secure hospital care). The caseload size of community forensic teams varies substantially, with a median size of 89. The teams are multidisciplinary in nature with individual "care coordinators" having caseloads of 12–20 patients and psychiatrists 30–100. Professional composition varies but includes psychiatry, psychology, nursing, social work, and occupational therapy.

Two different models for delivering specialist forensic care have been recognized and described; parallel and integrated. A parallel forensic service carries out separate assessments and case management to general (nonforensic) community mental health services. They have separate referral meetings, distinct caseloads, and funding. Alternatively, an integrated model involves professionals with forensic expertise working within general community mental health services.[17,18] One disadvantage of the integrated model is a lack of clarity about who is ultimately responsible for the patient. However, the advantages may include the aim to spread relevant forensic skills through general psychiatric services and allow forensic patients better access to community psychiatric resources with less of a stigmatized, separate position in mental health management.[16] The latter may be particularly important given the markedly different distributions of ethnicity between the general and forensic mental health teams in which black and other minority group patients are more likely to be found.[19]

The distinction between parallel and integrated models is a comparison which has been made as a retrospective description, however. In practice, community forensic mental health services have developed in an ad hoc manner, without well-defined theoretical models or a robust evidence base. The advantages and disadvantages of the parallel and integrated models remain discussed and debated but with little consensus reached.[20]

By 2004, approximately half of mental health trusts in England and Wales had some form of community forensic mental health team. Eighty percent of these reported that they used a parallel model, although in reality the approaches were mixed much of the time. In a completely parallel system, patients discharged from forensic services would never return to general psychiatric services but always be managed in the community by forensic services.[21] This is very rarely the case in practice and to see the models as mutually exclusive is probably erroneous.

Since 2019, many forensic community teams have includedf elements of both parallel and integrated models of working in their service, providing case management and treatment for their own forensic community patients as well as consultancy work for general community services, in the form of one-off assessments and advice and guidance. The Royal College of Psychiatrists *Standards for Community Forensic Mental Health Services* suggest the following core functions (abbreviated):[22]

Core Functions of Community Forensic Mental Health Services

- Case management of a defined caseload, particularly those leaving secure care. Case management may be long term.
- Treatment is provided within a recognized framework.
- The team provide liaison, advice, specialist interventions, educational and skills development.
- Active involvement in care pathway management into and out of secure settings and prison.
- Liaison with multiagency public protection arrangements (MAPPA).
- Links with criminal justice liaison and court diversion services.

Patient Entry to Community Forensic Services

There is no consensus on the entry criteria a mental health patient should meet to enter the care of a forensic mental health team as opposed to a general mental health team. Individual services will usually develop operationalized criteria that will include consideration of: risk, legal status, location prior to discharge (prison, secure hospital), specialist treatment needs (sex offending, stalking), gravity of offending.

For every 15 patients with a history of violence in a forensic mental health service there is one patient with a history of violence in general services. Those in forensic mental health services are more likely to be male and managed on long-acting injectable medication. This may be due to those under forensic mental health services being more likely to be subject to legal conditions (e.g. Section 37/41 of the Mental Health

Act 1983 – see below). Historic co-morbid substance misuse is more prevalent in the forensic than the general community teams, although current alcohol and substance misuse is similar.

Constraints may exist in funding arrangements that run contrary to what may make most sense clinically. For example, some community forensic services are commissioned to care for mentally disordered offenders in the community only after they have been discharged from a forensic hospital or referred from a community mental health team unable to contain the patient's risk of harm to others. Their funding may not commission them to accept referrals directly from prison. In this case, a person not previously known to psychiatric services who is diagnosed with a mental disorder in prison (who then receives treatment only in the prison) will not be eligible to directly enter a community forensic service caseload directly on leaving prison. Funding eccentricities such as this may contravene government strategies for personality disorder designed to demonstrate a "commitment to a consistent and coherent process of offenders moving along a range of different criminal justice and health interventions; starting in the community, moving through the sentence, and back to the community at the end of sentence."[23]

It has been argued that those with mental disorder who have a history of criminality and violence that is not connected to their mental disorder should not be managed by community forensic services, given that there is no proven intervention they can offer for criminality per se, with their acceptance onto the service case load incorrectly implying that mental health services can reasonably prevent further criminal acts not related to mental disorder.[24]

Whether a patient is accepted onto a forensic service's caseload or not is usually decided by the lead clinician of the team concerned, with multidisciplinary consultation. There are circumstances, however, in which they may not have complete control over this in practice. For example, if a patient in a medium secure hospital is judged by their inpatient team to be ready for discharge, an opinion from a community forensic service will be sought. The community forensic service may recommend further treatment to be completed before the patient is moved from the hospital into their care. However, if in the meantime the patient successfully argues to a Mental Health Tribunal that inpatient treatment is no longer the least restrictive means to manage their risks (to themselves or the public) then the tribunal can give a legally binding instruction to the hospital to release the patient without the consent of the community forensic service. In most cases, the community forensic service would then be required to take over their care.

When a general community mental health team feels unable to manage one of their patient's risks to others, they may refer a patient to a community forensic team to take over the patient's care. If the forensic team do not agree that the patient meets the threshold for entry into their service, they will still generally be expected to write a report on the patient containing advice on the patient's risk management. Some patients may be referred with only a request for advice. Some services will manage requests for advice with meetings between general and forensic community services.

Patient Exit from Community Forensic Services

An issue exists around what happens to patients who have remained stable in a community forensic service for many years who could be managed within general community mental health services if it was not for their past serious violence that will forever remain a static, historical risk factor for future violence. General community psychiatric services may sometimes be reluctant to take on these patients, either because of pressure in other areas or because of the historical risks. Debates about where the transfer point should be between the forensic and general community services and how the interface should be negotiated can lead to unhelpful tension between services. Whereas the validated, structured DUNDRUM needs assessment assists clinicians in when a patient should move between high, medium, low, or community level of security for mentally disordered offenders,[25] there is no such widely used instrument or set of guidelines for assisting in debates about when a patient should be moved from forensic to general community management.

Community Forensic Mental Health Services in Courts and Police Stations

The Bradley Report's most significant contribution has arguably been the development of liaison and diversion services. NHS England have commissioned liaison and diversion services over 83% of England. In the community, this involves the placement of mental health professionals in police stations and courts to assess alleged offenders for mental health problems and refer them for appropriate treatment and support where necessary. The main aim is to divert people away from the criminal justice system if their needs and the needs of the community would be better served by providing proper medical treatment rather than criminalizing and imprisoning. "Diversion schemes" refer to arrangements between magistrates' courts and mental health professionals whereby the professionals will attend regularly to assess those suspected of suffering from mental illness with the aim of diverting those with mental illness (where appropriate) out of the criminal justice system and into the healthcare system as early as possible.[26]

Court liaison services have received some criticism for being too orientated to male rather than female defendants.[27] Even in the presence of liaison and diversion services, people who are acutely mentally ill will still be missed and find themselves in prison.[28]

Police Services

In England and Wales, there are three main mental health interventions within the police system; liaison and diversion, street triage, and specialist staff embedded in police contact control rooms.[29]

Police station liaison services, like court liaison services, involve a mental health professional assessing those who report a mental health problem or who are flagged up to them by other concerned persons for assessment and diversion into the mental health system as soon as possible, where appropriate. Street triage capacities of police services will depend on the training level of each individual police officer and local arrangements.

Section 136 of the Mental Health Act 1983 allows police officers to remove members of the public suspected of mental health problems to a "place of safety" for assessment, without their consent, in circumstances where it is "in the interests of that person or for the protection of other persons in immediate need of care or control."

The specialist mental health professionals embedded in police control rooms are placed to triage telephone calls made to the police at their earliest stage. This service is not available in all police services. A recent systematic review of these different services did not find evidence of any of the three models being superior and recommended future research into models that integrate strategies together.

The need for mental health service provision in police stations was highlighted in a study of 1,092 referrals to a mental health service in London police stations which found high levels of mental illness, substance misuse, self-harm, and intellectual disability.[30]

Specialist Community Teams and Interagency Working

People with schizophrenia or other psychotic disorders who have committed serious violent offences are the core patient group for community forensic mental health services described above. Approximately 80% have a primary or secondary diagnosis of a schizophreniform disorder. There are, as expected, common co-morbidities amongst this patient group: personality disorder and drug or alcohol use disorders. The emphasis on schizophreniform disorders as the main focus of community teams has been associated with other groups being excluded from health services; the expectation being that they would remain the responsibility of justice services. Specialist services which have developed in a patchier way include those for children and young people and adults with a primary diagnosis of personality disorder or intellectual disability.

Probation Services

High risk offenders released into the community from prison or sentenced to community orders are managed by the National Probation Service (NPS).[31] The NPS is part of the National Offender Management Service (NOMS). In addition to the NPS, lower risk offenders are managed under community rehabilitation companies (CRCs). CRCs are controversial[32] private-sector organizations providing services previously delivered by public-sector Probation Trusts. The NPS and CRCs make up the entirety of the probation services in England and Wales. A recent announcement confirms that all probation will be taken back into public sector control in the near future.

The NPS is divided into regions with the same boundaries as the police (but different to NHS Trusts). As well as supervising released prisoners, probation services supervise and support offenders sentenced to community orders. On 30 September 2018, 258,157 offenders were on probation.[33] One of the few studies specifically examining people with mental health problems subject to probation found approximately 40% of people supervised by probation

have a mental disorder diagnosis.[34] Of those people with mental disorders, fewer than half were in receipt of mental health care. The data on mental disorder in probation samples are not of the same quality as comparative samples in prisons but it is probably reasonable to accept that this is a population with high levels of mental health morbidity. Practical barriers relating to the configuration of mental health services within the NHS persist. The organization of probation and mental health services is not along the same boundaries so it is common for offenders to find themselves placed in a particular region by probation and then unable to easily access local mental health services.

Children and Young People

There has been a significant reduction in the use of criminal justice sanctions for young people from arrest to conviction and custodial sentencing. Over the last 10 years the number of children and young people receiving a caution or sentence has fallen by 82%.[35] The rates of mental disorder amongst young offenders in the community are significantly higher than in the general population.[36] In 2017, 26,700 children and young people were cautioned or sentenced; 7% were sentenced to immediate custody. Reform of the youth justice system was driven by legislation passed in 1998. The legislation led to the formation of Youth Offending Teams (YOTs)[37] which, despite being a criminal justice initiative, included mental health professionals. Forensic child and adolescent mental health services (FCAMHS) have also been developed and there is a national initiative to develop regional services for children and young people with forensic mental health needs. The services which have developed tend to focus on the management of high-risk young people and so are not restricted to care for people who have already had contact with the justice system. They offer a range of services resembling those in adult teams. Comprehensive specialist teams are likely to include psychiatrists, clinical and forensic psychologists, nurses, social workers, occupational therapists, and other disciplines. As with adults, community forensic psychiatric provision for children and young people has lagged behind secure hospital provision. Services vary from comprehensive specialist teams to generic child and adolescent mental health services providing consultation to criminal justice services. There is also patchy provision of multisystemic therapy (MST).[38] Services remain fragmented and often poorly integrated. The national implementation for FCAMHS is intended to go towards addressing the current problems.[39]

Personality Disorder

Although personality disorder is highly prevalent amongst offenders, there were, until recently, relatively few community *health* services for offenders with a primary diagnosis of personality disorder. Previous attempts at involving health services in partnership with justice services to manage people with personality disorder – The Dangerous and Severe Personality Disorder program (DSPD) – were deemed unsuccessful overall.[40] The Offender Personality Disorder (OPD) Pathway[41] was initiated in 2011 as a partnership between departments of health and justice. It includes prison, hospital, and community services. There is clear partnership working between – in OPD community services – probation and health professionals. The overall aims include public protection and psychological health of offenders as well as producing a competent and trained workforce and efficient use of resources. Many of the services provided as part of this pathway are prison-based, but community services are included. The target population is higher risk offenders with severe personality pathology but without a strong emphasis on categorical diagnosis. Psychological formulation and joint casework is a core aim of the service as a basis for managing complex behavior and the main community provision of the community OPD service supports over 20,000 offenders, led by probation professionals.

In South London, the Forensic Intensive Psychological Treatment Service (FIPTS) was developed in 2004 as a partnership between health and justice services to treat and manage high risk offenders with personality disorder. It continues to function as a beacon of partnership working under the OPD umbrella managing a group of people historically excluded from health services. As well as providing community support it includes specialist community hostels.

Not all specialist community personality disorder services fall under the OPD pathway. In the West of England, *Pathfinder* is a multidisciplinary service working with individuals with personality disorder with a history of offending. They accept referrals from general mental health services, prisons, probation, and other mental health providers. Their model is closer to the integrated model described above; they provide consultation and advice to teams managing higher risk people with personality disorder.

Intellectual Disability

People with intellectual disability have been the focus of scrutiny after some high-profile incidents of abuse in hospitals and care homes. Arguably, the institutionalization of people with intellectual disability continued after other people were released from these institutions and there are now extensive attempts to rectify this situation.[42] These measures include consideration of people who may have had contact with the criminal justice system. However, community services for high-risk people with intellectual disability are relatively few. Where services exist, the model is similar to that which has already been described, with multidisciplinary teams providing treatment and supervision as well as consultation and liaison.[43] Most people under the care of these teams have co-morbid mental disorders and their intellectual disability is usually mild.

Other Specialist Services

The National Stalking Clinic is based in North London. It is an NHS service providing assessment, treatment, and advice on the management of stalkers. They also provide assessment and treatment of stalking victims. They accept referrals from health and justice agencies.

The Fixated Threat Assessment Centre (FTAC) is a joint police/NHS service. It was established in 2006. Their role is to assess risks posed to public figures by people who are suspected to have mental disorders. People are drawn to their attention because they have sent threatening or harassing communications or made approaches to high profile people. Their role will usually consist of assessing and then diverting people to appropriate mental health services. They receive approximately 1,000 referrals a year, with approximately half requiring any further action. In their own analysis of 100 consecutive cases, 57% of people were admitted to hospital and 26% were taken on by community services. Most of their cases were people with psychotic disorders.[44]

Recently, the Stalking Threat Assessment Centre (STAC) has been commissioned for a two-year pilot with the aim of reducing reoffending and improving public safety. The initiative is a partnership between criminal justice and health staff.

Interagency Risk Management

Legislation introduced from the mid 1990s sequentially got "tougher on crime" and in particular on people who had committed sexual offences, with longer sentences, longer probation periods, and a decrease in the rights of offenders to confidentiality and privacy. Multiagency public protection arrangements (MAPPA) came into effect in 2001 and represented an attempt to minimize the harm caused by high-risk violent and sexual offenders in the community.[45] The legislation placed a duty on police, probation, and prison services (as the "responsible authority") in each region, to set up risk management arrangements, involving relevant agencies, with a focus on information sharing. The aim of MAPPA is not primarily to manage mentally disordered offenders but equally people with mental disorder are not excluded from their remit. Their initial introduction was followed by subsequent legislation, imposing a "duty to cooperate" on health and social care organizations. A duty that continues to cause uncertainty for psychiatrists and other health professionals.

Offenders eligible for MAPPA consideration are divided into three categories according to their offending: (1) sexual offences (the largest group), (2) murder or other serious violent offences, (3) other people determined to be at risk of causing serious harm (possibly people with convictions for more minor offences but deemed to be higher risk). People are managed with reference to three levels: level 1 only involves one agency and is deemed ordinary risk management (this is likely to include people managed by health services); level 2 involves more than one agency but not at the most senior level, and level 3 concerns the small number of very high risk offenders who require senior involvement. Level 2 and 3 offenders are discussed at multiagency public protection panels (MAPPP) where their risk management is coordinated. These are hosted and chaired by the police or probation but with health professionals attending and participating by giving advice, contributing, and sharing information on cases where health services are involved, and contributing to decision-making about risk management strategies. There are approximately 4,500 level 2 and 3 offenders currently managed in the community. There is no data as to the proportion of those who are involved with mental health services.

The "duty to cooperate" is somewhat vaguely defined but causes most controversy in relation to sharing information. Duties associated with confidentiality for psychiatrists are not automatically over-ridden and so there is balancing of competing duties before deciding on what information to share. The Royal College of Psychiatrists provides guidance for psychiatrists.[46] For a psychiatrist, the usual involvement will be in relation to a convicted offender managed under mental health services where they are then requested to share information with other agencies. Disagreements about what information is shared do occur and these often arise out of the clash between professional or ethical duties and in particular the way that these differ from criminal justice professionals, whose expectations may be exaggerated. Ultimately, employers will have arrangements to resolve these issues so that the individual professional is not necessarily bound to breach their professional duties.

Attempts to study outcomes for MAPPA eligible offenders have found some support that these arrangements reduce rates of reoffending.[47]

Legislation and Its Application to Mentally Disordered Offenders in the Community

In broad terms, mentally disordered offenders may be subject to restrictions and conditions arising out of either mental health or criminal justice legislation. There are some circumstances where both can apply. Mental health law procedures all arise from one act of parliament, The Mental Health Act 1983 (amended in 2007). The Criminal Justice Act 2003 is the source of law as it applies to offenders who have been granted parole but there are other examples of specific legislation contributing to risk management strategies, particularly for sexual offenders. The Mental Capacity Act 2005 (MCA) enshrines the principle that treatment and care should be voluntary unless the person is unable to make decisions for themselves and it is in their best interest to treat them without consent.

Whilst patients may be subject to restrictions in the community, they cannot be forced to receive treatment, although it may be argued that treatment is nevertheless coerced because recall to hospital or prison is a possibility if conditions are breached.

Mental Health Act 1983 (MHA), as Amended in 2007

The MHA is law which is predominantly concerned with the detention of people for assessment and treatment of mental disorder in England and Wales. However, there are several relevant provisions which apply to people after they have been discharged from detention in hospital.

Hospital Order with Restrictions (Section 37/41)

The "restricted hospital order" ("section thirty-seven, forty-one" in common parlance) is the most prevalent form of detention for people in secure psychiatric hospitals. People convicted of an offence for which they may be sentenced to prison for one year or more may be "disposed of" by way of a hospital order (Section 37). This is an indefinite order which will always result in admission to a psychiatric hospital. If it is considered *necessary for the protection of the public from serious harm,* a restriction order (Section 41) may also be imposed. The overall effect of the restriction order is to give the Secretary of State for Justice powers over granting leave, transfer, and discharge of patients. In practice, these orders require the existence of a department in the Ministry of Justice specifically devoted to "restricted patients": The Mental Health Casework Section. This department has responsibility for considering requests for leave etc. from their responsible psychiatrists.

Arguably, the most significant aspect of this order is that almost all patients, when discharged from hospital, are discharged "conditionally" so that although they are no longer liable to be deprived of their liberty or detained, they do have conditions imposed on their discharge. In addition to these conditions, they are liable to be recalled to hospital. In practice, it is only after several years of cooperation with mental health treatment, an absence of reoffending, and convincing evidence of likely ongoing cooperation that "absolute discharge" will be granted. After being absolutely discharged, any ongoing treatment is fully voluntary, restrictions are removed, and the power of recall falls away. Although these conditions often mandate treatment with medication, they do not provide authority to treat people compulsorily in their own home; there is no power to restrain people and administer medication.

The use of Section 37/41 has steadily increased so that there were 4,811 detained patients in 2017 and 2,611 conditionally discharged patients. Seventy-five patients were "converted" from being conditionally discharged to being absolutely discharged.[48] Of those 2,611 people, 1,514 had been convicted of violent offences, 379 criminal damage and arson, and 235

sexual offences; 220 people were recalled to hospital in 2017.

> **Conditions Commonly Associated with Section 37/41 Conditional Discharge**
>
> - Residence at a specific place
> - Cooperation with prescribed medication
> - Abstinence from drugs and/or alcohol
> - Mandatory drug testing
> - Cooperation with care plans
> - Exclusion from specified areas (usually at the request of victims)
> - Prohibition on contact with victims or their families

Community Treatment Orders (Section 17a MHA 1983)

The MHA was amended in 2007 in an atmosphere of fear about the risks posed by mentally disordered people. The amendments on the whole reflected this and moved away from autonomy towards greater paternalism. A new power was inserted into the MHA – albeit already in existence in other countries around the world – which allowed for conditions to be imposed on people after their discharge from detention in hospital: the *community treatment order* (Section 17a). In many ways, it provided similar powers to those already associated with conditional discharge under Section 37/41. Section 17a is *not*, however, ordered by a judge, it is recommended by the treating psychiatrist for patients who usually have not committed any offence; it is a "civil" order. There is no oversight from the Ministry of Justice, although there is a similar power of recall at the discretion of the responsible clinician. Despite the initial hope that community treatment orders (CTOs) would address the issue of "revolving door patients," no clear benefit of CTOs has been shown in decreasing readmission rates or any outcome measure studied to date.[49] However, CTO use has been maintained.[50]

Other MHA Provisions

Guardianship (Section 7) is a rarely used order which has three powers requiring: (1) residence at a specific place; (2) attendance for treatment, education, training, or work; and (3) the patient to allow access to their home. Very few guardianship orders are made, even though they could theoretically be used as an alternative disposal for offenders who have committed minor offences.

Section 117 of the MHA applies to any patient who has been detained in hospital for treatment and comes into effect after they are released from detention. It places a duty on health and social care organizations to provide aftercare. It does not place any burden on the patient to cooperate with treatment offered.

Criminal Justice Orders

Community Orders

Sentences served in the community are referred to as community orders. These are not orders which are specific to mentally disordered offenders. Community orders as a sentence have undergone various revisions, the most recent in 2003 legislation.[51] They are available where imprisonment is a possibility (but not mandated) and the offence is sufficiently serious to warrant it. There are 13 requirements which may be imposed including unpaid work, offender programs, and curfews. The orders have the scope to offer punishment, reparation, and rehabilitation components and the judge is able to create their own "menu" of requirements.

There is the option of imposing a mental health treatment requirement (MHTR) (with the offender's consent) and drug or alcohol treatment requirements. Community orders with MHTRs are rarely used, although there have been recent attempts to increase their use and pilots continue. The court effectively have this option open when compulsory hospitalization (under powers in the MHA) is not necessary but treatment in the community is judged to be necessary. MHTRs do not depend on a psychiatrist recommendation and will usually be recommended by the probation officer or court diversion professional after liaison with mental health services. There must be willingness on the part of the offender to comply with the mental health treatment. There can be a requirement for treatment in a hospital, care home, or in another place. The court will not impose specific requirements in terms of treatment. The orders can be made for up to three years and are overseen by a responsible officer from the probation service. If the offender withdraws their consent then the court have powers to impose sanctions, including fines and custodial sentences. The total number of MHTRs made annually is in the hundreds, representing less than 1% of the total number of community orders; 90,618 community orders were made in 2018 for all offences. Barriers to the making of MHTRs include:[52]

- Lack of clarity about who the order is suitable for
- Poor understanding and awareness of the order amongst all professionals involved in the process of making the orders
- Difficulties in obtaining agreement from mental health services

License

People who receive a sentence of one year or longer serve half of their sentence in the community "on license." Their license will be supervised by the probation services but will include conditions. Their conditions may include mental health treatment but these conditions do not have the effect of compelling health services to offer treatment to the offender. If the offender breaches any of their conditions then they may be recalled to prison and serve more of their sentence in custody.

Other Measures to Manage Risky Offenders

There are several other legal measures to manage high risk offenders in the community, often related to sex offenders. The Sex Offenders Act 1997 introduced requirements for sex offenders to notify the police of their address and any travel. Sexual harm prevention orders (SHPOs) are imposed by a court on individuals who have been convicted of or found to have committed an act within specific sections of sexual offences legislation – essentially serious offences. They are not necessarily made at the time of conviction but can be made later; the police have the option of applying for them. The name is self-explanatory but will likely include conditions tailored to the individual. For example, restrictions on travel, association with specific people, internet use, or employment. They are unlikely to include any mental health requirements. Breaches can result in imprisonment; 5,931 SHPOs were imposed in 2016/17.

Outcomes for Mentally Disordered Offenders in the Community

The effectiveness of different models of community care for mentally disordered offenders is underevaluated. The evidence that does exist does not support the development of specialist community forensic services.

A systematic review of outcomes for patients discharged from secure hospitals included 18 studies from England and Wales.[53] They examined mortality, readmission, and repeat offending as outcomes. They found increased mortality rates when compared to released prisoners but similar rates to patients with schizophrenia, suggesting mental illness (with its associations with mortality) was the main contributor to the increased mortality. English and Welsh studies did not find such high mortality rates when compared to the rest of the world. Readmission rates were substantially varied between studies. Repeat offending was also markedly varied between studies. Comparisons with released prisoners suggested lower reoffending rates overall. Specialist forensic community services were formed on the assumption that staff who are specifically trained in the management of mentally disordered offenders would achieve better outcomes both clinically for patients and in terms of public protection. However, the evidence for this assumption remains limited. Many homicides by patients discharged from psychiatric hospitals take place after noncompliance with medication (particularly oral medication). For patients who have only been violent in the context of noncompliance with treatment for a major mental disorder, some may argue that any team that secures medication compliance will be adequate to contain risk to the public, regardless of any expertise in forensic matters.

Coid et al.[54] compared outcomes in a sample of 1,061 patients discharged from medium secure units, depending on whether they were case managed by a forensic community service or general community mental health services during their first seven years in the community. They found that forensic services did not supervise more high-risk patients in the community than the general mental health teams. They also found that following discharge from medium secure services there were no differences in outcomes – criminal convictions, hospital readmissions, and deaths – when comparing general and forensic services. Weaknesses of the study included that input and advice from forensic services to those initially discharged to a general psychiatry team could not be taken into account in the study design.

Humber et al. looked at a variety of measures including the HCR-20 risk assessments in a sample of 639 mental health patients comparing those managed by a general service with a forensic service. Predictably they found significantly higher mean HCR-20 scores in the forensic than general patients for the historical scale. They found no significant difference on the clinical and risk management scale scores. It is not reasonable to extrapolate that this implies that forensic services successfully contain dynamic risk factors to the extent that forensic patients become more comparable to general psychiatric patients. The same result could be used to argue that forensic patients do not require a specialist service.

Controversy and Conclusions

Forensic mental health services are well developed in England and Wales. Their development in the late twentieth century resulted from substantial investment and the secure hospital system continues to demand the lion's share of the budget. The natural evolution of services has meant that community services have developed last, with a more recent emphasis on integration of different agencies to manage the health and risks of mentally disordered offenders in the community. It is probably uncontroversial to state that the emphasis has shifted towards risk management so that clinicians are facing more complex ethical decisions in relation to the welfare of their patients. Overall, forensic psychiatry services in England and Wales are high-cost and treat few people. The development of forensic psychiatry – specifically the secure hospitals – was criticized in an editorial in *The Lancet* in 2011[55] largely because of this ratio. The authors emphasized the cost of secure services and also their perception of the need to concentrate resources in other areas including community teams with multiagency involvement and integration of justice and health. The authors also touched on what they saw as an unhealthy separation of general and forensic mental health services which has been a persistent problem in the development of community forensic services.

Turner and Salter concentrated on the distinction between general and forensic services[56] and emphasized the absence of evidence for the benefits of community forensic psychiatric services (and, in their opinion, the absence of special skills of forensic psychiatrists) and also highlighted the "unhappy result of [forensic psychiatry's] evolution into a separate specialist domain." They suggested that forensic community psychiatry should fall foul of the absence of evidence of benefit. Correspondence by the same authors a few years earlier set out their position on community forensic services. Albeit this may be an unreasonable reduction of the nuance of their argument they essentially posed the question, What's the point?[57] There is an ongoing debate within clinical services about the meaning of the term "forensic patient." It is not a legal term or a clinically agreed term. The decision about which team looks after which patients is therefore at risk of being arbitrary and variable across the country. There may be local agreements about the transfer of patients from forensic to general care, but these rarely prevent debates.

The near future is likely to be characterized by a demand to provide more services for less money and community and diversion forensic services offer an opportunity, if successful, to reduce the need for secure hospital services. The secure hospitals are expensive so community services that even modestly reduce the need for secure hospitals are likely to be welcomed. NHS England have responded to evaluation of the impact of community forensic service provision on length of stay

in secure hospitals by seemingly making community forensic psychiatry development a priority. Whilst community forensic psychiatry has been something of an afterthought in the development of treatment services for mentally disordered offenders in England and Wales, it is now moving towards the front of the minds of clinicians, commissioners, and managers.[58]

Disclosure

Richard Latham and Hannah Kate Williams have nothing to disclose.

References

1. Department of Health. *National Service Framework for Mental Health: Modern Standards and Service Models.* London: HMSO; 1999.

2. Killaspy H, Bebbington P, Blizard R, et al. The REACT study: randomised evaluation of assertive community

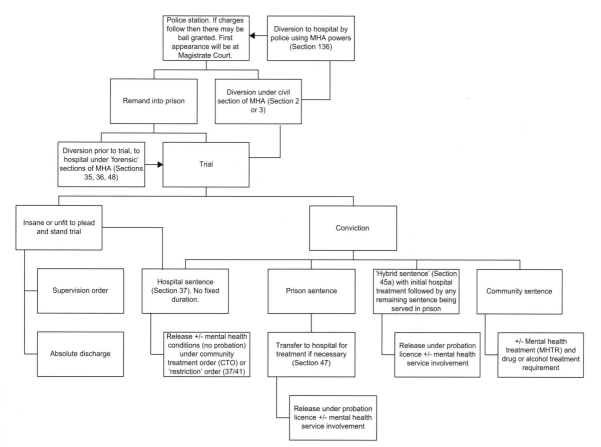

Pathways for mentally disordered offenders in England and Wales suspected of criminal offences.

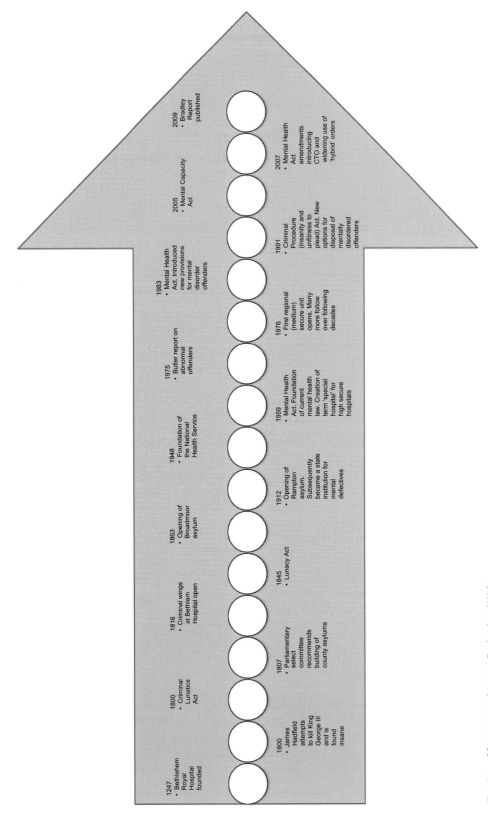

1247
• Bethlehem Royal Hospital founded

1800
• Criminal Lunatics Act

1816
• Criminal wings at Bethlem Hospital open

1863
• Opening of Broadmoor asylum

1948
• Foundation of the National Health Service

1975
• Butler report on abnormal offenders

1983
• Mental Health Act. Introduced new provisions for mental disorder offenders

2005
• Mental Capacity Act

2009
• Bradley Report published

1800
• James Hadfield attempts to kill King George III and is found insane

1807
• Parliamentary select committee recommends building of county asylums

1845
• Lunacy Act

1912
• Opening of Rampton asylum. Subsequently became a state institution for mental defectives

1959
• Mental Health Act. Foundation of current mental health law. Creation of term 'special hospital' for high secure hospitals

1976
• First regional (medium) secure unit opens. Many more follow over following decades

1991
• Criminal Procedure (insanity and unfitness to plead) Act. New options for disposal of mentally disordered offenders

2007
• Mental Health Act amendments introducing CTO and widening use of 'hybrid' orders

Timeline of forensic psychiatry in England and Wales

treatment in North London. *Br Med J.* 2006; **332**: 815–820.

3. Allderidge, PH. Criminal insanity: Bethlem to Broadmoor. *Proc R Soc Med.* 1974; **67**(9): 897–904.

4. Criminal Lunatics Act 1800.

5. Home Office and the Department of Health and Social Security. *Report of the Committee on Mentally Disordered Offenders (The Butler Report) (Cmnd 6244).* London: HMSO; 1976.

6. Killaspy H. From the asylum to community care: learning from experience. *Br Med Bull.* 2006; **79–80** (1): 245–258.

7. Coid J, Maden T. Should psychiatrists protect the public?: a new risk reduction strategy, supporting criminal justice, could be effective. *Br Med J.* 2003; 406–407.

8. Hallam A, Hallam A. Media influences on mental health policy: long-term effects of the Clunis and Silcock cases. *Int Rev Psychiatry.* 2002; **14**(1): 26–33.

9. Royal College of Psychiatrists. *Summary of workforce census;* 2017.

10. Thornicroft G. Deinstitutionalisation: from hospital closure to service development. *Br J Psychiatry.* 1989; **155**: 739–753.

11. Eastman NLG. Forensic psychiatric services in Britain: a current review. *Int J Law Psychiatry.* 1993; **16**(1–2): 1–26.

12. Grounds A. Forensic psychiatry for the millennium. *J Forensic Psychiatry.* 2008; **7**(2): 221–227.

13. Walker J, Amos T, Knowles P, et al. Putting a price on psychiatric care. *Health Serv J.* 2012; **122** (6296): 22–24.

14. Rutherford M, Duggan S. Forensic mental health services: facts and figures on current provision. *Br J Forensic Pract.* 2008; **10**(4): 4–10.

15. Bradley K. *Lord Bradley's Review of People with Mental Health Problems or Learning Disabilities in the Criminal Justice System.* London: House of Lords; 2009.

16. Whittle M, Scally M. Model of forensic psychiatric community care. *Psychiatr Bull.* 1998; **22**: 748–750.

17. Mohan R, Slade M, Fahy T. Clinical characteristics of community forensic mental health services. *Psychiatr Serv.* 2004; **55**(11): 1294–1298.

18. Gunn J. Management of the mentally disordered offender: integrated or parallel. *Proc R Soc Med.* 1977; **70**(12): 877–880.

19. Humber N, Hayes A, Wright S, et al. A comparative study of forensic and general community psychiatric patients with integrated and parallel models of care in the UK. *J Forens Psychiatry Psychol.* 2011; **22**: 183–202.

20. Buchanan A. The relationship between generic and forensic psychiatric services. *Crim Behav Ment Health.* 2001; **11**: 90–94.

21. Khosla V, Davidson P, Gordon H, et al. The interface between general and forensic psychiatry: the present day. *B J Psych Adv.* 2014; **20**: 359–365.

22. Kenney-Herbert J, Taylor M, Puri R, et al. *Standards for Community Forensic Mental Health Services.* London: Royal College of Psychiatrists; 2013.

23. NHS England, National Offender Management Service. *The Offender Personality Disorder Pathway Strategy.* 2015.

24. Dowsett J. Measurement of risk by a community forensic mental health team. *Psychiatr Bull.* 2005; **29**: 9–12.

25. Kennedy HG, O'Neill C, Flynn G, Gill P, Davoren M. The Dundrum Toolkit V1.0.30. Dangerousness, understanding, recovery and urgency manual (the Dundrum Quartet). Structured professional judgement instruments for admission triage, urgency, treatment completion and recovery assessments. Dublin: TARA; 2016: 1–141.

26. Blumenthal S, Wessely S. National survey of current arrangements for diversion from custody in England and Wales. *Br Med J.* 1992; **305**: 1322–1325.

27. Hean S, Heaslip V, Warr J, et al. A women's worker in court: a more appropriate service for women defendants with mental health issues? *Perspect Public Health.* 2010; **130**(2): 91–96.

28. Slade K, Samele C, Valmaggia L, et al. Pathways through the criminal justice system for prisoners with acute and serious mental illness. *J Forensic Leg Med.* 2016; **44**: 162–168.

29. Kane E, Evans E, Shokraneh F. Effectiveness of current policing-related mental health interventions in England and Wales and Crisis Intervention Teams as a future potential model: a systematic review. *Crim Behav Ment Health.* 2017; **28**(2): 108–119.

30. Forrester A, Samele C, Slade K, et al. Demographic and clinical characteristics of 1092 consecutive police custody mental health referrals. *J Forens Psychiatry Psychol.* 2017; **28**(3): 295–312.

31. Bourne R, Rajpur R, Field F. Working with probation services and mentally disordered offenders. *B J Psych Adv.* 2015; **21**: 273–280.

32. Ministry of Justice, HM Prison & Probation Service. *Transforming Rehabilitation: Progress Review.* 2019.

33. Ministry of Justice. *Offender Management Statistics Bulletin, England and Wales.* 31 January 2019.

34. Brooker C, Sirdifield C, Blizard R, et al. An investigation into the prevalence of mental health disorder and patterns of health service access in a probation population. *J Forens Psychiatry Psychol.* 2011; **23**(4): 522–537.

35. Ministry of Justice. *Youth Justice Statistics England and Wales.* Youth Justice Board January 2018.

36. Chitsabesan P, Kroll L, Bailey S, et al. Mental health needs of young offenders in custody and in the community. *Br J Psychiatry.* 2006; **188**: 534–540.

37. Crime and Disorder Act 1998. Section 39.

38. Butler S, Baruch G, Hickey N, et al. A randomized controlled trial of multisystemic therapy and a statutory therapeutic intervention for young offenders. *J Am Acad Child Adolesc Psychiatry.* 2011; **50**(12): 1220–1235.

39. Hindley N, Lengua C, White O. Forensic mental health services for children and adolescents: rationale and development. *B J Psych Adv.* 2017; **23**(1): 36–43.

40. Völlm B, Konappa N. The dangerous and severe personality disorder experiment – review of empirical research. *Crim Behav Ment Health.* 2012; **22**(3): 165–180.

41. Joseph N, Benefield N. A joint offender personality disorder pathway strategy: an outline summary. *Crim Behav Ment Health.* 2012; **22**(3): 210–217.

42. Bubb S. Winterbourne View – time for change. Transforming the commissioning of services for people with learning disabilities and/or autism. 2014.

43. Lindsay WR, Steele L, Smith AH, et al. A community forensic intellectual disability service: twelve year follow up of referrals, analysis of referral patterns and assessment of harm reduction. *Legal Criminol Psychol.* 2006; **11**(1): 113–130.

44. James DV, Kerrigan TR, Forfar R, et al. The fixated threat assessment centre: preventing harm and facilitating care. *J Forens Psychiatry Psychol.* 2010; **21** (4): 521–536.

45. Yakeley J, Taylor R, Cameron A. MAPPA and mental health – 10 years of controversy. *Psychiatrist.* 2012; **36** (6): 201–204.

46. Taylor R, Yakeley J. *Working with MAPPA: guidance for psychiatrists in England and Wales (faculty report FR/FP/01).* London: Royal College of Psychiatrists; 2013.

47. Bryant S, Peck M, Lovbakke J. *Reoffending analysis of MAPPA eligible offenders.* Ministry of Justice; 2015.

48. Ministry of Justice. *Restricted Patients 2017 England and Wales.* Ministry of Justice Statistics Bulletin. London, UK. 2018.

49. Maughan D, Molodynski A, Rugkasa J, Burns T. A systematic review of the effect of community treatment orders on service use. *Soc Psychiatry Psychiatr Epidemiol.* 2014; **49**(4): 651–663.

50. Gupta S, Akyuz EU, Baldwin T, et al. Community treatment orders in England: review of usage from national data. *B J Psych Bull.* 2018; **42**(3): 119–122.

51. Criminal Justice Act 2003

52. Khanom H, Samele C, Rutherford MA. A missed opportunity? Community sentences and the mental health treatment requirement. Sainsbury Centre for Mental Health; 2009.

53. Fazel S, Fiminska Z, Cocks C, et al. Patient outcomes following discharge from secure psychiatric hospitals: systematic review and meta-analysis. *Br J Psychiatry.* 2016; **208**(1): 17–25.

54. Coid JW, Hickey N, Yang M. Comparison of outcomes following after-care from forensic and general adult psychiatric services. *Br J Psychiatry.* 2007; **190**(6): 509–514.

55. Wilson S, James D, Forrester A. The medium-secure project and criminal justice mental health. *Lancet.* 2011; **378**(9786): 110–111.

56. Turner T, Salter M. Forensic psychiatry and general psychiatry: re-examining the relationship. *Psychiatr Bull.* 2008; **32**(1): 2–6.

57. Turner T, Salter M. What is the role of a community forensic mental health team? *Psychiatr Bull.* 2005; **29** (9): 352.

58. NHS England. *NHS Mental Health Implementation Plan 2019/20–2023/24.* July 2019.

A Longitudinal Description of Incompetent to Stand Trial Admissions to a State Hospital

Barbara E. McDermott, Katherine Warburton, and Chloe Auletta-Young

Introduction

According to the US Supreme Court, all individuals charged with a crime must be competent to stand trial (CST). As defined in *Dusky v. US*,[1] competency requires that defendants have the ability to consult with their attorney with a reasonable degree of rationality and possess a rational as well as factual understanding of the legal proceedings. The precise number of CST evaluations conducted each year is unknown. The oft-reported figure of 60,000 provided by Bonnie and Grisso[2] is an estimate based on the number of felony indictments coupled with the estimated percentage of referrals for competency evaluations made by the courts in the 1990s. Later work has suggested a much higher number.[3] Using a similar method, Vitacco and colleagues examined surveys indicating the frequency with which the issue of competency is raised by defense attorneys[4] and arrest rates at the time of publishing. They deduced that a conservative estimate of the quantity of evaluations could be 700,000 annually.[3]

The National Dilemma

Consistent with Vitacco's estimates, reports suggest that the number of referrals for competency evaluations and subsequent restoration services are increasing nationally. The state of Washington experienced an 82% increase in referrals for competency evaluations between the years 2000 and 2011.[5] In Colorado, requests for competency evaluations increased 524% from 2000 to 2017; corresponding requests for restoration increased 931% in the same time frame.[6] Los Angeles County experienced an increase of 273% in competency referrals for misdemeanant offenders from 2010 to 2015.[7,8] In Michigan, the number of evaluations rose from 3,000 in 2010 to 4,500 in 2016.[9] In Metro Detroit alone, the number of evaluations ordered increased 20% from 2012 to 2016.[10] In California, referrals to the Department of State Hospital (DSH) system for competency restoration almost doubled from fiscal year 2013/2014 to 2015/2016.[11]

As the number of referrals and evaluations increase, so does the corresponding number of defendants determined to be incompetent. Research consistently suggests that between 25% and 30% of defendants referred for CST evaluations are adjudicated incompetent.[8,12] McDermott and colleagues estimated that this would translate to a range of 15,000–30,000 defendants found incompetent every year, with substantially more if the figures of evaluation referrals from Vitacco et al. are accurate.[3,13] In many jurisdictions, competency restoration occurs on an inpatient basis in state psychiatric hospitals[8] and evidence suggests that patients admitted as incompetent to stand trial (IST) comprise the largest proportion of forensic patients in hospitals throughout the nation.[14,15] According to recent reports, over 50% of the total patients in the California DSH were IST as of February 2016.[16]

There are many potential explanations for these observed increases, such as decreasing access to treatment for both mental illness and substance use in the community[17–19] and decreasing availability of inpatient psychiatric beds.[17] For example, Los Angeles has experienced a 30% decrease in the number of inpatient psychiatric beds from 1995 to 2010.[7] Others have postulated that the increased popularity of specialty courts, such as mental health and drug courts, contributes to an increase in competence referrals for defendants who are unable to comply with the guidelines stipulated by these courts because of their serious mental illness.[20] Some have suggested a more complex series of events as an explanation for the increasing numbers of IST commitments. The Director of Community Health and Integrated Programs at the Los Angeles County Department of Health Services was cited as believing that his city's rise in competency referrals is due to the combination of homelessness, increasing awareness of mental illness in the criminal justice system, and increasing methamphetamine use.[21]

An alternative explanation for the increase in IST referrals is the frequency of malingering of psychiatric or cognitive symptoms among defendants coupled with the relative infrequency of court-appointed evaluators to systematically assessing feigning.[13] Rates of malingering on competency evaluations have been estimated to be as high as 21%.[22] In a study reviewing 464 competency reports, only 194 (41.8%) of evaluators considered the legitimacy of the reported symptoms and of those, only 69 (14.9%) employed a structured assessment of feigning.[23] It follows that if referrals for evaluations are increasing, but evaluators are not assessing for possible malingering, there could be an increase in patients erroneously ruled incompetent.

Regardless of the source, it is clear that referrals for both competency evaluations and restoration services are increasing nationally. Although alternatives to inpatient psychiatric treatment for restoration recently have been suggested or implemented,[8] with no adequate explanation for the observed increases that might suggest a reasonable solution, this trend is likely to continue.

Characteristics of IST Offenders

In studies of IST populations, there is a distinction between individuals referred for competency evaluations versus individuals on whom competency decisions have been made after evaluation. Although not specifically designed to understand the reasons for rises in IST referrals, both for evaluation and restoration, sociodemographic data, such as age, gender, and race, are frequently gathered to better understand the IST population. For example, research has shown that defendants found IST tend to be older than competent defendants.[12,24–27] However, among an all-female sample studied by Kois and colleagues, age was not a significant characteristic in predicting competency,[28] suggesting that women may have unique characteristics in the criminal justice system. Study samples of patients referred for competency restoration indicate that most are male.[24,26,27] However, although men are more frequently evaluated for competency, not surprising given the higher numbers of men arrested, studies have found that

males and females are equally likely to be ruled incompetent in the US.[12]

In terms of race and ethnicity, research has shown that the over-representation of people of color in the criminal justice system may be mirrored in the forensic psychiatric system for competency restoration.[29] Research has shown that African Americans are more often referred for competency evaluations.[24,26,28,29] This discrepancy continues even after the competency decision is made. Pirelli and colleagues demonstrated that, in 22 studies that presented ethnicity data, minority defendants were 1.5 times more likely to be found incompetent than white defendants.[12] One contributing factor could be the higher likelihood of a diagnosis of a psychotic or mood disorder among African Americans and Hispanics respectively.[30,31]

In regards to symptomatology, defendants found incompetent are more likely to be diagnosed with a psychotic disorder or evidence symptoms of psychosis than competent defendants or those not referred for an evaluation.[12,24,26,32,33] Cognitive disabilities also are closely related to incompetency.[16,27,34] Diagnoses, therefore, can confound other variables associated with incompetency. Among the elderly community, the correlation between an older age and decreased competency to stand trial could be explained by a greater prevalence of cognitive disorders.[25,35] Defendants with personality disorders and/or substance use disorder diagnoses are less likely to be found IST.[24,26,32] Viljoen and Zapf[32] found that defendants referred for competency evaluations were less likely to have a primary substance abuse disorder and less likely to meet the criteria for antisocial personality disorder compared to those not referred, a result consistent with other research.[24,26]

Other well-studied variables among the IST population are restorability and length of stay, both related to the nature of the mental disorder. A patient's diagnosis, or how symptomatic the patient is, can determine if they are successfully restored and how long that process takes.[33] Research has shown that cognitive disability and psychotic symptomology are not just associated with findings of incompetency, but also with restorability and a prolonged length of stay.[36–39] Using records from 351 inpatient pre-trial defendants who underwent competence restoration at a state psychiatric hospital from 1995 through 1999, patients with prolonged psychotic disorders and irremediable cognitive disorders were less likely to be restored.[36] Similarly, Morris and DeYoung[39] found that among 455 male defendants admitted to a forensic treatment center for competency restoration, psychotic disorders and cognitive disability predicted unsuccessful restoration within three months of treatment. They also demonstrated that diagnoses of personality disorders and substance use might represent a higher likelihood of competence, as they were predictive of successful restoration. Anderson and Hewitt[40] found that both higher intelligence and being African American was predictive of restoration. Others have found no major difference in populations of patients who have been restored versus those who have not.[41]

Criminogenic factors also have been studied with respect to competency to stand trial, although research suggests this is closely intertwined with other variables, such as diagnosis. Previous work has demonstrated that violent crimes are more often associated with competency, while nonviolent offenses are associated with incompetency.[24,26,42,43] In contrast, Cochrane and colleagues found that violent charges were associated with high rates of incompetency findings.[34] However, when the authors controlled for diagnosis, the significance of the relationship disappeared. Kois and colleagues initially found that although nonfelony charges were more likely associated with incompetency, active psychotic symptoms were more predictive.[28] Similarly, Viljoen and Zapf reported no difference in charging offense between defendants referred for an evaluation and those not referred for an evaluation.[32] In contrast, Pirelli and colleagues, when evaluating rulings of competency, found that among the studies that discussed current criminal charges, defendants with a violent charge were more likely to be found competent.[12]

Importance

Regardless of the characteristics of the defendants found IST, the increasing numbers of these types of admissions is real and the impact has been detrimental. Patients in need of treatment can wait in jail for weeks for admission to a hospital.[8] Moreover, over-crowded forensic psychiatric institutions can risk staff safety and patient wellbeing. To better understand this growing population and to inform hospital administration, the University of California Davis, in partnership with the Department of State Hospitals' (DSH) facility in Napa (DSH-Napa) implemented a triage screening procedure for individuals admitted for restoration to competence. This study utilizes archival clinical data from these screenings for IST patients admitted from 2009 to 2016. In addition to describing the sociodemographic, psychiatric, and criminal variables and the inter-relationship between these factors, we examined changes over time to assess if any demographic or clinical factors were related to the observed increase in these types of commitments.

Method

This research was approved by all relevant institutional review boards. The details of the methods and procedures have been described in a previous paper.[13] Briefly, the study was conducted at DSH-Napa, a 1200-bed primarily forensic inpatient psychiatric facility located in northern California. Approximately 380 beds are allocated for the restoration of patients committed as IST. The records of patients found IST and admitted to DSH-Napa for restoration of competence between the dates of January 1, 2009 and December 31, 2016 were eligible for inclusion in the study.

Procedure

All patients were admitted directly from the referring county jails. One component of the admission screening was a brief interview conducted by a psychologist, psychiatrist, or research assistant coupled with structured assessments. Once the patient was interviewed and assessment tools were completed, the interviewer was asked to form judgments about the patient's overall competence and on both components of the California competency standard (understanding of criminal proceedings and ability to assist in their defense), potential for feigning of psychiatric symptoms or cognitive/memory deficits, and presence of possible cognitive deficits. These opinions were documented on a coding sheet that also included basic demographic information, clinical information (e.g. current medications, prior psychiatric treatment), criminal arrest information (e.g. most serious commitment offense, prior IST finding, number of prior arrests), as well as scores from the structured assessments. All interviewers were trained in these procedures. While inter-rater reliability was not conducted, all interviewers received extensive training in these screening procedures.

Measures

The M-FAST

The Miller Forensic Assessment of Symptoms Test[44] (M-FAST) was developed as a screening instrument designed to identify feigned psychopathology. It is a 25-item structured interview that can be administered in approximately five minutes. Although it contains multiple subscales, a total score of 6 or greater is suggested as indicative of a need for a more extensive assessment of feigning. Scores in the sample ranged from 0 to 25, with an average score of 4.41 and a standard deviation of 4.89. While the modal score was 0, 31.0% scored at or above 6, the cut score for suspected malingering.

The BPRS

The Brief Psychiatric Rating Scale[45] (BPRS) was used to quantify psychotic symptoms. The BPRS consists of 18 items rating psychiatric symptoms such as anxiety, depression, and hallucinations. It is a widely used assessment that includes affective symptoms and hostility as well as both positive and negative symptoms of a psychotic disorder. The four items quantifying positive psychotic symptoms were selected for the brief screen (i.e. thought disorganization, suspiciousness, hallucinations, and unusual thought content). Items are rated on a seven-point scale, with 1 indicating that the symptom was not observed and 7 indicating that the symptom was very severe. Scores in this sample ranged from 1 to 25, with higher scores indicating more severe psychotic symptoms. The mean score for the sample was 9.03 with a standard deviation of 4.79.

Competency Screening

Four items were selected from the Georgia Court Competence Test[46] (GCCT) to assess the patients' abilities to understand courtroom proceedings. The GCCT was designed as a screening tool for assessing competence specific to the criteria in the United States. It contains three sections, including knowledge of the physical locations of courtroom personnel and their roles as well as an assessment of the defendant's ability to assist in their defense. The four questions selected in this study included the defendant's understanding of the roles of four courtroom personnel (defense attorney, district attorney, judge, jury). An additional question asked the defendant to name their attorney and express their beliefs about the adequacy of their attorney's performance (e.g. "What do you think of your attorney? What has it been like to work with him/her?"). Each item was scored as 0, 1, or 2, with 2 indicating an adequate answer, 1 a partially correct answer, and 0 either no answer or a wrong or delusionally based response. Because there were five questions, scores ranged from 0 to 10. The average score was 5.74 with a standard deviation of 3.29.

Participants

There were a total of 3158 unduplicated IST admissions available during the specified time period. Women comprised 25.4% of the admissions (n = 802). Most admissions were White (n = 1352, 42.8%), with the remainder Black (n= 917, 29.0%), Hispanic (n = 583, 18.5%), Asian (n = 207, 6.6%), or of other ethnic descent (n = 98, 3.1%). The largest number of patients reported not completing high school (n = 1005, 43.1%), although many had a high school diploma or equivalent (n = 659, 28.3%), and a substantial number had some educational experience beyond high school (n = 668, 28.6%). The age of the patients on admission ranged from 18 to 89, with an average age of 38.77 (std = 13.07). The majority of patients reported at least one prior inpatient psychiatric admission as an adult (n = 1540, 60.5%), although many reported no prior psychiatric history, either inpatient or outpatient (n = 577, 22.7%). The remainder reported a history of mental health treatment only as a juvenile or as an outpatient (n = 427, 16.8%). Past psychiatric treatment was unavailable on 614 patients. Most admissions were English speaking (n =2793, 93.7%); language was a barrier in 5.6% of interviews conducted (n = 166). The most common commitment offense was assault/battery (n = 1048, 35.7%), followed by theft (n = 284, 9.7%), robbery (n = 278, 9.5%), a sex offense (n = 231, 7.9%), murder (n = 224, 7.6%), miscellaneous charges (e.g. vandalism, disorderly conduct; n = 194, 6.6%), criminal threats (n = 140, 4.8%), drug offenses (n = 140, 4.8%), weapons offenses (n = 121, 4.1%), arson (n = 103, 3.5%), resisting arrest (n = 72, 2.5%), and other (kidnapping, white collar crimes, major driving offenses, escape) (n = 97, 3.3%). For 226 (7.2%) of the admissions, the offense was not recorded. Only the most serious offense was recorded as the commitment offense.

Of the 3158 patient records reviewed during the specified time period, 87.3% (n = 2757) were returned to court as competent. Over 10% (10.8%, n = 342) were deemed not restorable and were either discharged or conserved as dangerous or gravely disabled, and 1.9% ($n = 59$) were transferred to another facility, were released by the court, died during their hospitalization, or were retained in the hospital for another forensic commitment, such as a not guilty by reason of insanity (NGRI) finding.

Of the 3158 admissions, 1099 (34.8%) could not be interviewed. Reasons for the inability to interview the patient varied. For example, some patients were too thought disordered to conduct an adequate interview ($n = 392$, 35.7%), some refused to cooperate with the interview ($n = 292$, 26.6%), some were unable to speak English ($n = 125$, 11.3%), some were too agitated or physically threatening ($n = 68$, 6.2%), and sometimes the interviews were not able to be completed due to the patients' dementia or medical problems ($n = 30$, 2.7%). One hundred and ninety-three patients (17.6%) were not interviewed for unknown reasons (not documented by the evaluator).

Data Analysis

Data were analyzed using SPSS version 25. Statistical analyses included frequency distributions to provide information regarding basic demographics. Chi-square and ANOVAs were conducted to assess differences over time and interactions between various factors.

Results

As shown in Table 9.1, the number of IST admissions increased yearly throughout the course of this study. In 2009, 280 unique patients were admitted as IST compared to 539 in 2016. Additionally, a large number of factors exhibited statistically significant variability over time. Most notably, the number of admissions with more than 15 prior arrests increased significantly ($\chi^2 = 139.84$, $df = 28$, $p = 0.000$) from 17.7% in 2009 to 46.4% in 2016, depicted graphically in Figure 9.1. Multiple other variables evidenced changes over time, although often the statistically significant change was related to increases and decreases from year to year. For example, admissions that were thought to be already competent evidenced statistically significant differences over time ($\chi^2 = 93.36$, $df = 14$, $p = 0.000$), from a high of 24.6 in 2010 to a low of 10.7 in 2014.

One variable that evidenced a consistent decrease over time was the percent of patients reporting prior inpatient psychiatric hospitalization ($\chi^2 = 183.12$, $df = 14$, $p = 0.000$). The percentage of admissions reporting at least one past psychiatric hospitalization was over 76% in 2009 and decreased steadily to less than 50% in 2016. As seen in Figure 9.2, this decrease appeared primarily related to declines in hospitalizations reported by admissions diagnosed with unspecified schizophrenic spectrum and other psychotic disorder ($\chi^2 = 70.18$, $df = 14$, $p = 0.000$). Those diagnosed with a schizophrenia spectrum disorder (schizophrenia or schizoaffective disorder) reported slight decreases, especially in later years ($\chi^2 = 60.02$, $df = 14$, $p = 0.000$). Individuals with a diagnosis of bipolar disorder evidenced fluctuating rates of prior admissions from year to year ($\chi^2 = 27.89$, $df = 14$, $p = 0.015$), although there were notable drops in all diagnostic categories after 2013.

Admission diagnoses also evidenced an interesting trend, shown in Figure 9.3. Patients were more likely to receive a diagnosis of a schizophrenic spectrum disorder in 2009 through 2012 and more likely

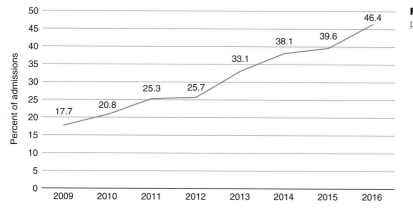

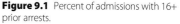

Figure 9.1 Percent of admissions with 16+ prior arrests.

Table 9.1 Changes in factors assessed over time

Categorical variables	Year of admission							
	2009 N (%)	2010 N (%)	2011 N (%)	2012 N (%)	2013 N (%)	2014 N (%)	2015 N (%)	2016 N (%)
Number of admissions	280	301	329	419	403	414	473	539
15 or more prior arrests	41 (17.7)	53 (20.8)	69 (25.3)	89 (25.7)	107 (33.1)	139 (38.1)	165 (39.6)	202 (46.4)
Possibly malingering	43 (18.2)	39 (15.0)	49 (18.2)	53 (15.1)	57 (17.7)	74 (20.0)	60 (14.9)	48 (14.7)
M-FAST over 5	75 (32.8)	65 (28.8)	76 (33.9)	86 (28.4)	78 (31.0)	90 (36.3)	89 (29.9)	66 (27.8)
Probably competent	45 (19.0)	61 (23.6)	66 (24.6)	75 (21.6)	58 (18.4)	39 (10.7)	72 (18.1)	49 (14.7)
Prior inpatient psychiatric	181 (76.1)	190 (73.4)	176 (64.2)	225 (64.7)	190 (61.3)	201 (59.3)	191 (50.0)	186 (47.2)
Schizophrenia spectrum[a]	144 (51.4)	153 (50.5)	147 (44.7)	169 (40.3)	144 (35.7)	163 (39.4)	178 (37.6)	191 (35.4)
Psychosis NOS[a]	39 (13.9)	57 (18.9)	81 (24.6)	102 (24.3)	125 (31.0)	140 (33.8)	115 (24.3)	173 (32.1)
Bipolar disorder[a]	20 (7.1)	30 (10.0)	37 (11.2)	67 (16.0)	64 (15.9)	45 (10.9)	50 (10.6)	60 (11.1)
Cognitive disorders[a]	8 (2.9)	9 (3.0)	18 (5.5)	18 (4.3)	11 (2.7)	13 (3.1)	3 (0.6)	4 (0.7)
Ethnic minorities	173 (61.8)	175 (58.1)	185 (56.2)	233 (55.6)	235 (58.3)	222 (53.6)	276 (58.4)	306 (56.9)
Female[b]	0 (0.0)	71 (23.6)	84 (25.5)	118 (28.2)	86 (21.3)	124 (30.0)	133 (28.1)	186 (34.5)
Continuous variables	2009 mean (std)	2010 mean (std)	2011 mean (std)	2012 mean (std)	2013 mean (std)	2014 mean (std)	2015 mean (std)	2016 mean (std)
BPRS	11.02 (5.17)	9.31 (5.29)	9.29 (4.94)	9.22 (4.85)	8.19 (4.48)	8.65 (4.11)	8.17 (4.10)	9.25 (5.20)
M-FAST score	4.69 (4.90)	4.21 (4.84)	4.58 (4.86)	4.21 (4.83)	4.48 (5.04)	4.98 (5.06)	4.37 (5.02)	3.8 (4.51)
Competency score	4.93 (3.16)	4.99 (3.39)	5.39 (3.38)	6.08 (3.20)	6.31 (3.37)	5.78 (3.39)	6.29 (3.02)	6.17 (3.04)
Age	37.83 (12.43)	39.12 (12.64)	39.22 (13.48)	40.00 (13.54)	37.94 (12.97)	40.18 (13.74)	38.61 (13.11)	37.49 (12.33)
LOS days – all admissions	304.57 (365.29)	265.63 (361.47)	243.56 (324.37)	207.13 (272.26)	201.76 (267.80)	217.03 (243.89)	205.69 (221.34)	169.87 (162.68)
LOS days for restored	203.18 (208.63)	170.31 (187.25)	165.35 (202.21)	141.98 (174.65)	125.83 (148.88)	153.58 (165.07)	152.09 (170.14)	158.23 (154.78)
LOS days for unrestorable	983.50 (492.05)	1002.97 (524.81)	1071.39 (209.87)	869.42 (204.09)	774.74 (293.47)	643.15 (269.79)	551.90 (223.50)	390.08 (161.32)

[a] Diagnoses on admission

[b] Women only admitted beginning in May 2010

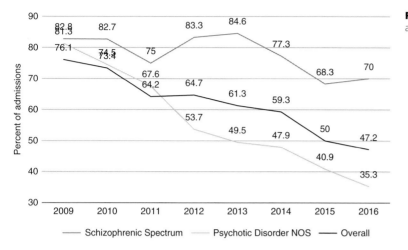

Figure 9.2 Percent of admissions reporting at least one prior hospitalization.

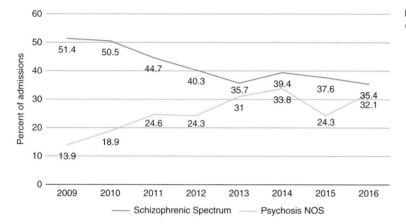

Figure 9.3 Change in admission diagnoses over time.

to receive a diagnosis of unspecified schizophrenic spectrum disorder (formerly psychotic disorder NOS) in later years ($\chi^2 = 214.15$, $df = 49$, $p = 0.000$). When these two diagnoses were combined, the percentage with this diagnosis did not evidence substantial differences over time ($\chi^2 = 21.63$, $df = 5$, $p = 0.000$). The highest percentage was 73.2 in 2014 with the lowest 61.9 in 2015.

As seen in Table 9.1, gender of the admissions fluctuated over time, even when removing the two years DSH-Napa did not admit females for the entire year (2009 and 2010; $\chi^2 = 60.02$, $df = 14$, $p = 0.000$). Generally speaking, the number of women admitted as IST increased over time.

Both age at admission and scores on the BPRS evidenced differences over time, although similar to

the competency variable, these changes were reflective of variations from year to year [$F(7,3150) = 2.50$, $p = 0.015$; $F(7,2566) = 10.24$, $p = 0.000$], rather than a steady increase or decrease over time. Age ranged from a low of 37.49 in 2016 to a high of 40.18 in 2014. Similarly, BPRS scores ranged from a low of 8.17 in 2015 to a high of 11.02 in 2009.

Length of stay also evidenced substantial changes over time, as shown in Table 9.1. The overall length of stay decreased from an average of 345.68 days in 2009 to 162.68 days in 2016 [$F(7,3112) = 8.48$, $p = 0.000$].

The changes were even more striking when the sample was divided into length of stay for those restored to competence versus those deemed not restorable [$F(7,2749) = 4.76$, $p = 0.000$; $F(7,305) = 19.45$, $p = 0.000$, respectively]. Admissions restored

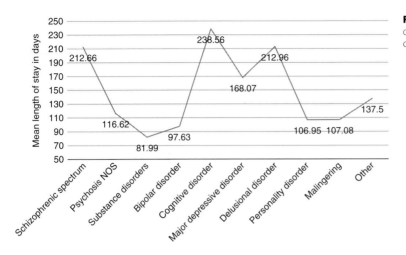

Figure 9.4 Length of stay by discharge diagnosis for patients restored to competence.

to competence showed a steady decrease in length of stay over time, with a slight increase beginning in 2014. In contrast, the length of stay for those determined to be unrestorable evidenced steady decreases, with the length of stay in 2016 almost a third the length of stay in 2009.

Length of stay also varied by diagnosis for admissions ultimately restored to competence, as seen in Table 9.2 [F(9,2415) = 28.10, p = 0.000]. Figure 9.4 provides a graphic depiction of these differences. Three diagnoses exhibited longer lengths of stay than most other diagnoses: schizophrenic spectrum disorders, cognitive disorders, and delusional disorders. Not surprisingly, substance use disorders evidenced the shortest lengths of stay, although their average length of stay was not significantly different from bipolar disorder, personality disorders, or individuals returned as malingering.

Multiple variables did not change over time. The percentage of admissions believed to be malingering did not evidence statistically significant differences, although the percentages fluctuated for a low of 14.7 in 2016 to a high of 20.0 in 2014 (χ^2 = 7.07, df = 7, p = 0.421). Consistent with this, both scores on the M-FAST and percentage of admissions scoring above the cut point did not evidence statistically significant differences over time [F(7,2009) = 1.28, p = 0.257; χ^2 = 7.25, df = 7, p = 0.403, respectively]. The ethnic distribution of the sample also did not vary over time (χ^2 = 5.72, df = 7, p = 0.573), with ethnic minorities representing close to 62% of admissions in 2009 and less than 54% in 2014.

Because we found significant increases in number of prior arrests each year, we examined the relationship between commitment offense and number of prior arrests, categorized as none, 1–2 priors, 3–5 priors, 6–15, and more than 15. As shown in Table 9.3 and depicted graphically in Figure 9.5, three commitment offenses in particular were associated with prior arrests. Patients committed for theft charges (robbery and theft) evidenced significantly more prior arrests; patients committed for homicide charges had fewer prior arrests (χ^2 = 154.46, df = 24, p = 0.000).

Table 9.4 provides the diagnoses for those restored to competence versus those who were deemed not restorable. Not surprisingly, two diagnostic categories were least likely to be restored: patients with a schizophrenic spectrum disorder and patients with a cognitive disorder. Over 40% of those diagnosed with a cognitive disorder were deemed unlikely to regain competence; almost 15% of those with a discharge diagnosis of a schizophrenic spectrum disorder were considered not restorable. These two diagnostic categories comprised almost 90% of the admissions ultimately determined to be unlikely to be restored to competence. Not surprisingly, all individuals discharged with diagnoses of either a personality disorder or malingering were restored to competence.

Discussion

Our data are consistent with previous studies documenting the characteristics of individuals

Table 9.2 Discharge length of stay if restored by diagnosis

Schizophrenic spectrum mean (std)	Psychosis NOS mean (std)	Substance mean (std)	Bipolar disorder mean (std)	Cognitive disorder mean (std)	MDD mean (std)	Delusional disorder mean (std)	PD mean (std)	Malingering mean (std)	Other mean (std)
212.66 (197.42)	116.62 (126.19)	81.99 (106.41)	97.63 (107.04)	238.56 (239.89)	168.07 (173.98)	212.96 (242.50)	106.95 (147.94)	107.08 (131.78)	137.50 (189.37)

Note: F(9.2415) = 28.10, p = 0.00

Table 9.3 Commitment offense by arrest rates

Offense	Number of prior arrests N (%)				
	None	**1–2**	**3–5**	**6–15**	**16+**
Murder	32 (17.2)	32 (11.3)	46 (11.4)	49 (5.5)	32 (3.7)
Assault and battery	63 (33.9)	107 (37.7)	155 (38.4)	307 (34.4)	305 (35.3)
Robbery	12 (6.5)	16 (5.6)	32 (7.9)	103 (11.5)	91 (10.5)
Sex offense	34 (18.3)	16 (5.6)	24 (5.9)	64 (7.2)	66 (7.6)
Theft	5 (2.7)	12 (4.2)	35 (8.7)	97 (10.9)	104 (12.0)
Drug offenses	3 (1.6)	8 (2.8)	10 (2.5)	54 (6.1)	53 (6.1)
All others	37 (19.9)	93 (32.7)	102 (25.2)	218 (24.4)	213 (24.7)

Note: $\chi^2 = 154.46$, $df = 24$, $p = 0.000$

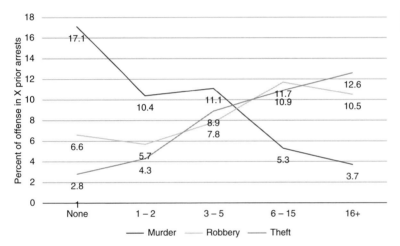

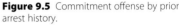

Figure 9.5 Commitment offense by prior arrest history.

found IST. They also provide additional insight into factors contributing to nationwide increases in IST admissions. Perhaps one of the most illuminating findings is the decreasing numbers of IST admissions reporting prior inpatient psychiatric treatment. This result is not surprising given the reported decreased numbers of psychiatric beds in the US, both state and community, since deinstitutionalization began in the 1950s. In 1955, there were over 500,000 state psychiatric hospital beds. As deinstitutionalization continued, by 1994, only 71,619 beds remained.[17] A recent count indicated that in the first quarter of 2016, slightly less than 38,000 beds remain, an astronomical decline of 96.5% in this 60-year time period.[47] Moreover, the majority of these state beds are forensic,[14] meaning that in order to be admitted

for treatment, you must commit a crime. Similar declines have been reported in community inpatient beds, to levels well below international standards and expert consensus guidelines.[17,48]

One relevant and likely related finding was the substantial increase over time of IST admissions with extensive criminal arrest histories. Although advancing age was considered as an explanation for this rise, as older defendants potentially have had more time in the community to offend, the age of admissions did not increase over time. As prior arrests accumulate, defendants face increasingly serious charges. In partial support of this notion, we found a significant relationship between number of prior offenses and the commitment offense. Defendants charged with homicide and sexual offenses were

Table 9.4 Discharge diagnoses by restoration status

Restoration Status	Discharge Diagnosis N (%)									
	Schizophrenic spectrum	Psychosis NOS	Substance	Bipolar disorder	Cognitive disorder	MDD	Delusional disorder	PD	Malingering	Other
Restored (percent restored)	1095 (85.1)	413 (96.0)	213 (98.6)	264 (98.9)	63 (55.8)	70 (95.9)	25 (89.3)	42 (100.0)	144 (100.0)	96 (97.0)
Not restorable (present in nonrestorable group)	191 (70.0)	17 (6.2)	3 (1.1)	3 (1.1)	50 (18.3)	3 (1.1)	3 (1.1)	0 (0.0)	0 (0.0)	3 (1.1)

Note: χ^2 = 241.33, df = 9, p = 0.000

much less likely to have extensive criminal arrest histories. In contrast, admissions charged with theft, robbery, or drug offenses all evidenced increasing numbers of prior arrests, a result entirely consistent with data reported by Torrey.[17] He noted that many individuals with serious mental illness are charged with relatively minor offenses, such as assault and theft.[49] Additionally, relatively minor offenses may become felonies as the number of prior arrests increase. For example, in California, petty theft becomes a felony when the individual has multiple prior arrests. As Figures 9.1 and 9.2 clearly depict, our data show that as arrest rates increase over time, percentages of admissions reporting prior hospitalizations decrease in the same time period.

While it remains unclear from our data if the increasing number of prior arrests and decreasing numbers of patients with prior psychiatric hospitalizations are related, both occurring coincidentally is consistent with the notion that the seriously mentally ill are now receiving services primarily from the criminal justice system, not from the mental health system. As recently as 2010, Torrey and colleagues conducted a study to ascertain where individuals with serious mental illness were receiving their treatment.[17] The evidence was clear: in the US, the odds of a person with a major mental disorder receiving treatment in a jail or prison instead of a psychiatric hospital was 3.2 to 1. Some states were substantially worse: in Nevada, the odds were 9.8 to 1, an almost 10 times greater likelihood that mental health treatment was provided in jails and prisons. This trend has been evident for the past several years. Combined with previous studies, our data provide information about an additional mechanism for the treatment of individuals with severe mental illness. While still receiving treatment via the criminal justice system, the setting is not a jail or prison; it is commitment in a state hospital.

Our data are entirely consistent with research on the impact of deinstitutionalization: individuals with serious mental illness released from institutions frequently receive mental health treatment via the criminal justice system. In the 1980s, Belcher found that a large number of patients released from a state hospital in Ohio were homeless within six months of discharge. Furthermore, almost 45% of those who were homeless had been arrested and incarcerated in that same time period.[50] Numerous studies have reported high percentages of inmates with major mental disorders,[51–53] with sheriffs across the country

lamenting the need to serve as de facto mental health institutions.[54] Consistent with Belcher's study, research has shown that homelessness has become a national problem[55–57] and a substantial number of these homeless individuals have a severe mental disorder.[57,58] Often these individuals are arrested for crimes associated with either their mental illness or homelessness. Once arrested, they are so ill due to their untreated disorder, they are found not competent to stand trial. Unfortunately, this cycle is perpetuated, as treatment for individuals found not competent typically is geared exclusively towards competence restoration.[59] Once competent, they are returned to jail and when released, no intervention is provided to keep them engaged in mental health treatment and out of the criminal justice system. The decrease in prior hospitalizations reported by our admissions is entirely consistent with the results of our national survey (reported in this issue). The number one reason identified by stakeholders across the country as an explanation for the surge in IST commitments is the lack of general mental health services in the community, followed closely by the lack of intensive community treatment and inpatient beds.

Interestingly, we found that increasing numbers of women were admitted as not competent to stand trial. It is unclear if this reflects an overall increase in the rate of findings of incompetence for women or increasing numbers of women entering the criminal justice system. A recent meta-analysis has shown that women and men are found IST at comparable rates.[12] However, the number of women involved in the criminal justice system is growing: between 1980 and 2017, the number of incarcerated women increased by 700%. In this same time period, incarceration rates of women grew 50% faster than they did for men.[60] It stands to reason if more women are entering the criminal justice system, even with steady rates of findings of incompetency, more women will be deemed IST. Moreover, Steadman and colleagues found that the rate of serious mental illness in incarcerated women is substantially higher than for men.[51,61] This finding, coupled with the increasing arrest rates of women, may be the reason for our observed increasing rates of admissions of women found IST.

Consistent with the literature, patients evidencing the longest time to restore were those with schizophrenic spectrum and cognitive disorders.[33,36–39] In addition, the majority of patients who could not be restored were those with a schizophrenic spectrum diagnosis (70%), followed closely by individuals with a cognitive disorder diagnosis (18.3%), indicating that almost 90% of patients determined to be nonrestorable fell under those two diagnostic categories. Furthermore, close to half (42.6%) of admissions with a cognitive disorder diagnosis were ultimately deemed unrestorable. Interestingly, patients returned to court as competent with a diagnosis of delusional disorder evidenced lengths of stay comparable to these two disorders. Initially considered a variant of schizophrenia with only delusions, delusional disorder has been the subject of minimal research, largely because of small sample sizes.[62] Hui and colleagues compared first episode patients with delusional disorder to first episode patients with schizophrenia and found numerous similarities.[63] In contrast, Marneros et al. conducted a longitudinal study of patients with delusional disorder and schizophrenia and found distinct patterns of response, symptoms, and outcomes between the two disorders.[64] Herbel and Stelmach demonstrated that the majority (77%) of patients with delusional disorder found IST were restored to competence, although over 50% of these required an extended period of time on medication.[65] In our sample, patients with a discharge diagnosis of delusional disorder evidenced a similar course of illness to patients with schizophrenic spectrum disorders, as well as a similar percentage who ultimately could not be restored. While our data did not compare characteristics between the two disorders, they suggest that the two diagnoses are comparable at least in regards to restorability and length of time to restoration.

Not surprisingly, individuals returned to court with a primary diagnosis of a personality disorder as well as those believed to be malingering evidenced very short restoration periods and all were "restored" to competence, a result consistent with the literature.[24,26] Two additional diagnostic groups evidenced the shortest length of stay: substance use disorders, typically a substance-induced psychotic disorder, and bipolar disorder. Research suggests that individuals receiving a diagnosis of bipolar disorder respond rapidly to medication,[66] which may explain their brief length of stay. Substance-induced psychotic disorders typically evidence a remission of symptoms once the substance is withdrawn.[67,68] Once psychotic symptoms have remitted, patients are generally able to understand criminal proceedings and assist their attorney.

Consistent with previous research, our data indicate that minorities, specifically Blacks, are overrepresented in our sample as compared to the ethnic distribution in CA. According to the 2017 census estimate, Blacks comprise 5.47% of the CA population. In our sample, almost 29% were Black, a result similar to the incarcerated population (27% Black).[47] In striking contrast, although Hispanics comprise over 39% of the CA population, they represented only 18.6% of our sample; in contrast, 41% of the incarcerated population is Hispanic. Perhaps more notably, although minorities represent the majority of our admissions, the single largest racial group in our sample was White, at 42.86%. While this is slightly higher than the 37% reported by the CA census, it is substantially lower than the 26% reported in CA jails and prisons. The reasons for these discrepancies are unclear. There is abundant evidence that Hispanics are less likely to seek mental health treatment for a variety of reasons, including mistrust and language barriers.[69] Additionally, Hispanics are slightly more likely to be homeless, at least compared to non-Hispanic Whites.[70] It is unclear if either of these factors is related to the decreased prevalence of Hispanics in our sample. Typically, competence is raised as an issue when the observed mental illness is so severe it impairs the individual's ability to understand or assist their attorney. Seeking a competency evaluation generally is not in the purview of the defendant.

The pattern of changes in diagnosing over time was of particular interest, most notable the increase in the unspecified schizophrenia diagnosis and the concurrent decrease in the schizophrenic spectrum diagnoses. One explanation for this pattern of diagnosing may lie in the change from the DSM-IV TR to the DSM-5. For this specific disorder, the change was primarily related to the name: psychotic disorder not otherwise specified was renamed unspecified schizophrenic spectrum and other psychotic disorder in DSM-5, although there were slight changes in the definition. A more likely explanation is that increasing substance use, particularly the use of methamphetamine, clouds the picture and course of the disorder, making a definitive diagnosis impossible. Interestingly, as depicted in Figure 9.2, the group most impacted by the decline in inpatient treatment was individuals diagnosed with unspecified schizophrenic spectrum disorder. This diagnosis is given when an individual is exhibiting psychotic symptoms but does not meet full criteria for schizophrenia. Previous research has suggested that this diagnosis often is associated with either a substance use disorder, specifically a substance-induced psychotic disorder, or malingering, a finding consistent with our data on length of stay.[71] Our survey findings indicate that some believe that the rising use of methamphetamine is related to increasing numbers of IST commitments. It is clear that co-morbid substance use disorders are prevalent in individuals with a schizophrenic spectrum disorder, which exacerbate psychotic symptoms.[72] With the dwindling availability of inpatient psychiatric beds, individuals presenting with psychotic symptoms and positive toxicology screens may not be admitted, at least until there is a definitive determination that the symptoms exhibited are not substance-induced. Increasingly literature is suggesting that there are discernable differences in substance-induced versus primary psychotic disorders[73] and one of these differences is involvement in the criminal justice system.[74]

Conclusions

Our data add to the body of literature on the potential causes of the nationwide increase in the competency referrals. Moreover, our results complement the extensive literature on the criminalization of individuals with mental illness since the closing of long-term state hospitals. The literature is clear that individuals with serious mental disorders are not accessing services in the community. Because of this, their mental illness remains untreated and often they are arrested. Jails and prisons are assuming the role of the nation's mental health provider. Unfortunately, as is generally the case with jails and prisons, once released from custody, very few mechanisms are in place to engage these individuals in community mental health treatment. Our data, and nationwide data, suggest that another system has assumed this role: state hospitals and other providers charged with restoring individuals to competence. It appears that what Belcher found in the 1980s is continuing: once released from a state hospital, individuals with serious mental disorders become (or return to) homelessness and are rearrested. And the cycle continues.

Acknowledgments

This research was conducted as part of a collaborative effort between DSH-Napa and UC Davis School of Medicine, Department of Psychiatry and Behavioral Sciences, funded by the California Department of State Hospitals.

Disclosure

Barbara McDermott, Katherine Warburton, and Chloe Auletta-Young have nothing to disclose.

References

1. *Dusky v. United States*, 362 402, 1960.

2. Bonnie R, Grisso T. Adjudicative competency and youthful offenders. In: Grisso T, Schwartz R, eds. *Youth on Trial: A Developmental Perspective on Juvenile Justice*. Chicago, IL: University of Chicago Press; 2000: 73–103.

3. Vitacco MJ, Rogers R, Gabel J. An investigation of the ECST-R in male pretrial patients: evaluating the effects of feigning on competency evaluations. *Assessment*. 2009; **16**(3): 249–257.

4. Melton G, Petrila J, Poythress N, Slobogin C. *Psychological Evaluation for the Courts: A Handbook for Mental Health Professionals*. 3rd edn. New York: Guilford; 2007.

5. *Trueblood v. Washington State Department of Social and Health Services, United States Court of Appeals, Ninth Circuit*. 2016.

6. Phillips N. Lawyers take Colorado DHS back to court over mental competency exam backlog. *The Denver Post*. June 14, 2018. www.denverpost.com/2018/06/14/colorado-competency-backlog/ (accessed June 2020).

7. Sewell A. LA County supervisors order report on unexplained surge in mental competency cases. *Los Angeles Times*. March 8, 2016. www.latimes.com/local/lanow/la-me-ln-mental-competency-cases-20160308-story.html (accessed June 2020).

8. Gowensmith WN, Frost LE, Speelman DW, Therson DE. Lookin' for beds in all the wrong places: outpatient competency restoration as a promising approach to modern challenges. *Psychol Public Policy Law*. 2016; **22**(3): 293–305.

9. Hinkley JA. Despite improvements, hundreds of criminal mental health evaluations still take too long. *Lansing State J*. 2018. www.lansingstatejournal.com/story/news/local/watchdog/2018/02/22/short-staffed-michiganpsychiatric-hospitals-delay-criminal-cases/323504002/ (accessed June 2020).

10. Brand-Williams O. Competency exam increase strains system in Detroit area. *The Detroit News*. June 16, 2017. https://eu.detroitnews.com/story/news/local/michigan/2017/06/16/competency-exams-detroit-courts-mental-evaluations/102938466/ (accessed June 2020).

11. Lowder J. Personal communication, 2017.

12. Pirelli G, Gottdiener WH, Zapf PA. A meta-analytic review of competency to stand trial research. *Psychol Public Policy Law*. 2011; **17**(1): 1–53.

13. McDermott BE, Newman WJ, Meyer J, Scott CL, Warburton K. The utility of an admission screening procedure for patients committed to a state hospital as incompetent to stand trial. *Int J Forensic Ment Health*. 2017; **16**(4): 281–292.

14. Wik A, Hollen V, Fisher WH. *Forensic Patients in State Psychiatric Hospitals: 1999–2016*. Alexandria, VA: National Association of State Mental Health Program Directors; 2017.

15. Miller RD. Hospitalization of criminal defendants for evaluation of competence to stand trial or for restoration of competence: clinical and legal issues. *Behav Sci Law*. 2003; **21**(3): 369–391.

16. Bartos BJ, Renner M, Newark C, McCleary R, Scurich N. Characteristics of forensic patients in California with dementia/Alzheimer's disease. *J Forensic Nurs*. 2017; **13**(2): 77–80.

17. Torrey EF, Kennard AD, Eslinger D, Lamb R, Pavle J. *More Mentally Ill Persons are in Jails and Prisons than Hospitals: A Survey of the States*. Arlington County, VA: Treatment Advocacy Center; 2010.

18. Lamb HR, Weinberger LE. The shift of psychiatric inpatient care from hospitals to jails and prisons. *J Am Acad Psychiatry Law*. 2005; **33**(4): 529–534.

19. Bondurant SR, Lindo JM, Swenson ID. Substance abuse treatment centers and local crime. *J Urban Econ*. 2018; **104**: 124–133.

20. Stafford KP, Sellbom MO. Assessment of competence to stand trial. In: Weiner I, Otto R, eds. *Handbook of Psychology, Volume 11. Forensic Psychology, 2nd edn*. Hoboken, NJ: John Wiley & Sons, Inc; 2012: 412–439.

21. Sewell A. Report on increase in mental competency cases leaves many unanswered questions. *Los Angeles Times*. May 25, 2016. www.latimes.com/local/lanow/la-me-ln-mental-competency-cases-20160525-snap-story.html (accessed June 2020).

22. Vitacco MJ, Rogers R, Gabel J, Munizza J. An evaluation of malingering screens with competency to stand trial patients: a known-groups comparison. *Law Hum Behav*. 2007; **31**(3): 249–260.

23. Homsy S, McDermott BE, Woofter C. *Competence to Stand Trial Reports Conducted by Community Psychiatrists and Psychologists: Does Quality Matter?* Seattle, Washington: American Psychology and Law Society; 2017.

24. Cooper VG, Zapf PA. Predictor variables in competency to stand trial decisions. *Law Hum Behav*. 2003; **27**(4): 423–436.

25. Frierson RL, Shea SJ, Shea ME. Competence-to-stand-trial evaluations of geriatric defendants. *J Am Acad Psychiatry Law*. 2002; **30**(2): 252–256.

26. Hubbard KL, Zapf PA, Ronan KA. Competency restoration: an examination of the differences between defendants predicted restorable and not restorable to competency. *Law Hum Behav*. 2003; **27** (2): 127–139.

27. Warren JI, Murrie DC, Stejskal W, et al. Opinion formation in evaluating the adjudicative competence and restorability of criminal defendants: a review of 8,000 evaluations. *Behav Sci Law*. 2006; **24**(2): 113–132.

28. Kois L, Pearson J, Chauhan P, Goni M, Saraydarian L. Competency to stand trial among female inpatients. *Law Hum Behav*. 2013; **37**(4): 231–240.

29. Pinals DA, Packer IK, Fisher W, Roy-Bujnowski K. Relationship between race and ethnicity and forensic clinical triage dispositions. *Psychiatr Serv*. 2004; **55**(8): 873–878.

30. Caldwell RM, Mandracchia SA, Ross SA, Silver NC. Competency to stand trial and criminal responsibility: an examination of racial and gender differences among African American and Caucasian pretrial defendants. *Am J Forensic Psychol*. 2003; **21** (3): 5–19.

31. Minsky S, Vega W, Miskimen T, Gara M, Escobar J. Diagnostic patterns in Latino, African American, and European American psychiatric patients. *Arch Gen Psychiatry*. 2003; **60**(6): 637–644.

32. Viljoen JL, Zapf PA. Fitness to stand trial evaluations: a comparison of referred and non-referred defendants. *Int J Forensic Ment Health*. 2002; **1**(2): 127–138.

33. Gay J, Vitacco M, Ragatz L. Mental health symptoms predict competency to stand trial and competency restoration success. *Legal Criminol Psychol*. 2017; **22**: 288–301.

34. Cochrane RE, Grisso T, Frederick RI. The relationship between criminal charges, diagnoses, and psycholegal opinions among federal pretrial defendants. *Behav Sci Law*. 2001; **19**(4): 565–582.

35. Lewis CF, Fields C, Rainey E. A study of geriatric forensic evaluees: who are the violent elderly? *J Am Acad Psychiatry Law*. 2006; **34**(3): 324–332.

36. Mossman D. Predicting restorability of incompetent criminal defendants. *J Am Acad Psychiatry Law*. 2007; **35**(1): 34–43.

37. Morris DR, Parker GF. Effects of advanced age and dementia on restoration of competence to stand trial. *Int J Law Psychiatry*. 2009; **32**(3): 156–160.

38. Colwell LH, Gianesini J. Demographic, criminogenic, and psychiatric factors that predict competency

restoration. *J Am Acad Psychiatry Law.* 2011; **39**(3): 297–306.

39. Morris DR, DeYoung NJ. Psycholegal abilities and restoration of competence to stand trial. *Behav Sci Law.* 2012; **30**(6): 710–728.

40. Anderson SD, Hewitt J. The effect of competency restoration training on defendants with mental retardation found not competent to proceed. *Law Hum Behav.* 2002; **26**(3): 343–351.

41. Advokat CD, Guidry D, Burnett DMR, Manguno-Mire G, Thompson JW, Jr. Competency restoration treatment: differences between defendants declared competent or incompetent to stand trial. *J Am Acad Psychiatry Law.* 2012; **40**(1): 89–97.

42. Rosenfeld B, Ritchie K. Competence to stand trial: clinician reliability and the role of offense severity. *J Forensic Sci.* 1998; **43**(1): 151–157.

43. Warren JI, Rosenfeld B, Fitch WL, Hawk G. Forensic mental health clinical evaluation: an analysis of interstate and intersystemic differences. *Law Hum Behav.* 1997; **21**(4): 377–390.

44. Miller HA. *Miller Forensic Assessment of Symptoms Test Professional Manual.* Odessa, FL: Psychologial Assessment Resources; 2001.

45. Overall JE, Gorham DR. The brief psychiatric rating scale. *Psychol Rep.* 1962; **10**: 799–812.

46. Johnson WG, Mullett N. Georgia Court Competency Test. In: *Dictionary of Behavioral Assessment Techniques.* New York: Pergamon Press; 1988.

47. Becker's Hospital Review. Amid shortage, number of psychiatric beds in US down 13% from 2010. www.beckershospitalreview.com/patient-flow/amid-shortage-number-of-psychiatric-beds-in-us-down-13-from-2010.html (accessed June 2020).

48. Bastiampillai T, Sharfstein SS, Allison S. Increase in US suicide rates and the critical decline in psychiatric beds. *J Am Med Assoc.* 2016; **316**(24): 2591–2592.

49. Torrey EF. Jails and prisons – America's new mental hospitals. *Am J Public Health.* 1995; **85**(12): 1611–1613.

50. Belcher JR. Are jails replacing the mental health system for the homeless mentally ill? *Community Ment Health J.* 1988; **24**(3): 185–195.

51. Steadman HJ, Osher FC, Robbins PC, Case B, Samuels S. Prevalence of serious mental illness among jail inmates. *Psychiatr Serv.* 2009; **60**(6): 761–765.

52. Trestman RL, Ford J, Zhang W, Wiesbrock V. Current and lifetime psychiatric illness among inmates not identified as acutely mentally ill at intake in Connecticut's jails. *J Am Acad Psychiatry Law.* 2007; **35**(4): 490–500.

53. Wilper AP, Woolhandler S, Boyd JW, et al. The health and health care of US prisoners: results of a nationwide survey. *Am J Public Health.* 2009; **99**(4): 666–672.

54. Ford M. America's largest mental hospital is a jail. *The Atlantic.* June 8, 2015. www.theatlantic.com/politics/archive/2015/06/americas-largest-mental-hospital-is-a-jail/395012/ (accessed June 2020).

55. Markowitz FE. Psychiatric hospital capacity, homelessness, and crime and arrest rates. *Criminology.* 2006; **44**(1): 45–72.

56. Martell DA, Rosner R, Harmon RB. Base-rate estimates of criminal behavior by homeless mentally ill persons in New York City. *Psychiatr Serv.* 1995; **46** (6): 596–601.

57. Roy L, Crocker AG, Nicholls TL, Latimer EA, Ayllon AR. Criminal behavior and victimization among homeless individuals with severe mental illness: a systematic review. *Psychiatr Serv.* 2014; **65** (6): 739–750.

58. Koegel P, Burnam MA, Farr RK. The prevalence of specific psychiatric disorders among homeless individuals in the inner city of Los Angeles. *Arch Gen Psychiatry.* 1988; **45**(12): 1085–1092.

59. Iglehart JK. Decriminalizing mental illness – the Miami model. *N Engl J Med.* 2016; **374**(18): 1701–1703.

60. Carson E. *Prisoners in 2014.* Washington DC: Bureau of Justice Statistics; 2015.

61. Teplin LA, Abram KM, McClelland GM. Prevalence of psychiatric disorders among incarcerated women. I. Pretrial jail detainees. *Arch Gen Psychiatry.* 1996; **53** (6): 505–512.

62. Peralta V, Cuesta MJ. Delusional disorder and schizophrenia: a comparative study across multiple domains. *Psychol Med.* 2016; **46**(13): 2829–2839.

63. Hui CL, Lee EH, Chang WC, et al. Delusional disorder and schizophrenia: a comparison of the neurocognitive and clinical characteristics in first-episode patients. *Psychol Med.* 2015; **45**(14): 3085–3095.

64. Marneros A, Pillmann F, Wustmann T. Delusional disorders – are they simply paranoid schizophrenia? *Schizophr Bull.* 2012; **38**(3): 561–568.

65. Herbel BL, Stelmach H. Involuntary medication treatment for competency restoration of 22 defendants with delusional disorder. *J Am Acad Psychiatry Law.* 2007; **35**(1): 47–59.

66. Harrison PJ, Cipriani A, Harmer CJ, et al. Innovative approaches to bipolar disorder and its treatment. *Ann N Y Acad Sci.* 2016; **1366**(1): 76–89.

67. McKetin R, Gardner J, Baker AL, et al. Correlates of transient versus persistent psychotic symptoms among dependent methamphetamine users. *Psychiatry Res.* 2016; **238**: 166–171.

68. McKetin R, Dawe S, Burns RA, et al. The profile of psychiatric symptoms exacerbated by methamphetamine use. *Drug Alcohol Depend.* 2016; **161**: 104–109.

69. De Luca SM, Blosnich JR, Hentschel EAW, King E, Amen S. Mental health care utilization: how race, ethnicity and veteran status are associated with seeking help. *Community Ment Health J.* 2016; **52**(2): 174–179.

70. Fusaro VA, Levy HG, Shaefer HL. Racial and ethnic disparities in the lifetime prevalence of homelessness in the United States. *Demography.* 2018; **55**(6): 2119–2128.

71. Scott CL, McDermott BE, Kile S. *Intoxication and Insanity: A Study of 500 NGRI Acquittees.* San Antonio, TX: American Academy of Psychiatry Law; 2003.

72. Hides L, Dawe S, McKetin R, et al. Primary and substance-induced psychotic disorders in methamphetamine users. *Psychiatry Res.* 2015; **226**(1): 91–96.

73. McKetin R, Baker AL, Dawe S, Voce A, Lubman DI. Differences in the symptom profile of methamphetamine-related psychosis and primary psychotic disorders. *Psychiatry Res.* 2017; **251**: 349–354.

74. Fraser S, Hides L, Philips L, Proctor D, Lubman DI. Differentiating first episode substance induced and primary psychotic disorders with concurrent substance use in young people. *Schizophr Res.* 2012; **136**(1–3): 110–115.

Jail Diversion: The Miami Model

Steven Leifman and Tim Coffey

The Problem

Every day, in every community in the United States, law enforcement agencies, courts, and correctional institutions are witness to a parade of misery brought on by untreated or under-treated mental illnesses. According to the most recent prevalence estimates, roughly 16.9% of jail detainees (14.5% of men and 31.0% of women) experience serious mental illness (SMI).[1] Considering that in 2018 law enforcement nationwide made an estimated 10.3 million arrests,[2] this suggests that more than 1.7 million involved people with SMIs. It is estimated that three-quarters of these individuals also experience co-occurring substance use disorders, which increases the likelihood of becoming involved in the justice system. On any given day, approximately 380,000 people with mental illnesses are incarcerated in jails and prisons across the United States.[3] Considering that as of 2016 there were only about 20,000 beds in civil state psychiatric hospitals,[4] this means there are 19 times as many people with mental illnesses in correctional facilities as there are in all civil state treatment facilities combined.

Although these national statistics are alarming, the problem is even more acute in Miami-Dade County, Florida. The county jail currently serves as the largest psychiatric institution in Florida and contains as many beds serving inmates with mental illnesses as all state civil and forensic mental health hospitals combined. On any given day, approximately 2,400 of the 4,200 individuals housed in the county jail (57%) are classified as having some mental health treatment need.[5] Based on a total per diem cost of $265 per bed, the estimated cost to taxpayers is $636,000 per day, or more than $232 million per year. On average, people with mental illnesses remain incarcerated eight times longer than people without mental illnesses arrested for the exact same charge, at a cost seven times higher.[6] With little treatment available, many individuals cycle through the system for the majority of their adult lives.

To illustrate the inefficient and costly consequences of the current system, researchers from the Florida Mental Health Institute at the University of South Florida examined arrest, incarceration, acute care, and inpatient service utilization rates among 97 individuals with SMIs participating in jail diversion programs in Miami-Dade County, Florida.[7] Individuals were selected for inclusion in the analysis based on their identification as frequent recidivists to the criminal justice system and acute care settings as defined by having been referred for diversion from jail to acute care crisis units on four or more occasions as the result of four or more discrete arrests. Total number of referrals for diversion services per individual ranged from 4 to 17, with an average of 7.1 referrals. Total number of lifetime bookings into the county jail ranged from 8 to 104, with an average of 36.6 bookings. As illustrated in Table 10.1, over a five-year period these individuals accounted for nearly 2,200 arrests, 27,000 days in jail, and 13,000 days in crisis units, state hospitals, and emergency rooms, at a cost to taxpayers of roughly $16 million.

The Solution

The Eleventh Judicial Circuit Criminal Mental Health Project (CMHP) was established 19 years ago to divert misdemeanor offenders with SMI, or co-occurring SMI and substance use disorders, away from the criminal justice system into community-based treatment and support services. Since that time the program has expanded to serve defendants that have been arrested for less serious felonies and other charges as determined appropriate. The program operates two components: pre-booking diversion consisting of crisis intervention team (CIT) training for law enforcement officers and post-booking diversion serving individuals booked into the jail and awaiting adjudication. All participants are provided with individualized transition planning, including linkages to community-based treatment and supports. Services available

Table 10.1 Miami-Dade County: heavy user data analysis (n = 97)

Event	Total events over 5 years	Average per individual	Average per diem cost	Estimated total cost
Arrests	2,172	22	–	–
Jail days	26,640	275	$265	$7 million
Baker Act initiations	710	8.6	–	–
Inpatient psychiatric days	7,000	72	$291	$2 million
State hospital days	3,200	33	$331	$1 million
Emergency room days	2,600	27	$2,338	$6 million
Total	39,440	407	–	$16 million

to program participants include supportive housing, supported employment, assertive community treatment (ACT), illness self-management and recovery (Wellness Recovery Action Planning, WRAP), trauma services, and integrated treatment for co-occurring mental health and substance use disorders.

Short-term benefits include reduced numbers of defendants with SMI in the county jail, as well as more efficient and effective access to housing, treatment, and wraparound services for individuals re-entering the community. This decreases the likelihood that individuals will re-offend and reappear in the criminal justice system, and increases the likelihood of successful mental health recovery. The long-term benefits include reduced demand for costly acute care services in jails, prisons, forensic mental health treatment facilities, emergency rooms, and other crisis settings; decreased crime and improved public safety; improved public health; decreased injuries to law enforcement officers and people with mental illnesses; and decreased rates of chronic homelessness. Most importantly, the CHMP is helping to close the revolving door which results in the devastation of families and the community, the breakdown of the criminal justice system, wasteful government spending, and the shameful warehousing of some of our community's most vulnerable and neglected citizens.

Program Development

Initial support for the development of the CMHP was provided in 2000 through a grant from the *National GAINS Center*[1] which enabled the court to convene

a two-day summit meeting of traditional and nontraditional stakeholders throughout the community. The purpose of the summit was to review the ways in which Miami-Dade County collectively responded to people with mental illnesses involved in the justice system. The GAINS Center provided technical assistance and helped the community map existing resources, identify gaps in services and service delivery, and develop a more integrated approach to coordinating care. Stakeholders included judges and court staff, law enforcement agencies and first responders, attorneys, mental health and substance abuse treatment providers, state and local social service agencies, consumers of mental health and substance abuse treatment services, and family members.

What was revealed was an embarrassingly dysfunctional system. Prior to the summit, it was readily apparent that people with mental illnesses were overrepresented in the justice system. What was not readily apparent, however, was the degree to which stakeholders were unwittingly contributing to and perpetuating the problem. Many participants were shocked to find that a single person with mental illness was accessing the services of almost everybody in the room including law enforcement, emergency medical services, mental health crisis units, emergency rooms, hospitals, homeless shelters, jails, and the courts. Furthermore, this was occurring over and over as individuals revolved between a criminal justice

---

[1] The National GAINS Center is a federally funded organization concerned with the collection and dissemination of information about the effective services for people with co-

occurring mental health and substance use disorders in contact with the justice system. GAINS is an acronym, which stands for *Gathering information, Assessing what works, Interpreting/integrating facts, Networking,* and *Stimulating change.* More information may be found at: http://gainscenter.samhsa.gov/

system that was never intended to handle overwhelming numbers of people with SMIs and a community mental health system that was ill-equipped to provide the necessary services to those most in need.

A common theme among summit participants was the frustration of repeatedly serving the same individuals with seemingly little that could be done to break the cycles of crises, homelessness, recidivism, and despair. Part of the problem was that stakeholders were largely disconnected from one another and no mechanisms were in place to coordinate resources or services. Everyone was so busy doing their jobs that no one was looking at the bigger picture to see the ways in which individual roles come together to impact the welfare of the system, and the individual, as a whole. The police were policing, the lawyers were lawyering, and the judges were judging. Treatment providers knew little about what went on when their clients were arrested and, because of barriers to accessing information and laws that prohibit reimbursement for services provided to people who are incarcerated, had little incentive to learn. For individuals who had no resources to pay for services (e.g. insurance, Medicaid), crisis units, hospitals, and the jail were often the only options to receive care. Ironically, while many individuals could not access the most basic prevention and treatment services in the community, they were being provided the costliest levels of crisis and emergency care over and over again.

The degree of fragmentation in the community not only prevented the mental health and criminal justice systems from responding more effectively to people with mental illnesses, but actually created increased opportunities for people to fall through the cracks. By the conclusion of the summit it became apparent that people with untreated SMIs are among the most expensive population in the community not because of their diagnoses, but because of the way the health care and justice systems treat them.

Using information generated from the summit meeting, program operations were initiated on a limited basis. Additional funding was secured from a local foundation to conduct a planning study of the mental health status and needs of individuals arrested and booked into the county jail, as well as the processes in place to link individuals to community-based services and supports. Information from this planning study was used to develop a more formal program design and to secure a federal grant in 2003 which enabled the CMHP to significantly expand its

staffing and operations. At the conclusion of the federal grant period, continuation of funding for all positions was assumed by the county. Because of the early success of the program and demonstrated outcomes, the CMHP was awarded another grant in 2007 by the State of Florida to further expand post-booking diversion operations to serve people charged with less serious felonies. In 2010, another state grant was awarded which was used to establish a specialized unit to expedite access to federal entitlement benefits. A 2016 grant supported the creation of jail in-reach team to streamline identification and assessment of program participants and support evidence-based re-entry planning. Finally, in 2018 the state funded a demonstration project to allow the CMHP to examine the impact of changes to state law allowing criminal court judges presiding over misdemeanor cases to leverage treatment compliance by ordering outpatient treatment under the state's civil commitment laws.

Since its inception the CMHP has received ongoing support from the Florida Department of Children and Families. In addition, since 2010, the CMHP has worked closely with Thriving Mind South Florida, which contracts with the state to administer non-Medicaid, mental health, and substance abuse treatment state funding for the uninsured and under-insured in Miami-Dade and Monroe Counties. Supplemented by additional federal, state, and county grants and contracts as well as philanthropic support, Thriving Mind manages a safety net system of care for the treatment of mental health and substance use disorders which is indispensable to the success of the CMHP.

The CMHP's success and effectiveness depend on the commitment, consensus, and ongoing effort of stakeholders throughout the community. To this end, the courts are in a unique position to bring together stakeholders who otherwise may not have opportunities to engage in such problem-solving collaborations. In establishing the CMHP, a mental health committee was established within the courts. In addition, a local chapter of the statewide advocacy organization, *Florida Partners in Crisis,* was formed. Both of these bodies are chaired by the judiciary and provide a venue and opportunity for discussion of issues that cut across community lines. This has been particularly effective in resolving problems that arise from poor communication and cross-systems fragmentation. Staff for the CMHP are employed through a combination of the Administrative Office of the Courts, Thriving Mind South Florida, and Community Health of South Florida, a local treatment provider, and work closely with all stakeholders in the community. Funding for staff positions comes from county, state, and federal sources and consists of a mix of general revenue and grant funding.

CMHP Program Overview

Pre-Booking Jail Diversion

The CMHP has embraced and promoted the CIT training model developed in Memphis, Tennessee in the late 1980s.[8] Known as the *Memphis Model,* the purpose of CIT training is to set a standard of excellence for law enforcement officers with respect to treatment of individuals with mental illnesses. CIT officers perform regular duty assignment as patrol officers, but are also trained to respond to calls involving mental health crises. Officers receive 40 hours of specialized training in psychiatric diagnoses, suicide intervention, substance abuse issues, behavioral de-escalation techniques, the role of the family in the care of a person with mental illness, mental health and substance abuse laws, and local resources for those in crisis.

The training is designed to educate and prepare officers to recognize the signs and symptoms of mental illnesses, and to respond more effectively and appropriately to individuals in crisis. Because police officers are often the first responders to mental health emergencies, it is essential that they know how mental illnesses can impact the behaviors and perceptions of individuals. CIT officers are skilled at de-escalating crises, while bringing an element of understanding and compassion to these difficult situations. When appropriate, individuals are assisted in accessing treatment in lieu of being arrested and taken to jail.

Because CIT programs are in operation in jurisdictions and municipalities countywide, and officers are called on to respond to a variety of situations ranging from relatively minor incidents to urgent crises, there is no single point of entry and no standard intervention provided. Rather, officers are trained to quickly assess situations and assist individuals in accessing a full array of crisis and non-crisis services and resources across the community. These include providing transportation to hospitals and crisis stabilization units in emergency situations, accessing the services of a mobile crisis team consisting of mental health professionals providing on-site assessment and referral services in the community, and providing informational resources to assist individuals in locating and accessing health and social services throughout the county.

The pre-booking diversion program has demonstrated tremendous results. To date, the CMHP has provided CIT training to more than 7,000 law enforcement officers from all 36 local municipalities in Miami-Dade County, as well as Miami-Dade Public Schools and the Department of Corrections and Rehabilitation. Countywide, CIT officers are estimated to respond to nearly 20,000 mental health crisis calls per year. As indicated in Table 10.2, since 2010 CIT officers from the Miami-Dade Police Department and City of Miami Police Department have responded to 91,472 mental health crisis calls resulting in 17,516 diversions from jail, 55,013 individuals assisted in accessing community-based treatment, and just 252 arrests. Since 2008, the number of annual jail bookings has decreased from roughly 118,000 to 53,000 last year (see Figure 10.1). The average daily population in the county jail system has dropped from 7,200 to 4,200 inmates today (see Figure 10.2), and the county has closed one entire jail facility at a cost-saving to taxpayers of $12 million per year.

Post-Booking Jail Diversion

The CMHP was originally established to divert non-violent misdemeanant defendants with SMI and possible co-occurring substance use disorders, from the criminal justice system into community-based treatment and support services. Since that time, the program has been expanded to serve defendants that have been arrested for less serious felonies and other charges as determined appropriate.

All defendants booked into the jail are screened for signs and symptoms of mental illnesses by correctional officers using an evidence-based screening tool. Additionally, defendants undergo medical screening by health care staff at the jail, which includes additional assessment of psychiatric functioning. Those who are identified as being in possible psychiatric distress are referred to corrections health services' psychiatric staff for more thorough evaluation.

In order to determine the appropriate level of treatment, support services, and community supervision, the CMHP screens each program participant in regards to mental health and substance use treatment

Table 10.2

Miami-Dade Police Dept and City of Miami Police Dept	2010	2011	2012	2013	2014	2015	2016	2017	2018*	Total	Rate per 1,000 CIT calls
CIT Calls	7,779	9,399	10,404	10,626	11,042	10,579	11,799	11,799	45,08,	91,472	–
Individuals transported to crisis	3,307	4,642	2,755	3,946	5,155	7,417	3,380	8,818	9,887	55,013	601.4
Individuals diverted from jail	1,940	3,563	2,118	1,215	1,871	1,633	1,694	1,860	1,622	17,516	191.5
Arrests made	4	45	27	9	24	10	119	11	3	252	1.7

* CIT data was not collected by City of Miami in 2018. Information reported reflects calls responded to by Miami-Dade Police Department only.

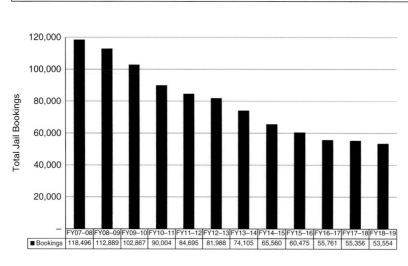

Figure 10.1 Annual County Jail Bookings FY2005-06 to FY2018-19.

	FY07–08	FY08–09	FY09–10	FY10–11	FY11–12	FY12–13	FY13–14	FY14–15	FY15–16	FY16–17	FY17–18	FY18–19
■ Bookings	118,496	112,889	102,867	90,004	84,695	81,988	74,105	65,560	60,475	55,761	55,356	53,554

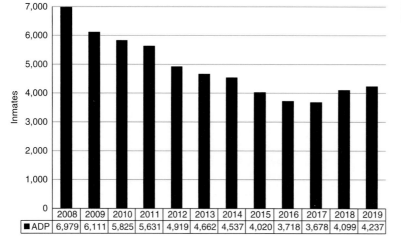

Figure 10.2 Average Daily Population (ADP) 2008–2019

	2008	2009	2010	2011	2012	2013	2014	2015	2016	2017	2018	2019
■ ADP	6,979	6,111	5,825	5,631	4,919	4,662	4,537	4,020	3,718	3,678	4,099	4,237

needs, as well as criminogenic risks factors. A two-page summary is developed that is used to develop an individualized transition plan aimed at reducing criminal justice recidivism and improved psychiatric outcomes, recovery, and community integration. The evidence-based screening tools include the Texas Christian University Drug Screen V[9] and the Ohio Risk Assessment: Community Supervision Tool.[10]

Upon stabilization, legal charges may be dismissed or modified in accordance with treatment engagement. Individuals who voluntarily agree to services are assisted with linkages to a comprehensive array of community-based treatment, support, and housing services that are essential for successful community re-entry and recovery outcomes. The CMHP utilizes the APIC Model to provide transition planning for all program participants.[11] This is a nationally recognized best practice model that provides a set of critical elements that improve outcomes for people with mental illnesses and co-occurring substance use disorders that are released from jails. CMHP staff *Assess, Plan, Identify,* and *Coordinate* transition plans that are individualized for each program participant. The goal is to support community living, reduce maladaptive behaviors, and decrease the chances that individuals will reoffend and reappear in the criminal justice system.

Misdemeanor Jail Diversion Program

Individuals charged with misdemeanors who meet involuntary examination criteria are transferred from the jail to a community-based crisis stabilization unit as soon as possible. Upon stabilization, legal charges may be dismissed or modified in accordance with treatment engagement. Individuals who agree to services are assisted with linkages to a comprehensive array of community-based treatment, support, and housing services that are essential for successful community re-entry and recovery outcomes. Program participants are monitored by CMHP for up to one year following community re-entry to ensure ongoing linkage to necessary supports and services. The vast majority of participants (75–80%) in the misdemeanor diversion program is homeless at the time of arrest and tends to be among the most severely psychiatrically impaired individuals served by the CMHP.

Felony Jail Diversion Program

Participants in the felony jail diversion program are referred to the CMHP through a number of sources including the Public Defender's Office, the State Attorney's Office, private attorneys, judges, corrections health services, and family members. All participants must meet diagnostic and legal criteria.[II] At the time a person is accepted into the felony jail diversion program, the state attorney's office informs the court of the plea the defendant will be offered contingent upon successful program completion. Similar to the misdemeanor program, legal charges may be dismissed or modified based on treatment engagement. All program participants are assisted in accessing community-based services and supports, and their progress is monitored and reported back to the court by CMHP staff.

Jail Diversion Program Outcomes

Recidivism rates among participants in the misdemeanor jail diversion program have decreased from roughly 75% to 20% annually. Individuals participating in the felony jail diversion program demonstrate reductions in jail bookings and jail days of more than 75%. Since 2008, total jail bookings and days spent in the county jail among felony jail diversion program participants decreased by 59% and 57% respectively, resulting in a difference of approximately 31,000 fewer days in jail (nearly 84 years of jail bed days).

Recovery Peer Specialists

Embedded in both the misdemeanor and felony jail diversion programs, recovery peer specialists are individuals diagnosed with mental illnesses who work as members of the jail diversion team. Due to their life experience they are uniquely qualified to perform the functions of the position. The primary function of the recovery peer specialists is to assist jail diversion program participants with community re-entry and engagement in continuing treatment and services. This is accomplished by working with participants, caregivers, family members, and other sources of support to minimize barriers to treatment engagement, and to model and facilitate the development of adaptive coping skills and behaviors. Recovery peer specialists also serve as consultants and faculty to the CMHP's Crisis Intervention Team (CIT) training program.

Access to Entitlement Benefits

Stakeholders in the criminal justice and behavioral health communities consistently identify lack of access to public entitlement benefits such as Supplemental Security Income (SSI), Social Security Disability Insurance (SSDI), and Medicaid as among the most significant and persistent barriers to successful community reintegration and recovery for individuals who experience SMIs and co-occurring substance use disorders. The majority of individuals served by the CMHP are not receiving any entitlement benefits at the time of program entry. As a result, many do not have the necessary resources to access adequate housing, treatment, or support services in the community.

In order to address this barrier and maximize limited resources, the CMHP developed an innovative plan to improve the ability to transition individuals from the criminal justice system to the community. Toward this goal, all participants in the program who are eligible to apply for Social Security benefits are provided with assistance utilizing a best practice model referred to as SSI/SSDI, Outreach, Access and Recovery (SOAR).[12] This is an approach that was developed as a federal technical assistance initiative to expedite access to social security entitlement benefits for individuals with mental illnesses who are homeless. Access to entitlement benefits is an essential element in successful recovery and community reintegration for many justice system involved individuals with SMIs.

[II] Legal criteria specify a current most serious charge of a third degree felony, with not more than three prior felony convictions.

The immediate gains of obtaining SSI and/or SSDI for these people are clear: it provides a steady income and health care coverage which enables individuals to access basic needs including housing, food, medical care, and psychiatric treatment. This significantly reduces recidivism to the criminal justice system, prevents homelessness, and is an essential element in the process of recovery.

The CMHP has developed a strong collaborative relationship with the Social Security Administration in order to expedite and ensure approvals for entitlement benefits in the shortest time frame possible. All CMHP participants are screened for eligibility for federal entitlement benefits, with staff initiating applications as early as possible utilizing the SOAR model. Current program data demonstrate that 78% of the individuals are approved on the initial application. By contrast, the national average across all disability groups for approval on initial application is 27%. In addition, the average time to approval for CMHP participants is approximately 40 days. This is a remarkable achievement compared to the ordinary approval process which typically takes between 9 and 12 months.

Forensic Hospital Diversion Program

Since August 2009, the CMHP has overseen the implementation of the Miami-Dade Forensic Alternative Center (MD-FAC) to divert individuals with mental illnesses committed to the Florida Department of Children and Families from placement in state forensic hospitals to placement in community-based treatment and forensic services. Participants include individuals charged with second and third degree felonies that do not have significant histories of violent felony offenses and are not likely to face incarceration if convicted of their alleged offenses. Participants are adjudicated incompetent to proceed to trial or not guilty by reason of insanity. The community-based treatment provider operating services for the project is responsible for providing a full array of residential treatment and community re-entry services including crisis stabilization, competency restoration, development of community living skills, assistance with community re-entry, and community monitoring to ensure ongoing treatment following discharge. The treatment provider also assists individuals in accessing entitlement benefits and other means of economic self-sufficiency to ensure ongoing and timely access to services and supports after re-entering the community. Unlike individuals

admitted to state hospitals, individuals served by MD-FAC are not returned to jail upon restoration of competency, thereby decreasing burdens on the jail and eliminating the possibility that a person may decompensate while in jail and require readmission to a state hospital. To date, the project has demonstrated more cost-effective delivery of forensic mental health services, reduced burdens on the county jail in terms of housing and transporting defendants with forensic mental health needs, and more effective community re-entry and monitoring of individuals who, historically, have been at high risk for recidivism to the justice system and other acute care settings.

Individuals admitted to the MD-FAC program are identified as ready for discharge from forensic commitment an average of 52 days (35%) sooner than individuals who complete competency restoration services in forensic treatment facilities, and spend an average of 31 fewer days (18%) under forensic commitment. The average cost to provide services in the MD-FAC program is roughly 32% less expensive than services provided in state forensic treatment facilities.

Miami Center for Mental Health and Recovery

Since 2006 the CMHP has been working with stakeholders from Miami-Dade County, the State of Florida, and the community on a capital improvement project to develop a first of its kind mental health diversion and treatment facility which will expand the capacity to divert individuals from the county jail into a seamless continuum of comprehensive community-based treatment programs that leverage local, state, and federal resources. The purpose of the Miami Center for Mental Health and Recovery is to create a comprehensive and coordinated system of care for individuals with SMIs who are frequent and costly recidivists to the criminal justice system, homeless continuum of care, and acute care medical and mental health treatment systems.

The building – which encompasses approximately 181,000 square feet of space and capacity for 208 beds – will include a central receiving center, an integrated crisis stabilization unit and addiction receiving facility, various levels of residential treatment, day treatment and day activity programs, outpatient behavioral health and primary care treatment services, vocational rehabilitation and supportive employment services, and classroom/educational spaces. The facility will also include a courtroom and space for social service agencies, such as housing providers, legal services, and immigration services that will address the comprehensive needs of individuals served.

Capital funding for the project is provided through the county's general obligation bond program, with additional support provided by the Jackson Health System – Public Health Trust. To expedite completion of the facility and contain costs, Miami-Dade County, with the support of the state, transferred the project to Thriving Mind South Florida for the purposes of providing oversight of the construction phase and eventual operations.

By housing a comprehensive array of services and supports in one location, and providing re-entry assistance upon discharge to the community, it is anticipated that many of the barriers and obstacles to navigating traditional community mental health and social services will be eliminated. The services planned for the facility will address critical treatment needs that have gone unmet in the past and reduce the likelihood of recidivism to the justice system, crisis settings, and homelessness in the future. Operation at the facility will begin in early 2021.

Conclusion

The CMHP has demonstrated substantial, cost-effective gains in the effort to reverse the criminalization of people with mental illnesses. The idea was not to create new treatment services which may duplicate existing services in the community, but rather to create more efficient and effective linkages to these services. The Project works by eliminating gaps in services and by forging productive and innovative relationships among all stakeholders who have an interest in the welfare and safety of one of our community's most vulnerable populations.

The CMHP offers the promise of hope and recovery for individuals with SMI that have often been misunderstood and discriminated against. Once engaged in treatment and community support services, individuals have the opportunity to achieve successful recovery, community integration, and reduce their recidivism to jail.

The CMHP provides an effective and cost-efficient solution to a community problem. Program results demonstrate that individualized transition planning to access necessary community-based treatment and services upon release from jail will ensure successful community re-entry and recovery for individuals with

mental illnesses, and possible co-occurring substance use disorders that are involved in the criminal justice system.

References

1. Steadman HJ, Osher FC, Robbins PC, Case B, Samuels S. Prevalence of serious mental illness among jail inmates. *Psychiatr Serv*. 2009; **60**(6): 761–765.

2. U.S. Department of Justice, Federal Bureau of Investigation. *Crime in the United States, 2018*. Clarksburg, WV; 2019.

3. Treatment Advocacy Center. *Serious Mental Illness (SMI) prevalence in jails and prisons*. Arlington, VA: Author; September 2016.

4. Fuller DA, Sinclair E, Geller J, Quanbeck C, Snook J. *Going, going, gone: trends and consequences of eliminating state psychiatric beds*, 2016. Arlington, VA: Treatment Action Center; 2016.

5. Jackson Health System, Corrections Health Services. *CHS Operational Statistics*. Unpublished raw data. Miami, FL; 2019.

6. Miami-Dade County Grand Jury. *Mental illness and the criminal justice system: a recipe for disaster/a prescription for improvement, Final Report of the Miami-Dade County Grand Jury; Spring Term 2004*. Miami, FL: Author; 2004.

7. Florida Mental Health Institute. *Miami-Dade County heavy user data analysis*. Unpublished raw data. Tampa, FL; 2010.

8. Dupont R, Cochran S. Police response to mental health emergencies – barriers to change. *J Am Acad Psychiatry Law*. 2000; **28**(3): 338–344.

9. Institute of Behavioral Research. *Texas Christian University Drug Screen 5*. Fort Worth: Texas Christian University: Author; 2017.

10. Latessa E, Smith P, Lemke R, Makarios M, Lowenkamp C. *Creation and validation of the Ohio Risk Assessment System: Final report*. Cincinnati, OH: University of Cincinnati, School of Criminal Justice, Center for Criminal Justice Research; 2009.

11. Osher F, Steadman HJ, Barr H. *A Best Practice Approach to Community Re-Entry from Jails for Inmates With Co-Occurring Disorders: The APIC Model*. Delmar, NY: The National GAINS Center; 2002.

12. Dennis D, Lassiter M, Connelly WH, Lupfer KS. Helping adults who are homeless gain disability benefits: the SSI/SSDI Outreach, Access, and Recovery (SOAR) program. *Psychiatr Serv*. 2011; **62**(11): 1373–1376.

Jail Diversion: A Practical Primer

Charles L. Scott

Introduction

The United States' incarceration rate of its national population is the highest in the world.[1] The percentage of incarcerated individuals with a mental illness is substantial, with 10% to 15% of inmates suffering from a serious mental illness (SMI).[2] Two-thirds of sentenced jail inmates met criteria for drug dependence or abuse.[3] Many inmates experience both mental illness and a substance use disorder as co-occurring conditions.

Multiple reasons account for the rise in the number of individuals with mental illness entering the criminal justice system. First, in the 1960s, a movement began to deinstitutionalize individuals with mental illness and discharge them from psychiatric hospitals to the least restrictive environment. As a result, large numbers of individuals previously treated in an inpatient setting were released into the community with a resulting decrease in inpatient psychiatric hospital beds. Second, during the 1970s, the United States increasingly turned to punishment of individuals with a drug offense rather than treatment. As a result, drug-related offenses increased with a subsequent rise in arrests and incarcerations. Third, during this same relative time period, judges were given less discretion in imposing sentence lengths as legislatures increasingly mandated determinate and fixed sentencing to demonstrate a "get tough on crime approach." Fourth, during the 1960s and mid-1970s, civil commitment laws were substantially reformed, making involuntary commitment of individuals with mental illness more difficult.[4] As a result of these, and other factors, a ballooning number of people with mental illness are finding their way into a jail or prison, rather than a hospital setting.

Criminalization of mental illness refers to the inappropriate diversion of those with mental problems to the criminal justice system rather than to treatment.[5]

To help address this mismatch of people and resources, public policy is shifting to finds ways to divert these individuals away from potentially long and costly incarcerations and into appropriate and effective treatment. An increasing use of the principle known as "therapeutic jurisprudence" is being utilized as an alternative approach to the mass incarceration of individuals with mental illness. Core concepts of therapeutic jurisprudence include the application of law in the most appropriate way to benefit all individuals, increasing therapeutic aspects of legal interventions while decreasing antitherapeutic aspects, and protecting the due process rights of both offenders and victims.[6]

In general, individuals eligible for diversion from the criminal justice system are those with a treatable mental and/or substance use disorder that can be safely maintained in the community. Munetz and Griffin[7] proposed the Sequential Intercept Model (SIM) as a useful framework to conceptualize a series of "points of interception" where individuals with a mental illness may be prevented from entering or progressing further into the criminal justice system. These authors acknowledge that individuals with mental illness who demonstrate criminal behavior unrelated to their mental illness should be held accountable for their behavior; however, people with mental illness should not be arrested or detained longer than others only because of their mental illness.[7] The five intercept points proposed by the SIM are summarized in Table 11.1.

This article focuses primarily on the first three SIM intercept points as related to jail diversion and reviews types of diversion programs, research outcomes for diversion programs, and important components that contribute to successful diversion.

Pre-booking Diversion Programs

The first intercept point involves the role of police in managing individuals in psychiatric crisis who

Table 11.1 Sequential intercept model interception points

Intercept 1: Law enforcement and emergency services
Intercept 2: Initial hearings and initial detention
Intercept 3: Jails and courts
Intercept 4: Re-entry from jails, prisons, and hospitals
Intercept 5: Community corrections and community support services

come to their attention with resolution of difficulties on site without further intervention. Persons with mental health (MH) problems may be referred to the police through concerns by family members, friends, or colleagues or through potentially law violating behaviors when police are called to the scene. Some research indicates that individuals with mental illness have more police contacts during their life than those without mental illness.

In his systematic review of nearly 330,000 cases involving police contacts, Livingston found that approximately 25% of people with mental disorders had a history of police arrest, nearly 10% had police involved in their pathway to MH care, and 1% of all police dispatches and encounters involved people with mental disorders.[8] Fisher et al.[9] compared the arrest rates for eight offense categories of nearly 11,000 individuals with severe and persistent mental illness to those of 3.3 million persons in the same age group (aged 18–54). These researchers found that individuals with mental illness had significantly higher odds of having at least one arrest across all charge categories. Except for charges of assault and battery against a police officer, the largest odds ratio for those with mental illness was for misdemeanor crimes.[9] Increased police contacts are not the only risk for individuals with a SMI. Research also indicates that nearly 25% of individuals fatally shot by the police are persons with a SMI.[10]

The police often serve as a gatekeeper in deciding whether or not an individual with MH problems enters the MH system, is taken to jail, or remains in their community without further intervention. In many situations, the person with a MH problem may be well known to the police through numerous contacts over time.[11] Moreover, police may serve as a peacekeeper or a provisional solution that helps reduce the likelihood of future interactions with the police.[12]

Numerous approaches to assist in the interactions between the police and individuals with MH problems and potentially divert these persons have been proposed and are summarized below.

Police-Based Specialized Police Response

As described above, police are often the first responders to situations involving individuals suffering from psychiatric symptoms. A major revamping of how police interact with individuals with mental illness stems from a fatal shooting by police in Memphis, TN. On September 24, 1987, Memphis police officers were called to the LeMoyne Gardens public housing project by a mother concerned about the mental state of her African-American 27-year-old son Joseph DeWayne Robinson. Mr. Robinson was reportedly diagnosed with schizophrenia and intoxicated on cocaine. By the time the police arrived, Mr. Robinson was holding an 8-in. butcher knife to his throat and threatening suicide. He had inflicted nearly 120 wounds over his body. When the police ordered him to put down his knife, he refused and allegedly lunged at the police. The surrounding four officers, all white, fired approximately 8 to 10 times and Mr. Robinson died of multiple gunshot wounds. As a result of this tragedy, the Memphis Mayor sought help from advocates from the National Alliance on Mental Illness and enlisted police, community MH professionals, hospital administrators, and church officials to develop a more effective way for the police to intervene with persons in the midst of a psychiatric crisis. Ultimately, Dr. Randolph Dupont and Major Sam Cochran developed a program known as "Crisis Intervention Training" (CIT) for frontline officers who volunteer for the training. The goal of CIT training is to enhance police's ability to better respond to individuals with mental illness and to find appropriate opportunities to connect the individual with treatment services rather than the criminal justice system. The CIT training developed has become known as the "Memphis Model."[13] The CIT Center at the University of Memphis has developed a national curriculum offered for selected officers within a police department who volunteer for the training. The 40-hour training involves six core areas as part of the curriculum delivered over a one-week period. The core areas include the following: MH didactics; community support and resources; de-escalation training; site visits of settings providing MH treatment; law enforcement issues related to police procedures and law enforcement liability; and research and systems with an emphasis on diversion strategies.[14] Subsequent research has demonstrated that delivering the training in segments over time produces similar results regarding officers' knowledge of mental illness and attitudes toward individuals with MH problems.[15] This segmented approach may provide an alternative approach to delivering CIT training thereby potentially increasing the availability of this training.

Over 3,000 programs in the United States have implemented CIT and approximately 20% of patrol officers in those programs receive the CIT training.[16] Those officers who volunteer for CIT training have better outcomes with regard to key attitudes toward individuals with mental illness, skills, and behaviors.[17,18] In his study of 46 police officers from 7 rural departments and 13 suburban departments, Strassle[19] also noted that officers who underwent CIT training had reductions in stigmatic attitudes toward individuals with mental illness.

Research that CIT decreases the arrest rate of persons with mental illness is mixed. Watson et al.[16] provided three possible reasons to explain why research on CIT programs outside of Memphis has not shown a decrease in arrest rates: (1) other programs do not adhere to the Memphis CIT program and therefore successful decrease in arrest rates cannot be duplicated; (2) officers without CIT training are arresting more people with mental illness but are not aware they are mentally ill thereby negating decrease arrest rate results from CIT trained officers; and (3) both non-CIT and CIT trained officers are decreasing their arrest of those with mental illness resulting in no appreciable difference in arrest rates between trained versus nontrained officers.[16] If a reduction in arrests of individuals with mental illness results from decreased arrests by both non-CIT and CIT trained officers, then this reduction nevertheless represents an overall success in preventing unnecessary arrests of individuals with SMIs.

Despite mixed evidence on CIT decreasing arrest rates, multiple studies have demonstrated that CIT programs increase the transport of individuals with mental illness to emergency treatment facilities and improve linkages to MH programs.[16] Steadman and Morrissette recommend a reframing of the CIT approach that focuses not only on what the police should do when they interact with a person in emotional distress but also on how police can be engaged as partners with community MH providers responsible for designing crisis treatment and interventions along the continuum.[20]

Police-Based Specialized MH Response Approach

Pre-arrest diversion can also be accomplished through a model where police and a MH professional work together to respond to a MH crisis. This model has been referred to as a "police-based specialized mental health response" or "police mental health street triage." This approach typically involves an on-site assessment by the police followed by a MH evaluation by a clinician who evaluates the level and nature of psychiatric distress. In some co-responder models, the MH professional assists remotely from a control room where they may have access to patient records and can help guide the officer on site. Compton et al.[21] describe a police–MH linkage system that illustrates one variation as to how remote assistance may help a police officer called to the scene. In this model, individuals with a SMI who receive community MH treatment and have a prior criminal history agree to be included in a database that can provide information in the event of future police encounters. If an officer has contact with a person enrolled in this system and runs a background check, the officer receives a text message that this person may be involved in the MH linkage system project. At this point, the officer can call a social worker employed at the community MH agency who can provide background information for the officer and assist him or her with how to manage certain behaviors and potential dispositions.[21]

Research indicates that this approach has achieved some success even though significant limitations on the quality of the research likely limit conclusive findings. In their review of the literature examining the effectiveness of co-response models, Puntis et al.[22] found that this co-responder approach was associated with decreased use of involuntary psychiatric referrals and detentions in police custody. Their review also notes that service users found this approach less distressing than a standard police response with quicker access to MH treatment during the crisis.[22]

Meehan et al.[23] followed 122 Australian individuals who had direct contact with the police–MH co-responder for two weeks to monitor subsequent emergency department presentations and inpatient admissions. Their research indicated that following the direct contact with the co-responder team, 67% of these individuals remained at their residence, 29% were transported to the emergency department, and only 4% were taken into custody by the police. These authors concluded that co-responded interventions helped resolve the immediate crisis for most of the contacts and likely diverted many away from the emergency room and inpatient treatment.[23]

MH-Based Specialized MH Response Programs

Like police-based specialized MH response programs described above, MH-based specialized MH response programs typically involve coordination between law enforcement and MH providers. However, in these programs, the MH clinician does the initial triage assessment with police back up as needed. These programs are often referred to as mobile crisis programs. The mobile crisis program of DeKalb County, Georgia illustrates several components of this approach summarized in Table 11.2.[24]

In a retrospective review of Dekalb County's mobile crisis program, Scott[24] examined the effectiveness and efficiency of this program in addressing 911 psychiatric emergency calls. In cases involving regular police intervention, 28% of the cases were managed without psychiatric hospitalization. In contrast, 55% of emergencies referred to the mobile crisis team avoided psychiatric hospitalization. Although this finding did not reach statistical significance, the average cost per case was 23% less for persons evaluated by the mobile crisis team. In addition, both consumers and police officers viewed the mobile crisis program positively.[24]

Specialized Crises Response Sites

Emergency rooms are unlikely settings to adequately address the needs of all individuals with mental illness

Table 11.2 Common components of mobile crisis programs

- Includes relationship with local community mental health agency
- Involves local advocacy groups and family members of those with mental illness for program input
- Includes police officers and mental health clinicians
- Provides response to 911 calls or suicide hot lines identified as psychiatric emergencies
- Has clinician conduct assessment with police back up as needed
- Has clinician determine referral to hospital or community services
- Provides team member to conduct follow-up via phone or home visits

who are detained by the police in lieu of jail. Challenges with emergency rooms serving the sole or primary avenue to address psychiatric crises include long periods of wait times for police in the emergency room setting, refusal of psychiatric admission due to the individual not meeting involuntary commitment criteria, and diversion of individuals who need MH assistance but do not represent a psychiatric emergency.[25] In addition, using the emergency room department to board psychiatric patients after medical clearance increases emergency room costs, diverts care from other psychiatric and medical emergencies, and creates an often loud and chaotic setting not equipped to appropriately manage psychiatric patients.

Specialized crisis response sites can serve an important role in pre-booking pre-trial diversion programs. Steadman et al.[25] outline basic principles that have been described as important to the role of these sites in assisting with the success of pre-trial diversion programs. First, the centralized site should be available 24 hours a day so that police can take a person in MH crisis to this location whenever needed. The MH and substance use services should be co-located at the site to minimize the responsibility of officers in determining the primary etiology of the person's acute symptoms and where the person should be taken. Second, the drop-off site should have "police friendly" procedures with a no-refusal policy for law enforcement referrals. The site should strive for a streamlined intake to expedite the officer's transport and transition of the individual so that they can quickly return to their work promoting public safety. Third, the site should have an established legal foundation to accept and hold persons who may also be facing a criminal charge. Fourth, training should be provided to both law enforcement and MH providers to address roles and responsibilities as well as any biases of either group. Finally, these specialized crisis sites should establish strong linkages to community services, including facilitating connections with both MH and substance abuse services. A responsible individual, referred to as a "boundary spanner," plays a crucial role in overcoming various institutional barriers to ease access to care. In their review of different pre-booking diversion models, these researchers found that having a psychiatric triage or drop-off center was a key factor in the success of pre-booking diversion, regardless of the diversion model.[25]

Post-Booking Diversion

Post-booking diversion involves a process where inmates with a mental illness who have been arrested and booked are identified and subsequently diverted to a treatment program outside of the jail setting. Three models of post-booking diversion described are pre-trial jail diversion programs, deferred prosecution programs (pre-arraignment or post-arraignment), and specialty courts. Each of these models is summarized below.

Jail-Based Post-Booking Diversion

In jail-based post-booking diversion programs, pre-trial service personnel or specialized jail personnel identify those jail inmates appropriate for community treatment with the agreement of the judge, prosecutor, and defense attorney. Proposed benefits of jail diversion include improvement of MH symptoms, reduction in overcrowded jails with insufficient resources to treat this population, fewer future contacts with police, and decreased criminal recidivism.[26]

In one of the few studies examining the outcomes specific to jail-based post-booking, Shafer et al.[27] followed 248 individuals with co-occurring disorders of SMI and substance use disorders who had been arrested and booked on misdemeanor charges. Numerous outcomes of individuals assigned to diversion or nondiversion were evaluated 12 months after their index offense. The authors found that diverted clients were significantly more likely to utilize emergency rooms for MH or substance use treatment and reported fewer symptoms of depression and anxiety than their nondiverted counterparts. However, they did not show any significant difference in their rearrest rate compared to nondiverted individuals, although they did have significantly lower rearrest for lower level misdemeanor crimes.[27]

Gill and Murphy[28] examined the outcomes of a unique jail-based diversion program coordinated by the county prosecutor's office. These researchers followed outcomes of 125 individuals diverted toward MH services over a five-year period. In contrast to earlier research, individuals who completed the program were a lower risk of being arrested and had fewer arrests. Although those who did not complete the diversion program also benefited in these same areas, their response was not as strong as diversion completers. Individuals who had a longer period of participation in active treatment demonstrated better outcomes, indicating that a lengthier period of follow-up care may be needed to sustain initial gains.[28]

Deferred Prosecution Programs

In deferred prosecution programs, the court refers a defendant charged with a crime to a community treatment program in lieu of prosecution. If the person successfully completes the proposed treatment, then the original charge may be dismissed and the arrest no longer appears on the defendant's record. Deferred prosecution has been a diversion tool for decades for individuals charged with driving while intoxicated (DWI). In a 1983 study of offenders charged with DWI in Washington State, DWI offenders who received deferred prosecution and concomitant alcoholism treatment had significantly *more* post-deferral alcohol-related traffic violations than did a control group of DWI offenders who received normal judicial sanctions. The authors suggested two possible reasons why those diverted to a treatment program had higher alcohol-related violations compared to those who were not referred. First, the deferred prosecution group may have accepted the treatment to avoid legal sanctions rather than to genuinely address their alcohol problem. Second, the alcoholism treatment offered to this group may not have been effective.[29] What constituted "alcoholism treatment" was not defined in this study making it difficult to know if the lack of benefit was due to a poor treatment, lack of motivation by those referred, or some other factor.

In 2007, the University of Washington State Institute for Public Policy studied the impact of deferred prosecution of driving under the influence (DUI) cases on recidivism. Recidivism was defined as filing of a subsequent DUI, criminal traffic, or alcohol-related case within three years of the original DUI filing. Under this Washington State statute, deferred prosecutions have strict requirements. In particular, the defendant must admit they have an alcohol, drug, or mental disorder that will likely result in reoffense without treatment, must attend a two-year substance abuse or MH treatment program, must attend two self-help meetings (e.g. alcoholic anonymous) every week for at least two years, must pay for treatment, and must continue under court monitoring for at least three additional years with no use of alcohol or nonprescribed drugs. Failure to meet any of these conditions results in prosecution of the DUI. Under these strict guidelines, individuals with a DUI deferred prosecution had lower adjusted recidivism rates than defendants with similar characteristics who pled guilty or were convicted of a DUI.[30] The results of this study suggest that rigid ongoing monitoring in deferred prosecution of cases involving substance use may be an essential component of success as defined by decreased recidivism of alcohol- or drug-related charges.

Problem Solving Courts

As with other forms of diversion, problem solving courts work to connect individuals with a mental illness who may be better served through community treatment as opposed to incarceration. A wide range of problem solving courts has developed and examples of such courts are listed in Table 11.3.

Miami-Dade drug treatment court (DTC) has often been cited as the first example of a problem solving court. This court was established in 1989 by Judge Herbert Klein. An important goal of this court was to address the escalating violence associated with cocaine trafficking in the Miami, FL area and failure of the criminal justice system and the "War on Drugs" to decrease drug use and arrests. Drug courts represent an example of therapeutic jurisprudence and restorative justice through utilization of treatment for the offender, intense supervision, regular court appearances, and the chance to make amends to victims and the community by becoming more productive citizens free from addiction. There are two general formats of drug courts. In a pre-adjudication drug court, the individual does not plead guilty but does waive his or her right to a jury trial, a speedy trial, and a right to confront witnesses. If the person successfully completes the program, charges are dismissed. In contrast, individuals who enter a drug court through a post-adjudication format plead guilty and are referred to drug court as a condition of probation. If the person does not complete the program, then probation can be revoked with sentencing and potential

Table 11.3 Problem solving court examples

- Drug court
- Mental health court
- Homeless court
- Veteran's court
- Domestic violence court
- Prostitution court
- Community court
- Gambling court
- Teen court

incarceration following.[31] Sanctions are an important component associated with decreased drug use and recidivism of drug court participants.[32] Sanctions can be wide ranging and include jail incarceration, increased treatment, performing community service, increased court appearances, verbal reprimands, and program termination.[33]

Research has demonstrated that individuals who complete the treatment program prescribed by the drug court have decreased recidivism. In his study of 381 subjects referred to a DTC, Fulkerson[34] noted that subjects in the DTC group had a significantly lower recidivism rate over a four-year period when compared to a traditional probation group. Successful completion of the program was a key factor, as those who withdrew or failed the DTC program experienced the same frequency of future arrests as those never referred to the DTC program.[34]

The goal of a mental health court (MHC), like other forms of jail diversion, is to decrease criminal recidivism while improving the MH of participants.[35] Although MHCs across the United States vary in how participants are selected and the length of time from identification to MHC referral, they generally have the following common characteristics: voluntary participation; separate docket for defendants with mental disorders; judicial oversight of treatment plans; regular appearance by the participant in court before the judge; nonadversarial team approach with both criminal justice and MH professionals involved in the decision-making, and defined conditions for successful completion.[36,37]

Redlich et al.[38] noted that MH courts have evolved since their first inception and describe differences between "first generation" MHCs and "second generation" MHCs. In their review, these authors note that most "first generation" courts accepted only individuals with a mental illness facing misdemeanor charges and all used sanctions when difficulties arose with compliance. Supervision models included primary responsibility resting with community providers, court staff, or probation officers, or joint supervision by both MH staff and probation.[38]

Although second generation MHCs also utilize a therapeutic jurisprudence model for inmates with mental illness, four dimensions have evolved when compared to first generation MHCs. These dimensions involve an increased acceptance of defendants facing felony charges, increased use of post-plea adjudication models, increased use of jail as a sanction, and increased use of criminal justice supervision as compared to supervision by community providers.[38]

Do MHCs work in their stated goals to decrease recidivism and improve quality of life for participants? Several studies have attempted to answer this question with some mixed results. In their study of a San Francisco MHC, McNeil and Binder[36] compared 170 people who entered a MHC after arrest with adults with mental disorders who were booked into the county jail but not referred to the MHC. These authors concluded that participation in the MHC program had the following positive outcomes: longer time without any new criminal charges; longer time without new charges for violent crime; and decreased recidivism and violence, even after graduates were no longer under the MHC supervision.[36]

In their meta-analytic investigation of studies examining recidivism rate for MHC participants, Lowder et al.[37] noted that participation in MHC had a small effect on recidivism compared with traditional criminal processing but appeared to be most effective at decreasing time spent in jail after exiting from MHC. These authors encouraged further research examining strategies that may improve outcomes and decrease recidivism such as more frequent status hearings and increased attention to addressing criminogenic risks and needs.[37]

Yuan and Capriotti[39] reviewed existing research in this area and concluded that the literature suggests that those who participate in MHC do have lower recidivism rates when compared with those who do not. Furthermore, individuals with mental illness who participated in MHCs demonstrated fewer post-court arrests, longer average time to arrest, and decreased offense severity when they did reoffend. In their review of the Sacramento County MHC, these same authors also found MHC graduates had fewer psychiatric hospitalizations than those who did not graduate from the MHC program.[39]

An important aspect of enhancing positive outcomes for participants in MHC treatment programs is the provision of care that matches the needs of the referrals. Pinals et al.[40] examined an approach for treating individuals with co-occurring disorders known as Maintaining Independence and Sobriety through Systems Integration, Outreach, and Networking-Criminal Justice (MISSION-CJ). MISSION-CJ utilizes six integrated evidence-based components outlined in Table 11.4.

Table 11.4 MISSION-CJ evidence-based components

- Critical time intervention case management
- Intensive in-community support that decreases in intensity over time
- Dual recovery therapy
- Peer support
- Vocational and educational support
- Trauma-informed care

In their review of 97 MHC participants followed up at six months, those MHC participants who received MISSION-CJ demonstrated a decrease in behavioral health symptoms, illegal drug use, trauma symptoms, and time incarcerated. This study reflects the relevance of addressing specific needs of referred individuals at a level of intensity sufficient to meet those needs.[40]

Summary

The success of jail-based diversion, whatever diversion model is used, depends in large part on the availability and quality of the community MH treatment provided.[27] In addition to matching treatment to the person's specific risks and needs, the success of the program depends on the selection of appropriate candidates for the specific diversion program, a trusted collaboration between MH community services, law enforcement, and the court, and the careful monitoring of program compliance with both rewards and sanctions used where appropriate. As individuals with SMI do not only commit crimes because of their mental illness, treatment programs should also attend to criminogenic factors unrelated to mental illness to maximize reductions in recidivism.

The need for continued research is substantial. Although many prior studies have attempted to examine the impact of diversion on decreasing recidivism in those with SMI, there are also numerous limitations when examining the literature at large. Challenges when drawing general conclusions from the research include varying definitions of SMI, different criteria qualifying an individual for diversion, a lack of uniformity in how risk assessments are conducted (if at all), the lack of a matched control population not diverted, the failure of some programs to address co-occurring substance use disorders, the failure of some programs to address criminogenic needs, the use of evidence-based treatment programs, and varying lengths of time to measure recidivism. Future research will be improved by addressing these limitations as well as evaluating how motivation versus coercion impacts outcome and the likely need for continued and ongoing long-term management.

In his foreword in the book titled *"Insanity Inside Out"*, Judge Bazelon addresses an individual's right to MH treatment. His poetic words of yesterday apply to the challenges we face today as a society striving to provide better care for those with mental illness who may be best served by diverting away from the criminal justice system. When discussing the need for the judicial and MH systems to work together toward this goal, he eloquently acknowledges, "These are large demands, but the problems cannot be met with less."[41]

Disclosure

The author has nothing to disclose.

References

1. Walmsley R. World prison population list. *World Prison Brief*. 12th edn. London, UK: Institute for Criminal Policy Research; 2018. www .prisonstudies.org (accessed August 10, 2019).

2. Hoge SK, Buchanan AW, Kovasznay MB, Roskes EJ. *Outpatient Services for the Mentally Ill Involved in the Criminal Justice System*. American Psychiatric Association Task Force Report: Washington, DC; 2009: 1–15.

3. Bronson J, Stroop J, Zimmer S, Berzofsky M. *Drug Use, Dependence, and Abuse Among State Prisoners and Jail Inmates, 2007–2009*. NCJ250546. Washington, DC: U.S. Department of Justice, Office of Justice Programs, Bureau of Justice Statistics; 2017.

4. Pinals DA. Forensic services, public mental health policy, and financing: charting the course ahead. *J Am Acad Psychiatry Law*. 2014; **42**(1): 7–19.

5. Dewa CS, Loong D, Grujillo A, Bonato S. Evidence for the effectiveness of police-based pre-booking diversion programs in decriminalizing mental illness: a systematic literature review. *PLoS One*. 2018; **13**(6): e0199368.

6. Winick B, Wexler DB. *Judging in a Therapeutic Key: Therapeutic Jurisprudence and the Court*. Durham, NC: Carolina Academic Press; 2003.

7. Munetz MR, Griffin PA. Use of the sequential intercept model as an approach to decriminalization of people with serious mental illness. *Psychiatr Serv*. 2006; **57**(4): 544–549.

8. Livingston JD. Contact between police and people with mental disorders: a review of rates. *Psychiatr Serv*. 2016; **67**(8): 850–857.

9. Fisher WH, Roy-Bujnowski KM, Grudzinskas A, et al. Patterns and prevalence of arrest in a statewide cohort of mental health care consumers. *Psychiatr Serv*. 2006; **56**(11): 1623–1628.

10. Fuller DA, Kamb HR, Biasotti M, Snook J. Overlooked in the undercounted: the role of mental illness in fatal law enforcement encounters. Treatment Advocacy Center; . www.treatmentadvocacycenter.org/evidence-and-research/studies.

11. Reuland M, Schwarzfeld M, Draper L. *Law Enforcement Responses to People with Mental Illnesses: A Guide to Research-Informed Policy and Practice*. New York, NY: Council of State Governments Justice Center; 2012.

12. Wood JD, Watson AC. Improving police interventions during mental health-related encounters: past, present and future. *Policing Soc*. 2017; **27**: 289–299.

13. Dupont R, Cochran MJ, Pillsbury S. *Crisis Intervention Team Core Elements*. The University of Memphis, School of Urban Affairs and Public Policy, Department of Criminology and Criminal Justice, CIT Center. 2007: 1–20.

14. Crisis Intervention Training. National Curriculum. University of Memphis, CIT Center. http://cit .memphis.edu/curriculuma.php?id-0 (accessed June 2020).

15. Cuddeback GS, Kurtz RA, Wilson AB, VanDeinse T, Burgin SE. Segmented versus traditional Crisis Intervention Team training. *J Am Acad Psychiatry Law*. 2016; **44**(3): 338–343.

16. Watson AC, Ottati VC, Morabito M, et al. Outcomes of police contacts with persons with mental illness: the impact of CIT. *Adm Policy Ment Health*. 2010; **37**: 302–317.

17. Compton MT, Bahor M, Watson AC, Oliva JR. A comprehensive review of extant research on Crisis Intervention Team (CIT) programs. *J Am Acad Psychiatry Law*. 2008; **36**(1): 47–55.

18. Compton MT, Bakeman R, Broussard B, D'Orio B, Watson AC. Police officers' volunteering for (rather than being assigned to) Crisis Intervention Team (CIT) training: evidence for a beneficial self-selection effect. *Behav Sci Law*. 2017; **35** (6–6): 470–479.

19. Strassle CG. CIT in small municipalities: officer level outcomes. *Behav Sci Law*. 2019; **37**(4): 342–352.

20. Steadman HJ, Morrissette D. Police responses to persons with mental illness: going beyond CIT training. *Psych Serv*. 2016; **67**(10): 1054–1056.

21. Compton MT, Halpern B, Broussard B, et al. A potential new form of jail diversion and reconnection to mental health services: 1. Stakeholders' views on acceptability. *Behav Sci Law*. 2017; **35**: 480–491.

22. Puntis S, Perfect D, Kirubarajan A, et al. A systematic review of co-responder models of police mental health 'street' triage. *BMC Psychiatry*. 2018; **18**(1): 1–11.

23. Meehan T, Brack J, Mansfield Y, Stedman T. Do police-mental health co-responder programmes reduce emergency department presentations or simply delay the inevitable? *Australas Psychiatry*. 2019; **27**(1): 18–20.

24. Scott RL. Evaluation of a mobile crisis program: effectiveness, efficiency, and consumer satisfaction. *Psychiatr Serv*. 2000; **51**(9): 1153–1156.

25. Steadman HJ, Stainbrook KA, Griffin P, et al. A specialized crisis response site as a core element of police-based diversion programs. *Psychiatr Serv*. 2001; **52**(2): 219–222.

26. Sirotich F. The criminal justice outcomes of jail diversion programs for persons with mental illness; a review of the evidence. *J Am Acad Psych Law*. 2009; **37**(4): 461–472.

27. Shafer MS, Arthur B, Franczak MJ. An analysis of post-booking jail diversion programming for persons with co-occurring disorders. *Behav Sci Law*. 2004; **22**: 771–785.

28. Gill KJ, Murphy AA. Jail diversion for persons with serious mental illness coordinated by a prosecutor's office. *Biomed Res Int*. 2017; **2017**: 7917616.

29. Salzberg PM, Klingberg CL. The effectiveness of deferred prosecution for driving while intoxicated. *J Stud Alcohol*. 1983; **44**(2): 299–306.

30. Barnoski R. Deferred prosecution of DUI cases in Washington State: evaluating the impact on recidivism, August 2008. www.wsipp.wa.gov (accessed August 21, 2019).

31. Fulkerson A, Keena LD, O'Brien E. Understanding success and nonsuccess in the drug court. *Int J Offender Ther Comp Criminol*. 2012; **57**(10): 1297–1316.

32. Harrell A, Roman J. Reducing drug use and crime among offenders: the impact of graduated sanctions. *J Drug Issues*. 2001; **31**: 207–232.

33. Lindquist CH, Krebs C, Lattimore PK. Sanctions and rewards in drug court programs: implementation, perceived efficacy, and decision making. *J Drug Issues*. 2006; **36**: 119–145.

34. Fulkerson A. Drug treatment versus probation: an examination of comparative recidivism rates. *Southwest J Crim Justice*. 2012; **8**: 30–45.

35. Goldkamp JS, Irons-Guynn C. Emerging judicial strategies for the mentally ill in the criminal caseload: mental health courts in Fort Lauderdale, Seattle, San Bernardino, and Anchorage. Washington, DC: Department of Justice, Office of Justice Programs, Bureau of Justice Assistance Monograph; 2000. Pub no. NCJ 182504.

36. McNeil DE, Binder RL. Effectiveness of a mental health court in reducing criminal recidivism and violence. *Am J Psychiatry*. 2007; **164**: 1395–1403.

37. Lowder EM, Rade CB, Desmarais SL. Effectiveness of mental health courts in reducing recidivism: a meta-analysis. *Psychiatr Serv*. 2018; **69**(1): 15–22.

38. Redlich AD, Steadman HJ, Monahan K, Petrila J, Griffin PA. The second generation of mental health courts. *Psychol Public Policy Law*. 2005; **11**(4): 527–538.

39. Yuan Y, Capriotti MR. The impact of mental health court: a Sacramento case study. *Behav Sci Law*. 2019; **37**: 452–467.

40. Pinals DA, Gaba A, Clary KM, et al. Implementation of MISSION – criminal justice in a treatment court: preliminary outcomes among individuals with co-occurring disorders. *Psychiatr Serv*. 2019; **70**(11): 1044–1048.

41. Bazelon D. Foreword. In: Donaldson K, *Insanity Inside Out*. New York: Crown University of Michigan; 1976.

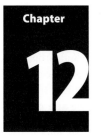

Chapter 12

Principles and Practices of Risk Assessment in Mental Health Jail Diversion Programs

Sarah L. Desmarais and Evan M. Lowder

Introduction

Efforts are underway across the United States to reduce the population of individuals in our jails and prisons, such as through mental health diversion programs. Mental health diversion programs are now among the most common interventions for individuals with mental health problems who come into contact with the criminal justice system. Briefly, these programs divert individuals with mental health problems from traditional case processing into community-based behavioral health treatment and alternative case processing. The Sequential Intercept Model describes the points of interception or opportunities for diversion across multiple stages of case processing, from initial police contact (pre-booking) through court appearance (post-booking) through sentencing (post-conviction) and, even, re-entry.[1] There are now hundreds of mental health jail diversion programs in operation across the United States,[2] including over 400 mental health courts.[3] We focus herein on post-booking mental health jail diversion programs, including but not limited to mental health courts.

Increasingly, and not without controversy, risk assessment tools are being discussed as one strategy that may be used to support criminal justice reforms and alternatives to traditional case processing, including mental health jail diversion programs.[4–6] Risk assessment can be defined as the process of estimating the likelihood of future adverse outcomes. In the context of mental health jail diversion programs, the adverse outcome of interest is typically danger or threat to public safety (although the specific definition differs across jurisdictions and programs). Eligibility criteria for participation in mental health jail diversion programs, whether formally written in statute or otherwise, specify that for individuals with mental health problems to be diverted from the criminal justice

system to alternative settings, including the community, they should not pose an unreasonable threat to public safety (see, for example, California Assembly Bill 1810). In other words, an individual should not be diverted from the criminal justice system to the community to the detriment of public safety.[7]

Traditionally, assessments regarding an individual's threat to public safety – and thus, eligibility for diversion or other alternative to incarceration programs – are made by judges based on the facts of the case, official records, and any other information presented in court.[8] This approach to risk assessment can be described as unstructured professional judgment because there is no validated checklist or protocol guiding what information should be considered and how this information should be combined or weighted to estimate threat to public safety. Instead, judges and other assessors relied on their professional training and experience to guide their identification, integration, and consideration of information to estimate an individual's risk to public safety. However, on average, unstructured risk assessments are both less accurate and less consistent than those completed using structured risk approaches.[9–11] The use of risk assessment tools also can lead to better public safety outcomes.[12–15] The use of risk assessment tools, then, may help improve decisions regarding an individual's appropriateness and eligibility for mental health jail diversion as a function of their estimated threat to public safety and the resources that would be required to mitigate that level of risk.[7] Their use in mental health jail diversion programs also may contribute to improved individual and public safety outcomes.

In this paper, we first describe the process and components of risk. We then consider the use of risk assessment tools in mental health jail diversion programs. In doing so, our goal is to provide an overview of the science and practice of risk assessment to inform decision-making and risk mitigation in the context of mental health jail diversion programs.

Process and Components of Risk Assessment

The process of risk assessment involves the gathering, consideration, and integration of information about characteristics of a person, their case, and their circumstances to estimate the risk they pose to public safety with the goal of informing decision-making and guiding risk management. There are four issues pertaining to the process of risk assessment in the context of mental health jail diversion programs that merit some elaboration and clarification before moving into a review of risk assessment tools and their components.

First, there will always be uncertainty regarding whether or not a person presents a threat to public safety, even if a risk assessment is completed. People and their behavior do not occur in a void; individual behavior, including violence, is influenced by a complex and nested system of individual, social, community, and societal level factors (see Figure 12.1).[16] Risk assessment tools can help identify and estimate risk associated with some, but not all of these influences; some will remain unknown, unanticipated, or unexpected. Even after a well-done risk assessment, we cannot say with 100% certainty that a person does or does not present a danger to the public or that they will or will not engage in future violence. Instead, the process of risk assessment can help us improve the consistency and accuracy, as well as the transparency, with which we estimate risk to public safety.

Second, the process of risk assessment will occur in the context of mental health jail diversion regardless of whether or not a risk assessment tool is used. That is,

every time a decision is made regarding the eligibility of an individual for mental health jail diversion, their threat to public safety will be considered. In the absence of the use of a risk assessment tool, a judge or other decision-maker will review and integrate the facts of the case, official records, and whatever other information may be presented in court to arrive at a decision regarding whether the individual poses an unreasonable and/or unmanageable threat to public safety. Instead of replacing the exercise of judicial discretion, risk assessment tools provide information that can be used to inform these decisions.[6] The information they produce should be considered within the full range of eligibility criteria, some – or even most – of which will *not* be addressed in the risk assessment process (e.g. diagnostic criteria, evidence regarding the role mental health problems played in the charged offense[s]).

Third, the process of risk assessment should be distinguished from other types of screening or assessment processes that may occur in mental health jail diversion programs. For instance, risk assessment should be distinguished from risk screening, which differs in terms of both the process and goals. The goal of risk *screening,* on the one hand, is to quickly identify individuals who are *potentially* at heightened risk of threat to public safety and should receive a more in-depth risk assessment.[17] Risk screening tools comprise just a handful of items that can be scored through a short interview, based on information readily available in records, or even self-administered. The process of risk *assessment,* on the other hand, involves a more comprehensive evaluation to inform an estimate regarding the risk they pose to public safety and how this risk can be managed (or not). Risk

Society	
Social and cultural norms, and health, economic, educational, and social policies	• Mental health stigma • Funding for public mental health services
Community	
Social and physical environments	• Few recreational opportunities • Limited work opportunities • Neighborhood disorganization
Social	
Closest social circle, including peers, partners, and family	• Antisocial friends and family • Relationship instability • Social isolation
Individual	
Personal characteristics, beliefs, or behaviors	• Mental health symptoms • Substance abuse • Antisocial attitudes • Homelessness

Figure 12.1 Nested levels of factors relevant to threat to public safety among mental health jail diversion program participants.

Note: Adapted from the Centers for Disease Control and Prevention's Social-Ecological Model of violence prevention.[82] Factors listed at each level are examples and are not exhaustive.

assessment will typically require more intensive data gathering efforts, more time, and a greater degree of training and expertise than risk screening, but it also should provide more in-depth and accurate information. For jurisdictions facing a high rate of bookings, risk screening might represent an efficient strategy for reducing the number of people for whom a full risk assessment is needed.[17] To do so, risk screening would be conducted as soon as possible to screen in those who require further evaluation.

Fourth, risk assessment should be distinguished from assessments of specific characteristics, behaviors, or domains of functioning, such as personality, substance use, cognitive functioning, or criminal thinking. As for risk assessment, assessments of specific characteristics, behaviors, or functioning may be completed via unstructured professional judgment or using clinical, behavioral, personality, and criminal thinking assessment tools. Such instruments were not designed to assess risk to public safety, even though their results may be statistically associated with risk to public safety[18] and they may be used for this purpose in practice.[19,20] To be clear, results of these assessments can provide information relevant to understanding an individual's threat to public safety, but they do not provide the full picture.

Risk and Protective Factors

Risk assessment tools are comprised of items that measure characteristics of a person, their case, and their circumstances. Some items are associated with increases in their risk to public safety. In the context of risk assessment, these characteristics are often referred to as risk factors. Other terms, such as precipitating or aggravating factors, may be used in other settings or contexts with similar (but not exactly the same) meaning. Some items included in risk assessment tools may be associated with decreases in their risk to public safety. Although there is some discussion and debate regarding their exact definition and function, such characteristics are often referred to as protective factors. As for risk factors, protective factors may be referred to using different terms with similar but not exactly the same meaning, such as mitigating factors, buffers, resources, or strengths.

Even though the term *risk factor* is frequently applied in the context of risk assessment, a characteristic must meet two criteria to be appropriately labeled a risk factor. The first criterion is that the characteristic correlates (statistically) with the outcome of interest, in this case, threat to public safety. The second criterion is that it occurs before the outcome of interest.[21] For example, assuming violent recidivism is our working definition of threat to public safety, drug use is a risk factor *if* drug use is statistically correlated with violent recidivism *and* it occurs before the new violent crime is perpetrated. If the drug use occurs after perpetrating a new violent crime, then it is a correlate of violent recidivism but not a risk factor. The characteristic, in this example drug use, may be related to a person's threat to public safety, but it does not *predict* or *cause* it. Kraemer and colleagues[21] further distinguish between types of risk factors that can and cannot change, a distinction we return to later.

There have been many different conceptualizations of the relationship between risk and protective factors.[22] Protective factors have been described as qualitatively distinct from risk factors, showing direct and independent associations with key negative outcomes, including threat to public safety.[23,24] For instance, the absence of a history of child abuse does not necessarily indicate the presence of a warm, supportive relationship with an adult caregiver during childhood. As another example, the absence of unemployment does not necessarily suggest the presence of stable, ongoing employment that would mitigate risk. Protective factors also have been described as mitigating factors that dampen the effect of a risk factor but do not directly predict negative outcomes.[4,25] To demonstrate, a supportive family environment may buffer the severity of the impact of a risk factor, such as substance abuse, on criminal behavior by affording opportunities for symptom monitoring in the community and facilitating treatment engagement. However, this definition may be limiting when one considers that a supportive family environment – even in the absence of problematic substance use – also may directly reduce an individual's risk of criminal justice involvement. Though risk and protective factors may be correlated, research shows they contribute relevant and distinct information that improves the predictive accuracy of risk assessments,[26,27] and in mental health jail diversion settings specifically.[28,29]

Further, in high risk and high need populations, such as mental health jail diversion program participants, protective factors may better discriminate between individuals than risk factors because the latter show *ceiling effects*. That is, mental health jail diversion program participants may have many – if not most – risk factors included in a given tool, there is greater variability in terms of the presence and strength of protective factors. To demonstrate, one investigation of 95 mental health jail diversion program participants showed that protective factors, as operationalized by Short-Term Assessment of Risk and Treatability (START)[30] assessments, were stronger predictors of rearrests and jail days relative to risk factors across multiple follow-up periods (ranging from 3 to 18 months). In the same study, protective factors showed less evidence of differential predictive validity as a function of race relative to risk factors.[29] Other work shows that participants who succeed in mental health diversion programs often attribute their success to positive changes in their lives, such as increased participation in prosocial activities, improved family relationships, and greater community engagement.[31] Overall, research suggests protective factors capture distinct information regarding an individual's threat to public safety and should be considered in the context of mental health jail diversion programs.

Type and Timing of Factors

Understanding the different types and timing of risk and protective factors as they relate to an individual's threat to public safety can improve the specificity, accuracy, and practical utility of risk assessment tools in the context of mental health jail diversion programs. Risk and protective factors can be either static or dynamic, as a function of the degree to which they can change. *Static factors* are historical or otherwise unchangeable characteristics, such as the age of first offense or the current charge(s). *Dynamic factors* are characteristics that may change over time or when targeted in treatment,[32] such as prosocial activities, employment, housing, or substance use. Dynamic factors can be either *stable,* changing relatively slowly, or *acute,* changing relatively quickly. For instance, procriminal attitudes or antisocial peers are potentially dynamic in nature but may be relatively stable, changing over time at a relatively slow rate.

Other characteristics, such as an individual's neighborhood, may be dynamic but stable due to external or systemic barriers (e.g. poverty). At the same time, factors such as mental health symptoms or substance use may change more quickly, especially under stressful conditions such as release from jail into a community treatment setting. Community re-entry, in particular, has been shown to trigger substance use relapse and to exacerbate mental health symptoms.[33] As such, static, stable dynamic, and acute dynamic factors would have different program implications and need to be addressed and monitored in different ways in the context of mental health jail diversion. Further, static factors may be more relevant to decisions regarding *inter*individual risk level, such as appropriateness for diversion, whereas dynamic factors may be more relevant to decisions regarding *intra*individual risk, including specific risk management strategies.[34]

Risk and protective factors can also be distal or proximal, depending on when they occur. *Distal factors* are those factors that occurred in the more distant past, such as child abuse or a history of drug use, whereas *proximal factors* are those factors that occurred more recently or are currently present. Research suggests that distal factors are more relevant to outcomes over the longer term, spanning several months to years, and that proximal factors are more relevant to outcomes over the shorter term, such as the coming days to weeks.[35,36] To demonstrate, a person may have a history of drug use but has been clean for several years. This history of drug use may elevate risk for perpetrating crime years into the future, but risk for perpetrating new violent crime over the coming months may be low (or, at least, be unaffected by this risk factor).

Further, there may be events that limit the relevance of historical factors, such as physical incapacity, setting, relationships, employment, intervention, or the passage of time.[37] These distinctions are not just relevant to forecasting threat to public safety, but also mitigating risk.

Finally, a distinction is often made between factors that reflect *risk* versus *need*. Risk factors, as defined earlier, are associated with increased threat to public safety, but the association between needs and threat to public safety is more complicated. *Criminogenic needs* represent the intervention target(s) of identified dynamic risk factors.[38] For instance, if an individual has antisocial attitudes, then intervention should aim to reduce antisocial cognition, increase recognition of risky thinking and feeling, and promote anticriminal, less risky thinking and feeling. As another example, if an individual has substance use problems, then intervention could be focused on reducing substance misuse, managing cravings, and reducing substance-use related interpersonal supports and behaviors. *Noncriminogenic needs,* on the other hand, may represent important areas for treatment and intervention, such as emotional distress, that do not directly contribute to risk to public safety. Noncriminogenic needs are sometimes referred to as *treatment* or *clinical needs*.

In the context of mental health jail diversion programs, however, treatment needs may in fact be criminogenic in nature. Specifically, eligibility criteria for participation in mental health jail diversion programs often include evidence that the mental disorder played a significant role in the commission of the charge(s) and that treatment of the mental health disorder would reduce an individual's risk of recidivism.[7] While there is much debate in the field, methodologically rigorous studies show that some symptoms of serious mental disorders can be causally related to violence risk.[39] There are also large-scale studies demonstrating that psychiatric treatment, including medication and outpatient treatment, reduces recidivism rates among persons with serious mental disorders[40,41] (see Figure 12.2). At the same time, there may be multiple factors contributing to risk to public safety among persons with serious mental disorders.[42] As such, treatment of mental health *and* criminogenic needs may be necessary to ultimately – and effectively – reduce risk. Indeed, research demonstrates the importance of criminogenic factors in predicting noncompliance and rearrest among mental health jail diversion participants[43] and suggests that programs targeting general risk factors, such as cognitive behavioral therapy, are more effective in reducing recidivism than is mental health treatment alone.[44]

Predicting Outcomes

Risk assessment tools differ not only in their content, but also in their intended outcome. Not all risk assessment tools predict the same outcomes over the same period of time using the same strategies. By and large, risk assessment tools estimate threat to public safety in one of two ways: (1) the application of algorithms and actuarial tables, or (2) structured professional judgment. Actuarial risk assessment involves scoring items, and then weighting and combining these scores to arrive at total risk scores. The methods through which item ratings are weightened and combined differ, but generally reflect the degree to which the items are related to the outcome of interest and the statistical association between the items in the development sample(s). The risk scores, then, are cross-referenced with actuarial tables to identify the estimated outcome probabilities and assign a risk level.[45] Some actuarial risk assessment tools have been developed and calibrated using machine learning, while others have used less complicated methods. Structured professional judgment tools, in comparison, guide assessors to consider conceptually relevant and evidence-based factors. Even though items may be given numerical scores, assessors ultimately estimate the risk level based on their professional judgment rather than using total scores.[46] Research reviews show that both approaches predict public safety risks with comparable levels of consistency and accuracy.[47] Some risk assessment tools use a hybrid approach that combines features of the actuarial and structured professional judgment approaches. Specifically, these instruments provide the assessor with the option to over-ride the statistically estimated level of risk to assign a higher or lower final risk estimate. Research on the predictive validity of over-rides is limited and the findings that do exist are mixed.[48,49]

Some risk assessment tools are designed to predict general recidivism risk, including committing a new crime (nonviolent and violent) and violating conditions of probation or parole. More than 60 such risk assessment tools have been identified as being used in criminal justice settings in the United States.[50] Other tools are designed to forecast violence risk, which may or may not qualify as violent *recidivism* (e.g. a first instance of violence or behavior that is violent in nature but does not meet standards to be prosecuted as a crime). Such tools forecast violence risk over different periods of time and among different

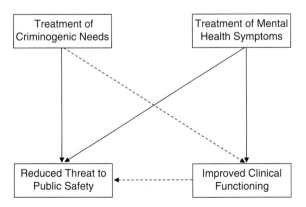

Figure 12.2 Treatment of criminogenic and mental health needs among mental health jail diversion program participants.

Note: Solid lines represent direct effects; dashed lines represent indirect effects.

populations, including adults with mental health problems. Other tools are designed to estimate risk of specific forms of violence or offending, including sexual violence, domestic violence, drug offenses, or traffic offenses. Most recently, in the wake of a new wave of bail reform, there has been renewed focus on risk assessment tools that are designed to estimate risk of failure to appear in court and perpetration of a new (violent) crime during the pre-trial period.[6] Other tools, still, estimate risk for multiple adverse outcomes, including but not limited to threats to public safety.

Risk assessment tools also differ in the degree to which they are designed to inform risk management.[51] Some risk assessment tools, referred to as the second generation of risk assessment, conceptualize risk prediction as the goal of risk assessment. Thus, their results – or the item ratings at least – are not intended to guide risk management and treatment planning through the identification of intervention targets.[51] Given the emphasis of mental health jail diversion programs on community-based risk management and treatment, second generation risk assessment tools may have limited utility. Other risk assessment tools, referred to as the third generation of risk assessment, include dynamic factors that are relevant to risk management and treatment. Though they do include treatment-relevant factors, they do not explicitly (or automatically) incorporate assessment results into a risk management plan. Finally, some risk assessment tools, referred to as the fourth generation of risk assessment, explicitly integrate case planning and risk management into the risk assessment process, with the goal of enhancing treatment and supervision.

Predictive Validity

To date, only a handful of studies have reported on the predictive validity of risk assessments conducted in mental health jail diversion programs, specifically. In a sample of 175 jail diversion participants with co-occurring mental health and substance use problems in New York City, for example, Broner and colleagues[52] examined the predictive validity of risk assessments completed using the Historical-Clinical-Risk Management 20 (HCR-20)[53] vis-à-vis program compliance and recidivism, defined as new jail bookings and felony rearrests. The HCR-20 assessments demonstrated validity in predicting these outcomes, but were a stronger predictor of felony rearrests than jail bookings. In another study, Barber-Rioja and

colleagues[54] examined the predictive validity of HCR-20 assessments with respect to any diversion noncompliance and reincarceration in 131 mental health jail diversion participants. Findings revealed good validity in predicting outcomes assessed 12 months following the start of diversion program participation.

Two more recent investigations have examined the predictive validity of Level of Service Inventory-Revised (LSI-R)[55] assessments in 146 mental health court participants[56] and 95 mental health jail diversion participants,[29] respectively. In the study of mental health court participants, LSI-R total scores were associated with likelihood of program termination, after controlling for offense characteristics, prior violations, prior jail days, and time in program.[56] (Recidivism was not examined as an outcome in this study.) In the study of mental health jail diversion program participants, LSI-R total scores predicted rearrests and jail days across 3- to 12-month follow-up periods, whereas the LSI-R risk classifications (i.e. categorizations from very low to very high) predicted rearrests and jail days up to 18 months after assessment. This study also examined the validity of START assessments in predicting criminal justice outcomes. Results showed that START vulnerability total scores predicted rearrests and jail days across 6- to 18-month follow-up periods, whereas the START strength total scores predicted rearrests and jail days across all follow-up periods (up to 18 months). In fact, strength total scores were the strongest predictor of recidivism across follow-up periods and outcomes. START general offending risk estimates (piloted in this study) predicted jail days across all follow-up periods, but only predicted rearrests at 12-month follow-up. In a final study of 550 mental health jail diversion program participants,[28] START strength total scores predicted both rearrests and jail days 12 months following the date of assessment and after controlling for mental health diagnosis and demographic characteristics, whereas START vulnerability total scores predicted jail days but not rearrests.

Taken together the extant research suggests assessments completed using structured risk assessment tools – and the HCR-20, LSI-R, and START, in particular – can be used to evaluate risk of recidivism and other key program outcomes with good predictive validity among mental health jail diversion program participants. However, the number of published studies reporting on the predictive validity of risk assessments completed in jail diversion programs, mental health or otherwise, is relatively small. Consistent with implementation best practices,[57] there should be local, pilot implementation and evaluation of risk assessment tools prior to full-scale implementation. Pilot implementation and evaluation will afford the opportunity to establish jurisdiction-specific validity and to identify local barriers to and facilitators of implementation with fidelity.[58]

Using Risk Assessment Tools in Mental Health Jail Diversion Programs

The use of risk assessment tools in and of itself will not improve decisions and mitigate risk in the context of mental health jail diversion programs. Instead, risk assessment tools must be implemented with fidelity and their results must inform decisions and case planning in meaningful ways. Moreover, the resources to manage the identified threat to public safety and treat identified needs also must be available in the community. Finally, the risk assessments should be routinely reviewed and amended throughout the duration of an individual's participation in the mental health jail diversion programs. We delve into these issues in more detail in the sections that follow.

Implementation

Done well, implementation of a risk assessment tool – in the context of mental health jail diversion programs or otherwise – is a time and resource intensive process. It is also key to promoting public safety. Many factors can affect the fidelity with which risk assessment tools are implemented in mental health jail diversion programs. To demonstrate, a recent systematic review of 11 studies evaluating the implementation of violence risk assessment tools in psychiatric and correctional settings identified four categories of factors that affected implementation outcomes: (1) characteristics of the risk assessment instrument itself (e.g. adaptability, perceived utility); (2) characteristics of the assessors (e.g. knowledge, attitudes, and beliefs); (3) characteristics of the setting (e.g. size and complexity of the organization, staff turnover); and (4) the implementation process (e.g. implementation plan, stakeholder engagement, implementation leaders).[59] A detailed discussion of evidence-based strategies to support implementation of risk assessment tools in mental health jail diversion programs is beyond the scope of this paper. Readers are referred to the guidebook developed by Vincent, Guy, and Grisso[57]

to support the implementation of risk assessment tools in juvenile justice settings. Many of the strategies and resources provided therein could be adapted and applied to the context of mental health jail diversion programs.

There is scant research examining the implementation of risk assessment tools in mental health jail diversion programs. In a paper describing the implementation of START in the Miami-Dade Criminal Mental Health Project's misdemeanor and felony pretrial diversion programs,[60] results showed that the modal number of missing item ratings and missing risk estimates was zero, supporting the feasibility of completing START assessments in this setting. Further, START strength and vulnerability total scores, as well as risk estimates, related with each other and differed in the expected directions across the misdemeanor and felony programs, suggesting that START assessments can be completed with fidelity in mental health jail diversion programs. However, this study did not report on other implementation outcomes, such as acceptability, adoption, penetration, and sustainability.[61] Additionally, Levin and colleagues' review[59] raised concerns about the quality of risk assessment implementation studies more generally. Specifically, the authors rated just 2 of the 11 studies as being good quality; most studies were rated as inconsistent or poor in quality. As such, rigorous evaluation of the implementation of risk assessment tools in mental health jail diversion programs is an important avenue for future research.[62]

Informing Decisions

The Risk-Need-Responsivity model provides a framework for how to use the results of risk assessment tools to inform decisions and case planning in mental health jail diversion programs. The *risk principle* describes the calibration of supervision and resources with an individual's level of risk; the greater the level of risk, the greater the supervision and resources, and vice versa.[38] For mental health jail diversion programs, this principle speaks to two issues: (1) the appropriateness of an individual for diversion, and (2) frequency and intensity of supervision and intervention. First, an individual must pose a level of risk that is simultaneously high enough to warrant the level of resources, supervision, and intervention that will be afforded through participation in a mental health jail diversion program. There is a tendency to assume that lower risk individuals should be diverted and higher risk individuals should be detained; however, mental health jail diversion programs may be most appropriate for individuals who pose heightened risk to public safety, *if resources are available to manage that risk in the community.* Mental health jail diversion programs may represent a level of intervention that is too high for low risk individuals.[63–65] In fact, overintervening with low risk individuals can actually *increase* threat to public safety by increasing risk factors and reducing protective factors.[66]

Second, the frequency and intensity of supervision and intervention in mental health jail diversion programs should be calibrated with risk. Persons at lower risk to public safety should receive less frequent and less intense supervision and services, while those who pose greater risk to public safety should be assigned more frequent and more intense supervision and services. In practice, such calibration may occur in the context of mental health jail diversion programs through conditions and supervision strategies (e.g. house arrest, electronic monitoring), frequency of supervision meetings or court appearances, and treatment dosage (both pharmacological and psychosocial). There are no universal standards or guidelines regarding the type and numbers of hours of supervision or treatment required as a function of a given level of risk to public safety. As noted earlier, some risk assessment tools provide case management recommendations that could include such guidance. There also have been efforts to develop recommendations regarding frequency and intensity of intervention that are not tool-specific, including a five-level risk and needs system that includes guidance regarding approximate number of hours of supervision per level.[67] However, neither the tool-generated nor five-level risk and needs system guidelines have been evaluated in the context of mental health jail diversion programs. In practice, guidelines regarding the frequency and intensity of supervision and services vis-à-vis the results of a risk assessment tool should be developed prior to implementation.

The *need principle* asserts that interventions should target criminogenic needs. Much has been written about the "central eight" risk/needs factors that are major predictors of criminal behavior at a population level: criminal history, antisocial personality pattern, procriminal attitudes, antisocial peers, substance abuse, family/marital relationships, school/work, and leisure activities.[68] Even though these central eight factors may increase risk across a population, they may or may not increase

risk for a given person. As such, interventions should target needs that increase public safety risk *for that individual.* The reasons and motivations for criminal behavior may differ from person to person; one person may be heavily influenced by antisocial peers and have few prosocial contacts, while another person may have antisocial peers, but is not negatively influenced by their antisocial attitudes, beliefs, or behaviors. An intervention focused on positive peer support may have greater effectiveness in reducing risk in the former than latter case. Risk assessment tools that include at least some dynamic factors will provide critical, person-specific information regarding behaviors, beliefs, or other factors to be targeted in treatment.

There has been relatively limited investigation of the risk and need principles in the context of mental health jail diversion programs. In one study of 107 mental health court participants, Campbell and colleagues[69] examined the program's adherence to the risk and need principles using the Level of Service Inventory/Risk-Need-Responsivity (LSI/RNR)[70] tool. Findings showed higher LSI/RNR total scores were associated with greater receipt of behavioral health interventions, providing support for adherence to the risk principle. The authors examined adherence to the need principle in a subset of 48 participants. Results showed that only one in every three needs were targeted in case plans, suggesting relatively poor adherence to the need principle (also referred to as "treatment match"). Yet, as the number of identified needs that were targeted through case plans increased, the rate of new offenses following exit from the mental health court decreased. Research conducted in other community-based, justice-involved populations has similarly demonstrated that implementation of risk assessment tools does not uniformly increase treatment match, but that increases in treatment match are associated with reductions in risk to public safety.[13,14,71] Although applying the need principle in practice may be challenging, when it is done well, there are observable improvements in public safety.

Finally, the *responsivity principle* describes the importance of tailoring risk management and treatment strategies to a person's abilities, motivation, and strengths. There are two types of responsivity: general and specific. *General responsivity* refers to the use of cognitive social learning methods, such as prosocial modeling, reinforcement, and problem solving.[72] *Specific responsivity* refers to the adaptation of interventions to take into account a person's strengths, personality, motivation, and social characteristics (e.g. race, gender, culture). Evidence supporting the use of culturally appropriate,[73] gender responsive,[74] and trauma-informed interventions[75] in criminal justice settings speaks to the importance of responsivity vis-à-vis risk reduction. Further, interventions focused on enhancing motivation could promote service utilization and engagement, as well as overall treatment response.[76,77] No study, to our knowledge, has examined responsivity – general or specific – in the context of mental health jail diversion programs specifically. Nonetheless, responsivity may be the key to reducing public safety risk and improving outcomes among justice-involved persons with mental health problems. In particular, the severity of mental health problems that are often required to meet diversion eligibility criteria may represent a degree of cognitive impairment that necessitates treatment modifications to promote accessibility, acceptability, feasibility, and relevance.[78,79]

Beyond application of the RNR principles, risk assessment results must be reviewed and amended over time to promote their utility and effectiveness in mental health jail diversion programs. A fundamental assumption of mental health jail diversion programs is that an individual's risk to public safety can – and will – change over time as a result of intervention. As noted earlier, a person's risk to public safety at any given time reflects a complex interplay of diverse factors that will be affected by changes in their circumstances.[37] For these reasons, risk assessments will have a shelf life. Though research has demonstrated that dynamic factors do change over time,[80,81] there is limited evidence regarding the optimal period of time for reassessment and review.[23] In practice, optimal periods for review and reassessment may differ per person as a function of their case characteristics, current functioning, and circumstances. Mechanisms should be put in place to afford reassessment of a person's threat to public safety, as well as policies and protocols that specify the circumstances that would trigger reassessment during their participation in mental health jail diversion programs. These may include but are not limited to regularly scheduled reviews (e.g. every three months during community supervision meetings), major life events (e.g. loss of a loved one, change in employment or housing status), or transitions (e.g. re-entry from a treatment center into the community).

Conclusion

Risk assessment tools were developed to support consistency and accuracy, as well as transparency, in criminal justice decisions, including those pertaining to supervision, release, and case management. To that end, risk assessment tools are increasingly being used in mental health jail diversion settings to inform decisions regarding an individual's appropriateness and eligibility for mental health jail diversion programs as a function of their estimated threat to public safety and the strategies that may be successful in mitigating risk. Even though there have been relatively few studies of risk assessment tools in the context of mental health jail diversion programs, specifically, what research does exist suggests that they can be implemented with fidelity and that their results predict a variety of relevant public safety outcomes, including recidivism and program completion, with good accuracy. That said, questions remain regarding the impact that risk assessment tools may have on mental health jail diversion program participation and outcomes. Given the unique considerations of mental health jail diversion programs and the typically high risk and high need nature of program participants, risk assessment tools that consider protective factors may be particularly well suited to support decision-making that leads to improved outcomes in this context.

Disclosures

Dr. Sarah L. Desmarais is a co-author of the risk assessment tool, the Short-Term Assessment of Risk and Treatability (START). Dr. Evan M. Lowder has nothing to disclose.

References

1. Munetz MR, Griffin PA. Use of the Sequential Intercept Model as an approach to decriminalization of people with serious mental illness. *Psychiatr Serv*. 2006; **57**(4): 544–549.

2. Case B, Steadman HJ, Dupuis SA, Morris LS. Who succeeds in jail diversion programs for persons with mental illness?: a multi-site study. *Behav Sci Law*. 2009; **27**(5): 661–674.

3. US Department of Health & Human Services. Adult mental health treatment court locator. SAMHSA's GAINS Center; 2019. www.samhsa.gov/gains-center/mental-health-treatment-court-locator/adults (accessed June 2020).

4. Monahan J, Skeem JL. Risk assessment in criminal sentencing. *Annu Rev Clin Psychol*. 2016; **12**: 489–513.

5. Casey PM, Warren RK, Elek JK. *Using Offender Risk and Needs Assessment Information at Sentencing: Guidance for Courts from a National Working Group*. Williamsburg, VA: National Center for State Courts; 2011.

6. Desmarais SL, Lowder EM. *Pretrial Risk Assessment Tools: A Primer for Judges, Prosecutors, and Defense Attorneys*. Chicago, IL; 2019.

7. Barber-Rioja V, Rotter M, Schombs F. Diversion evaluations: a specialized forensic examination. *Behav Sci Law*. 2017; **35**(5–6): 418–430.

8. Talesh S. Mental health court judges as dynamic risk managers: a new conceptualization of the role of judges. *DePaul L Rev*. 2007; **57**: 93.

9. Ægisdóttir S, White MJ, Spengler PM, et al. The meta-analysis of clinical judgment project: fifty-six years of accumulated research on clinical versus statistical prediction. *Couns Psychol*. 2006; **34**(3): 341–382.

10. Grove WM, Meehl PE. Comparative efficiency of informal (subjective, impressionistic) and formal (mechanical, algorithmic) prediction procedures: The clinical-statistical controversy. *Psychol Public Policy Law*. 1996; **2**(2): 293–323.

11. Grove WM, Zald DH, Lebow BS, Snitz BE, Nelson C. Clinical versus mechanical prediction: a meta-analysis. *Psychol Assess*. 2000; **12**(1): 19.

12. Mamalian CA. *State of the Science of Pretrial Risk Assessment*. Washington, DC: U.S. Bureau of Justice Assistance; 2011.

13. Singh JP, Desmarais SL, Sellers BG, et al. From risk assessment to risk management: matching interventions to adolescent offenders' strengths and vulnerabilities. *Child Youth Serv Rev*. 2014; **47**: 1–9.

14. Vieira TA, Skilling TA, Peterson-Badali M. Matching court-ordered services with treatment needs: predicting treatment success with young offenders. *Crim Justice Behav*. 2009; **36**(4): 385–401.

15. Vincent GM, Paiva-Salisbury ML, Cook NE, Guy LS, Perrault RT. Impact of risk/needs assessment on juvenile probation officers' decision making: importance of implementation. *Psychol Public Policy Law*. 2012; **18**(4): 549–576.

16. Krug EG, Mercy JA, Dahlberg LL, Zwi AB. The world report on violence and health. *Lancet*. 2002; **360** (9339): 1083–1088.

17. Cartwright JK, Desmarais SL, Johnson KL, Van Dorn RA. Performance and clinical utility of a short violence risk screening tool in U.S. adults with mental illness. *Psychol Serv*. 2018; **15**(4): 398–408.

18. Dolan M, Doyle M. Violence risk prediction: clinical and actuarial measures and the role of the Psychopathy Checklist. *Br J Psychiatry*. 2000; **177**: 303–311.

19. Singh JP, Desmarais SL, Hurducas C, et al. International perspectives on the practical application of violence risk assessment: a global survey of 44 countries. *Int J Forensic Ment Health*. 2014; **13**(3): 193–206.

20. Viljoen JL, McLachlan K, Vincent GM. Assessing violence risk and psychopathy in juvenile and adult offenders: a survey of clinical practices. *Assessment*. 2010; **17**(3): 377–395.

21. Kraemer HC, Kazdin AE, Offord DR, et al. Coming to terms with the terms of risk. *Arch Gen Psychiatry*. 1997; **54**(4): 337–343.

22. Klepfisz G, Daffern M, Day A. Understanding protective factors for violent reoffending in adults. *Aggress Violent Behav*. 2017; **32**: 80–87.

23. Webster CD, Nicholls TL, Martin ML, Desmarais SL, Brink J. Short-Term Assessment of Risk and Treatability (START): the case for a new structured professional judgment scheme. *Behav Sci Law*. 2006; **24**(6): 747–766.

24. Rogers R. The uncritical acceptance of risk assessment in forensic practice. *Law Hum Behav*. 2000; **24**(5): 595–605.

25. Rutter M. Psychosocial resilience and protective mechanisms. *Am J Orthopsychiatry*. 1987; **57**(3): 316–331.

26. Desmarais SL, Nicholls TL, Wilson CM, Brink J. Using dynamic risk and protective factors to predict inpatient aggression: reliability and validity of START assessments. *Psychol Assess*. 2012; **24**(3): 685–700.

27. Serin RC, Chadwick N, Lloyd CD. Dynamic risk and protective factors. *Psychol Crime Law*. 2016; **22**(1–2): 151–170.

28. Lowder EM, Desmarais SL, Rade CB, Coffey T, Van Dorn RA. Models of protection against recidivism in justice-involved adults with mental illnesses. *Crim Justice Behav*. 2017; **44**(7): 893–911.

29. Lowder EM, Desmarais SL, Rade CB, Johnson KL, Van Dorn RA. Reliability and validity of START and LSI-R assessments in mental health jail diversion clients. *Assessment*. 2019; **26**(7): 1347–1361.

30. Webster CD, Martin M-L, Brink J, Nicholls TL, Desmarais SL. *Manual for the Short-Term Assessment of Risk and Treatability (START)*. 1.1 edn. Coquitlam, Canada: British Columbia Mental Health and Addiction Services; 2009.

31. Yuan Y, Capriotti MR. The impact of mental health court: a Sacramento case study. *Behav Sci Law*. 2019; **37**(4): 452–467.

32. Douglas KS, Skeem JL. Violence risk assessment: getting specific about being dynamic. *Psychol Public Policy Law.* 2005; **11**(3): 347–383.

33. Osher F, Steadman HJ, Barr H. A best practice approach to community reentry from jails for inmates with co-occurring disorders: the APIC model. *Crime Delinq.* 2003; **49**(1): 79–96.

34. Douglas KS, Skeem JL. Violence risk assessment: getting specific about being dynamic. *Psychol Public Policy Law.* 2005; **11**(3): 347.

35. Johnson KL, Desmarais SL, Grimm KJ, et al. Proximal risk factors for short-term community violence among adults with mental illnesses. *Psychiatr Serv.* 2016; **67**(7): 771–778.

36. Sadeh N, Binder RL, McNiel DE. Recent victimization increases risk for violence in justice-involved persons with mental illness. *Law Hum Behav.* 2014; **38**(2): 119–125.

37. Buchanan A, Binder R, Norko M, Swartz M. Psychiatric violence risk assessment. *Am J Psychiatry.* 2012; **169**(3): 340.

38. Andrews DA, Bonta J. Rehabilitating criminal justice policy and practice. *Psychol Public Policy Law.* 2010; **16**(1): 39–55.

39. Van Dorn RA, Grimm KJ, Desmarais SL, et al. Leading indicators of community-based violent events among adults with mental illness. *Psychol Med.* 2017; **47**(7): 1179–1191.

40. Van Dorn RA, Andel R, Boaz TL, et al. Risk of arrest in persons with schizophrenia and bipolar disorder in a Florida Medicaid program: the role of atypical antipsychotics, conventional neuroleptics, and routine outpatient behavioral health services. *J Clin Psychiatry.* 2011; **72**(4): 502–508.

41. Van Dorn RA, Desmarais SL, Petrila J, Haynes D, Singh JP. Effects of outpatient treatment on risk of arrest of adults with serious mental illness and associated costs. *Psychiatr Serv.* 2013; **64**(9): 856–862.

42. Skeem JL, Winter E, Kennealy PJ, Louden JE, Tatar JR. Offenders with mental illness have criminogenic needs, too: toward recidivism reduction. *Law Hum Behav.* 2014; **38**(3): 212–224.

43. Honegger LN, Honegger KS. Criminogenic factors associated with noncompliance and rearrest of mental health court participants. *Crim Justice Behav.* 2019; **46**(9): 1276–1294.

44. Skeem JL, Steadman HJ, Manchak SM. Applicability of the risk-need-responsivity model to persons with mental illness involved in the criminal justice system. *Psychiatr Serv.* 2015; **66**(9): 916–922.

45. Hilton NZ, Harris GT, Rice ME. Sixty-six years of research on the clinical versus actuarial prediction of violence. *Couns Psychol.* 2006; **34**(3): 400–409.

46. Guy LS, Packer IK, Warnken W. Assessing risk of violence using structured professional judgment guidelines. *J Forensic Psychol Pract.* 2012; **12**(3): 270–283.

47. Fazel S, Sing JP, Doll H, Grann M. Use of risk assessment instruments to predict violence and antisocial behaviour in 73 samples involving 24 827 people: Systematic review and meta-analysis. *Br Med J.* 2012; **345**: e4692.

48. Guay J-P, Parent G. Broken legs, clinical overrides, and recidivism risk: an analysis of decisions to adjust risk levels with the LS/CMI. *Crim Justice Behav.* 2018; **45**(1): 82–100.

49. Schmidt F, Sinclair SM, Thomasdóttir S. Predictive validity of the youth level of service/case management inventory with youth who have committed sexual and non-sexual offenses: the utility of professional override. *Crim Justice Behav.* 2016; **43**(3): 413–430.

50. Desmarais SL, Johnson KL, Singh JP. Performance of recidivism risk assessment instruments in U.S. correctional settings. *Psychol Serv.* 2016; **13**(3): 206–222.

51. Skeem JL, Monahan J. Current directions in violence risk assessment. *Curr Dir Psychol Sci.* 2011; **20**(1): 38–42.

52. Broner N, Mayrl DW, Landsberg G. Outcomes of mandated and nonmandated New York City jail diversion for offenders with alcohol, drug, and mental disorders. *Prison J.* 2005; **85**(1): 18–49.

53. Webster C, Douglas K, Eaves D, Hart S. *HCR-20: Assessing Risk for Violence (Version 2).* Burnaby, Canada: Mental Health Law, and Policy Institute, Simon Fraser University; 1997.

54. Barber-Rioja V, Dewey L, Kopelovich S, Kucharski LT. The utility of the HCR-20 and PCL: SV in the prediction of diversion noncompliance and reincarceration in diversion programs. *Crim Justice Behav.* 2012; **39**(4): 475–492.

55. Andrews DA, Bonta J. *Level of Service Inventory-Revised (LSI-R): User's Manual.* Toronto: Multi-Health Systems; 2001.

56. Bonfine N, Ritter C, Munetz MR. Exploring the relationship between criminogenic risk assessment and mental health court program completion. *Int J Law Psychiatry.* 2016; **45**: 9–16.

57. Vincent GM, Guy LS, Grisso T. *Risk Assessment in Juvenile Justice: A Guidebook for Implementation.* Chicago, IL: John D. and Catherine T. MacArthur Foundation; 2012.

58. Desmarais SL. Commentary: risk assessment in the age of evidence-based practice and policy. *Int J Forensic Ment Health.* 2017; **16**(1): 18–22.

59. Levin SK, Nilsen P, Bendtsen P, Bulow P. Structured risk assessment instruments: a systematic review of implementation determinants. *Psychiatr Psychol Law.* 2016; **23**(4): 602–628.

60. Desmarais SL, Van Dorn RA, Telford RP, Petrila J, Coffey T. Characteristics of START assessments completed in mental health jail diversion programs. *Behav Sci Law*. 2012; **30**(4): 448–469.

61. Proctor E, Silmere H, Raghavan R, et al. Outcomes for implementation research: conceptual distinctions, measurement challenges, and research agenda. *Adm Policy Ment Health*. 2011; **38**(2): 65–76.

62. Nonstad K, Webster CD. How to fail in the implementation of a risk assessment scheme or any other new procedure in your organization. *Am J Orthopsychiatry*. 2011; **81**(1): 94–99.

63. Hanley D. Appropriate services: examining the case classification principle. *J Offender Rehabil*. 2006; **42**(4): 1–22.

64. Spring B. Sound health care economics: provide the treatment needed (not less, not more). *Health Psychol*. 2019; **38**(8): 701–704.

65. Andrews DA, Dowden C. Risk principle of case classification in correctional treatment: a meta-analytic investigation. *Int J Offender Ther Comp Criminol*. 2006; **50**(1): 88–100.

66. Lowenkamp CT, Latessa EJ, Holsinger AM. The risk principle in action: what have we learned from 13,676 offenders and 97 correctional programs? *Crime Delinq*. 2006; **52**(1): 77–93.

67. Hanson KR, Bourgon G, McGrath RJ, *et al. A Five-Level Risk and Needs System: Maximizing Assessment Results in Corrections through the Development of a Common Language*. New York: Council of State Governments Justice Center; 2017.

68. Andrews DA, Bonta J, Wormith JS. The recent past and near future of risk and/or need assessment. *Crime Delinq*. 2006; **52**(1): 7–27.

69. Campbell MA, Canales DD, Wei R, et al. Multidimensional evaluation of a mental health court: adherence to the Risk-Need-Responsivity model. *Law Hum Behav*. 2015; **39**(5): 489–502.

70. Andrews DA, Bonta J, Wormith JS. *The Level of Service/ Risk, Need, Responsivity (LS/RNR) Manual*. Toronto: Multi-Health Systems; 2008.

71. Nelson RJ, Vincent GM. Matching services to criminogenic needs following comprehensive risk assessment implementation in juvenile probation. *Crim Justice Behav*. 2018; **45**(8): 1136–1153.

72. Dowden C, Andrews DA. The importance of staff practice in delivering effective correctional treatment: a meta-analytic review of core correctional practice. *Int J Offender Ther Comp Criminol*. 2004; **48**(2): 203–214.

73. Vergara AT, Kathuria P, Woodmass K, Janke R, Wells SJ. Effectiveness of culturally appropriate adaptations to juvenile justice services. *J Juv Justice*. 2016; **5**(2): 85.

74. Covington SS, Bloom BE. Gender responsive treatment and services in correctional settings. *Women Ther*. 2007; **29**(3–4): 9–33.

75. Levenson JS, Willis GM. Implementing trauma-informed care in correctional treatment and supervision. *J Aggress Maltreatment Trauma*. 2019; **28**(4): 481–501.

76. Heilbrun K, Pietruszka V, Thornewill A, Phillips S, Schiedel R. Diversion at re-entry using criminogenic CBT: review and prototypical program development. *Behav Sci Law*. 2017; **35**(5–6): 562–572.

77. Van Dorn RA, Desmarais SL, Rade CB, et al. Jail-to-community treatment continuum for adults with co-occurring substance use and mental disorders: study protocol for a pilot randomized controlled trial. *Trials*. 2017; **18**(1): 365.

78. Skeem JL, Manchak S, Peterson JK. Correctional policy for offenders with mental illness: creating a new paradigm for recidivism reduction. *Law Hum Behav*. 2011; **35**(2): 110–126.

79. Young S, Chick K, Gudjonsson G. A preliminary evaluation of reasoning and rehabilitation 2 in mentally disordered offenders (RR2M) across two secure forensic settings in the United Kingdom. *J Forens Psychiatry Psychol*. 2010; **21**(3): 336–349.

80. Wilson CM, Desmarais SL, Nicholls TL, Hart SD, Brink J. Predictive validity of dynamic factors: assessing violence risk in forensic psychiatric inpatients. *Law Hum Behav*. 2013; **37**(6): 377–388.

81. Sellers BG, Desmarais SL, Hanger MW. Measurement of change in dynamic factors using the START: AV. *J Forensic Psychol Pract*. 2017; **17**(3): 198–215.

82. National Center for Injury Prevention and Control, Division of Violence Prevention. The social-ecological model: a framework for prevention. Updated January 16, 2019. Accessed August 24, 2019.

Decriminalization in Action: Lessons from the Los Angeles Model

Kristen Ochoa, Oona Appel, Viet Nguyen, and Elizabeth Kim

The insane criminal has nowhere any home: no age or nation has provided a place for him. He is everywhere unwelcome and objectionable. The prisons thrust him out; the hospitals are unwilling to receive him. And yet humanity and justice, the sense of common danger, and a tender regard for a deeply degraded brother-man, all agree that something should be done for him—that some plan must be devised different from, and better than any that has yet been tried, by which he may be properly cared for, by which his malady may be healed, and his criminal propensity overcome.
Jarvis E. Criminal insane: Insane transgressors and insane convicts. Am J Psychiatry. *1857;13:195–231.*

Introduction

A home and treatment. And not giving up on anybody. That is what we do in Los Angeles to decriminalize mental illness. Our model stands on philosophies of harm reduction and housing first. It is an admittedly basic approach, but has worked to remove thousands of persons with serious mental disorders from our vast jail system. This approach asserts that many persons are in jail because of a systematic failure to adequately care for them. It is an approach that recreates systems to provide permanent care, without rationing, for the lifetime of the patient. To accomplish this, the new system must say "Yes" with the same veracity and availability of a jail bed, and with the same ease and routine of a jail booking. It has to be flexible and forgiving; it has to be a commitment to "care first, jail last."

This is not to say that we are not realists. We understand that not everyone can avoid jail, for some have crimes too serious. We also understand that, if sufficient community services existed, more than half of the jail mental health population could be released. On any given day, Los Angeles jails over 16,000 people. More than 5,000 of those reside in the mental health section of the jail. Providing an alternative place for those with serious mental disorders to live and thrive is a tremendous undertaking. Los Angeles has only begun to build a continuum of care to accommodate this need, but the concept proves that thoughtfully removing persons with serious mental disorders from the jail is possible and necessary for the health of both patients and community.

In addressing one of the greatest public health problems of our time, we can learn from other scientists. Consider ecologists, who are concerned with inter-relationships and their impact on the environment. When ecologists create reserves, they reconnect habitats that have been fragmented, allowing them to function as a whole rather than as a set of independent pieces. The Los Angeles model works to create that "reserve" through the Office of Diversion and Reentry (ODR), which connects institutions and justice partners on clinical matters and public health solutions. Through elaborate clinical interventions on behalf of persons with serious mental disorders in custody, connections are made between jail and court, community and hospital, clinic and housing, and back again.

ODR's Community-Based Programs

At the time of this writing, ODR has diverted more than 3,800 persons with serious mental disorders from the Los Angeles County Jail system. Within ODR, diversion is conceptualized as circumventing or significantly reducing jail time through linkage to housing and community treatment services. All ODR programs consist of three primary interventions: jail in-reach services, enhanced treatment efforts provided by ODR clinical staff (additional clinical assessments and initiation of medications, as indicated), and immediate interim housing upon release in anticipation of permanent supportive housing (see Figure 13.1).

The ODR Housing program provides permanent supportive housing to individuals who are homeless, have a serious mental health disorder, and who are incarcerated in the Los Angeles County Jail. This program, offered in partnership with the Los Angeles County Superior Court, is available to pre-trial defendants who have criminal felony cases. ODR Housing attempts to resolve these felony cases early and divert defendants through a grant of probation. Clients in the ODR Housing program are assigned an Intensive Case Management Services (ICMS) provider who works with the client as they transition from custody to community. ICMS providers serve as the core point of contact for supportive services including medical and mental health treatment. See Figure 13.2 for preliminary data on permanent supportive housing.

There are two programs that divert individuals found incompetent to stand trial; one program for those charged with misdemeanors, and one for those charged with felonies. These defendants are diverted into community-based settings for competency restoration treatment. Settings are tailored to meet the needs and clinical acuity of the clients; placements range from acute inpatient to open residential settings.

California Assembly Bill 1810 and Senate Bill 215 amended the California Penal Code (PC 1001.36) to create a pathway for courts to authorize pre-trial diversion. ODR's specialized use of PC 1001.36 is funded by the Department of State Hospitals (DSH), and diverts clients who are charged with felonies, have a serious mental disorder, and who may be found incompetent to stand trial if there were no clinical intervention. This program, called DSH Diversion, provides supportive housing, intensive case management, medical and mental health treatment, and specialized pre-trial probation services. Upon completion of this program, the charge(s) will be dismissed.

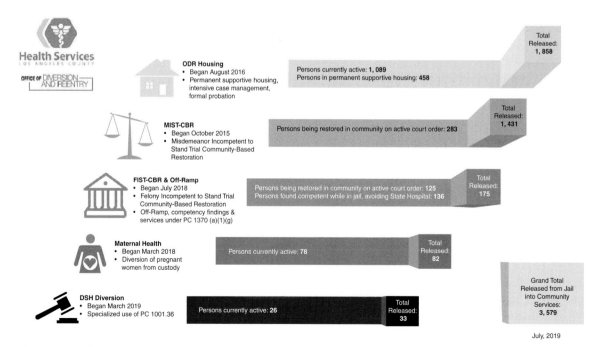

Figure 13.1 Office of Diversion and Reentry diversion dashboard.

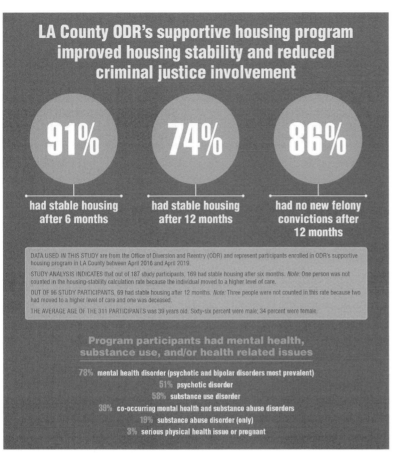

Figure 13.2 Preliminary data on ODR's permanent supportive housing program.[6]

Under the directive of the Los Angeles County Board of Supervisors, ODR created the Maternal Health Program. This program diverts pregnant women from jail to community through providing housing and supportive services. The majority of pregnant women served by ODR reside in specialized interim housing settings that allow women to remain with their children until they are moved to permanent supportive housing.

Jail diversion of people with serious mental disorders requires a continuum of care in the community. Currently, ODR's highest level of care is a dedicated psychiatric inpatient unit at Olive View-UCLA Medical Center (OVMC). Patients in this 18-bed unit are transported directly from the jail through ODR's clinical and court interventions. Prior to transport, they are among those with the highest symptom acuity in the jail, and are typically waiting for admission to the jail's psychiatric inpatient unit. Once a patient is transferred from the jail and stabilized at OVMC, they are moved to one of ODR's community-based programs.

Complex clinical and court interventions are required to divert people into the aforementioned programs. ODR's team works across spaces and disciplines to support the adversarial legal process, provide direct clinical care, and conduct forensic evaluations to hasten and expand diversion efforts.

Adversarial Process

ODR's clients have serious mental disorders, are homeless but for their jail bed, and are involved in pre-trial legal proceedings. A client's admission to an ODR program is done through court order, thus legal components are intrinsic to the work. The ODR Housing program currently operates out of two different courts ("Hubs"), which receive cases from courthouses in nearby jurisdictions ("Feeder Courts"). After a defense attorney refers a client, ODR conducts a brief review of the case and ensures it is in the correct legal posture to proceed. Through reviewing both jail and community medical records, ODR's clinical team then completes a comprehensive assessment to identify the presence of a serious mental disorder and/or serious medical need. When it remains unclear whether the client meets clinical eligibility criteria, ODR staff meets with the client in jail and/or gathers information from additional collateral sources. This understanding of the client's clinical needs informs ODR's legal interventions. If a client is deemed initially eligible clinically, ODR submits a recommendation to the court and a hearing for legal suitability is calendared. Legal suitability hearings dictate the actual disposition of a case and are by definition adversarial. However, the parties have a common goal of diverting clients with serious mental disorders from jail into appropriate treatment. When the prosecutor and defense attorney do not agree on diversion, or the judge requests a better understanding of the client, ODR serves as a neutral advisor to all parties in the courtroom. As neutral advisor, ODR helps legal partners transcend the adversarial proceedings to inform a truly collaborative effort.

Clinical Courtrooms

The role of the ODR psychiatrist is unique. They are differentiated from the correctional health psychiatrist, who often has no stake in the patient's release into the community, and additionally differentiated from the traditional forensic expert, who has no involvement in treatment. The ODR psychiatrist evaluates and manages treatment by first envisioning the patient's circumstances out of custody, then ensuring they are stable for community treatment, and finally liaising and consulting with community partners to ensure stability after release. To effectively identify, evaluate, and manage patients with serious mental disorders, the ODR psychiatrist must collaborate with justice partners, the Sheriff's department, correctional health services, and Los Angeles County's public mental health system.

Patients cannot fully engage with community services if their symptoms, often exacerbated within the jail, are not treated and stabilized prior to release. The ODR psychiatrist plays an important role in treating and stabilizing identified clients through providing evidenced-based, high-quality treatment within the correctional setting prior to release. Given that treatment adherence is a common issue when patients are in the community, the use of long-acting injections (LAIs) is prudent. In large cohort studies, LAIs have been shown to reduce mortality in patients with schizophrenia,[1] in addition to reducing relapse in symptoms compared with oral agents.[2] Along with permanent supportive housing, LAIs are a crucial part of a typical ODR client's treatment plan.

For the ODR Housing program, ODR psychiatrists are present in specialized courts that serve the entirety of Los Angeles County's criminal court system. Once candidates have gone through the initial legal and clinical screening, they present to court. In the court's lock-up area, ODR psychiatrists evaluate patients who are potentially unstable in the jail, have questionable medication regimens, are not prescribed medications at all, or whose difficulty following the rules and conditions of probation could be addressed by a medication evaluation (e.g. oral medication noncompliance in the community). ODR psychiatrists have remote access to the jail electronic medical record, and can place orders in real time after a client's case has been resolved.

Moving clinical care and treatment to the courtroom allows for enhanced collaboration between justice partners, ODR, and the patient. In addition to evaluating and potentially treating candidates, the ODR psychiatrist provides clinical expertise to the court in helping create individualized treatment plans inclusive of housing, linkage to outpatient mental health treatment, and other rehabilitative services. Likewise, probation terms can be tailored to individual needs if there is clinical expertise advising the court. This collaborative process is critical in helping ODR successfully divert patients with serious clinical needs into the community.

Forensic Evaluations

As highlighted above, ODR's work is at the intersection of mental health and the law. In addition to providing court consultation and direct clinical services, ODR staff conducts both traditional forensic evaluations (e.g. competency to stand trial) and quasi-forensic evaluations (e.g. jail diversion evaluations) to assist in diversion efforts. ODR's evaluators, including a forensically trained psychiatrist and psychologist, maintain core principles of forensic evaluation including objectivity and awareness of relevant law and ethics. Simultaneously, evaluations align with ODR's fundamental mission to reduce the population of those with serious mental disorders in the jails. ODR uses forensic evaluations as one tool in recreating the public mental health system, allowing practitioners to think more broadly about how their work impacts individuals and communities.

In California, as in many states, there has been a marked increase in defendants found incompetent to stand trial. It is well established that defendants found incompetent to stand trial languish in local jails while awaiting appropriate treatment.[3-5] Those found incompetent on felony charges in California join a lengthy waitlist for admission to DSH. To address this waitlist, ODR and DSH created new pathways for felony defendants found incompetent to stand trial. The Felony Incompetent to Stand Trial Community-Based Restoration (FIST-CBR) program was created in an effort to divert felony defendants with serious mental disorders out of the jail and into community care while under court supervision. FIST-CBR provides housing, competency restoration treatment, case management, individual and group therapy, and medication management. This small-scale deinstitutionalization effort treats defendants in the community rather than in the penal or state hospital system.

Additionally, in 2018 ODR worked with legal partners to amend the California Penal Code. The amendment, PC 1370(a)(1)(g), states that if the symptoms of a defendant found incompetent to trial "have changed to such a degree as to create a doubt in the mind of the judge as to the defendant's current mental incompetence, the court may appoint a psychiatrist or a licensed psychologist to opine as to whether the defendant has regained competence." Subsequent to this amendment, ODR staff evaluates incompetent felony defendants who may have regained competency while waiting for DSH placement. If defendants are competent, these evaluations help move their cases forward while also decreasing the burden on DSH. Moreover, by not sending competent defendants to DSH for restoration, more state hospital beds are open for patients who truly need that higher level of care.

ODR also submits competency evaluations for the most psychiatrically acute defendants in jail. These defendants often miss court due to symptom acuity, and are left with their cases being continued, resulting in prolonged detention for those with serious mental disorders. ODR tracks the legal proceedings of the most psychiatrically acute defendants in jail, and intervenes by evaluating these defendants in jail if they miss their competency-related court dates. Through these evaluations, ODR assists in hastening psychiatric treatment while also moving criminal proceedings forward. Moreover, those defendants whom ODR opines incompetent to stand trial become eligible for transfer to ODR's psychiatric inpatient unit at OVMC. Once stabilized on the inpatient unit, the defendants are transitioned to community-based restoration in an open residential setting.

Conclusion

It will take years of work to stem the tide of mass incarceration and create the necessary community resources to divert those who are homeless with serious mental disorders. Recognizing this staggering challenge, Los Angeles now has a large-scale and effective alternative to incarceration through the work of ODR. A growing commitment to scale diversion may radically decriminalize and deinstitutionalize the largest jailed population in the United States.

Disclosures

Kristen Ochoa, Oona Appel, Viet Nguyen, and Elizabeth Kim do not have anything to disclose.

References

1. Taipale H, Mittendorfer-Rutz E, Alexanderson K, et al. Antipsychotics and mortality in a nationwide cohort of 29,823 patients with schizophrenia. *Schizophr Res.* 2018; **197**: 274–280.

2. Tiihonen J, Mittendorfer-Rutz E, Majak M, et al. Real-world effectiveness of antipsychotic treatments in a nationwide cohort of 29 823 patients with schizophrenia. *JAMA Psychiatry.* 2017; **74**(7): 686–693.

3. Wortzel H, Binswanger IA, Martinez R, Filley CM, Anderson, CA. Crisis in the treatment of incompetence to proceed to trial: harbinger of a systemic illness. *J Am Acad Psychiatry Law.* 2007; **35**(3): 357–363.

4. Gowensmith NW, Frost LE, Speelman DW, Therson DE. Lookin' for beds in all the wrong places: outpatient competency restoration as a promising approach to modern challenges. *Psychol Public Policy Law.* 2016; **22**(3): 293–305.

5. Torrey EF, Kennard AD, Eslinger D, Lamb R, Pavle J. More mentally ill persons are in jails and prisons than hospitals: a survey of the states. Treatment Advocacy Center Arlington, VA and National Sheriff's Association; 2010. www.treatmentadvocacycenter.org /storage/documents/final_jails_v_hospitals_study.pdf (accessed June 2020).

6. Hunter SB, Scherling A. *Los Angeles County Office of Diversion and Reentry's Supportive Housing Program: A Study of Participants' Housing Stability and New Felony Convictions.* Santa Monica, CA: RAND Corporation; 2019. www.rand.org/pubs/research_re ports/RR3232.html (accessed June 2020).

Economics of Decriminalizing Mental Illness: When Doing the Right Thing Costs Less

Darci Delgado, Ashley M. Breth, Shelley Hill, Katherine Warburton, and Stephen M. Stahl

Are We Getting Our Money's Worth Treating Serious Mental Illness as a Crime?

U.S. health care costs are staggering, with spending at $3.5 trillion dollars in 2017.[1] Additionally, criminal justice system expenditures are estimated at $270 billion dollars.[2] Our nation's most at-risk individuals are falling through the cracks and entering a vicious cycle of incarceration and temporary institutionalization, which only exacerbates these costs.

In Figure 14.1, the movement of a person through the criminal justice system is represented by squares for each institution or system that provides an individual with mental health treatment and include: county jail,

state hospital, and prison. Within each of these institutions, costs for mental health treatment are staggering (Table 14.1). Estimates place jail treatment for individuals with mental illness at anywhere from $33,000 to $168,000 per person per year nationally.[3,4] Additionally,

Table 14.1 Cost of treatment per person per year

Treatment locale	Per person per year cost range
Local county jail[4,15]	$33,000–$168,000
State prison inpatient treatment bed[7]	$300,000–$550,000
State hospital treatment bed[5,6]	$242,000–$255,000
State prison outpatient treatment bed[7]	$80,000–$100,000
Community diversion[3,11]	$35,000–$47,000

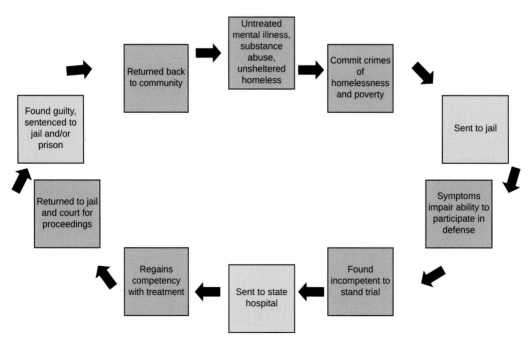

Figure 14.1 Cycle of the criminal justice system for a person with mental illness.

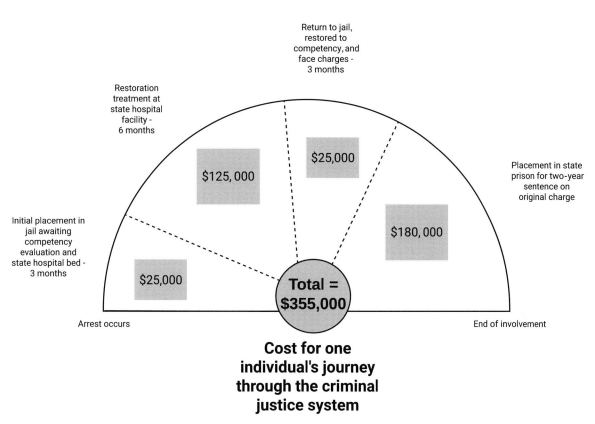

Figure 14.2 Example of estimated cost of one individual's journey through the criminal justice system.

once placed in state hospital treatment this cost increases to an average of $242,000 per patient per year in the United States (email correspondence, S. Melching, April 10, 2019).[5] The cost of a subsequent placement in state prison depends on whether an individual's mental health treatment necessitates outpatient or inpatient treatment. The former costs are noted at approximately $80,000 to $100,000 per inmate per year while the range increases substantially if inpatient mental health treatment is required: $300,000 to $550,000 per inmate per year (email correspondence, L. Koushmaro, August 30, 2018). Even with utilizing the most conservative numbers, an individual who commits a crime, undergoes competency restoration, and serves a two-year prison sentence will cost taxpayers somewhere in the range of $355,000 (Figure 14.2).

Doing Well (for the Budget) While Doing Good (for the Forensic Patient)

While these economic costs become astronomical when multiplying by the massive number of people who travel through the criminal justice system, the potential for change and fiscal improvement is equally considerable. The Sequential Intercept Model (SIM; Figure 14.3) conceptualizes how systemic interventions can break this cycle.[6] SIM provides a way for policies and programs to divert individuals out of the criminal justice system and into mental health treatment, long-term housing, and overall stability. Initial studies show promising cost savings when implementing diversion programs.[7,8] As shown in Table 14.1, the annual cost of providing mental health treatment and housing to a person in the community ranges anywhere from $35,000 to $47,333.[3,9] By successfully implementing diversion with even a small group of individuals, cost-savings could be significant. Two recent examples of the potential cost savings of these programs to communities are in San Antonio, Texas and Miami, Florida where diversion programs have saved taxpayers $10 million and $12 million per year, respectively.[3]

Consider the potential fiscal outcomes of implementing mental health diversion programs across the

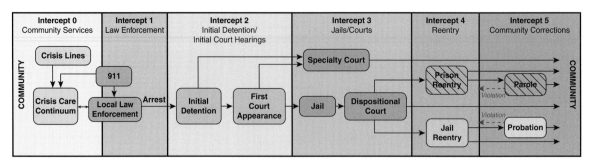

Figure 14.3 Sequential Intercept Model.[8]

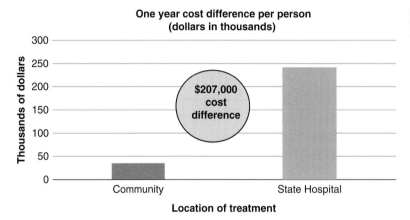

Figure 14.4 Prospective cost differences in one year of utilizing mental health diversion for one individual.

United States. These hypothetical programs could specifically target individuals who, if not for an untreated or undertreated mental illness, would not be in jail. These individuals could receive treatment for their mental illness in the community, thereby breaking the cycle of inconsistent treatment providers across multiple systems (jails, prison, state hospitals).

Given these figures, conservative estimates can be drawn on the potential fiscal savings for implementing a mental health diversion program. Estimates of community mental health treatment costs indicate that mental health diversion would cost approximately $35,000 per person per year,[3] while a forensic state hospital bed in the United States averaged $242,000 per person per year.[5] The mental health diversion of only one person could potentially save $207,000 (Figure 14.4). When including the estimated state costs of diversion participation to the annual cost of incarceration in a state prison for individuals with serious mental illnesses, the potential savings to the state are even greater Figure 14.5.

A mental health diversion program would not have difficulty finding participants within the large cohort of individuals with mental illness in the criminal justice system; a recent study[10] found that over half (56%) of the mental health population in a large U.S. jail system could be safely treated in the community if sufficient services were available. In 2016 alone, 13,734 individuals were admitted to state hospital beds around the country for competency.[5] If even 50% of these individuals (half of the 13,734 individuals admitted = 6867 people) could have instead been diverted and safely treated in the community, with a cost savings of $207,000 each, the criminal justice system would have saved a staggering $1,421,469,000 (Figure 14.5). Over $1.4 billion dollars saved, and as a bonus, individuals with mental illness receive the treatment they deserve – in the community.

Conclusions

Mental health diversion programs are a promising solution to the difficulties resulting from a combination of deinstitutionalization and state/federal funding cuts in the community behavioral healthcare system.[11] States across this country are grappling with the deluge of people suffering from serious mental illnesses who

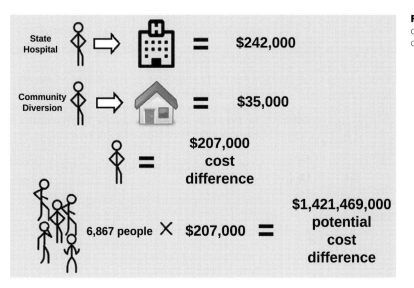

Figure 14.5 Prospective cost differences of state hospital treatment versus community diversion treatment.

often have no recourse for their illness except incarceration. The costs of this public policy problem to taxpayers is enormous and is exponentially higher for the people who cannot access needed treatment and for their families, friends, and communities. Diversion programs are an attempt to change that – to provide treatment resources in the community that stabilize these individuals, allow them to function effectively in society, and break the cycle of recidivation. Not only can diversion programs improve both criminal justice and mental health outcomes,[12,13–15] it is a fiscally responsible way to provide much-needed mental health treatment to a vulnerable population. For diversion programs to be successful, adequate financial resources must be provided during implementation and sustainability phases. Repeating past failures in community-based mental health treatment can be avoided by the provision of fiscal support for diversion programs. Such support is an investment in the future, as broad estimates demonstrate the potential for a one-year cost saving of over $1.4 billion dollars from diverting treatment out of state hospitals and into the community.

Disclosures

Dr. Delgado, Ms. Breth, Ms. Hill, and Dr. Warburton have no conflicts of interest to disclose. Over the past 36 months, Dr. Stahl has served as a consultant to Acadia, Adamas, Alkermes, Allergan, Arbor Pharmaceuticals, AstraZeneca, Avanir, Axovant, Axsome, Biogen, Biomarin, Biopharma, Celgene, Concert, ClearView, DepoMed, Dey, EnVivo, EMD Serono, Ferring, Forest, Forum, Genomind, Innovative Science Solutions, Intra-Cellular Therapies, Janssen, Jazz, Lilly, Lundbeck, Merck, Neos, Novartis, Noveida, Orexigen, Otsuka, Pam Labs, Perrigo, Pfizer, Pierre Fabre, Reviva, Servier, Shire, Sprout, Sunovion, Taisho, Takeda, Taliaz, Teva, Tonix, Trius, Vanda, Vertex, and Vifor Pharma; Dr. Stahl has been a board member of RCT Logic and Genomind; he has served on speakers bureaus for Acadia, AstraZeneca, Dey Pharma, EnVivo, Eli Lilly, Forum, Genentech, Janssen, Lundbeck, Merck, Otsuka, Pam Labs, Pfizer Israel, Servier, Sunovion, and Takeda and he has received research and/or grant support from Acadia, Alkermes, Arbor Pharmaceuticals, AssureX, AstraZeneca, Avanir, Axovant, Biogen, Braeburn Pharmaceuticals, BristolMyer Squibb, Celgene, CeNeRx, Cephalon, Dey, Eli Lilly, EnVivo, Forest, Forum, Genmmind, GlaxoSmithKline, Intra-Cellular Therapies, ISSWSH, Janssen, JayMac, Jazz, Lundbeck, Merck, Mylan, Neurocrine, Neuronetics, Novartis, Otsuka, Pam Labs, Pfizer, Reviva, Roche, Sepracor, Servier, Shire, Sprout, Sunovion, TMS NeuroHealth Centers, Takeda, Teva, Tonix, Vanda, Valeant, and Wyeth.

References

1. Martin AB, Hartman M, Washington B, Catlin A, Team NHEA. National health care spending in 2017: growth slows to post-great recession rates; share of GDP stabilizes. *Health Aff.* 2019; **38**(1): 05085.

2. White House Council of Economic Advisors. *Economic Perspectives on Incarceration and the Criminal Justice System.* Washington DC: Penny Hill Press; 2016.

3. Giliberti M. NAMI Website. -Executive-Director/May-2015/Treatment,-Not-Jail-It's-Time-to-Step-Up. 2015.

4. Salas N. *NYC Jail's Population: Who's There and Why.* New York, NY: New York City Independent Budget Office, Department of Correction; 2012.

5. Lutterman T, Shaw R, Fisher W, Manderscheid R. *Trend in Psychiatric Inpatient Capacity, United States and Each State, 1970 to 2014.* Alexandria, VA: National Association of State Mental Health Program Directors; 2017.

6. Munetz MR, Griffin PA. Use of the Sequential Intercept Model as an approach to decriminalization of people with serious mental illness. *Psychiatr Serv.* 2006; 57(4): 544–549.

7. Cowell AJ, Hinde JM, Broner N, Aldridge AP. The impact on taxpayer costs of a jail diversion program for people with serious mental illness. *Eval Program Plann.* 2013; 41: 31–37.

8. Broner N, Mayrl DW, Landsberg G. Outcomes of mandated and nonmandated New York City jail diversion for offenders with alcohol, drug, and mental disorders. *Prison J.* 2005; 85(1): 18–49.

9. Department of State Hospitals. *DSH Diversion Funding Program.* Sacramento, CA; 2018.

10. *An Estimate of Persons in the Jail Mental Health Population Likely to be Appropriate for Safe Release into Community Services.* Los Angeles County, CA: Health Services; 2019.

11. Miller JE. *Too Significant to Fail: the Importance of State Behavioral Health Agencies in the Daily Lives of Americans with Mental Illness, for Their Families, and for Their Communities.* Alexandria, VA: National Association of State Mental Health Program Directors; 2012.

12. Hoff RA, Baranosky MV, Buchanan J, Zonana H, Rosenheck RA. The effects of a jail diversion program on incarceration: a retrospective cohort study. *J Am Acad Psychiatry Law.* 1999; 27(3): 377–386.

13. Tyuse SW. The effectiveness of a jail diversion program in linking participants to federal entitlements and stable housing. *Calif J Health Promot.* 2005; 3: 84–98.

14. Steadman HJ, Naples M. Assessing the effectiveness of jail diversion programs for persons with serious mental illness and co-occurring substance use disorders. *Behav Sci Law.* 2005; 23(2): 163–170.

15. Henrichson C, Joshua R, Delaney R. *The price of jails: measuring the taxpayer cost of local incarceration.* New York, NY: Vera Institute of Justice; 2015.

Decriminalizing Severe Mental Illness by Reducing Risk of Contact with the Criminal Justice System, Including for Forensic Patients

Kimberlie Dean, Sara Singh, and Yin-Lan Soon

Introduction

Amongst those with mental illness and a history of contact with the criminal justice system (CJS), "forensic patients," constitute a small but significant subgroup. They typically have severe mental illnesses and have been charged with serious violent offences. As a group, they characteristically have complex mental health and other needs,[1] and concern about their risk of reoffending is a key consideration for those tasked with oversight of their treatment and detention. As a result, forensic patients often spend long periods in secure mental health facilities[2] and are often subject to high levels of supervision once judged to be safe to return to the community.

In many ways, the existence of this group of patients represents a failure of preventative mental health care – a criminalization of those with mental illness that lies at the extreme end of a spectrum of such criminalization. While diversion away from the CJS into mental health care following a serious index offence is a common outcome for those with severe mental illness, it can be seen as an act of diversion that has come late and at great cost, including for the victims of the serious violent offences typically committed. This review will consider the decriminalizing potential of efforts to prevent both initial and repeat contact with the CJS for those with severe mental illness, particularly for the subgroup of forensic patients.

Prevention of Initial CJS Contact for Those with Severe Mental Illness

There is a well-established association between mental illness, particularly severe mental illness, and risk of contact with the CJS. Studies conducted over the last several decades in prison, clinical, and population-based samples have confirmed the increased risk of CJS contact for those with severe mental illness.[3,4] More recent research has identified a wide range of potential explanatory factors, including the co-occurrence of substance use problems,[5] the consequences of social disadvantage,[6] and the presence of untreated symptoms.[7] In addition, there is evidence that mental illness is a risk factor for repeated contact with the criminal justice system – for recurrent and cumulative criminalization.[8] In this context, decriminalization is likely to necessitate successfully identifying those with mental illness at increased risk of CJS contact as well as intervening to address the factors underlying the increased risk, but there has been limited research focused on testing approaches to the prevention of CJS contact, including initial contact, amongst those with severe mental illness.

A number of intervention studies intended to improve other clinical and functional outcomes in psychosis have, however, considered violence or other offending behavior as a secondary outcome. For example, trials of intensive or assertive community care,[9] outpatient commitment,[10] and administration of specific psychotropic medications[11] have considered measures of CJS contact and offending outcomes, with varying results. In a systematic review of nonpharmacological interventions for reducing aggression and violence in serious mental illness (with the majority of identified studies focused on forensic patient or other mentally disordered offender samples) the quality of evidence to support any interventions was found to be poor.[12] It is also of note that many of these intervention studies have involved participants with chronic psychosis, many of whom have already had CJS contact. While the "early intervention

137

in psychosis" literature is extensive, few studies have focused on preventing violence or CJS contact as an outcome.

Testing early assertive and specialized community care for individuals with first episode psychosis in Denmark, the OPUS trial found evidence of benefits for a range of clinical and social outcomes.[13] Subsequently, trial participants were linked to official criminal records in order to examine the impact of the intervention, and its established benefits, on risk of subsequent contact with the CJS.[14] Unfortunately, no impact on CJS contacts was seen over either the two years of the intervention or the subsequent three years of follow-up. The results of this study undermine the notion that gold standard early intervention for first episode psychosis reduces CJS contact, perhaps indicating that a targeted rather than universal approach is needed, that intervention needs to be offered even earlier than the first episode of psychosis (in the Danish study many had already offended prior to recruitment to the study), and/or that the intervention needs to be specifically focused on reducing criminality. In this context it is important to note that there is evidence that the risk of violence for those with serious illness might well be greatest during the earliest phases of illness,[15] particularly prior to treatment, and perhaps even in the prodromal or at-risk period.[16]

While the index offences of forensic patients, being typically serious violent offences, represent a relatively rare outcome that is not ideal as a focus of prevention, it is clear that the clinical and service-contact narratives of individual forensic patients commonly present apparent "missed opportunities" for intervention. In a study of individuals found Not Guilty by reason of Mental Illness in NSW over 25 years, over 80% were noted to have had contact with mental health services at some point prior to the index offence.[17] In addition, the early phases of psychosis may not only represent a high-risk time for offending behavior and CJS contact, but for risk of serious violent offending in particular.[18] Whether attempts to identify and intervene as early as possible in the course of emerging psychosis can prevent CJS contact, including for the type of serious violence that defines the forensic patient group, remains unknown.

Reoffending Rates amongst Released Forensic Patients

While diversion away from the CJS and into mental health services in order to meet the significant mental health needs of forensic patients is a common approach internationally, the precise manner in which this is done varies considerably between jurisdictions. While the M'Naghten rules that underlie a complete mental health defence against a criminal charge arose from English case law, they are now more commonly applied in jurisdictions outside than inside the UK. In Australia, for example, modified versions of the M'Naghten rules are still relied upon in several jurisdictions.

If diversion of forensic patients away from the CJS into mental health services is to be fully realized as a tool of decriminalization, one of the key outcomes must be a reduction in the risk of post-release reoffending. Beginning in the early 1990s, many studies following forensic patients after release from secure care have now been conducted. A recent systematic review and meta-analysis of such studies,[19] identified 35 studies from 10 countries (18 from England and Wales). The pooled estimate of post-release reoffending for the 30 studies providing data on this outcome was 4,484 per 100,000 person years (95% CI 3,679–5,287). Substantial heterogeneity across studies was found in relation to reported reoffending rates but the only factor found to provide any explanation was the association between the age of studies and reoffending rate reported. Table 15.1 provides a summary of the included studies and an update on studies published since the review.

Judgments about whether or not the rates of reported recidivism for released forensic patients are low or high rests on the nature of comparison groups. No study to date has undertaken a formal case-control analysis, in part because of the inherent difficulty in identifying a suitable comparison group, but many have made comparisons to local prison-release reoffending rates. In the systematic review described, 10 of the 30 recidivism studies reported rates for comparison populations and in all cases forensic patients were noted to have a lower rate of reoffending.[19] In one of the Australian studies included in the review, a study of 197 forensic patients in NSW, the reconviction rate for conditionally released patients (followed up for 8.4 years on average) was 11.8% for any offence and 3.1% for any violent offence.[20] While a comparison group was not included, in a study of 661 nonforensic offenders charged with serious but nonlethal violent offence in the same jurisdiction, over half of those diagnosed with psychotic illness had returned to prison during the follow-up period,

Table 15.1 Studies of post-release reoffending in samples of forensic patients

Author/Year published	Jurisdiction	Sample	Follow-up period	Recidivism outcomes	Risk factors for recidivism
Pasewark et al. (1982)[i]	US (New York)	148 not guilty by reason of insanity (NGRI) acquittees (111 males and 22 females had been released into the community; and 15 males had escaped)	Total follow-up period was not reported. Average time spent in hospital and average time following release/escape from hospital and end of study was reported: e.g. males released into the community average days in hospital=670 days and average days following release=1809 days, females released into the community average days in hospital=642 days and average days following release=1929 days	Males released into the community: 31.5% were arrested following hospitalization. Females released into the community: 13.6% were arrested following hospitalization	N/A
Black (1982)[ii]	UK	128 male patients discharged from Broadmoor Hospital	5 years	Of the 125 patients for whom follow-up data were available, 22.4% were imprisoned following discharge and 39.2% had further court appearances	Predictors of recidivism include: having a previous history of offending, and having a non-homicide index offence
Bogenberger et al. (1957)[iii]	US (Hawaii)	107 individuals found not responsible for a criminal act due to insanity	Unclear. Sample comprised individuals who were acquitted from Jan 1, 1970 to June 30, 1976, with the cut-off period for the study being June 30, 1984	67.2% rearrested following acquittal	Individuals who had been hospitalized following acquittal had more arrests for offences against the person and property combined, than for public order and drug offences combined, as compared to individuals who were released conditionally or unconditionally following acquittal
Silver et al. (1989)[iv]	US (Maryland)	127 individuals found NGRI who had been released into the community; a matched control group of 127 individuals on parole; and a comparison group of 135 mentally disordered offenders who had received hospital treatment, and who were later released on parole	Mean follow-up period for NGRI group=10.5 years (range=7–17 years) Mean follow-up period for control group=10.8 years (range=7–16 years) Mean follow-up period for comparison group=7.9 years (range=4–16 years)	5 years following release: 54.3% of the NGRI group were rearrested within 5 years following release. The control and comparison groups had higher rearrest rates during that time period at 65.4% and 73.3% respectively Across total follow-up period: at the end of the follow-up period 65.8% of the NGRI group, 75.4% of the control group, and 78.5% of the comparison group had been rearrested	N/A

Table 15.1 (cont.)

Author/Year published	Jurisdiction	Sample	Follow-up period	Recidivism outcomes	Risk factors for recidivism
Rice et al. (1990)[v]	Canada	253 NGRI patients in a maximum security institution; and a comparison group made up of 210 convicted men who had been admitted to same institution for brief pre-trial psychiatric assessments	Mean follow-up period of 78.2 months	NGRI group had lower recidivism rate than comparison group General recidivism General recidivism rate was 40.7% for the NGRI group and 54.4% for the comparison group Violent recidivism Violent recidivism rate was 20.1% for the NGRI group and 29.4% for the comparison group	Factors associated with recidivism for NGRI group include school maladjustment, being arrested at a young age (i.e. <16 year old), having a personality disorder diagnosis, alcohol abuse, and higher Level of Supervision Inventory (LSI) score
McGreevy et al. (1991)[vi]	US (New York)	331 NGRI acquittees granted conditional release	Mean follow-up period of 3.8 years	22.7% rearrested	N/A
Nicholson et al. (1991)[vii]	US (Oklahoma)	30 NGRI acquittees discharged from forensic unit	Mean follow-up period of 960.5 days	33.3% rearrested	Acquittees who left the forensic unit AWOL were more likely to be rearrested than those who were discharged at their first court review or after completing treatment
Tellefsen et al. (1992)[viii]	US (Maryland)	36 NGRI acquitees directly released from forensic hospital into community ("non-regionalized group"); and 24 NGRI acquitees discharged into state mental hospitals before subsequently being released into community ("regionalized group")	5 years	62.5% of regionalized group and 47.2% of non-regionalized group rearrested	Rearrests in the regionalized group associated with the following factors: being between the ages of 25 and 35 years old at admission, lower GAF score at discharge, and less favorable clinical assessment at discharge Rearrests in non-regionalized group associated with the following factors: heroin addiction, younger age at admission (<35 years), more severe index offence, having more prior arrests, and poor adjustment in hospital
Bailey and Macculloch (1992)[ix]	UK	106 male forensic patients released from special hospital (6 patients were readmitted, bringing the total number of cases analyzed to 112)	Mean follow-up period of 6 years (range=5 months–14 years)	36.6% of cases were convicted of an offence following release	Individuals who had a Mental Health Act classification of psychopathic disorder were significantly more likely to have been convicted following release than those with a classification of mental illness. Individuals who were absolutely discharged (as opposed to conditionally discharged), and individuals who had a personality disorder (as opposed to patients without) were also significantly more likely to be convicted post-release

Study	Country	Sample	Follow-up period	Reoffending/reconviction	Factors associated
Komer and Galbraith (1992)[x]	Canada	32 individuals detained under Lieutenant-Governor warrant who had spent time living in community	Mean follow-up period of 8.5 years	18.8% had new charges and 6.3% had new convictions	Factors associated with new charges/convictions include having a primary diagnosis of personality disorder, having a greater number of prior convictions or jail sentences, and having more breaches of the warrant
Wiederanders (1992)[xi]	US (California)	191 forensic patients released on condition that they attend community aftercare program; and a comparison group of 44 forensic patients who were unconditionally released with no aftercare	Mean follow-up period of 706.6 days (range=181–1097 days)	Patients released on condition that they attend aftercare were significantly less likely to be rearrested in follow-up period than those unconditionally released with no aftercare (5.8% vs. 27.3%)	Conditional release to community after program associated with lower likelihood of rearrest
Macculloch et al. (1993a,[xii] 1993b)[xiii]	UK	112 forensic patients discharged from special hospital	Mean follow-up period of 6 years (range=5 months–14 years)	36.6% convicted of a new offence 16.9% reconvicted for serious offence (i.e. homicide, assault, rape, indecent assault, robbery, arson)	N/A
Cope and Ward (1993)[xiv]	UK	51 patients discharged from Special Hospital	Mean follow-up period of 5.3 years (range=6 months–10 years)	11.4% of the 35 patients who were discharged into the community or local psychiatric hospitals were reconvicted	N/A
Russo (1994)[xv]	Italy	91 patients released from maximum security special hospital	Mean follow-up period of 5 years (range=1 year and 3 months–10 years and 10 months)	22.0% were rearrested following release, with 7.7% rearrested for at least one violent crime	Patients who were younger (<45 years) had a diagnosis of psychopathy or oligophrenia, had a previous criminal record, had early criminal experiences (i.e. engaged in criminal behavior as a juvenile), had been hospitalized for short periods (<4 years), came from a family with criminal records, had never received intermediate forms of treatment, and had an index of offence that was a property or violent offence that was not murder were more likely to be rearrested
Reiss et al. (1996)[xvi]	UK	49 patients with a Mental Health Act classification of psychopathy disorder who were treated at the Young Persons Unit of Broadmoor Hospital	Data for follow-up following release into the community were only available for 28 patients. Mean follow-up period for this group was 4.7 years. The remaining 12 patients were still in hospital at the end of follow-up. Mean time spent in hospital was 12.5 years	20.4% of the total sample reoffended, with 16.3% reoffending in the community	Factors associated with reoffending include: being in foster care as a child, engaging in fighting or bullying when under the age of 12, having a previous conviction for assault or actual bodily harm, having a previous conviction for a sex offence, and having a lower IQ score Patients who had stronger employment records and relationship histories before their hospital admission were less likely to reoffend

Table 15.1 (cont.)

Author/Year published	Jurisdiction	Sample	Follow-up period	Recidivism outcomes	Risk factors for recidivism
Wiederanders et al. (1997)[xvii]	US (California, Oregon, New York)	Comparison of three studies conducted in three different states (California [n=331]; Oregon [n=366]; and New York [n=888]) of NGRI patients conditionally released	Authors calculated annualized rearrest rates of each study	Annualized rearrest rates: New York: 7.8% Oregon: 5.8% California: 3.4%	N/A
Green and Baglioni (1998)[xviii]	Australia (Queensland)	574 patients admitted to secure hospital.	Follow-up period ranged from approximately 2.5–8.5 years	Of the 571 patients released, transferred, granted leave, or offended in hospital, 19.8% reoffended. 11.2% were charged with a violent offence Of the 194 patients who were insanity acquittees who had been released, transferred, or granted leave, 19.6% reoffended. 11.9% violently reoffended	N/A
Steels et al. (1998)[xix]	UK	75 men and 20 women with a psychopathic disorder; and a comparison group of 70 men and 19 women with mental illness. Both groups had been discharged from special hospital with a restriction order	Follow-up period ranged from 16–18 years for men, and 1418 years for women	Men 60.0% of men in the psychopathic disorder group, and 20.0% of men in the mental illness group were reconvicted after discharge Women 40.0% of women in the psychopathic disorder group and 15.8% of women in the mental illness group were reconvicted after discharge	Men were more likely to be reconvicted and to commit more offences following discharged compared to women. Individuals with a previous conviction or sentence of imprisonment were significantly more likely to be reconvicted
Luettgen et al. (1998)[xx]	Canada	109 not criminally responsible (NCR) patients treated at a forensic hospital	Mean follow-up period of 6.7 years	Of the 74 patients who were released into the community, 10.8% were convicted of an offence during the follow-up period	N/A
Buchanan (1998)[xxi]	UK	425 patients discharged from special hospital	10.5 years	5.5 years after discharge 24% convicted of any offence. 9% convicted of serious offence. 8% convicted of violent offence 10.5 years after discharge 31% convicted of any offence. 14% convicted of serious offence. 14% convicted of violent offence	Reconviction associated with factors such as, being younger at time of discharge, having more prior convictions, and having a legal classification of psychopathic disorder

Study	Country	Sample	Follow-up period	Recidivism outcome	Associated factors / notes
Friendship et al. (1999)[xxii]	UK	234 patients discharged from medium security unit	Mean follow-up period of 6.6 years (range=6 months–14 years)	23.9% convicted during follow-up period. 12.4% convicted of serious offence	Younger age at first admission, shorter length of admission, and greater number previous convictions predicted reconviction
Maden et al. (1999)[xxiii]	UK	234 patients discharged from medium secure unit	Mean follow-up period of 6.6 years (range=6 months–almost 14 years)	24.0% convicted of any offence. 14.1% convicted of violent offence	Those who were reconvicted tended to be younger, have more prior convictions, and shorter admission lengths
Baxter et al. (1999)[xxiv]	UK	63 patients with schizophrenia discharged from a medium security unit	Mean follow-up period of 3.9 years (range=0.3–8.75 years)	30.2% reconvicted for violent offence	Factors associated with reconviction include young age, having a conduct disorder, having substance use problem (alcohol problems, and poly-drug abuse), and absence of a restriction order
Kravitz and Kelly (1999)[xxv]	US (Illinois)	43 NGRI patients in outpatient treatment	Length of time in the outpatient treatment program ranged from 4.9 months–18.4 years	18.6% reoffended (rearrested or committed new offence)	Reoffending associated with having unimproved or worse symptoms as the outcome of most recent episode
Falla et al. (2000)[xxvi]	UK	85 patients discharged from a medium secure regional psychiatric unit	Mean follow-up period of 3 years and 5 months	16.4% were reconvicted following discharge, with only 7.1% reconvicted of a serious offence (i.e. assault, arson, sexual offences)	N/A
Edwards et al. (2002)[xxvii]	UK	225 first admissions to a medium secure unit	2 and 5 years following admission	2 years after admission Of the 66 patients who had spent some time in the community by the end of the 2-year follow-up period, 10.6% had been reconvicted 5 years after admission Of the 104 patients who had a 5-year follow-up period and who had spent some time in the community by the end of that period, 9.8% were reconvicted	N/A
Livingston et al. (2003)[xxviii]	Canada	200 not criminally responsible on account of mental disorder (NCRMD) individuals discharged to community	2 years following discharge	18.0% charged with new offence. 7.5% convicted	N/A
Lee (2003)[xxix]	US (California)	Sample includes 74 NGRI individuals treated in community	11 years	Of the 57 insanity acquittees included in recidivism analysis, 50.8% reoffended	N/A
Parker (2004)[xxx]	US (Ohio)	83 NGRI acquittees conditionally released to community treatment	5 years	4.8% rearrested. Estimated annual rearrest rate was 1.4%	Length of potential conditional release positively associated with rearrest/hospitalization, while a diagnosis of paranoid schizophrenia was negatively associated with rearrest/hospitalization

Table 15.1 (cont.)

Author/Year published	Jurisdiction	Sample	Follow-up period	Recidivism outcomes	Risk factors for recidivism
Bertman-Pate et al. (2004)[xxxi]	US (Louisiana)	119 NGRI and incompetent to proceed in community forensic aftercare conditional release program	Study examined rearrests amongst clients whilst they were engaged in the program. Mean length of stay in program was 22.6 months	10.1% arrested for any charge whilst engaged in the program – 2.4% arrested for felony charges, and 7.6% arrested for misdemeanor charges	N/A
Maden et al. (2004)[xxxii]	UK	959 patients discharged from medium secure units	2 years	15.1% convicted. 6.3% convicted of violent offences	Factors associated with offending include having more previous convictions, having a history of substance misuse, losing contact
Jamieson and Taylor (2004)[xxxiii]	UK	204 patients discharged from high security hospitals	12 years	36.3% convicted following discharge. 25.5% convicted of serious offences.	Factors associated with reconviction associated with being detained under the legal classification of psychopathic disorder, having a greater number of previous court appearances, and being younger at discharge
Jamieson and Taylor (2005)[xxxiv]	UK	223 patients discharged from high security hospital in 1984, and 212 discharged in 1996	5 years	1984 cohort Of the 197 patients included in the reconviction analysis, 31.0% were reconvicted within the 5-year follow-up period. 18.8% were reconvicted of a serious offence 1996 cohort Of the 167 patients included in the reconviction analysis, 21.0% were reconvicted within the 5-year follow-up period. 14.4% were reconvicted of a serious offence	1984 cohort Patients with a legal classification of psychopathic disorder, and who were discharged to prison were more likely to be reconvicted 1996 cohort Patients who were discharged to prison were more likely to be reconvicted than those who were discharged to the community or other setting Serious reconviction Patients who were discharged to the community were more likely to be reconvicted of a serious offence than patients who were discharged to prison, court, or other setting
Alexander et al. (2006)[xxxv]	UK	Two cohorts of patients discharged from a medium secure unit for individuals with intellectual disability (cohort 1=27 patients; cohort 2=37 patients)	Range=1–13 years	29.7% had police contact. 10.9% received cautions. 10.9% were reconvicted	Patients who were younger (< 27 years old), had a history of theft/burglary, or a personality disorder diagnosis were more likely to be reconvicted. Having a diagnosis of schizophrenia was a protective factor against reconviction
Simpson et al. (2006)[xxxvi]	New Zealand	105 forensic patients discharged from in-patient care to forensic community services	Mean follow-up period of 21.7 months	Of those who were discharged from forensic community services (n=48), 18.8% were rearrested, 12.5% were reconvicted, and 10.5% were imprisoned	N/A

Study	Country	Sample	Follow-up	Reconviction rates	Findings
Skipworth et al. (2006)[xxxvii]	New Zealand	135 NGRI individuals released into community	Maximum follow-up period was 27.5 years	2 years after discharge 15% reconvicted of any offence. 5.7% reconvicted of violent offence 10 years after discharge 40% reconvicted of any offence	Violent reconviction associated with younger age at discharge (< 35 years old), Maori ethnicity, and more prior offences with services, and being a survivor of sexual abuse
Coid et al. (2007)[xxxviii]	UK	1344 patients (1167 men; 177 women) discharged from medium secure forensic psychiatry services	Mean follow-up period of 6.2 years (range=<1 month–9.9 years)	34.3% of men and 15.3% of women convicted of any offence. 18.1% of men and 5.1% of women convicted of violent offence	Factors associated with violent reconviction include younger age, being male, belonging to minority ethnic group, having more previous violent convictions, having a primary diagnosis of personality disorder, having a primary/comorbid diagnosis of antisocial personality disorder, and having a legal classification of psychopathic disorder. Greater length of admission (>2 years) was a protective factor
Davies et al. (2007)[xxxix]	UK	542 patients discharged from medium secure unit	Mean follow-up period of 9.4 years	48.7% reconvicted during entire follow-up period. 14.4% convicted of a grave offence (i.e. offences with a maximum sentence of life imprisonment, and arson not endangering life)	Reconviction associated with having a legal classification of psychopathic disorder
Yoshikawa et al. (2007)[xl]	Japan	489 individuals found not responsible or to have diminished responsibility for an offence. Individuals received psychiatric treatment before being released into community	Median follow-up period of 10.8 years (range=0.1–14.5 years)	10.6% arrested/convicted of violent offences	Violent reoffending associated with the presence of a substance use disorder, prior violent offending, homelessness, and shorter length of admission (<6 months). Older age (>45 years old) was a protective factor
Vitacco et al. (2008)[xli]	US (Wisconsin)	363 NGRI individuals released into community	Mean follow-up period of 2.85 years (range=2–6 years)	7.1% had conditional release revoked due to new offence. 3.7% had conditional release revoked due to violent offence	N/A
Blattner and Dolan (2009)[xlii]	UK	72 patients from a high secure psychiatric hospital who were transferred to and subsequently discharged from a medium secure unit	Study examined reconvictions amongst patients released directly into the community. Mean follow-up period for this group was 4.9 years (range=0.08–12.17 years)	20.5% of patients released directly into the community were reconvicted. 15.4% were reconvicted of a serious offence (e.g. indecent assault of a child, malicious/intended wounding, assault, burglary, robbery)	Patients with a legal classification of psychopathic disorder were more likely to be reconvicted

Table 15.1 (cont.)

Author/Year published	Jurisdiction	Sample	Follow-up period	Recidivism outcomes	Risk factors for recidivism
Sahota et al. (2009)[xliii]	UK	163 patients discharged from medium secure unit (70 discharged to specialized community forensic services; 93 to generic service)	Mean follow-up period of 10 years	53% of patients discharged to community forensic services, and 45% of patients discharged to generic service were reconvicted	Discharge to generic service (as opposed to specialized community forensic service) associated with longer time to reconviction
Ong et al. (2009)[xliv]	Australia (Victoria)	25 individuals found unfit to stand trial for homicide	3 years	3 years after release 4% reoffended	N/A
Bjørkly et al. (2010)[xlv]	Norway	38 forensic patients discharged from maximum security forensic unit	Mean follow-up period of 8.23 years	34.2% reconvicted. 13.2% convicted for serious violent crime (i.e. GBH), and 7.9% convicted for less serious violent crime	Factors associated with reconviction include having a history of drug abuse, being a survivor of childhood sexual abuse, and being subject to a restriction order following discharge
Miraglia and Hall (2011)[xlvi]	US (New York)	386 NGRI patients released into the community	Mean follow-up period of 14 years (range=<1 year–>26 years)	3 years after release 11% arrested for any offence. 3% arrested for violent offence 5 years after release 16% rearrested for any offence. 7% rearrested for violent offence Entire follow-up period 21% rearrested for any offence. 11% rearrested for violent offence	Predictors of rearrest include younger age, being male, and having an antisocial personality disorder diagnosis
Nilsson et al. (2011)[xlvii]	Sweden	99 violent and/or sexual offenders who were court-referred for pre-trial forensic psychiatric investigations – 46 were subsequently sentenced to forensic psychiatric care and 53 were sentenced to prison	Mean time spent at liberty was 30.9 months (range=0–72 months)	14.1% (3.0% of the forensic psychiatric care group and 20.7% of the prison group) were reconvicted for a violent offence during conditional release or after discharge	N/A (study did not report on predictors of recidivism for psychiatric care group and prison group separately)
Green et al. (2011)[xlviii]	Australia (Queensland)	1647 individuals who appeared before the Mental Health Tribunal for determinations relating to soundness of mind or fitness to stand trial	Mean follow-up period of 7.2 years (range=0.8–17.1 years)	Any offending 30.8% of individuals found to be of unsound mind, and 10.8% of individuals found not fit to stand trial reoffended Violent offending 11.9% of individuals found to be of unsound mind, and 1.5% of individuals found not fit to stand trial reoffended in a violent way	Previous violent offending was positively associated with violent reoffending, while age was negatively associated with violent reoffending

Study	Country	Sample	Follow-up	Findings	Factors associated with reoffending
Tabita et al. (2012)[xlix]	Sweden	88 forensic patients discharged from medium security unit (only 63 patients included in recidivism analyses)	Mean follow-up period of 9.4 years (range=15 months–17 years)	38.1% reoffended. 16.7% of those who reoffended had committed serious violent crimes (i.e. sexual offence, homicide).	Factors associated with reoffending include having a substance-related diagnosis, and having a diagnosis of PD.
Lund et al. (2013)[l]	Sweden	349 male offenders who were court-referred for pre-trial forensic psychiatric evaluation – 169 were subsequently ordered to forensic psychiatric treatment, 126 were sentenced to prison, and 54 received non-institutional sanctions	13–30 years. Note that follow-up began from time of sanction to end of study period	Violent reconvictions The three offender groups did not differ significantly in terms of violent reconvictions – 46.0% of the forensic psychiatric treatment group, 46.7% of the prison group, and 50.0% of the non-institutional sanctions group were reconvicted of a violent offence Nonviolent reconvictions The forensic psychiatric treatment group had the lowest rate of nonviolent reconvictions (17.2% vs. 27.5% for the prison group and 21.2% for the non-institutional sanctions group)	N/A (study did not report on predictors of recidivism for each group separately)
Howard et al. (2013)[li]	UK	53 men treated in a secure personality disorder unit, and who were subsequently released into the community	Mean follow-up period of 200.7 weeks	62.2% reconvicted during follow-up period. Mean time to first reconviction was 121.7 weeks	APD/BPD comorbidity, higher PCL-R factor 2 score, and having the risk factor combination of APD/BPD comorbidity, severe conduct disorder in childhood, and substance dependence were associated with significantly shorter time to reconviction
Hayes et al. (2014)	Australia (NSW)	364 NGMI forensic patients in NSW	Mean follow-up period of 91 months	Conditionally released patients: 18.0% of patients on conditional release were charged with new offence, and 11.8% were convicted. 8.7% were charged with a violent offence, and 3.1% were convicted Unconditionally released patients: 12.5% of patients who had been unconditionally released were charged with new offence, and 9.4% were convicted. 6.3% were charged with a violent offence, and 4.7% were convicted	Reoffending associated with the following factors: being Indigenous, being younger at time of first offence, having previous convictions, having been imprisoned previously, having a substance abuse disorder, having APD, and being unemployed at time of conditional release

Table 15.1 (cont.)

Author/Year published	Jurisdiction	Sample	Follow-up period	Recidivism outcomes	Risk factors for recidivism
Charette et al. (2015)[iii]	Canada	1800 offenders found NCRMD (1768 followed for 3 years following index verdict; 1319 followed for 3 years following conditional discharge; and 949 followed for 3 years following absolute discharge)	Mean follow-up period of 5.7 years (range=approximately 3–8 years)	At 3 years after index verdict: 16.7% recidivated with new conviction or CRMD finding At 3 years after conditional discharge: 20.3% recidivated At 3 years after absolute discharge: 21.3% recidivated	Recidivism associated with the following factors: having a comorbid substance use disorder, having comorbid PD, having a less severe index offence, having prior criminal convictions or NCRMD verdicts, and not being under the Review Board's supervision
Nagtegaal and Boonmann (2016)[iii]	The Netherlands	447 forensic patients on conditional release	Data on patients' outcomes were recorded for the period of time during which they were on conditional release, as well as at 2 and 5 years following unconditional release.	Of the 256 patients included in analysis on reoffending while on conditional release, 3.5% were reconvicted 2 years after conditional release, 29.5% of those who had been granted conditional release contrary to experts' recommendations and 16.0% of those who had been granted conditional release consistent with experts' recommendations had reoffended. At 5 years, the rates had increased to 46.4% and 26.7% respectively	Factors associated with recidivism include having more prior convictions and being younger at the time of TBS order (a TBS order is a sentence imposed by courts in the Netherlands in relation to individuals found to be unaccountable for their offending due to a mental disorder)
Norko et al. (2016)[liv]	US (Connecticut)	177 NGRI acquittees granted conditional release; 196 NGRI acquittees unconditionally discharged	Study examines individuals NGRI acquittees granted conditional or unconditional release during the 30-year existence of the Connecticut Psychiatric Security Review Board	Conditionally released patients: 2.3% of those who had been on conditional release were rearrested Unconditionally released patients: 16.3% of those who had been unconditionally released were rearrested	Those who had been on conditional release prior to being unconditionally discharged, longer hospital stays, and spent more time under the Review Board's supervision were less likely to be rearrested
Krona et al. (2017)[lv]	Sweden	125 offenders sentenced to forensic psychiatric in-patient treatment	Median follow-up period of 6.2 years (range=0.6–9.7 years)	24.0% reconvicted during follow-up period. 13% reconvicted of violent crime	General recidivism associated with the following factors: low educational attainment, younger age at first sentence, having a first degree relative that has a major mental disorder, and not having a Special Court Supervision (SCS) order attached to treatment Violent recidivism associated with the following factors: low educational attainment, low GAF score, having a cluster B personality disorder, and not having an SCS order attached to treatment

Study	Country	Sample	Follow-up	Recidivism	Factors
Simpson et al. (2018)[lvi]	Canada	60 NCRMD patients who had been absolutely discharged	12 months following absolute discharge	16.7% reoffended	Factors associated with recidivism: having a psychotic disorder, having a comorbid substance use disorder, not being assessed as low risk under the HCR-20, and having more previous criminal charges
Richer et al. (2018)[lvii]	Canada	528 people found Not Criminally Responsible on Account of Mental Disorder (NCR) and placed under the jurisdiction of the Alberta Review Board (ARB)	The follow-up period was 1 to 35 years.	19.7% reoffended	This study found an inverse relationship between a severe mental disorder and recidivism In terms of criminological traits this study found that criminal history was a good predictor of recidivism

i Pasewark, RA, Bieber, S, Bosten, KJ, et al. Criminal recidivism among insanity acquittees. *International Journal of Law and Psychiatry.* 1982;5(3–4):365–375.

ii Black, D. A 5-year follow-up study of male patients discharged from Broadmoor hospital. In: Gunn J and Farrington D, eds. *Abnormal Offenders, Delinquency, and the Criminal Justice System.* Chichester, New York: Wiley; 1982:307–323.

iii Bogenberger, RP, Pasewark, RA, Gudeman, H, et al. Follow-up of insanity acquittees in Hawaii. *International Journal of Law and Psychiatry.* 1987;10(3):283–295.

iv Silver, SB, Cohen, MI, Spodak, MK. Follow-up after release of insanity acquittees, mentally disorder offenders, and convicted felons. *Bulletin of the American Academy of Psychiatry and the Law.* 1989;17(4):387–400.

v Rice, M, Harris, G, Lang, C, et al. Recidivism among male insanity acquittees. *The Journal of Psychiatry & Law.* 1990;18(3–4):379–403.

vi McGreevy, M, Steadman, H, Dvoskin, J, et al. New York state's system of managing insanity acquittees in the community. *Hospital and Community Psychiatry.* 1991;42(5):512–517.

vii Nicholson, R, Norwood, S, Enyart, C. Characteristics and outcomes of insanity acquittees in Oklahoma. *Behavioral Sciences and the Law.* 1991;9(4):487–500.

viii Tellefsen, C, Cohen, M, Silver, S, et al. Predicting success on conditional release for insanity acquittees: Regionalized versus nonregionalized hospital patients. *Bulletin of the American Academy of Psychiatry and the Law.* 1992;20(1):87–100.

ix Bailey, J, Macculloch, M. Patterns of reconviction in patients discharged directly to the community from a special hospital: Implications for aftercare. *Journal of Forensic Psychiatry.* 1992;3(3):445–461.

x Komer, B, Galbraith, D. Recidivism among individuals detained under a warrant of the Lieutenant-Governor living in the community. *Canadian Journal of Psychiatry.* 1992;37(10):694–698.

xi Wiederanders, M. Recidivism of disordered offenders who were conditionally vs. unconditionally released. *Behavioral Sciences and the Law.* 1992;10(1):141–148.

xii Macculloch, M, Bailey, J, Jones, C, et al. Nineteen male serious reoffenders who were discharged direct to the community from a special hospital: I. General characteristics. *The Journal of Forensic Psychiatry.* 1993a;4(2):237–248.

xiii Macculloch, M, Bailey, J, Jones, C, et al. Nineteen male serious reoffenders who were discharged direct to the community from a special hospital: II. Illustrated clinical issues. *The Journal of Forensic Psychiatry.* 1993b;4(3):451–469.

xiv Cope, R, Ward, M. What happens to special hospital patients admitted to medium security? *The Journal of Forensic Psychiatry.* 1993;4(1):13–24.

xv Russo, G. Follow-up of 91 mentally ill criminals discharged from the maximum security hospital in Barcelona P.G. *International Journal of Law and Psychiatry.* 1994;17(3): 279–301.

xvi Reiss, D, Grubin, D, Meux, C. Young 'psychopaths' in special hospital: Treatment and outcome. *British Journal of Psychiatry.* 1996;168(1):99–104.

xvii Wiederanders, M, Bromley, D, Choate, P. Forensic conditional release programs and outcomes in three states. *International Journal of Law and Psychiatry.* 1997;20(2):249–257.

xviii Green, B, Baglioni, A. Length of stay, leave and re-offending by patients from a Queensland security patients hospital. *Australian and New Zealand Journal of Psychiatry.* 1998;32(6):839–847.

xix Steels, M, Roney, G, Larkin, E, et al. Discharged from special hospital under restrictions: A comparison of the fates of psychopaths and the mentally ill. *Criminal Behavior and Mental Health.* 1998;8(1):39–55.

xx Luettgen, J, Chrapko, W, Reddon, J. Preventing violent re-offending in not criminally responsible patients: An evaluation of a continuity of treatment program. *International Journal of Law and Psychiatry.* 1998;21(1):89–98.

xxi Buchanan, A. Criminal conviction after discharge from special (high security) hospital: Incidence in the first 10 years. *British Journal of Psychiatry.* 1998;172(6):472–476.

xxii Friendship, C, McClintock, T, Rutter, S, et al. Re-offending: Patients discharged from a regional secure unit. *Criminal Behaviour and Mental Health.* 1999;9(3):226–236.

xxiii Maden, A, Rutter, S, McClintock, T, et al. Outcome of admission to a medium secure psychiatric unit: I. Short- and long-term outcome. *British Journal of Psychiatry.* 1999;175(4):313–316.

xxiv Baxter, R, Rabe-Hesketh, S, Parrot, J. Characteristics, needs and reoffending in a group of patients with schizophrenia formerly treated in medium security. *Journal of Forensic Psychiatry.* 1999;10(1):69–83.

xxv Kravitz, H, Kelly, J. An outpatient psychiatry program for offenders with mental disorders found not guilty by reason of insanity. *Psychiatric Services.* 1999;50(12):1597–1606.

xxvi Falla, S, Sugarman, P, Roberts, L. Reconviction after discharge from a regional secure unit. *Medicine, Science, and the Law.* 2000;40(2):156–157.

xxvii Edwards, J, Steed, P, Murray, K. Clinical and forensic outcome 2 years and 5 years after admission to a medium secure unit. *Journal of Forensic Psychiatry.* 2002;13(1):68–87.

xxviii Livingston, J, Wilson, D, Tien, G, et al. A follow-up study of persons found not criminally responsible on account of mental disorder in British Columbia. *The Canadian Journal of Psychiatry.* 2003;48(6):408–415.

xxix Lee, D. Community-treated and discharged forensic patients: An 11-year follow-up. *International Journal of Law and Psychiatry.* 2003;26(3):289–300.

xxx Parker, G. Outcomes of assertive community treatment in an NGRI conditional release program. *Journal of the American Academy of Psychiatry and the Law.* 2004;32(3):291–303.

xxxi Bertman-Pate, L, Burnett, D, Thompson, J, et al. The New Orleans forensic aftercare clinic: A seven year review of hospital discharged and jail diverted clients. *Behavioral Sciences and the Law.* 2004;22(1):159–169.

xxxii Maden, A, Scott, F, Burnett, R, et al. Offending in psychiatric patients after discharge from medium secure units: Prospective national cohort study. *British Medical Journal.* 2004;328(7455):1534.

xxxiii Jamieson, L, Taylor, P. A re-convictions study of special (high security) hospital patients. *The British Journal of Criminology.* 2004;44(5):783–802.

xxxiv Jamieson, L, Taylor, PJ. Patients leaving English high security hospitals: Do discharge cohorts and their progress change over time? *International Journal of Forensic Mental Health.* 2005;4(1):71–87.

xxxv Alexander, R, Crouch, K, Halstead, S, et al. Long-term outcome from a medium secure service for people with intellectual disability. *Journal of Intellectual Disability Research.* 2006;50(4):305–315.

xxxvi Simpson, A, Jones, R, Evans, C, et al. Outcome of patients rehabilitated through a New Zealand forensic psychiatry service: A 7.5 year retrospective study. *Behavioral Sciences and the Law.* 2006;24(6):833–843.

xxxvii Skipworth, J, Blinded, P, Chaplow, D, et al. Insanity acquittee outcomes in New Zealand. *Australia and New Zealand Journal of Psychiatry.* 2006;40(11–12):1003–1009.

xxxviii Coid, J, Hickey, N, Kahtan, N, et al. Patients discharged from medium secure forensic psychiatry services: Reconvictions and risk factors. *British Journal of Psychiatry.* 2007;190(3):223–229.

xxxix Davies, S, Clarke, M, Hollin, C, et al. Long-term outcome after discharge from medium secure care: A cause for concern. *British Journal of Psychiatry.* 2007;191(1):70–74.

xl Yoshikawa, K, Taylor, P, Yamagami, A, et al. Violent recidivism among mentally disordered offenders in Japan. *Criminal Behaviour and Mental Health.* 2007;17(3):137–151.

xli Vitacco, M, Van Rybroek, G, Rogstad, J, et al. Developing services for insanity acquittees conditionally released into the community: Maximizing success and minimizing recidivism. *Psychological Services.* 2008;5(2):118–125.

xlii Blattner, R, Dolan, M. Outcome of high security patients admitted to a medium secure unit: The Edenfield Centre study. *Medicine, Science, and the Law.* 2009;49(4):247–256.

xliii Sahota, S, Davies, S, Duggan, C, et al. The fate of medium secure patients discharged to generic or specialised services. *The Journal of Forensic Psychiatry & Psychology.* 2009;20(1):74–84.

xliv Ong, K, Carroll, A, Reid, S, et al. Community outcomes of mentally disordered homicide offenders in Victoria. *Australian and New Zealand Journal of Psychiatry.* 2009;43(8):775–780.

xlv Bjørkly, S, Sandli, C, Moger, T, et al. A follow-up interview of patients eight years after discharge from a maximum security forensic psychiatry unit in Norway. *International Journal of Forensic Mental Health.* 2010;9(4):343–353.

xlvi Miraglia, R, Hall, D. The effect of length of hospitalization on re-arrest among insanity plea acquittees. *Journal of the American Academy of Psychiatry and the Law.* 2011;39(4):524–534.

xlvii Nilsson, T, Wallinius, M, Gustavson, C, et al. Violent recidivism: A long-term follow-up study of mentally disordered offenders. *PLoS One.* 2011;6(10):e25768.

xlviii Green, B, Stedman, T, Chapple, B, et al. Criminal justice outcomes of those appearing before the Mental Health Tribunal: A follow-up study. *Psychiatry, Psychology and Law.* 2011;18(4):573–587.

xlix Tabita, B, de Santi, M, Kjellin, L. Criminal recidivism and mortality among patients discharged from a forensic medium secure hospital. *Nordic Journal of Psychiatry.* 2012;66(4):283–289.

l Lund, C, Hofvander, B, Forsman, A, et al. Violent criminal recidivism in mentally disordered offenders: A follow-up study of 13–20 years through different sanctions. *International Journal of Law and Psychiatry.* 2013;36(3–4):250–257.

lii Howard, R, McCarthy, L, Huband, N, et al. Re-offending in forensic patients released from secure care: The role of antisocial/borderline personality disorder co-morbidity, substance dependence and severe childhood conduct disorder. *Criminal Behaviour and Mental Health*. 2013;23(3):191–202.

liii Charette, Y, Crocker, A, Seto, M, et al. The national trajectory project of individuals found not criminally responsible on account of mental disorder in Canada. Part 4: Criminal recidivism. *Canadian Journal of Psychiatry*. 2015;60(3):127–134.

liiii Nagtegaal, M, Boonmann, C. Conditional release of forensic psychiatric patients consistent with or contrary to behavioural experts' recommendations in the Netherlands: Prevalence rates, patient characteristics and recidivism after discharge from conditional release. *Behavioral Sciences and the Law*. 2016;34(2–3):257–277.

liiv Norko, M, Wasser, T, Magro, H, et al. Assessing insanity acquittee recidivism in Connecticut. *Behavioral Sciences and the Law*. 2016;34(2–3):423–443.

lv Krona, H, Nyman, M, Andreasson, H, et al. Mentally disordered offenders in Sweden: Differentiating recidivists from non-recidivists in a 10-year follow-up study. *Nordic Journal of Psychiatry*. 2017;71(2):102–109.

lvi Simpson, A, Chatterjee, S, Duchcherer, M, et al. Short-term outcomes for forensic patients receiving an absolute discharge under the Canadian Criminal Code. *The Journal of Forensic Psychiatry & Psychology*. 2018;29(6):867–881.

lvii Richer, K, Cheng, J, Haag, AM. Historical recidivism rates of Alberta's not criminally responsible population. *Journal of Community Safety and Well-Being*. 2018;3(2):59–64.

suggesting that even compared to a psychotic offender control group, forensic patients may have lower rates of recidivism.[21] In a follow-up to the NSW forensic patient study, with an increased sample size of 477, 12-month post-release reconviction rates were reported in order to make a comparison with routinely reported prison-release reoffending rates in the same jurisdiction.[17] Only 6.3% of the forensic patient sample were found to have committed "proven" offences in the 12 months following release, compared to 41% reported for released prisoners in NSW for the 12 months of 2015.[22] The explanation for the relatively low rate of reoffending for forensic patients released from secure care is unclear but the consistency of findings on this point arguably support the notion that forensic mental health services, typically supported by formal supervision/monitoring frameworks, are successfully contributing to the decriminalization of forensic patients. The specific ingredients of the complex models of forensic mental health care that give rise to this impact are, however, unknown.

Risk Factors for Reoffending Following Release from Secure Care

While rates of reoffending appear to be relatively low for forensic patients released from secure care, it is important to understand the drivers of reoffending in this group if efforts at further reducing post-release contact with the CJS are to be successful.

Table 15.1 summarizes the post-release reoffending predictors reported in published studies of forensic patient samples (from 1982 to 2018). Factors related to previous CJS contact, such as the number and type of previous charges, as well as age of first offence, were highlighted by many studies. Some studies identified measures related to service or organizational interventions, such as failures of prior supervision or restriction. A few studies found that length of hospital admission was associated with risk of post-release reoffending but there was no consistency with regard to the direction of the association. Few studies commented on positive factors associated with reduced risks (e.g. employment).

With regard to clinical risk factors, two key factors are commonly identified as important predictors of post-release reoffending. Somewhat related to the importance of measures of prior criminality and supervision failures, a recorded co-morbid diagnosis of personality disorder, particularly of antisocial type

has been identified as an important clinical predictor of post-release reoffending in a number of forensic patient samples. A 36-year study of 6,520 patients released from forensic hospitals in Sweden found that a diagnosis of personality disorder, either as the only diagnosis or co-morbid with a psychotic illness or substance use disorder, was associated with a higher rate of violent reoffending.[23] Similarly, in the expanded NSW forensic patient study described earlier, the presence of a recorded clinical diagnosis of co-morbid personality disorder was found to be the only independent predictor of post-release reoffending.[17] The importance of co-morbid antisocial personality disorder in predicting adverse outcomes for forensic patients supports the calls for "criminogenic needs" to be a stronger focus of the interventions provided by forensic mental health services,[24] although even in the non-forensic literature, the evidence of benefit for the current approaches to recidivism reduction remains limited.[25]

Substance use problems have also been identified as clinical targets for intervention in forensic patient studies,[26] but there have been few evaluations of substance use interventions in forensic settings. In one recent study of an inpatient intervention adapted for forensic patients, substance-related knowledge and self-reported relapse prevention skills were increased in completers compared to noncompleters,[27] but there was no impact on time-to-first substance use or on rates of positive urine screening during follow-up. The impact on reoffending behavior was not examined.

The extent to which identified predictors of post-release reoffending can be useful targets for intervention depends on their dynamic nature, as well as on the availability of evidence-based and targeted interventions. Beyond treating severe mental illness, the interpersonal and emotion regulation problems characteristic of co-morbid personality disorder, and the persistence of substance use problems appear to be the key targets for forensic mental health services to address if post-release reoffending is to be further reduced. Developing an evidence base to support such efforts needs to be prioritized.

Conclusions

Whilst they may be a relatively small subgroup, forensic patients should not be neglected in the development of strategies to decriminalize mental illness, particularly in light of the complex and costly nature of their care and the seriousness of their offences. The prevention of CJS contact for individuals with emerging severe mental illnesses may require a targeted approach, challenging the assumption that optimal mental health treatment will inevitably improve the full spectrum of potential outcomes for all. Preventing repeat CJS contact for forensic patients released from secure care is an important outcome for forensic mental health services and should be considered amongst the range of decriminalization strategies. The relatively low reoffending rates consistently reported for released forensic patients are encouraging but further work is needed to develop the evidence base required to address the factors repeatedly identified as predicting post-release reoffending.

Disclosure

Kimberlie Dean, Sara Singh, and Yin-Lan Soon do not declare any conflicting interests in relation to this publication.

References

1. Segal A, Daffern M, Thomas S, Ferguson M. Needs and risks of patients in a state-wide inpatient forensic mental health population. *Int J Ment Health Nurs.* 2010; **19**(4): 223–230.

2. Shah A, Waldron G, Boast N, Coid JW, Ullrich S. Factors associated with length of admission at a medium secure forensic psychiatric unit. *J Forens Psychiatry Psychol.* 2011; **22**(4): 496–512.

3. Fazel S, Seewald K. Severe mental illness in 33 588 prisoners worldwide: systematic review and meta-regression analysis. *Br J Psychiatry.* 2012; **200**(5): 364–373.

4. Fazel S, Gulati G, Linsell L, Geddes JR, Grann M. Schizophrenia and violence: systematic review and meta-analysis. *PLoS Med.* 2009; **6**(8): e1000120.

5. Short T, Thomas S, Mullen P, Ogloff JRP. Comparing violence in schizophrenia patients with and without comorbid substance-use disorders to community controls. *Acta Psychiatr Scand.* 2013; **128**(4): 306–313.

6. Sariaslan A, Larsson H, Lichtenstein P, Fazel S. Neighborhood influences on violent reoffending risk in released prisoners diagnosed with psychotic disorders. *Schizophr Bull.* 2017; **43**(5): 1011–1020.

7. Keers R, Ullrich S, DeStavola B, Coid J. Association of violence with emergence of persecutory delusions in untreated schizophrenia. *Am J Psychiatry.* 2014; **171**(3): 332–339.

8. Fazel S, Yu R. Psychotic disorders and repeat offending: systematic review and metaanalysis. *Schizophr Bull.* 2011; **37**(4): 800–810.

9. Walsh E, Gilvarry C, Samele C, et al. Reducing violence in severe mental illness: randomised controlled trial of intensive case management compared with standard care. *Br Med J.* 2001; **323**(7321): 1093.

10. Swanson JW, Swartz MS, Borum R, et al. Involuntary out-patient commitment and reduction of violent behaviour in persons with severe mental illness. *Br J Psychiatr.* 2000; **176**: 324–331.

11. Swanson JW, Swartz MS, Elbogen EB, Van Dorn RA. Reducing violence risk in persons with schizophrenia: olanzapine versus risperidone. *J Clin Psychiatry.* 2004; **65**(12): 1666–1673.

12. Rampling J, Furtado V, Winsper C, et al. Non-pharmacological interventions for reducing aggression and violence in serious mental illness: a systematic review and narrative synthesis. *Eur Psychiatry.* 2016; **34**: 17–28.

13. Petersen L, Nordentoft M, Jeppesen P, et al. Improving 1-year outcome in first-episode psychosis: OPUS trial. *Br J Psychiatry Suppl.* 2005; **48**: s98–s103.

14. Stevens H, Agerbo E, Dean K, Mortensen PB, Nordentoft M. Reduction of crime in first-onset psychosis: a secondary analysis of the OPUS randomized trial. *J Clin Psychiatry.* 2013; **74**(5): e439–e444.

15. Nielssen OB, Malhi GS, McGorry PD, Large MM. Overview of violence to self and others during the first episode of psychosis. *J Clin Psychiatry.* 2012; **73**(5): e580–e587.

16. Brucato G, Appelbaum PS, Lieberman JA, et al. A longitudinal study of violent behavior in a psychosis-risk cohort. *Neuropsychopharmacology.* 2018; **43**(2): 264–271.

17. Dean K, Singh S, Kemp R, Johnson A, Nielssen O. Profile and post-release-reoffending patterns in a 25-year Australian cohort of male and female Forensic Patients. *Submitted.* 2019

18. Nielssen O, Large M. Rates of homicide during the first episode of psychosis and after treatment: a systematic review and meta-analysis. *Schizophr Bull.* 2010; **36**(4): 702–712.

19. Fazel S, Fiminska Z, Cocks C, Coid J. Patient outcomes following discharge from secure psychiatric hospitals: systematic review and meta-analysis. *Br J Psychiatry.* 2016; **208**(1): 17–25.

20. Hayes H, Kemp RI, Large MM, Nielssen OB. A 21-year retrospective outcome study of New South Wales forensic patients granted conditional and unconditional release. *Aust N Z J Psychiatry.* 2014; **48**(3): 259–282.

21. Nielssen O, Yee NY, Dean K, Large M. Outcome of serious violent offenders with psychotic illness and cognitive disorder dealt with by the New South Wales criminal justice system. *Aust N Z J Psychiatry*. 2019; **53**(5): 441–446.

22. Bureau of Crime Statistics and Research. Re-offending statistics for NSW. NSW Bureau of Crime Statistics and Research (NSW Justice); 2017.

23. Fazel S, Wolf A, Fiminska Z, Larsson H. Mortality, rehospitalisation and violent crime in forensic psychiatric patients discharged from hospital: rates and risk factors. *PLoS One*. 2016; **11**(5): e0155906.

24. Skeem JL, Winter E, Kennealy PJ, Louden JE, Tatar JR, 2nd. Offenders with mental illness have criminogenic needs, too: toward recidivism reduction. *Law Hum Behav*. 2014; **38**(3): 212–224.

25. MacKenzie DL, Farrington DP. Preventing future offending of delinquents and offenders: what have we learned from experiments and meta-analyses? *J Exp Criminol*. 2015; **11**(4): 565–595.

26. Monson CM, Gunnin DD, Fogel MH, Kyle LL. Stopping (or slowing) the revolving door: factors related to NGRI acquittees' maintenance of a conditional release. *Law Hum Behav*. 2001; **25**(3): 257–267.

27. Milosevic A, Ahmed AG, Adamson D, et al. Evaluation of a substance use treatment program for forensic psychiatric inpatients. *J Subst Use*. 2018; **23**(6): 640–647.

Chapter 16

The Cal-DSH Diversion Guidelines

Michael A. Cummings (Editor), Charles Scott, Juan Carlos Arguello, Ai-Li W. Arias, Ashley M. Breth, Darci Delgado, Philip D. Harvey, Jonathan M. Meyer, Jennifer O'Day, Megan Pollock, George J. Proctor, Tiffany Rector, Benjamin Rose, Eric Schwartz, Helga Thordarson, Katherine Warburton, and Stephen M. Stahl (Academic Advisor)

Introduction

Nearly three times as many people detained in a jail have a serious mental illness (SMI) when compared to community samples.[1] Once an individual with SMI gets involved in the criminal justice system, they are more likely than the general population to stay in the system, face repeated incarcerations, and return to prison more quickly when compared to their non-mentally ill counterparts.[2] Confronted with this harsh reality, the inevitable question must be posed:

> Is there a better way to intervene with individuals with a SMI who become involved in the criminal justice system?

By the 1970s, the concept of "diversion" emerged in response to the increasing number of individuals with a mental illness who became incarcerated. Diversion models attempt to identify those detained individuals with an SMI who may be better served outside the justice system through linkage to community-based treatment.[3] Although definitions of SMI may vary, the National Institute of Mental Health's definition of SMI typifies many organizations' definition and reads as follows:

> **Serious mental illness (SMI)** is defined as a mental, behavioral, or emotional disorder resulting in serious functional impairment, which substantially interferes with or limits one or more major life activities.[4]

Some states add specific diagnoses to the broader definition provided above. For example, the New York City jail system notes that jail inmates diagnosed with schizophrenia spectrum and other psychotic disorders, bipolar spectrum disorders, depressive disorders, and post-traumatic stress disorder all qualify for SMI.[5]

Ideally, a diversion program would identify all individuals with an SMI who may be eligible for their program. There are a range of different screening mechanisms utilized to identify individuals with mental illness who may be appropriate for diversion. Some jails have a screening questionnaire that includes only one question about the person's mental health history, whereas other jails incorporate more extensive questionnaires that include observations by transporting officers, booking staff, and mental health staff. Many jails utilize empirically validated screening questionnaires, such as the Brief Jail Mental Health Screen (BJMHS).[6] The BJMHS is completed by booking officers and includes eight "yes/no" questions about the person's mental health history and symptoms.[7] Because there are concerns that the BJMHS does not sufficiently identify SMI in women, Kessler et al. recommend the use of the mental health screening instrument known as the Kessler Psychological Distress Scale (K6). The K6 includes six broad screening questions that ask the individual to rate the severity of their symptoms over the past month. The questions ask if the person has been: (1) nervous; (2) hopeless; (3) restless or fidgety; (4) so depressed that nothing can cheer you up; (5) everything was an effort; and (6) feeling worthless.[8,9] In their study examining the use of the K6 in a jail setting, Bronson and Berzofksy determined that 26% of jail inmates met current criteria for a mental health problem.[10]

In a subsequent study examining screening procedures in New York Jail, Kubiak et al. found that 20% of inmates scored positive for mental health problems on the K6 with an additional 16% identified through staff identification. These findings indicate that best practices for screening likely include both a structured questionnaire combined with identification of those with a likely SMI by jail staff.[6] Once an individual with an SMI is identified, their appropriateness in a community diversion treatment program can be considered.

Diversion programs have a goal of decreasing criminal recidivism. Therefore, understanding why individuals with SMI become involved with criminal justice is critical to the success of diversion interventions. Two key theories have evolved to help explain the relationship of individuals with SMI to criminal offending. The first theory is known as the "criminalization of the mentally ill" hypothesis. According to this hypothesis, several factors increase the risk that individuals with SMI will be involved in the criminal justice system. These factors include stricter involuntary commitment laws with fewer psychiatric patients receiving inpatient care, poorly funded community mental health treatment services with undertreatment of mental illness, and the discharge of large numbers of psychiatric patients from psychiatric hospitals into the community with limited treatment resources.[11] Based on this "criminalization of the mentally ill" theory, untreated mental illness is the primary explanation as to why those with SMI are involved in the criminal justice system.

Under this hypothesis, enhanced mental health programs were developed and included diversion programs, mental health courts, forensic assertive community treatment (FACT) teams, and re-entry programs. These approaches have been called "first-generation" criminal justice interventions.[12] If a causal relationship between the lack of mental health treatment and criminal involvement by those with SMI exists, then programs primarily focused on treating mental illness would be expected to have fewer criminal arrests from persons enrolled in their program. Despite these first-generation diversion programs assisting in the treatment of individuals with SMI, the evidence does not indicate that these programs have had a lasting impact on decreasing criminal recidivism. Likewise, research evidence does not indicate that dual-diagnosis treatment programs for this population have resulted in a decrease in involvement in the criminal justice system.[11]

One noted concern is that the "criminalization of the mentally ill hypothesis" does not adequately explain or address nonclinical factors that result in

individuals with mental illness becoming involved in the criminal justice system.[11] In fact, only 10–20% of criminal behavior committed by individuals with mental illness symptoms has been attributed to mental illness symptoms.[13,14]

Clearly mental health and substance use treatment is an important component of any diversion program for individuals with a SMI. However, to further reduce criminal recidivism, is there another perspective that should be considered? The answer to this question is a strong "yes." More recently, research has emerged emphasizing the importance of risk factors for criminal justice involvement that play a primary role for individuals both with and without a SMI. This approach is known as the "criminogenic risk perspective."[11] Andrews and Bonta proposed a model known as the Risk–Need–Responsivity (RNR) model and this model has served as an important foundation for the criminogenic risk perspective. Under the RNR rehabilitation model, treatment interventions address each person's identified risks, their dynamic treatment needs, and their responsivity to treatment.[15] Eight criminogenic risk factors have been identified under the RNR model and are listed in Table 16.1.

The first four criminogenic risk factors listed in Table 16.1 are known as the "Big Four" as they have demonstrated the strongest relationship to future criminal offending.[15] These criminogenic risk factors are relevant to individuals with and without a SMI. The remaining four risk factors have a moderate, though less robust, association with criminal justice involvement. To further improve outcomes for individuals enrolled in diversion programs, addressing criminogenic needs in addition to utilization of evidence-based treatments for both mental illness and substance use are more likely to be effective than standard community mental health treatment alone. This combined intervention approach represents a "second generation" of services and is relevant for

Table 16.1 Central eight criminogenic risk factors[15]

1. Established criminal history
2. Antisocial personality pattern
3. Antisocial cognition
4. Antisocial associates
5. Substance abuse
6. Employment instability
7. Family problems
8. Low engagement in prosocial leisure pursuits

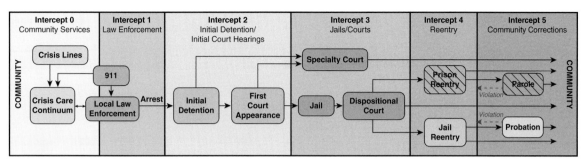

Figure 16.1 The Sequential Intercept Model.

delivery of care at all stages of a person's involvement with the criminal justice system.[11]

An important component to assist in diverting individuals with SMI away from the criminal justice system is identifying various stages where alternative programs can be introduced to either prevent involvement in the criminal justice system or provide programming to keep persons with SMI from returning to jail or prison. One recognized model in identifying such intercepts is known as the Sequential Intercept Model (SIM).[16]

The SIM covers six different intercepts, numbered 0–5, each of which identifies an alternative solution or strategy that can be offered to divert someone with mental illness out of the criminal justice system.

The basic assumption of the SIM is that criminalization of the mentally ill can be curtailed by recognizing points of interception "at which intervention can be made to prevent individuals from entering or penetrating deeper into the criminal justice system."[16] Early identification of psychiatric disorders allows individuals to be diverted into appropriate community care where symptoms can be treated and behaviors that invite criminal justice involvement can be reduced.

This continuum includes programs such as Crisis Intervention Training (CIT) to help police officers communicate and interact with individuals with mental illness (Intercept 1) to improved parole/probation contacts for individuals with mental illness (Intercept 5). Empirical studies of the interventions across the six intercepts demonstrate varying levels of effectiveness, with some community-based alternative services showing strong support, such as FACT teams, while others require further evaluation.

The SIM can also help guide policy development by providing a framework for stakeholders to understand what gaps exist in their provision of services and programs for individuals with mental illness and

criminal justice involvement. Communities are encouraged to review local SIMs with pertinent stakeholders, including but not limited to county behavioral health departments, district attorneys, public defenders, judicial representatives, probation, and local law enforcement. These stakeholders could utilize the SIM to assess and identify where improvements can be made in service provision to increase the likelihood of positive change with criminal justice-involved persons with mental illness.

This article summarizes 10 key aspects of suggested treatment goals and interventions for diversion programs that can be incorporated throughout the SIM stages to maximize treatment of diverted individuals and minimize their risk for future involvement in the criminal justice system. These treatment goals and the methods to achieve them are summarized in Table 16.2.

Prescribe Appropriate Psychotropic Medications

Diversion programs have been historically recognized to involve a critical transition of individuals from jails or detention centers to community treatment settings.[17,18] While many factors can affect the continuum of care of diverted forensic patients, e.g. communication of information among involved clinicians, timely transmission of relevant documents, active coordination of services, etc., availability of formularies aligned with respect to pivotal medications, such as clozapine and long-acting injectable (LAI) antipsychotics, and coordinated pharmacy services plays a central role in patients continuing to receive appropriate medications.[19] A critical element in the successful completion of such transfers and continued stability of the diverted patient's mental disorders is the ongoing availability of the pharmacological agents that provided stabilization of the

Table 16.2 Ten key aspects of diversion treatment

Treatment goal	Methods
Prescribe appropriate psychotropic medications	Continue or initiate evidence-based treatments for serious mental illness Use long-acting injectable antipsychotic medications for treatment responsive patients Use clozapine for treatment-resistant patients as indicated
Treat substance abuse disorders	Engage individuals in substance abuse treatment, using motivational techniques Use pharmacological supports to reduce harm Use peer supports to maintain engagement Monitor individual's progress
Provide trauma-informed interventions	Carefully screen for trauma history Provide TIC interventions throughout SIM stages
Address the "Big Four" criminogenic risk factors	Use established scales to evaluate criminogenic risks and antisocial cognitions Provide treatment targeted for antisocial personality patterns Provide CBT-type treatments for antisocial cognitions Encourage prosocial contacts and discourage antisocial contacts
Provide cognitive and social cognitive training	Computerized interventions are inexpensive and easy to deliver with demonstrated efficacy Adherence and engagement with these interventions can be monitored
Provide functional skills training and vocational rehabilitation	Initially target skills required to sustain independent residence in the community Enhance employment related skills
Provide social skills training	Recognize the importance of social interactions Adopt a systematic social skills training approach Use social networks to reinforce progress in diversion
Provide family psychoeducation	Provide relevant family members with education regarding mental illness, recognition of warning signs of relapse, and the association between relapse and re-involvement in the criminal justice system Enlist family members in patient monitoring and patient support
Obtain housing	Explore temporary versus permanent housing options
Utilize a court liaison	Engages with diverted individual, the court, and community programs to maximize community success

patient, including long-acting second-generation injectable antipsychotics. Formulary restrictions that restrict the use of evidence-based medications may result in greater rates of decompensation and greater long-term costs.[20] Indeed, failure to continue medications has been identified as the most common cause of relapse among persons suffering from chronic mental illness.[21]

Mood stabilizers, antipsychotics, and antidepressants are the mainstay medications when considering likely diagnoses in diverted individuals. In their study of New York's jail diversion program, Gill and Murphy reviewed the diagnoses in all individuals diverted from jail over a five-year period. The most common diagnosis was bipolar disorder (40%), followed by schizophrenia or schizoaffective disorder (33%), depression (17%), and anxiety (5%). The authors also found that 57% met criteria for a dual drug and/or alcohol diagnosis.[22] Overall, schizophrenia spectrum disorders (schizophrenia, schizoaffective disorder) and bipolar I disorder, combined with substance use disorders, are the most prevalent

diagnoses enrolled in diversion programs; therefore, treating clinicians must have expertise in managing these disorders using evidence-based options.[23]

Schizophrenia spectrum and other psychotic disorders afflict the bulk of chronically mentally ill individuals who are arrested and jailed.[24] Thus, antipsychotic medications form the core of pharmacological treatment in diverted forensic populations.[25] Unfortunately, adherence to oral antipsychotics in outpatient settings, even when defined as taking only 80% of prescribed doses, is consistently less than 50%.[26,27] Due to enhanced adherence, LAI antipsychotics have proven superior to their oral counterparts in reducing crime and violence.[28–31] Obtaining plasma antipsychotic and mood stabilizer levels can also assist the practitioner in monitoring compliance as well as adjustments to assist in achieving a therapeutic response.

An estimated 30% of schizophrenia spectrum patients are deemed treatment-resistant by having failed to respond adequately to two nonclozapine antipsychotics despite verified adherence; moreover, recent community samples indicate that up to 50% may be classified as having treatment-resistant schizophrenia.[32,33] Clozapine is an essential medication for stabilizing patients with treatment-resistant schizophrenia and schizoaffective disorder.

In these treatment-resistant schizophrenia patients, the response rate to clozapine is approximately 50%, while response rates to other antipsychotics are under 5%, and for olanzapine 7–9%.[34] Clozapine also has data supporting use in treatment-resistant mania associated with bipolar I disorder, and for reduction in suicidality and treatment of persistent aggression in schizophrenia spectrum patients.[35–37] In addition, research data demonstrate that extended delays in clozapine prescribing are also associated with decreased response rates.[38] Moreover, jurisdictions that demonstrate a persistent pattern of clozapine underutilization also risk administrative or legal actions from overseeing bodies or patient advocacy groups.[39]

A complete discussion of all aspects of clozapine prescribing, monitoring for and treatment of hematological and nonhematological adverse effects is extensive and beyond the scope of these guidelines. For this reason, the reader should consult published resources,[40] and consider registering at smiadviser.org to receive answers to clinical questions.

Treat Substance Abuse Disorders

As summarized above, in a five-year study of inmates diverted from New York county jails to the community, 57% had a co-occurring alcohol and/or drug diagnosis.[22] This high rate of co-occurrence further complicates the treatment needs for individuals interfacing with diversion programs and plays a significant role in a person's entrance into and successful diversion from the criminal justice system. Due to the intricate nature of factors that either contribute to or are the result of substance abuse, treatment is often multifaceted, as shown in Figure 16.2, as adapted from the National Institute on Drug Abuse.[41]

Many of these areas are consistent with general approaches to providing comprehensive, wraparound treatment of diversion participants: intake processing/assessment, clinical and case management, and overall treatment planning. Unique factors specific to targeting substance use include pharmacotherapy, contingency management interventions, and self-help/peer support groups.[41] Best practices for each of these four categories are described in the following paragraphs, but note that a multisystemic, multipronged approach (such as Medicated-Assisted Treatment for opioid use disorder)[42] shows the greatest efficacy in improved treatment outcomes.[43]

Pharmacotherapeutic interventions can be used to supplement psychosocial treatments depending on the diverted individual's drug of choice. Specifically, practice guidelines have been developed for practitioners treating individuals with opioid use disorders.[44] Readers are referred to these guidelines given the nuanced recommendations for the use of methadone, buprenorphine, and naltrexone. Similarly, Connor and colleagues produced guidelines for use of medications in the treatment of and abstinence maintenance of alcohol use. This document reviews the efficacy of medications for acute management of withdrawal (i.e.

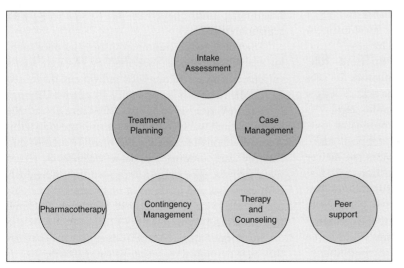

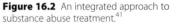

Figure 16.2 An integrated approach to substance abuse treatment.[41]

benzodiazepines) and relapse prevention (naltrexone, acamprosate, and disulfiram).[45]

In addition to substance treatment programs and pharmacological interventions, contingency approaches also may be used to support substance abuse rehabilitation. Contingency management (CM) interventions are the provision of tangible, voucher, or monetary incentives/rewards when an individual demonstrates objective behavioral goals. This could include, for example, provision of gift cards to a local grocery store when a person has negative urine drug screenings. A thorough review of 69 studies examining CM for various substance use disorders found moderate to large effect sizes.[46] These findings were consistent with previous meta-analyses of CM interventions which found them to be efficacious in decreasing substance use during and, to a lesser degree, after treatment cessation.[47,48]

Therapy and counseling should adhere to principles of Motivational Interviewing and the Stages of Change Model,[49] especially when treated individuals also experience severe mental illness.[50] These principles include assessment and recognition of the different phases of a person's decision-making when considering behavioral changes in their substance use: pre-contemplation, contemplation, preparation, action, maintenance, and termination. Using Motivational Interviewing in individual therapy sessions can reduce the frequency of a person's substance use compared to those who do not receive Motivational Interviewing techniques.[51] Traditional cognitive behavior therapy (CBT) interventions have also been found to improve outcomes for individuals with substance use disorders, including decreased substance use,[52] as have other CBT-based treatment modalities such as Acceptance and Commitment Therapy,[53] and Dialectical Behavior Therapy.[54]

Peer support also plays an important role. Outcomes research shows positive outcomes for peer support in substance use treatment, but acknowledges that most studies lack strong scientific rigor.[55,56] Nonetheless, existing studies show promising outcomes using "peer coaches," "peer support staff," and/or "substance abuse peer counselors" to deliver either short-term or long-term interventions with targeted populations.[55] The use of peer support services also appears to be embedded in many larger service-based provisions programs, as a means of developing more consistent, long-term relationships to aid in the treatment of chronic substance abuse conditions.[57]

Additionally, 12-step recovery programs have been shown to be effective in decreasing substance use in three-year longitudinal studies,[58] highlighting the importance of social support as a protective factor in relapse prevention.[59]

Provide Trauma-Informed Care

Recent studies show 88% to 96% of men and women already in jail diversion programs reported significant trauma history prior to incarceration.[60,61] According to the Substance Abuse and Mental Health Services Administration (SAMHSA), trauma is "an almost universal experience among people who use public mental health, substance abuse, and social services, as well as people who are justice-involved or homeless."[62] Multiple studies demonstrate that a significant number of individuals with a serious mental disorder (SMI) also warrant a diagnosis of post-traumatic stress disorder (PTSD), although a minority are diagnosed with any trauma-related co-occurring disorder. Under-recognition of PTSD in the presence of a "primary" psychiatric disorder is common. In one multisite study, 43% of 275 patients with SMI qualified for a diagnosis of PTSD upon evaluation, but only 2% were identified with the disorder per the medical record.[63]

Diagnosis of PTSD in the presence of a serious psychiatric disorder can be challenging. Severe trauma symptoms may be misinterpreted as evidence of personality disorder and/or psychosis. Additionally, trauma symptoms may exacerbate expression of co-morbid conditions: co-occurring PTSD has been associated with increased psychopathology, positive symptoms, neurocognitive impairment, and lower general functioning and quality of life in patients with schizophrenia.[64]

The link between trauma exposure and poor mental health outcomes is supported by research across various healthcare settings. In individuals diagnosed with SMI, trauma is associated with increased symptom severity, relapse, co-morbid substance abuse, violence risk, and worsened prognosis over the long term. A growing body of research also reveals a relationship between early trauma and later violence. A recent meta-analysis, for example, indicated that individuals with psychosis and histories of maltreatment in childhood were twice as likely to be violent as psychotic individuals lacking that history.[65]

Some traumatized SMI persons engage in behaviors that have developed over time as survival strategies or fear responses, which may take them to unwanted contact with the criminal justice system.[66–70] Applied to diversion, a trauma-informed lens offers the opportunity to identify and address trauma-related sequelae that may contribute to individuals' psychiatric and behavioral instability, substance use, poor treatment response, relapse, unwanted contact with law enforcement agencies, recidivism, and other poor outcomes. Embedding trauma-informed care (TIC) principles into the intercept model can alleviate the effects of trauma on individuals, minimize retraumatization, and stem the flow of individuals with SMI into the criminal justice system by addressing primary or contributory sources of problem behavior.

Systems that fail to recognize and acknowledge the role of trauma contribute to retraumatization, disengagement, relapse, behavioral incidents, and an overly criminalized view of multiply determined behaviors. Broad-based benefits have been demonstrated in settings where relationship-based care is provided in a trauma-informed milieu and supported by congruent policies and procedures. TIC experts therefore advocate for a comprehensive approach that informs screening, assessment, crisis intervention, treatment programming, risk management, milieu development, and provision of primary medical care.

SAMHSA's Treatment Improvement Protocol defines TIC as "a strengths-based framework that is grounded in an understanding of and responsiveness to the impact of trauma, that emphasizes physical, psychological, and emotional safety for both providers and survivors, and one that creates opportunities for survivors to rebuild a sense of control and empowerment."[71–73] In trauma-informed systems, the impact of trauma is recognized at all levels and proactive policies/procedures are employed to mitigate harm and reduce the risk of retraumatization. TIC is associated with improved mental health outcomes, more effective behavior management, and enhanced safety for consumers and their care providers. Specifically, implementation of TIC has been linked to marked reductions in violence, fewer containment-related injuries, less frequent use of seclusion and restraint, and increased positive outcomes in public and private mental health settings. For example, a review of TIC programs found: reduced utilization of seclusion and restraint; reduced use of sedative hypnotics; improved measures of patient stress; increased patient satisfaction, compliance, and participation rates; decrease in trauma-related symptoms; increased effectiveness of coping skills; and decrease in substance usesexually risky behaviors after trauma-informed practices were adopted across various settings.[74]

In recent years, SAMHSA established the GAINS Center for Behavioral Health and Justice Transformation to provide information and skills training at local, state, and national levels. The overarching goal of the center is to enhance partnerships between the mental health and criminal justice systems to avoid retraumatizing individuals, increase community safety, reduce the risk of criminal recidivism, and link individuals with trauma-informed services and treatment.

Bratina highlights the fact that the sequential intercept model is "anchored at both ends" by community, and interagency collaboration is needed at all intercepts.[68] Therefore, trauma-informed intervention for individuals at later intercepts (i.e. state hospitals, jails/prisons, community re-entry programs, probation, parole) is also needed to interrupt cycles of involuntary hospitalization, incarceration, and community-based correctional supervision.

Address the "Big Four" Criminogenic Risk Factors

As highlighted in the introduction, criminogenic factors play a substantial role in reoffending behaviors of individuals involved in the criminal justice system. The four criminogenic risk factors with the greatest association with recidivism are known as the "Big Four." Brief definitions of these criminogenic risk factors and suggested evaluation/interventions are summarized below:[15,75]

1. Established criminal history – This factor includes a person's past criminal history.
   Intervention: As the best predictor of future behavior is past behavior, the evaluator should review self-reported history of law violations and aggression, rap sheets, and obtain collateral information from third parties (i.e. family or other knowledgeable persons) to gain as accurate an understanding as possible of a person's criminal past. Reviewing factors that increase the risk of future violence should be noted and include age of offending onset, diversity of offending behaviors, and failing probation and/or conditional release.

2. Antisocial personality pattern – Andrews, Bonta, and Wormith describe the individual with this

criminogenic factor as one who has poor self-control, is aggressive, and focuses on self-pleasure.[76]

Intervention: Provide programs that focus on problem-solving, anger management, and impulsive control along with interventions that address problematic personality traits.[75]

3. Antisocial cognition, and antisocial associates – These individuals have attitudes that support their criminal behavior and they generally feel justified in violating the law or the rights of others. They may also feel entitled to special treatment or material items that they want and often interpret innocent comments as threats.[75,76]

Interventions: Evaluators should consider using self-report instruments to help assess antisocial cognition. Two known scales include the Psychological Inventory of Criminal Thinking Scale (PICTS) and the Criminal Sentiments Scale.[75] Morgan et al. utilized these scales to evaluate the percentage of inmates with mental illness that endorsed antisocial cognitions. They found that 66% of this sample self-reported thoughts and attitudes that supported a criminal belief system, indicating that this way of thinking is very common in offenders with mental illness.[77] Providers should implement CBT programs that address the criminogenic thinking in individuals who have antisocial cognitions. Validated CBT programs for this purpose include reasoning and rehabilitation,[78] moral reconation therapy,[79] and thinking for a change.[80]

4. Antisocial associates – Spending time with other individuals involved in criminal behavior.

Intervention: Clinicians can work with diversion participants to identify primary social networks that may include antisocial associates and work to develop a network of people who engage in prosocial behavior. Some diversion programs also utilize prosocial peers as part of the support and programming for enrolled individuals.[75]

Provide Cognitive Rehabilitation

Individuals with SMI commonly find themselves trapped in an extended cycle of arrests, incarceration, abbreviated psychiatric treatment, release to the community, and rearrest. Unaided, this cycle is often very difficult for SMI individuals to break. The cycle requires completion of complex legal tasks, adherence to psychological treatments, and coordinated improvements

in psychosocial organization to reassure the criminal justice system that the individual can safely return to living in the community. Unfortunately, individuals with SMI typically have cognitive and social cognitive deficits that impede them from securing and then sustaining the requisite supports to extricate them from the criminal justice system. Research has demonstrated that after adjustment for pre-morbid intellectual functioning, essentially everyone with schizophrenia shows some degree of cognitive impairment.[81,82] For individuals with SMI in the criminal justice system, there are major problems associated with having decreased cognitive abilities, including: reduced effectiveness of evidenced-based psychosocial treatments,[83,84] reduction in community functioning,[85,86] and increased aggressive behaviors.[87]

Social cognition describes an individual's cognitive abilities to understand, process, and respond to social situations. These core abilities have been parsed in various ways, but the majority of theories approximate the model put together by Horan, Roberts, and Holshausen,[88] which describe the major domains of social cognition as: emotion processing, social perception, mentalizing (theory of mind), and social cognitive bias. Social cognitive deficits, commonly seen in SMI individuals, are associated with impairments in various community outcomes, including: independent living, relationships, obtaining and maintaining work, and engaging in recreational pursuits. The main influence of social cognitive deficits is in the domain of interpersonal functioning. As criminal justice involvement typically involves interpersonal challenges, social cognition is a critical treatment target. Further, social cognition and neurocognition are closely linked,[89] but nearly all domains of social cognition exert influences on social outcomes beyond the influences of neurocognition. Social cognitive deficits can contribute to aggression[90,91] and subsequent risk for involvement in the criminal justice system. In addition, O'Reilly et al.[92] found that when social cognition is looked at in conjunction with neurocognition, social cognition has an independent effect on aggression and also mediates the relationship between neurocognition and aggression.

Computerized cognitive training (CCT) is now widely accepted as having efficacy for improving cognitive performance in schizophrenia. Several studies have suggested that CCT can reduce violent incidents, even in forensic populations. These interventions, like virtual reality assessments, can be administered by individuals with reduced levels of professional credentials. Further, these interventions are very low cost, as subscriptions for individuals receiving training cost less than $10.00 per month on average.

Social cognitive training is also available in computerized formats as well as in personal manualized treatment strategies. Social cognitive training has also been shown to be associated with reductions in violent behavior on the part of people with severe mental illness. In addition, combining social cognitive and computerized cognitive training has been shown to lead to greater benefits in both domains compared to either intervention alone. This is likely because social cognitive tasks also require neurocognitive skills and that enhancement of these skills may speed the acquisition of the typically more complex social cognitive tasks. Computerized social cognition training (CSCT) interventions have the benefits of convenience and co-administration with CCT.

Provide Functional Skills Training and Vocational Rehabilitation

Functional skills training has typically been delivered in person, such as in supported employment programs, social skills training, and other teach-type interventions such as functional adaptation skills training (FAST). While these interventions may be feasible in forensic inpatient settings, the lack of access to these interventions on an outpatient basis is one of the major clinical problems in the treatment of severe mental illness. It is estimated, for example, that less than 1% of the people with schizophrenia in America are enrolled in individualized placement and support (IPS), the best evidence-based strategy to support work outcomes. Often skills training interventions are only available in academic medical centers and even there they are often restricted to randomized clinical trials. This deficiency should be corrected because it is well known that working is associated with better outcomes in many domains, including substance abuse, homelessness, psychotic symptoms, cognition, and relapse. Although there are technology-based interventions available to improve functional skills, they are not commonly used in jail diversion programs.[93]

Vocational rehabilitation has been one of the mainstays of community-based treatment for SMI

and with good reason. In reviews of SMI individuals engaged in vocational rehabilitation programming, results indicated an improvement in global functioning, reduced depressive symptoms, increased self-esteem, and improvement in quality of life.[94–96] Results have not only been seen on assessment instruments but also in the experience of the individuals with SMI. When individuals with schizophrenia were surveyed about what would define recovery, 62% reported that independence in self-care and returning to work as the factors most important to them. Further, the majority of SMI patients report a desire to work.[97] In addition, work by itself has been shown to be beneficial for cognitive abilities as people age or go through a debilitating disease.[98]

Despite the benefits that come from vocational rehabilitation, the employment rates for SMI individuals remains relatively low.[99,100] In a systematic review of the barriers for SMI individuals' involvement in vocational rehabilitation, Tsang et al. found that cognitive functioning was a significant predictor for enrollment and success within vocational rehabilitation services.[101] Liberman and Green also described information processing problems as "rate-limiting" factors in successful social and occupational functioning.[102]

To address the role cognitive deficits have in vocational rehabilitation, many clinicians and researchers have employed cognitive remediation programs to improve outcomes in vocational rehabilitation settings. Van Duin et al. recently completed a meta-analysis of combined cognitive remediation and rehabilitation programs.[103] Results indicated significant improvement in employment rates, hours worked, job duration, and quality of performance in work. One of the most important studies on cognitive remediation and supported employment demonstrated that the addition of cognitive rehabilitation to supported employment interventions increased hours worked and wages earned in competitively obtained employment.[104]

Provide Social Skills Training

Social skills references how individuals interact with each other. Societies develop their own general guidelines as to what is considered normal or socially sanctioned behaviors. Such behaviors ran the gamut of human interaction and involve how a person talks, what they say, how they express their emotions, and even what interpersonal distance is considered appropriate.[105] Although a range of mental disorders can impair the individual's social skills, diagnosis of social dysfunction in schizophrenia is very common, fairly stable across the lifetime, and often remains when other symptoms are stabilized such as hallucinations and delusions.[106] Social skills deficits account for a large variance in a person's ability to fulfill meaningful roles, such as the ability to establish and maintain social and intimate relationships and sustain employment.[105,106] Some examples of these social deficits may include difficulty with conversations, trouble expressing one's needs, and in interpersonal behaviors that others may consider odd.

Two specific treatment recommendations to assist with social skills for persons diagnosed with a schizophrenia spectrum disorder are Social Skills Training (SST) for schizophrenia, and Cognitive Behavioral Social Skills Training (CBSST) for schizophrenia. The Schizophrenia Patient Outcomes Research Team (PORT) and the U.S. Department of Health and Human Services recommend SST and CBSST as evidenced-based psychosocial interventions for schizophrenia.[107]

SST is an evidence-based practice for improving social functioning for people with schizophrenia and related severe mental illnesses and is based on social learning theory. It is a structured format for teaching interpersonal skills that incorporates modeling, roleplays, and other behavioral learning activities. SST is skill-based and designed to create a fun and supportive environment. It targets three inter-related functions: (1) social perception: the ability to accurately perceive social cues, (2) social problem-solving: the ability to correctly analyze the social situation and identify an effective response, and (3) behavioral competence: the ability to effectively implement the response. SST covers nine key social skills, which include: (1) basic social skills, (2) conversation skills, (3) assertiveness, (4) conflict management, (5) communal living, (6) friendship and dating, (7) health maintenance/communicating with provider, (8) vocational/work, and (9) coping skills for drug and alcohol use. Within these nine broad categories are very specific practical exercises. The approach has followed the same format since its inception.

CBSST is a newer treatment than SST, developed in the early 2000s. CBSST is a recovery-oriented psychosocial rehabilitation intervention, targeting improved functioning and negative symptoms that combines CBT, SST, and problem-solving.[108] Taking into consideration the potential efficacy of both CBT and SST for schizophrenia, a combined approach was developed. CBSST is manualized treatment with three modules: Cognitive Skills, Social Skills, and Problem-Solving. Each module begins with a goal-setting session and the modules are six sessions in length. For many patients completing the treatment program twice is recommended.[108]

There continues to be ongoing research on CBSST. More recently, CBSST was implemented individually within ACT (assertive community treatment) teams in San Diego County Mental Health System and two private multiservice behavioral health agencies located in the southwestern metropolitan area.[108,109] Publications thus far on this integration of services has focused on treatment implementation factors. Recent research on implementing CBSST on ACT teams offers some additional implementation strategies. Researchers assessed how well CBSST and ACT were expected to fit using the Tool for Integrating Multiple Interventions (TIMI).[109] The TIMI looks at six intervention domains to determine how likely services are to align. These six domains include: (1) target population, (2) intervention content, (3) frequency/duration, (4) context/setting, (5) service delivery format, and (6) primary outcomes. Findings from stakeholder feedback suggested that it is crucial to access structural fit of CBSST within the ACT model and warrant modifications as needed and the implementation must have organizational support.[109] This research study highlighted the importance of tailoring to specific systems and organizations. This includes the needed elements for successful implementation: leadership buy-in, effective embedding mechanisms, flexibility, training supports, and adaptations to the practice and system when needed. These implementation recommendations are likely beneficial for the integration of varied interventions.[110]

Provide Family Psychoeducation

Family psychoeducation (FPE) is an umbrella term describing one facet of family involvement in the treatment of mental illness. Unlike family therapy, FPE targets the illness itself rather than the family as the focus of treatment.[111] The foundation of FPE is a collaboration between consumer, family, and professional aimed at assisting the consumer in his/her recovery. The goal is to equip families by teaching day-to-day skills for managing mental illness, and providing support on topics such as grief and burden.[112] FPE models vary from brief to long term, and between single family or multifamily formats. Sessions typically involve education about mental disorders, early warning signs, and relapse prevention strategies, as well as skills coaching in the areas of goal setting, communication, coping, and problem-solving.[113,114] Other family education programs exist which are peer-led rather than facilitated by treatment professionals, such as the National Alliance on Mental Illness (NAMI) Family-to-Family program available throughout the U.S.[113,115] Programs of this nature, in combination with professionally led FPE, should be included in any program designed to maintain people with mental illness in the community.

For individuals with serious and persistent mental illness, family psychoeducation and support can be effective complementary interventions to decrease the risk of psychiatric relapse.[116] A meta-analysis reviewing 53 randomized or quasi-randomized control trials found that family interventions for people with schizophrenia can not only decrease psychiatric relapse, but may also reduce hospital admissions and improve medication compliance.[117] These findings are likely generalizable to a diversion setting for individuals treated in the community with family members or caregivers willing to participate. Although initial family psychoeducation and support studies in the 1980s and 1990s indicated the primary goal of this treatment was to decrease high expressed emotion,[118] recent adaptations move toward a CBT-based model of providing family members with coping, communication, and problem-solving skills.[119] Additionally, recent literature review suggests pairing supportive interventions from both professionals and family members with lived experience (e.g. NAMI) may provide the most overall benefit.

Obtain Housing

Providing housing for individuals in diversion programs is critical to their achieving success. Literature identifies two major paradigms for providing housing to homeless individuals: the linear model[120] and the Housing First model.[121,122] The linear model provides temporary housing and operates along a continuum that includes emergency shelters and transitional housing programs, any of which may lead to independent housing. A key feature of the linear model is its requirement for individuals to maintain participation in substance abuse and mental health treatments.[123] In the linear model, individuals with mental illness who are re-entering the community from hospitals, jails, or prisons are placed in shelter or group homes first. The three basic types of group homes are transitional housing, supportive housing, and supported housing.[124] *Transitional housing* is a classic group home where the individual lives in one house or building with other residents and staff and is usually up to 24 months in duration.[62] The residents are supervised and receive medication assistance, daily living skills, meals, assistance paying bills, transportation, and treatment management. The goal is for residents to learn skills needed for independent living. *Supportive housing* includes rental units in one location that typically maintain on-site around-the-clock crisis support services. Additionally, the residents have access to other off-site support. These residents can generally perform daily living tasks for themselves, but staff visit frequently. Residents in supportive housing can have part-time jobs or participate in a day treatment program. *Supported housing* consists of individual apartments that are part of the same program, but not in the same location. The residents live mostly independently. They receive limited assistance and infrequent visits by staff members but can contact staff if needed. The linear model has been criticized for requiring sobriety and treatment engagement. Studies have found little or no evidence that these requirements affect outcome.[125,126]

The Housing First model provides permanent housing for individuals, but sobriety and participation in treatment is not a requirement.[122] Two models of Housing First are *rapid rehousing* and *permanent supportive housing* (PSH).[127] Rapid rehousing is used for people and families to quickly obtain housing. In rapid rehousing, the housing may be initially temporary, but the goal is to provide services and keep the participants permanently housed. Housing First PSH is used more commonly with homeless individuals with substance abuse and/or severe mental illness. Housing First PSH is diverse, from multiunit dwellings to scattered sites, and individuals live along with housing staff. Housing First PSH addresses mental health and medical needs through community-based teams such as ACT or intensive case management (ICM).[122] Sobriety or active participation in mental health treatment is not required so that if individuals relapse, they do not lose their housing. Housing is also put on hold for individuals if they leave housing for short periods of time.[128] Pathways to Housing in 1992 was the initial model for Housing First. Pathways to Housing was initially located in

New York and required patients to pay 30% of their income and to participate in two case management visits per month.[128] Participants in the Housing First PSH achieved better housing outcomes and showed faster improvements in community functioning and quality of life than treatment as usual.[122] The improvement in community functioning and quality of life was seen in Housing First programs that used ACT,[129] but not seen in those that utilized ICM.[130]

Utilize a Court Liaison

The role of a court liaison can vary tremendously depending on the unique factors of any given court. Broadly, a court liaison engages with diverted individuals to facilitate engagement in mental health treatment with the ultimate goal of remaining out of the criminal justice system.[131] In some courts, a liaison functions independently with limited engagement aside from providing treatment resources. Alternatively, court liaisons can be embedded within larger diversion programs and/or function on interdisciplinary teams, e.g. FACT teams, providing in-depth wrap-around services to diverted individuals.[132]

General tasks of a court liaison include organizing and ensuring communication of court activities to diverted individuals. Other administrative tasks can include providing referrals for housing, employment, substance abuse treatment, mental health treatment, or any other social services that could improve a diverted individual's quality of life.[131] There is no specific discipline or minimum level of education/classification for a court liaison, but a working knowledge of the law, court proceedings, and mental health services is imperative. Programs often utilize social workers and/or staff associated with local law enforcement to serve in court liaison positions.[133]

Holistic defense programs are an expanded and comprehensive variation of court liaison utilization. Counties that support holistic defense programs offer interdisciplinary teams to deliver both legal and social services[134] to provide stabilization. In these programs, a clinician (i.e. social worker) pairs directly with a public defender to provide services to support individuals in the criminal justice system. This could include provision of employment support, housing, social service linkage. Outcomes studies have found that holistic defense programs support safe release of individuals into the community

without increasing recidivism rates, and decreasing taxpayer costs for jail days.[131]

Community Management and Support of Diverted Individuals

The range of services and interventions outlined above represent general approaches for diversion programs with the dual goal of decreasing the mental health distress burden and risk for future offending of those diverted. These services can be provided through intensive case management, assertive community treatment, or some combination of both.

Intensive Case Management (ICM) for severely mentally ill individuals has its origins in two models of care: Assertive Community Treatment (ACT) and Case Management.[135] In ICM the services are provided by a single case manager while in ACT the services are provided by an interdisciplinary team.[136] The goal of ICM is to provide community-based services to prevent hospitalization to patients that are more functional than those receiving services with ACT. An intensive case manager typically has a small case load of patients and is responsible for assessing the patient's needs, developing a plan of care and connects the patient with community services. The case managers usually see their patients frequently, as determined by their current clinical needs. ICM aims to develop the patient's functional autonomy, personal skills, social skills, and community living. When ICM is compared to standard care, ICM reduces hospitalizations, improves social function, and increases patient involvement with care, but it is less clear what effects it has on mental state and quality of life.[137] A strong case manager–patient alliance appears to be associated with reduction of symptoms and improved global functioning.[138] Forensic Intensive Case Management (FICM) provides the same services as ICM but has the additional goal of preventing the patient from having further involvement with the criminal justice system.[139]

ACT is an outpatient evidence-based program for chronically ill, often severely ill, mental health patients.[136] In many settings, ACT programs dedicated to the criminal justice population are termed Forensic Assertive Community Treatment (FACT) programs. Overall, however, ACT is the most common name for this outpatient, multidisciplinary, individualized, holistic, and intensive intervention for severely ill mental health patients with criminal justice involvement.[136]

The ACT model consists of a multidisciplinary team that works together and provides services around the clock to severely mentally ill individuals who are at high risk for relapse, rehospitalization, and housing instability.[136] The ACT teams are mobile and usually include a psychiatrist or other licensed prescriber, a nurse, and several master-level clinicians or psychologists. The team provides community-based services, in which they collaborate closely and have low staff-to-patient ratios. Services provided by the team include treatment of the psychiatric disorder, treatment of medical illnesses, support with practical living needs, rehabilitation, and psychosocial interventions. The team ensures that the patient receives the appropriate treatment for their psychiatric disorder, often involving adherence to psychotropic medications. The team also addresses co-occurring substance use disorders. The team nurse collaborates closely with primary care to treat the patient's medical co-morbid illnesses. Practical living services include helping and teaching the patient to pay bills, shopping for food and clothing, using public transportation and maintaining their residence. Psychosocial intervention includes social skills training and managing living with mental illness.

The goal is to maintain the patient living in the community and receiving community-based treatments. The team typically meets daily to discuss the needs and progress of each patient. The team then prioritizes which member will be seen based on severity of symptoms and functional capacity. The ACT team provides services 24/7 and has contact with the patients usually daily but at least weekly. As noted above, an adaptation of ACT that is used with justice-involved patients is called Forensic Assertive Community Treatment (FACT). One approach that has gained significant support examines not only the patient's mental health needs but also their specific criminogenic needs and risks. This dual-targeted approach matches the patient's intensity of services to the most prevalent treatment goals present: clinical impairment or criminogenic behaviors.[140] Studies have shown that after participation in ACT, the rates of ambulatory mental health follow-up increased while rates of psychiatric inpatient hospitalizations decreased.[141] ACT patients have fewer convictions for new crimes, less time in jail and more time in outpatient treatment among justice-involved patients than those receiving treatment as usual.[142]

Table 16.3 The Stepping Up Initiative Key Questions

1. Is our leadership committed?
2. Do we conduct timely screening and assessments?
3. Do we have baseline data?
4. Have we conducted a comprehensive process analysis and inventory of services?
5. Have we prioritized policy, practice, and funding improvements?
6. Do we track progress?

Summary

Diversion programs represent a meaningful opportunity to improve the lives of individuals with SMI involved in the criminal justice system as well as decreasing unnecessary and potential harmful incarcerations. As diversion programs have evolved, the need for multimodal interventions in addition to good mental health care has become clear. In addition, counties should consider the six questions noted in Table 16.3 provided by The Stepping Up Initiative when developing diversion programs.[143]

Progress has been realized by diversion programs yet more progress can be achieved. First- and second-generation research gives directions that are critical to moving forward. Our guidelines utilize 10 key principles that serve as a roadmap to help achieve that desired destination – a diversion program that works to improve the life of individuals with SMI and a diversion approach that reflects a society willing to treat the vulnerable with dignity and hope.

References

1. Steadman HJ, Osher FC, Robbins PC, et al. Prevalence of serious mental illness among jail inmates. *Psychiatr Serv.* 2009; **60**: 761–765.

2. Baillargeon J, Binswanger AI, Penn JV, Williams BE, Murray OJ. Psychiatric disorders and repeat incarcerations: the revolving prison door. *Am J Psychiatry.* 2009; **166**: 103–109.

3. Steadman HJ, Barbera SS, Dennis DL. A national survey of jail diversion programs for mentally ill detainees. *Hospital and Community Psychiatry.* 1994; **45**: 1109–1113.

4. National Institute of Mental Health. Serious Mental Illness. www.nimh.nih.gov/health/statistics/mental-illness.shtml#:~:text=Serious%20mental%20illness%20(SMI)%20is,or%20more%20major%20life%20activities (accessed June 2020).

5. Ford EB, Silverman KD, Solimo A, et al. Clinical outcomes of specialized treatment units for patients

with serious mental illness in the New York City jail system. *Psychiatr Serv.* 2020; **71**: 547–555.

6. Kubiak S, Comartin EB, Hanna J, Swanson L. Identification, referral, and services for individuals with serious mental illness across multiple jails. *J Correct Health Care.* 2020; **26**(2): 168–182.

7. Steadman HJ, Scott JE, Osher F, Agnese TK, Robbins PC. Validation of the brief jail mental health screen. *Psychiatr Serv.* 2005; **56**: 816–822.

8. Kessler RC, Andrews G, Colpe LJ, et al. Short screening scales to monitor population prevalences and trends in nonspecific psychological distress. *Psychol Med.* 2002; **32**: 959–976.

9. Kessler RC, Barker PR, Colpe LJ, et al. Screening for serious mental illness in the general population. *Arch Gen Psychiatry.* 2003; **60**: 184–189.

10. Bronson J, Berzofsky M. Indicators of mental health problems reported by prisoners and jail inmates, 2011–2012 (NCJ 250612). US Department of Justice, Bureau of Justice Statistics; 2017. www.bjs.gov/content/pub/pdf/imhprpji1112.pdf (accessed June 2020).

11. Bonfine N, Wilson AB, Munetz MR. Meeting the needs of justice-involved people with serious mental illness within community behavioral health systems. *Psychiatr Serv.* 2020; **71**: 355–363.

12. Epperson MW, Wolff N, Morgan RD, et al. Envisioning the next generation of behavioral health and criminal justice interventions. *Int J Law Psychiatry.* 2014; **37**: 427–438.

13. Peterson J, Skeem JL, Hart E, Vidal S, Keith F. Analyzing offense patterns as a function of mental illness to test the criminalization hypotheses. *Psychiatr Serv.* 2010; **61**: 1217–1222.

14. Peterson J, Skeem JL, Kennealy P, Bray B, Zvonkovic A. How often and how consistently do symptoms directly precede criminal behavior among offenders with mental illness. *Law Hum Behav.* 2014; **39**: 439–449.

15. Andrews DA, Bonta J. *The Psychology of Criminal Conduct, 5th edn.* New Providence, NJ: Anderson; 2010.

16. Munetz MR, Griffin PA. Use of the Sequential Intercept Model as an approach to decriminalization of people with serious mental illness. *Psychiatr Serv.* 2006; **57**: 544–549.

17. Steadman HJ, Morris SM, Dennis DL. The diversion of mentally ill persons from jails to community-based services: a profile of programs. *Am J Public Health.* 1995; **85**: 1630–1635.

18. Steadman HJ, Deane MW, Morrissey JP, et al. A SAMHSA research initiative assessing the effectiveness of jail diversion programs for mentally ill persons. *Psychiatr Serv.* 1999; **50**: 1620–1623.

19. Karel LI, Delisle DR, Anagnostis EA, Wordell CJ. Implementation of a formulary management process. *Am J Health Syst Pharm.* 2017; **74**: 1245–1252.

20. Hawthorne WB, Folsom DP, Sommerfeld DH, et al. Incarceration among adults who are in the public mental health system: rates, risk factors, and short-term outcomes. *Psychiatr Serv.* 2012; **63**: 26–32.

21. Berge D, Mane A, Salgado P, et al. Predictors of relapse and functioning in first-episode psychosis: a two-year follow-up study. *Psychiatr Serv.* 2016; **67**: 227–233.

22. Gill KJ, Murphy AA. Jail diversion for persons with serious mental illness coordinated by a prosecutor's office. *Biomed Res Int.* 2017; **2017**: 7917616.

23. Comartin E, Kubiak SP, Ray B, Tillander E, Hanna J. Short- and long-term outcomes of mental health court participants by psychiatric diagnosis. *Psychiatr Serv.* 2015; **66**: 923–929.

24. Gottfried ED, Christopher SC. Mental disorders among criminal offenders: a review of the literature. *J Correct Health Care.* 2017; **23**: 336–346.

25. Cummings MA, Proctor GJ, Arias AW. Dopamine antagonist antipsychotics in diverted forensic populations. *CNS Spectr.* 2020; **25**(2): 128–135.

26. Garcia S, Martinez-Cengotitabengoa M, Lopez-Zurbano S, et al. Adherence to antipsychotic medication in bipolar disorder and schizophrenic patients: a systematic review. *J Clin Psychopharmacol.* 2016; **36**: 355–371.

27. de Haan L, Lavalaye J, van Bruggen M, et al. Subjective experience and dopamine D2 receptor occupancy in patients treated with antipsychotics: clinical implications. *Can J Psychiatry.* 2004; **49**: 290–296.

28. Ostuzzi G, Barbui C. Comparative effectiveness of long-acting antipsychotics: issues and challenges from a pragmatic randomised study. *Epidemiol Psychiatr Sci.* 2016; **25**: 21–23.

29. Mohr P, Knytl P, Vorackova V, Bravermanova A, Melicher T. Long-acting injectable antipsychotics for prevention and management of violent behaviour in psychotic patients. *Int J Clin Pract.* 2017; **71**: 1–7.

30. Stevens GL, Dawson G, Zummo J. Clinical benefits and impact of early use of long-acting injectable antipsychotics for schizophrenia. *Early Interv Psychiatry.* 2016; **10**: 365–377.

31. Taipale H, Mittendorfer-Rutz E, Alexanderson K, et al. Antipsychotics and mortality in a nationwide cohort of 29,823 patients with schizophrenia. *Schizophr Res.* 2018; **197**: 274–280.

32. Howes OD, McCutcheon R, Agid O, et al. Treatment-Resistant Schizophrenia: Treatment Response and Resistance in Psychosis (TRRIP) working group

consensus guidelines on diagnosis and terminology. *Am J Psychiatry*. 2017; **174**(3): 216–229.

33. Beck K, McCutcheon R, Stephenson L, et al. Prevalence of treatment-resistant psychoses in the community: a naturalistic study. *J Psychopharmacol*. 2019; **33**(10): 1248–1253.

34. Meyer JM, Stahl SM. *The Clozapine Handbook*. New York, NY: Cambridge University Press; 2019.

35. Meyer JM, Cummings MA, Proctor G, Stahl SM. Psychopharmacology of persistent violence and aggression. *Psychiatr Clin North Am*. 2016; **39**: 541–556.

36. Suppes T, Webb A, Paul B, et al. Clinical outcome in a randomized 1-year trial of clozapine versus treatment as usual for patients with treatment-resistant illness and a history of mania. *Am J Psychiatry*. 1999; **156**: 1164–1169.

37. Meltzer HY, Alphs L, Green AI, et al. Clozapine treatment for suicidality in schizophrenia: International Suicide Prevention Trial (InterSePT). [erratum appears in *Arch Gen Psychiatry*. 2003; **60**(7): 735]. *Arch Gen Psychiatry*. 2003; **60**(1): 82–91.

38. Yoshimura B, Yada Y, So R, Takaki M, Yamada N. The critical treatment window of clozapine in treatment-resistant schizophrenia: secondary analysis of an observational study. *Psychiatry Res*. 2017; **250**: 65–70.

39. Sheitman BB, Catlett TL, Zarzar TR. Limited availability and use of clozapine in state prisons. *Psychiatr Serv*. 2019; **70**: 256.

40. Meyer JM. Monitoring and improving antipsychotic adherence in outpatient forensic diversion programs. *CNS Spectr*. 2020; **25**(2): 136–144.

41. National Institute on Drug Abuse. Principles of drug addiction treatment: a research-based guide, 3rd edn. 2018. www.drugabuse.gov/publications/principles-drug-addiction-treatment-research-based-guide-third-edition (accessed June 2020).

42. Connery HS. Medication-assisted treatment of opioid use disorder: review of the evidence and future directions. *Harv Rev Psychiatry*. 2015; **23**: 63–75.

43. Crowley RA, Kirschner N. The integration of care for mental health, substance abuse, and other behavioral health conditions into primary care: executive summary of an American College of Physicians position paper. *Ann Intern Med*. 2015; **163**(4): 298–299.

44. Kampman K, Jarvis M. American Society of Addiction Medicine (ASAM) national practice guideline for the use of medications in the treatment of addiction involving opioid use. *J Addict Med*. 2015; **9**(5): 358–367.

45. Connor JP, Haber PS, Hall WD. Alcohol use disorders. *Lancet*. 2016; **387**: 988–998.

46. Davis DR, Kurti AN, Skelly JM, et al. A review of the literature on contingency management in the treatment of substance use disorders, 2009–2014. *Prev Med*. 2016; **92**: 36–46.

47. Higgins ST, Sigmon SC, Heil SH. Contingency management in the treatment of substance use disorders: trends in the literature. In: Ruiz P, Strain E., eds. *Lowinson and Ruiz's Substance Abuse: a Comprehensive Textbook*. Philadelphia, PA: Lippincott Williams & Wilkins; 2011: 603–621.

48. Lussier JP, Heil SH, Mongeon JA, Badger GJ, Higgins ST. A meta-analysis of voucher-based reinforcement therapy for substance use disorders. *Addiction* 2006; **101**: 192–203.

49. Prochaska JO, DiClemente CC. *The Transtheoretical Approach: Crossing Traditional Boundaries of Therapy*. Florida, US: Krieger Pub Co; 1994.

50. DiClemente CC, Nidecker M, Bellack AS. Motivation and the stages of change among individuals with severe mental illness and substance abuse disorders. *J Subst Abuse Treat*. 2008; **34**(1): 25–35.

51. Smedslund G, Berg RC, Hammerstrøm KT, et al. Motivational interviewing for substance abuse. *Cochrane Database Syst Rev*. 2011; (5): CD008063.

52. McHugh RK, Hearon BA, Otto MW. Cognitive behavioral therapy for substance use disorders. *Psychiatr Clin*. 2010; **33**: 511–525.

53. Lee EB, An W, Levin ME, Twohig MP. An initial meta-analysis of Acceptance and Commitment Therapy for treating substance use disorders. *Drug Alcohol Depend*. 2015; **155**: 1–7.

54. Stotts AL, Northrup TF. The promise of third-wave behavioral therapies in the treatment of substance use disorders. *Curr Opin Psychol*. 2015; **2**: 75–81.

55. Bassuk EL, Hanson J, Greene RN, Richard M, Laudet A. Peer-delivered recovery support services for addictions in the United States: a systematic review. *J Subst Abuse Treat*. 2016; **63**: 1–9.

56. Reif S, Braude L, Lyman DR, et al. Peer recovery support for individuals with substance use disorders: assessing the evidence. *Psychiatr Serv*. 2014; **65**: 853–861.

57. Committee on Crossing the Quality Chasm: Adaptation to Mental Health and Addictive Disorders, Board on Health Care Services, Institute of Medicine, National Academy of Sciences. *Improving the Quality of Health Care for Mental and Substance-Use Conditions (Quality Chasm)*. Washington, DC: National Academies Press; 2006.

58. Bond J, Kaskutas LA, Weisner C. The persistent influence of social networks and alcoholics anonymous on abstinence. *J Stud Alcohol*. 2003; **64**(4): 579–588.

59. Stevens E, Jason LA, Ram D, Light J. Investigating social support and network relationships in substance use disorder recovery. *Subst Abus*. 2015; **36**(4): 396–399.

60. Redlich AD, Steadman HJ, Monahan J, Petrila J, Griffin PA. The second generation of mental health courts. *Psychol Public Policy Law*. 2005; **11**: 527–538.

61. Jaggi LJ, Mezuk B, Watkins DC, Jackson JS. The relationship between trauma, arrest, and incarceration history among Black Americans: findings from the national survey of American life. *Soc Ment Health*. 2016; **6**: 187–206.

62. US Department of Health & Human Services. Housing and Shelter. SAMHSA; 2019. www .samhsa.gov/homelessness-programs-resources/hpr-resources/housing-shelter (accessed June 2020).

63. Mueser K, Goodman L, Trumbetta S, et al. Trauma and posttraumatic stress disorder in severe mental illness. *J Consult Clin Psychol*. 1998; **66**(3): 493–499.

64. Seow LSE, Ong C, Mahesh MV, et al. A systematic review on comorbid post-traumatic stress disorder in schizophrenia. *Schizophr Res*. 2016; **176**: 441–451.

65. Green K, Browne K, Chou S. The relationship between childhood maltreatment and violence to others in individuals with psychosis: a systematic review and meta-analysis. *Trauma Violence Abuse*. 2019; **20**: 358–373.

66. Guarino K, Bassuk E. Working with families experiencing homelessness: understanding trauma and its impact. *Zero to Three J*. 2010; **30**: 11–20.

67. Ko S, Ford J, Kassam-Adams N, et al. Creating trauma-informed systems: child welfare, education, first responders, health care, juvenile justice. *Prof Psychol Res Pr*. 2008; **39**(4): 396–404.

68. Bratina MP. *Forensic Mental Health: Framing Integrated Solutions*. New York and Abingdon, UK: Routledge; 2017.

69. Fowler PJ, Farrell AF. Housing and child well being: implications for research, policy, and practice. *Am J Community Psychol*. 2017; **60**(1–2): 3–8.

70. Roy L, Crocker AG, Nicholls TL, Latimer E, Isaak CA. Predictors of criminal justice system trajectories of homeless adults living with mental illness. *Int J Law Psychiatry*. 2016; **49**: 75–83.

71. Center for Substance Abuse Treatment (US). *Trauma Informed Care in Behavioral Health Services. Treatment Improved Protocol (TIP) Series, No. 57*. Rockville, MD: Substance Abuse and Mental Health Services Administration; 2014.

72. US Department of Health and Human Services. SAMHSA's Concept of Trauma and Guidance for a Trauma-informed Approach. SAMHSA's Trauma and Justice Strategic Initiative; 2014. https://store .samhsa.gov/sites/default/files/d7/priv/sma14-4884 .pdf (accessed June 2020).

73. Thompson-Lastad A, Yen IH, Fleming MD, et al. Defining trauma in complex care management: safety-net providers' perspectives on structural vulnerability and time. *Soc Sci Med*. 2017; **186**: 104–112.

74. Muskett C. Trauma-informed care in inpatient mental health settings: a review of the literature. *Int J Ment Health Nurs*. 2014; **23**: 51–59.

75. Skeem JL, Peterson JK. Major risk factors for recidivism among offenders with mental illness. 2011. http://risk-resilience.berkeley.edu/journal-article/major-risk-factors-recidivism-among-offenders-mental-illness (accessed June 2020).

76. Andrews D, Bonta J, Wormith JS. *Level of Service/ Case Management Inventory (LC/CMI): an offender assessment system. User's manual*. Toronto: Multi-Health Systems. 2004.

77. Morgan RD, Fisher WH, Duan N, Mandracchia JT, Murray D. Prevalence of criminal thinking among state prison inmates with serious mental illness. *Law Hum Behav*. 2010; **43**: 324–336.

78. Ross R, Fabiano E, Ewles C. Reasoning and rehabilitation. *Int J Offender Ther Comp Criminol*. 1988; **32**: 29–35.

79. Little GL, Robinson KD. Moral Reconation Therapy: a systematic step-by-step treatment system for treatment resistant clients. *Psychol Rep*. 1998; **62**: 135–151.

80. Bush J, Glick B, Taymans J. *Thinking for a Change: Integrated Cognitive Behavior Change Program*. Washington DC: National Institute of Corrections, US Department of Justice; 1997 (revised 1998).

81. Kurtz MM, Donato J, Rose J. Crystallized verbal skills in schizophrenia: relationship to neurocognition, symptoms, and functional status. *Neuropsychology*. 2011; **25**: 784–791.

82. Wilk CM, Gold JM, McMahon RP, et al. No, it is not possible to be schizophrenic yet neuropsychologically normal. *Neuropsychology*. 2005; **19**: 778–786.

83. Kern RS, Green MF, Satz P. Neuropsychological predictors of skills training for chronic psychiatric patients. *Psychiatry Res*. 1992; **43**: 223–230.

84. Mueser KT, Bellack AS, Douglas MS, Wade JH. Prediction of social skill acquisition in schizophrenic and major affective disorder patients from memory and symptomatology. *Psychiatry Res*. 1991; **37**: 281–296.

85. Green MF, Kern RS, Braff DL, Mintz J. Neurocognitive deficits and functional outcome in

schizophrenia: are we measuring the 'right stuff'? *Schizophr Bull.* 2000; **26**: 119–136.

86. Green MF, Kern RS, Heaton RK. Longitudinal studies of cognition and functional outcome in schizophrenia: implications for MATRICS. *Schizophr Res.* 2004; **72**: 41–51.

87. Reinharth J, Reynolds G, Dill C, Serper M. Cognitive predictors of violence in schizophrenia: a meta-analytic review. *Schizophr Res: Cogn.* 2014; **1**(2): 101–111.

88. Horan W, Roberts DL, Holshausen K. Integrating social cognitive training. In: Medalia A, Bowie C, eds. *Cognitive Remediation to Improve Functional Outcomes.* New York: Oxford University Press; 1995: 194–210.

89. Deckler E, Hodgins G, Pinkham A, Penn D, Harvey PD. Social cognition and neurocognition in schizophrenia and healthy controls: intercorrelations of performance and effects of manipulations aimed at increasing task difficulty. *Front Psychiatry.* 2018; **9**: 356.

90. Jones MT, Harvey PD. Neurocognition and social cognition training as treatments for violence and aggression in people with severe mental illness. *CNS Spectr.* 2020; **25**(2): 145–153.

91. Picchioni M, Harris S, Surgladze S, Reichenberg AVI, Murphy D. A neuro-psychological model of violence propensity in schizophrenia. *Eur Psychiatry.* 2015; **30**: 28–31.

92. O'Reilly K, Donohoe G, Coyle C, et al. Prospective cohort study of the relationship between neuro-cognition, social cognition and violence in forensic patients with schizophrenia and schizoaffective disorder. *BMC Psychiatry.* 2015; **15**: 155.

93. Silberstein JM, Pinkham AE, Penn DL, Harvey PD. Self-assessment of social cognitive ability in schizophrenia: association with social cognitive test performance, informant assessments of social cognitive ability, and everyday outcomes. *Schizophr Res.* 2018; **199**: 75–82.

94. Burns T, Catty J, White S, et al. The impact of supported employment and working on clinical and social functioning: results of an international study of individual placement and support. *Schizophr Bull.* 2009; **35**: 949–958.

95. Mueser KT, Becker DR, Torrey WC, et al. Work and nonvocational domains of functioning in persons with severe mental illness: a longitudinal analysis. *J Nerv Ment Dis.* 1997; **185**: 419–426.

96. Luciano A, Bond GR, Drake RE. Does employment alter the course and outcome of schizophrenia and other severe mental illnesses?: a systematic review of longitudinal research. *Schizophr Res.* 2014; **159**: 312–321.

97. Tsang HWH, Chen EYH. Perceptions on remission and recovery in schizophrenia. *Psychopathology.* 2007; **40**(6): 469.

98. Vance DE, Bail J, Enah CC, Palmer JJ, Hoenig AK. The impact of employment on cognition and cognitive reserve: implications across diseases and aging. *Nurs: Res Rev.* 2016; **6**: 61–71.

99. Anthony WA, Cohen M, Farkas M, Gagne C. *Psychiatric Rehabilitation, 2nd edn.* Boston, MA: Center for Psychiatric Rehabilitation, Sargent College of Health and Rehabilitation Sciences, Boston University; 2002.

100. Cook JA, Leff HS, Blyler CR, et al. Results of a multisite randomized trial of supported employment interventions for individuals with severe mental illness. *Arch Gen Psychiatry.* 2005; **62**: 505–512.

101. Tsang HW, Leung AY, Chung RC, Bell M, Cheung WM. Review on vocational predictors: a systematic review of predictors of vocational outcomes among individuals with schizophrenia: an update since 1998. *Aust N Z J Psychiatry.* 2010; **44**: 495–504.

102. Liberman RP, Green MF. Whither cognitive-behavioral therapy for schizophrenia? *Schizophr Bull.* 1992; **18**: 27–35.

103. van Duin D, de Winter L, Oud M, et al. The effect of rehabilitation combined with cognitive remediation on functioning in persons with severe mental illness: systematic review and meta-analysis. *Psychol Med.* 2019; **49**: 1414–1425.

104. McGurk SR, Mueser KT, Pascaris A. Cognitive training and supported employment for persons with severe mental illness: one-year results from a randomized controlled trial. *Schizophr Bull.* 2005; **31**: 898–909.

105. Bellack A, Mueser KT, Gingerich S, Agresta J. *Social Skills Training for Schizophrenia: a Step by Step Guide, 2nd edn.* New York and London: Guildford Press; 2004: 3.

106. Tenhula WN, Bellack AS. Social skills training. In: Mueser KT, Jeste DV, eds. *Clinical Handbook of Schizophrenia.* New York and London: Guildford Press; 2008: 241–248.

107. Dixon LB, Dickerson F, Bellack AS, et al. The 2009 schizophrenia PORT psychosocial treatment recommendations and summary statements. *Schizophr Bull.* 2010; **36**: 48–70.

108. Granholm E, McQuaid JR, Holden J. *Cognitive Behavioral Social Skills Training for Schizophrenia:*

a Practical Treatment Guide. New York and London: Guildford Press; 2016.

109. Sommerfeld DH, Aarons GA, Naqvi JB, et al. Stakeholder perspectives on implementing cognitive behavioral social skills training on assertive community treatment teams. *Adm Policy Ment Health*. 2019; **46**(2): 188–199.

110. Sommerfeld DH, Granholm E, Holden J, et al. Concept mapping study of stakeholder perceptions of implementation of cognitive-behavioral social skills training on assertive community treatment teams. *Psychol Serv*. 2019; 10.1037/ser0000335.

111. Dixon L, Adams C, Lucksted A. Update on family psychoeducation for schizophrenia. *Schizophr Bull*. 2000; **26**: 5–20.

112. Rosenberg SJR, Rosenberg J. *Community Mental Health: Challenges for the 21st Century, 3rd edn*. New York, NY: Routledge, Taylor & Francis Group; 2018.

113. Toohey MJ, Muralidharan A, Medoff D, Lucksted A, Dixon L. Caregiver positive and negative appraisals: effects of the national alliance on mental illness family-to-family intervention. *J Nerv Ment Dis*. 2016; **204**: 156.

114. Hayes L, Harvey C, Farhall J. Family psychoeducation for the treatment of psychosis. *InPsych*. 2013; **35**: 16–17.

115. Brister T, Cavaleri MA, Olin SS, et al. An evaluation of the NAMI basics program. *J Child Fam Stud*. 2012; **21**: 439–442.

116. McFarlane WR. Family interventions for schizophrenia and the psychoses: a review. *Fam Process*. 2016; **55**(3): 460–482.

117. Pharoah F, Mari J, Rathbone J, Wong W. Family intervention for schizophrenia. *Cochrane Database Syst Rev*. 2010; (12): CD000088.

118. Hooley JM. Expressed emotion: a review of the critical literature. *Clin Psychol Rev*. 1985; **5**: 119–139.

119. Harvey C. Family psychoeducation for people living with schizophrenia and their families. *BJPsych Adv*. 2018; **24**(1): 9–19.

120. Padgett DK. There's no place like (a) home: ontological security among persons with serious mental illness in the United States. *Soc Sci Med*. 2007; **64**(9): 1925–1936.

121. Kertesz SG, Crouch K, Milby JB, Cusimano RE, Schumacher JE. Housing first for homeless persons with active addiction: are we overreaching? *Milbank Q*. 2009; **87**(2): 495–534.

122. Aubry T, Nelson G, Tsemberis S. Housing first for people with severe mental illness who are homeless: a review of the research and findings from the At Home – Chez Soi demonstration project. *Can J Psychiatry*. 2015; **60**: 467–474.

123. Tsemberis S, Eisenberg RF. Pathways to housing: supported housing for street-dwelling homeless individuals with psychiatric disabilities. *Psychiatr Serv*. 2000; **51**(4): 487–493.

124. Peterson T. Finding group homes for mentally ill adults. Healthy Place; 2019. www .healthyplace.com/other-info/mental-illness-overview/finding-group-homes-for-mentally-ill-adults (accessed June 2020).

125. Mares AS, Kasprow WJ, Rosenheck RA. Outcomes of supported housing for homeless veterans with psychiatric and substance abuse problems. *Ment Health Serv Res*. 2004; **6**: 199–211.

126. Tsai J, Rosenheck RA, Kasprow WJ, McGuire JF. Sobriety as an admission criterion for transitional housing: a multi-site comparison of programs with a sobriety requirement to programs with no sobriety requirement. *Drug Alcohol Depend*. 2012; **125**(3): 223–229.

127. National Alliance to End Homelessness. Fact sheet: Housing First. 2016. http://endhomelessness.org/wp-content/uploads/2016/04/housing-first-fact-sheet.pdf (accessed June 2020).

128. Pearson CL. The applicability of Housing First models to homeless persons with serious mental illness. United States Department of Housing and Urban Development – Office of Policy Development Research; 2007. www.huduser.gov/Publications/pdf/hsgfirst.pdf (accessed June 2020).

129. Aubry T, Tsemberis S, Adair CE, et al. One-year outcomes of a randomized controlled trial of housing first with ACT in five Canadian cities. *Psychiatr Serv*. 2015; **66**: 463–469.

130. Stergiopoulos V, Hwang SW, Gozdzik A, et al. Effect of scattered-site housing using rent supplements and intensive case management on housing stability among homeless adults with mental illness: a randomized trial. *J Am Med Assoc*. 2015; **313**: 905–915.

131. Anderson JM, Buenaventura M, Heaton P. The effects of holistic defense on criminal justice outcomes. *Harv Law Rev*. 2019; **132**(3): 819.

132. Grudzinskas AJ, Jr., Clayfield JC, Roy-Bujnowski K, Fisher WH, Richardson MH. Integrating the criminal justice system into mental health service delivery: the Worcester diversion experience. *Behav Sci Law*. 2005; **23**(2): 277–293.

133. Buchanan S, Nooe RM. Defining social work within holistic public defense: challenges and implications for practice. *Soc Work*. 2017; **62**(4): 333–339.

134. Steinberg R. Heeding Gideon's call in the twenty-first century: holistic defense and the new public defense paradigm. *Washington Lee L Rev.* 2013; **70**: 961.

135. Dieterich M, Irving CB, Bergman H, et al. Intensive case management for severe mental illness. *Cochrane Database Syst Rev* 2017; **1**(1): CD007906.

136. Bond GR, Drake RE, Mueser KT, et al. Assertive community treatment for people with severe mental illness. *Dis Manage Health Outcomes.* 2001; **9**(3): 141–159.

137. Dieterich M, Irving CB, Bergman H, et al. Intensive case management for severe mental illness. *Schizophr Bull.* 2017; **43**: 698–700.

138. Neale MS, Rosenheck RA. Therapeutic alliance and outcome in a VA intensive case management program. *Psychiatr Serv.* 1995; **46**: 719–721.

139. US Department of Health and Human Services. Adult mental health treatment court locator. SAMHSA's GAINS Center; 2019. www.samhsa.gov /gains-center/mental-health-treatment-court-locator/adults (accessed June 2020).

140. Skeem JL, Manchak S, Peterson JK. Correctional policy for offenders with mental illness: creating a new paradigm for recidivism reduction. *Law Hum Behav.* 2011; **35**: 110–126.

141. Huz S, Thorning H, White CN, et al. Time in assertive community treatment: a statewide quality improvement initiative to reduce length of participation. *Psychiatr Serv.* 2017; **68**: 539–541.

142. Lamberti JS, Weisman RL, Cerulli C, et al. A randomized controlled trial of the Rochester Forensic Assertive Community Treatment Model. *Psychiatr Serv.* 2017; **68**: 1016–1024.

143. Haneberg R, Fabelo T, Osher F, Thompson M. Reducing the number of people with mental illnesses in jail: six questions county leaders need to ask. The Stepping Up Initiative; 2017. https://stepuptogether .org/wp-content/uploads/2017/01/Reducing-the-Number-of-People-with-Mental-Illnesses-in-Jail_Six-Questions.pdf (accessed June 2020).

Decriminalizing Mental Illness: Specialized Policing Responses

Charles Dempsey, Cameron Quanbeck, Clarissa Bush, and Kelly Kruger

Introduction

The criminalization of persons suffering from a mental illness continues to be a urgent public health concern, a resource-draining criminal justice problem, and an overarching societal issue, not only in the state of California, but also across the United States and the world. With the advent of deinstitutionalization, which was codified by the Lanterman–Petris–Short Act (Cal. Welf and Inst. Code, sec. 5000 et seq.) in 1967 in the State of California and subsequent legislation across the nation, states could no longer simply lock a person with mental illness away in a mental health facility or sanitarium, which violated their constitutional right to due process. The intent of the Lanterman–Petris–Short Act was to move away from the numerous state-run institutions and create a community-based treatment model, providing mental health services in least restrictive environments. Although the intent of deinstitutionalization had its merits, it created an unfunded mandate, and then a capacity crisis at most psychiatric emergency departments and medical emergency rooms across the country. Deinstitutionalization shifted access to mental health services and treatment predominantly to "first responders," who became the primary means by which persons in a mental health crisis were contacted, de-escalated, detained, and transported for mental health treatment.[1]

Law Enforcement/First Responder Diversion Models

Many states modified their laws giving law enforcement the power to detain and involuntarily transport those persons with a serious mental illness from their homes or the street to facilities in order to treat their mental illness.[2] Across the United States and in many other nations, these powers are based in the legal standard of probable cause, wherein the person contacted is believed to be suffering from a mental disorder that is acute, and as a result the person is a danger to self, others, and/or gravely disabled and unable to care for their basic needs. The shift to deinstitutionalization has led to the criminalization of those with a serious mental illness and the role law enforcement plays in this process is well documented. Most law enforcement agencies, who were now codified by state laws to handle calls involving persons with mental illness, were ill-prepared to manage this shift of responsibility. The lack of promised community supports and services left officers with few choices in the management of these calls involving persons with serious mental illness, resulting in their arrests and subsequent housing in jails and prisons.[3]

This shift in the role of the first responder in managing crisis mental health calls ultimately led to several tragedies in which a person with a mental illness died as a result of the involvement of law enforcement. These tragedies led to the inception of two law enforcement-based response strategies or specialized policing responses.[4]

The first strategy is the crisis intervention team (CIT) model (more commonly known as the "Memphis Model"), a "first responder" law-enforcement based model. This model (developed in 1988 in Memphis, Tennessee) is widely accepted nationally and has become an important safety net and crisis intervention strategy in many communities, where access to mental health services or the lack thereof has fallen on first responders.[5] Now available in 2,700 communities nationwide, CIT programs create connections between law enforcement, other first responders (e.g. paramedics, dispatchers), mental health professionals, and persons suffering from a serious mental illness and their family members. A typical CIT program involves an intensive 40 hour/ week training during which participants learn how to recognize symptoms of major mental illness, interact, and gain perspective from those who have experienced mental health crises and their families, engage in role-playing exercises that help enhance verbal de-escalation skills, and visit sites in the community where follow-up care is provided after a law enforcement referral is made for treatment services.

Research on the effectiveness of CIT training has examined changes in outcomes before and after CIT training and compared outcomes of crisis calls for officers with CIT training to those without training. CIT training increases the likelihood that an officer will divert a person suffering from a mental illness who has committed low-level offenses to mental health services as opposed to jail.[6–8] Referrals for treatment rather than arrest can be effective in re-establishing regular mental health contact in persons experiencing mental health crises, many of whom have disengaged from mental health care in the year prior to the crisis.[9] Diverting and reconnecting individuals to community mental health services rather than making an arrest is cost-effective because it avoids expensive inpatient referrals from a jail to a psychiatric facility for competency restoration.[10]

Research has shown that CIT training changes officer attitudes more favorably toward persons with a mental illness,[6] enhances knowledge about mental health conditions,[7] and improves skill in de-escalating crisis situations using verbal engagement and negotiation.[8] These important learning strategies are designed to increase empathy toward persons suffering from a mental illness. When dealing with persons exhibiting psychotic agitation, CIT-trained officers have increased awareness that physical interventions are likely to be ineffective and are less likely to use force[11,12] as well as an appreciation that the behaviors exhibited by persons with schizophrenia have biological causes.[13] A training approach that is widely accepted as effective in CIT training programs are role-playing exercises during which police officers interact with actors presenting with psychiatric-related behaviors commonly encountered in the field.[14] Law enforcement officers who have received feedback during role-playing exercises have an increased ability to recognize mental health issues as a reason for a call, deal with mental health issues more efficiently, and decrease their use of weapons use physical force in interactions with persons with mental illness.[15]

Although the CIT training model has been a useful tool in diversion of persons with serious mental illness from criminal justice settings, a major limitation is the CIT officer's lack of formal mental health training. In a study comparing ability to recognize signs and symptoms of mental illness in a variety of clinical scenarios, graduate students in mental health fields recognized the presence of mental disorders twice as often as CIT-trained officers.[16] Furthermore, CIT officers do not have clinical backgrounds and connections to mental health resources in the community that can facilitate linking the appropriate treatment to an individual with mental illness encountered in the field. Lastly, even when officers recognize the symptoms of a mental illness and are familiar with the resources within their communities, it is the lack of those resources which can limit the ability of officers to divert the person who is suffering from a mental illness from the criminal justice system.

The second law enforcement response strategy that evolved shortly after CIT is known as the "Co-Responder Team (CRT)." This is a "secondary" response model, in which a specially trained officer and a mental health clinician respond to the person in crisis, after being contacted by uniformed patrol officers. Typically, these teams are dispatched and ride together in a police vehicle. This strategy was first employed by the Los Angeles County Sheriff's Department in 1992, known as Mental Evaluation Team, and in 1993 by the Los Angeles Police Department (LAPD), when it began deploying the Systemwide Mental Assessment Response Teams (SMART).[17] CRT provides emergency assessment and referral for individuals with mental illness who come to the attention of law enforcement through phone calls from community members or in-field law enforcement requests for emergency assistance.

Table 17.1 Proposed levels of care of the Behavioral Health Justice Center: diversion of mentally ill individuals from the criminal justice system into treatment in San Francisco

Level 1	Emergency Mental Health Reception Center and Respite Beds. A 24-hour venue for police to bring individuals experiencing a mental health episode for an initial mental health assessment.
Level 2	Short-term (2–3 wk) transitional housing and on-site residential treatment.
Level 3	Long-term Residential Dual Diagnosis Treatment. Longer-term intensive residential psychiatric care and substance abuse treatment in an unlocked setting.
Level 4	Secure Inpatient Transitional Care Unit. Short-term, voluntary inpatient treatment for persons with mental illness transitioning to community-based residential treatment programs.

The mental health clinician has access to the information from the community's mental health system and the law enforcement officer can access past contacts with law enforcement and the local jail. The CRT evaluates the crisis, assesses the individual's mental health condition and current needs, and, as indicated, transports persons to a hospital, or refers them to a community-based resource or treatment program.

The addition of a skilled and experienced mental health clinician at the scene of a crisis call has been shown to enhance positive outcomes for persons with mental illness. Compared to police-only interactions with those in mental health crises, CRT interactions had lower rates of injury and arrest, more voluntary transports to a hospital, less time at the hospital during handover to staff,[18] as well as less time spent on-scene.[19] In contrast to police-only response, CRT teams can admit individuals directly to inpatient psychiatric units[20,21] and are significantly better able to manage mental health crises in outpatient mental health settings, avoiding unnecessary hospitalization.[18]

Service users of CRTs see the benefit of a joint mental health professional/police officer team response to crisis calls in the community.[22] Compared to the police-only response, CRTs offered improved communication, de-escalation skills, information sharing, interagency collaboration, and a greater likelihood of consumers achieving a preferred outcome to their mental health crisis.[20] A Los Angeles County study examined differences in treatment outcomes of 15,454 mentally ill individuals encountered by LAPD patrol officers and LAPD's CRT (SMART) over a one-year time period. The overwhelming majority (90%) of persons with mental illness contacted by LAPD patrol officers were taken to Los Angeles County psychiatric facilities; in contrast, 60% of those in a mental health crisis seen by SMART were taken to a private psychiatric facility or urgent care center.[23] This clearly demonstrates the ability of CRTs to provide better placements for those experiencing a mental health crisis. CIT and co-responder models are widely accepted as "best practices" across the United States and the world in the ongoing effort to reduce the population of those suffering from a serious mental illness from being housed in our city jails and prisons. Unfortunately, despite these successes, the criminalization rate of persons with mental illness has continued to rise over time.

Sequential Intercept Model/ Community-Based Mapping

As communities continued to struggle with this insidious public health and public safety issue, there was no clear understanding of how, when, and where persons with a serious mental illness engaged, entered into, traversed, and exited the criminal justice system (usually worse off than before criminal justice involvement). It was at this point that the Sequential Intercept Model was introduced (Figure 17.1),[23] developed as a conceptual model to inform community-based responses to the involvement of people with mental and substance use disorders in the criminal justice system. Developed over several years in the early 2000s by Mark Munetz, M.D. and Patricia A. Griffin, Ph.D., along with Henry J. Steadman, Ph.D., of Policy Research Associates, Inc. the Sequential Intercept Model identified five key intercepts in which an individual suffering from a mental illness intersects and navigates the criminal justice system. Intercept 1 is law enforcement in the community setting, which involves the initial 911 call for service and a law enforcement response. Intercept 2 is the initial arrest/detention and first court appearance. Intercept 3 is the process through the jails and courts to include sentencing. Intercept 4 is re-entry from jail or prison. Finally, Intercept 5 involves community correction, such as probation and parole.

The Sequential Intercept Model became the road map many communities utilized, for those who were engaged in the process of diversion, assuming that diversion begins with Intercept 1 and a law enforcement contact. Recently, the developers of the Sequential Intercept Model added an Intercept 0, which focused on community-based services being the first or preferred contact with a person who is suffering from a serious mental illness, hopefully in a pre-crisis situation (Figure 17.2).[24] By adding Intercept 0, this reinforced the pre-law enforcement contact and understanding that community engagement is a valid intercept, preventing that initial law enforcement contact in the first place. Early intervention points in the community include crisis hotlines, coordination of community dispatchers with law enforcement, mobile and peer crisis services, devoted psychiatric emergency rooms, and short-term crisis residential stabilization units.

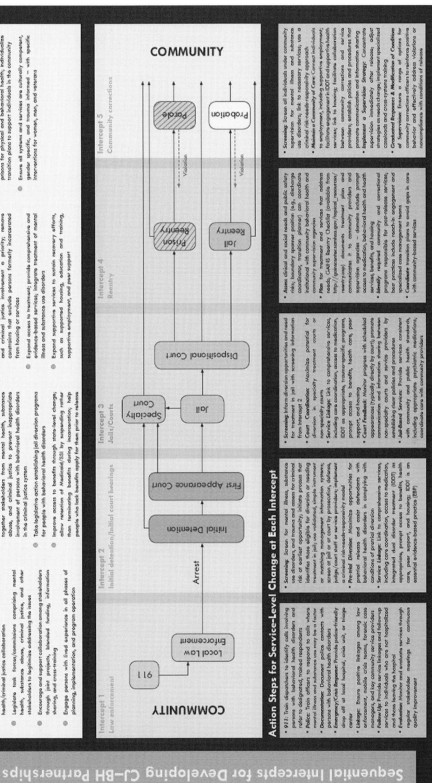

Figure 17.1 The Sequential Intercept Model at first identified five key intercepts: Intercept 1 – law enforcement; Intercept 2 – initial detention/initial court hearings; Intercept 3 – jails/courts; Intercept 4 – re-entry; and Intercept 5 – community corrections.

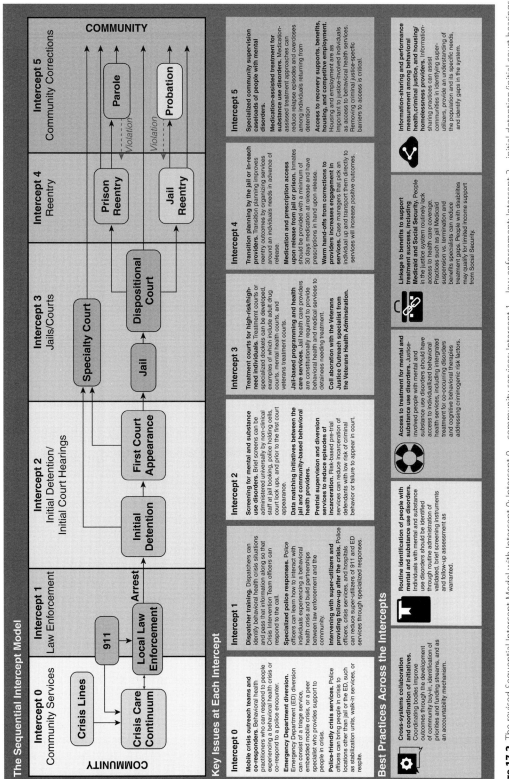

Figure 17.2 The revised Sequential Intercept Model with Intercept 0: Intercept 0 – community services; Intercept 1 – law enforcement; Intercept 2 – initial detention/initial court hearings; Intercept 3 – jails/courts; Intercept 4 – re-entry; and Intercept 5 – community corrections.

Community Education

In his Master's thesis paper titled "A Descriptive Study of LAPD's Co-Response Model for Individuals with Mental Illness," Hector Lopez made a fascinating observation. He noted that the African-American community in the City of Los Angeles disproportionately relied on 911 to access mental health services, and usually after a crisis had occurred.[22] What he discovered was that (in an effort to promote public safety) governments and communities have created a default response to mental health-related crises, thus assuring a de facto first responder/law enforcement response to all community mental health-related situations. This, in turn, leads the public to believe that this is the appropriate best response. Because of this finding, the LAPD, with the cooperation of the Los Angeles County Department of Mental Health (LACDMH) and with feedback from the National Alliance on Mental Illness (NAMI), created its 911 checklist. This checklist provided the community and family members three basic messages: (1) if they must call 911, what information the dispatcher needs; (2) what to expect when the police respond; and (3) if it is not a true emergency refrain from calling 911. In addition to the 911 checklist, they are also provided the LAPD–LACDMH Community Mental Health Resource Guide.[25] These are distributed by responding officers to 911-related mental health crisis calls, at community meetings, and at NAMI support group meetings. Los Angeles is not alone in this effort of educating communities; others such as Dallas and Houston have developed similar efforts and tools.[26–29] The goal is to educate community members, families, and others to address the needs of a person suffering from a mental illness in the community pre-crisis setting, Intercept 0. It is believed that collaboration, awareness, and education of the community and families will result in fewer contacts between law enforcement and those suffering from a serious mental illness and increase awareness of those community mental health and housing resources available to those who suffer from a serious mental illness.

911 Call Diversion and Other Non-Law Enforcement Strategies

In addition, some communities such as Houston and Harris County, Texas have come to realize that not all mental health crisis calls are equal, and many do not require the response of law enforcement. The Houston Police Department has partnered with the Harris County Crisis Line, having a crisis worker housed in the public safety answering point who triages and manages many calls that would have previously been dispatched to uniformed officers.[30] Lieutenant Brian Bixler, the Mental Illness Project Coordinator for the LAPD and Officer in Charge of the Crisis Response Support Section was quoted in an article, stated, "What if somebody called 911, and we had [the person speak to someone] who could de-escalate [the situation] or talk to them in an appropriate way to get them the help they needed, instead of sending a police car?"[31] Other communities such as Eugene and Portland, Oregon have similar programs, diverting calls from police response, utilizing dispatch questionnaires and algorithms to determine if the call can be diverted to a crisis line or community crisis response team.[32] Crisis Assistance Helping out on the Streets, which is a unique program in Eugene, Oregon is funded through the police departments general budget to provide an outreach and engagement team, consisting of a social worker and emergency medical technician. This program, which is primarily for homeless outreach, has been in existence for over 20 years and is positively received by the community, families, and those who suffer from a mental illness.[33]

De-escalation of the Incident by Disengaging Law Enforcement from the Crisis

The strategic disengagement of barricaded persons, who have been determined to be a danger only to themselves, is another successful method of diverting persons suffering from a mental illness away from the criminal justice system. There are some 911 calls which require an immediate response and tactical management by law enforcement, while others allow officers the opportunity to communicate with the suspect/subject, refine tactical plans, and call for additional resources.[33] The actions of first responders will be weighed against the information known, the gravity of the situation, the subject's actions, and efforts to de-escalate the situation. Tactical disengagement is a strategy that may be considered when continued contact may result in an undue safety risk to the suspect/subject, the public, and/or department members, especially in situations involving a barricaded suspect, a suicidal subject, or a person suspected of experiencing a mental health crisis. In conjunction with this tactical disengagement, it is prudent to develop a plan to re-engage that person at a later time or date, when the crisis has passed, to refer and/or provide them with mental health services. This is an important concept, understanding that the continued engagement by law enforcement may escalate the situation and result in a person committing a crime, such as battery on a peace officer, or a justifiable use of force by officers, creating a "Lawful but Awful" outcome.[34]

The focus of the effort to decriminalize those suffering from a serious mental illness has its greatest impact at Intercept 0, community services. This is accomplished by educating the community, caregivers, families, and those with a mental illness on how to access those promised community-based services, without relying on the 911 system. In those communities, which lack services, the leveraging of existing resources and advocacy for additional resources must be included in the overall strategy. In California with the passage of Proposition 63 and the establishment of the Mental Health Services Act, dedicated funding for these services was established. Proper screening of 911 calls for service and diverting those, when appropriate, to crisis lines prevents unnecessary law enforcement responses. Lastly, when law enforcement is engaged, weighing the necessity of that response to the seriousness of the incident, and developing protocols to disengage, when appropriate, and providing the person in crisis an opportunity to calm down and to de-escalate, allows for the possibility of contacting the person at a later date for follow-up, and then connecting the person to mental health services.

The criminalization of persons suffering from a serious mental illness, and their journey through the criminal justice system is a symptom of the lack of those community-based mental health services and the funding that was promised years ago, when the deinstitutionalization of persons with a serious mental illness from state-run hospitals began. Continuing to heavily invest in the design and development of law enforcement-based first responder strategies as opposed to funding these critical community-based services, is like treating a fever; it may temporarily alleviate the symptom, but does not address the underlying illness.

Assisted Outpatient Treatment: A Community-Based Approach

In 2011, a national online survey of more than 2,400 senior law enforcement officials was conducted

querying the officials as to how their interaction with persons with mental illness has changed over the course of their careers.[35] The vast majority of respondents agreed that over the course of their careers: the amount of time their department spends on calls for service involving persons with mental illness has increased, that officers spend more time on calls involving mental illness compared to noncrisis calls – especially when violent behavior is involved, that the population of persons with mental illness has been steadily growing over time and become more criminal-justice involved, and that most police officer injuries and fatalities that occur in the line of duty involve encounters with persons experiencing symptoms of mental illness at the time of the incident.

When asked what they attribute the increase in law enforcement resources devoted to calls involving persons with mental illness, most respondents cited two primary root causes: the inability to get acutely ill people into the hospital and/or to keep them there until they are stable enough to rejoin the community, and, that the public doesn't have access to effective referral routes into mental health treatment programs. Notably, one survey respondent commented that law enforcement officials will often arrest and book persons with mental illness to give them access to mental health treatment: "Our jail system provides more bed space for mentally ill subjects than the local state services. Law enforcement recognize the potential for individuals to access these services if the subject is booked for a crime, particularly when other treatment resources are unavailable."

When asked about the main obstacles that prevent them from making a referral into effective treatment that would prevent future crisis contacts with a mentally ill person, the respondents mentioned their inability to refer obviously psychotic persons to treatment programs unless they meet the "danger to self or others" criteria and the limited or lack of availability of mental health services in the field (for example, mobile crisis teams, community crisis teams, and other community-based services) as primary reasons. The author further elaborates on the consequences of waiting until an obviously psychotic person becomes dangerous before detaining and transporting them for treatment, "The vast majority of individuals in the early stages of psychiatric crisis or in a nonviolent psychiatric crisis are required to deteriorate to a point at which they are notably dangerous or until they enter the criminal justice system as a result of antisocial behavior, which may include acts of violence and/or self-harm, crimes against property, misdemeanors such as vagrancy, or any of a variety of other chargeable offenses. Because immediate family members most commonly call for emergency services to intervene in a psychiatric emergency and are typically rebuffed pending the development of danger, family members are often at risk of becoming victims of violence, and the individual in crisis is left at risk of self-harm."

The significant difficulty the senior law enforcement officials reported in getting subjects with serious mental illness in their communities into effective mental health treatment reflects a feature of serious mental illnesses that is now widely accepted. Approximately 50% of persons with a serious mental illness (schizophrenia, schizoaffective, and severe bipolar disorder) lack insight into their illness.[36-40] Lack of insight is a cardinal feature of serious mental illness that prevents the sufferer from understanding they are ill and that the symptoms they are experiencing are part of the illness. It is the single largest reason why people with serious mental illness refuse medications and fail to seek out treatment voluntarily. Without awareness of the illness, declining treatment appears rational, no matter how clear the need for treatment might be to others.

In 2000, the American Psychiatric Association recognized that lack of insight into illness is a prevalent feature of serious mental illness and that those who lack insight have a poorer prognosis than those who do not. In Schizophrenia and Related Disorders Section of the *Diagnostic and Statistical Manual of Mental Disorders, Fourth Edition, Text Revision* (DSM-IV-TR, APA Press, 2000): "Most individuals with schizophrenia have poor insight regarding the fact that they have a psychotic illness. Evidence suggests that poor insight is a manifestation of the illness rather than a coping strategy. It may be comparable to the lack of awareness of neurological deficits seen in stroke, termed anosognosia. This symptom predisposes the individual to noncompliance with treatment and has been found to be predictive of higher relapse rates, increased number of involuntary hospital admissions, poorer psychosocial functioning, and a poorer course of illness," page 304, DSM-IV (American Psychiatric Association Press, 2000).[41] Subsequent research has clearly demonstrated that persons with a serious mental illness and poor insight are likely to be nonadherent to

psychiatric medications and go untreated for a longer period of time than those who retain insight.[42-49] Fortunately, insight can improve if treatment is initiated and sustained over time.[50-52] Over the past decade, a number of research studies have been conducted comparing the brains of individuals with a serious mental illness with and without anosognosia. The results have demonstrated that anosognosia has a neurological cause involving damage to a network of brain structures including the anterior insula, anterior cingulate cortex, medial frontal cortex, and inferior parietal cortex.[53]

Further, though most individuals living with a serious mental illness do not engage in violent behavior and are more likely to be victims rather than perpetrators of violence, those with the most severe forms of illness are at increased risk of violence when not in treatment and are experiencing specific symptoms, specifically paranoid delusions with or without command auditory hallucinations. Lack of insight or anosognosia is associated with nonadherence to psychiatric treatment, physical aggression, and violent offending, criminal conviction, and recidivism.[54] Law enforcement first responders repeatedly encounter persons with a serious mental illness who lack insight when responding to calls for service and it is important they understand these individuals are suffering from a brain disease.

The survey's findings and high prevalence of persons with a serious mental illness who lack insight into their illness helps inform the types of services and programs that should be made available in Intercept 0 in the new Sequential Intercept Model that may help prevent persons with mental illness from becoming entangled in the criminal justice system. The senior law enforcement officials' concerns that they can't refer obviously psychotic persons for inpatient treatment unless they meet the strict "danger to self and others" criterion and the public's inability to find care referrals for persons with mental illness could be addressed through expanded use of assisted outpatient treatment (AOT). AOT is a form of civil commitment that mandates adherence to mental health treatment in the community. The overarching purpose of this intervention is to prevent psychotic decompensation, criminal justice and hospital recidivism, and other outcomes associated with nonadherence to treatment, including violent behaviors.[55] Because AOT is a civil commitment that aims to prevent criminal justice involvement, it is an

Intercept 0 intervention in the recently updated Sequential Intercept Model. AOT programs target adults with a serious mental illness who have a history of nonadherence to psychiatric treatment that has resulted in repeated hospitalizations, jailing, and/or violent behavior (see Figure 17.3 for New York's AOT criteria). Mental health professionals, family members, co-habitants, and a peace, parole, or probation officer assigned to supervise a person with mental illness can make an AOT referral. AOT program participants are primarily comprised of seriously mentally ill persons diagnosed with schizophrenia, schizoaffective, and bipolar I disorder who lack insight into their illness and decline recommended voluntary outpatient treatment despite clear evidence they would likely benefit from it.[56] AOT programs attempt to engage this challenging population who would otherwise not agree to voluntary care by using a multidisciplinary treatment team combined with judicial oversight to ensure that the program participant and providers are following the treatment plan.

Multiple research studies have demonstrated that, compared to standard outpatient care, AOT programs produce positive outcomes for participants including the following: less frequent hospitalizations, shorter lengths of stay if hospitalized, fewer days spent homeless, a reduced risk of violence behavior and criminal arrest, decreased harmful behaviors, a reduced risk of being victimized, and significantly improved medication adherence.[57–61] The positive outcomes that AOT programs produce continue to increase the longer a participant remains engaged in AOT or continues in intensive outpatient services after the court order expires (based on data comparing outcomes at six months to one year after entering the program).[62,63] Cost-analysis studies have found AOT programs to be cost-effective for public mental health systems by shifting the pattern of service utilization from psychiatric emergency care, acute psychiatric hospitalizations, arrest, and jailing to routine outpatient encounters.[64,65] Most of the research on the effectiveness of AOT was based on program outcomes in New York and North Carolina. In 2013, California passed Senate Bill 585 which provided a funding source of AOT programs; consequently, 20 of California's 58 counties have implemented AOT, for example, "Laura's Law" programs, including the majority of California's most populous counties. A recent report found that in all California AOT programs for which outcome data are available, program participants have experienced significant decreases in psychiatric hospitalizations, crisis contacts, homelessness, as well as arrests and jailings.[66]

Many believe that the positive outcomes of AOT programs are largely due to enhanced community services as opposed to the fact that the services are judicially mandated. Several recent studies have shown that it is not just the lack of enhanced intensive care services that prevents some people with a serious mental illness from accepting and benefitting from mental health treatment.[67] A study compared the severity of psychotic symptoms in people with a serious mental illness participating in intensive outpatient services in an AOT program to those receiving the same services on a voluntary basis. Those in the AOT program had greater improvement in the severity of their symptoms and greater use of mental health services than those receiving the same services voluntarily. Other recent studies demonstrated that most people with a serious mental illness who had been offered and failed to adhere to assertive community treatment alone became adherent to the same services after a judicial order was introduced into their treatment plan. Another study showed that patients in an AOT program were more likely to accept both mental health as well as physical health care compared to patients engaged in voluntary treatment. Some individuals with a serious mental illness may not need intensive outpatient services coupled with AOT to derive benefits; a 2019 study found that AOT combined with standard outpatient clinic care experienced significantly reduced hospitalizations and fewer hospital days during and after the court order.[68]

The federal government has given broad support to AOT programs. The Office of Justice Programs, an agency of the United States Department of Justice, has designated AOT "an effective crime prevention intervention" for people living with a serious mental illness.[69] In 2016, the Substance Abuse and Mental Health Services Administration (SAMHSA) and Interdepartmental Serious Mental Illness Steering Committee announced plans to award $54 million to fund 17 new AOT programs nationwide for four years with the goal of "improving the health and wellbeing of those with a serious mental illness and to identify evidence-based practices to reduce psychiatric emergency care, hospitalizations, homelessness, and interactions with the criminal justice system."[70]

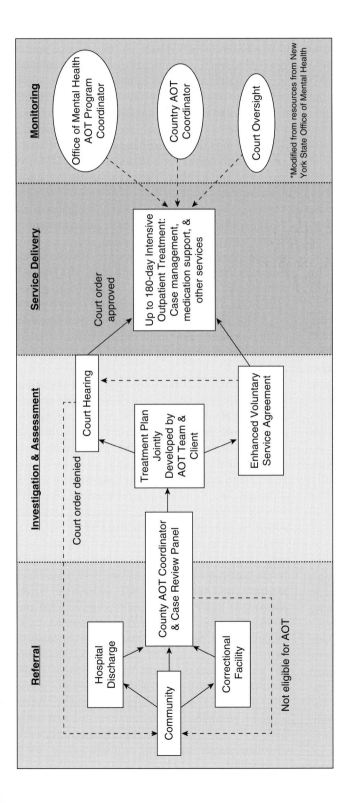

New York AOT Eligibility Criteria (New York Mental Hygiene Law, Section 9.60)

1. At least 18 years old and suffering from mental illness.
2. Clinical determination needs to indicate that they are unlikely to survive safely in the community without supervision.
3. History of lack of compliance with treatment for mental illness that has significantly contributed to at least two hospitalizations or incarcerations within the last 36 months, or one or more acts of serious violent behavior in the last 48 months.
4. Unlikely to voluntarily participate in outpatient treatment that would enable him or her to live safely in the community.
5. Considering treatment history and current behavior, is in need of assisted outpatient treatment in order to prevent a relapse or deterioration which would likely result in serious harm to self/others.
6. Likely to benefit from assisted outpatient treatment.
7. Previously executed health care proxies shall be taken into account by the court in determining the written treatment plan.

Figure 17.3 New York-assisted outpatient treatment process and eligibility criteria.

Meldrum et al. used a qualitative design and analysis to describe the actual operation of AOT programs in practice nationally in 2014.[71] Twenty states had active, operational, and documented AOT programs. The study found that people were referred to AOT via three pathways: (1) community gateway into services or advocates trying to engage a person into treatment who is having difficulties; (2) hospital transition or discharge into an AOT program from an involuntary inpatient hospitalization or jailing; and (3) as method of community surveillance or monitoring persons thought to be a danger to others. The hospital transition gateway was the best studied and most effective way a participant entered an AOT program; the community gateway and surveillance pathways were not as well studied. Nearly all states cited inadequate resources as barrier in the implementation of AOT, with only four state legislatures having authorized devoting funding for AOT programs. The study also identified a lack of communication and coordination between mental health agencies, law enforcement, and the courts as a major problem area. Resistance of providers to accepting AOT patients, courts declining cases due to overloaded dockets, and inadequate monitoring of participants were also noted to be problematic. Despite these challenges, when properly implemented and resourced, AOT has been shown to be a useful tool to improve treatment adherence, reduce relapse and rehospitalization, and decrease likelihood of dangerous behavior or deterioration among the subset of patients with a serious mental illness who lack insight. Data collected from AOT programs funded by the 2016 SAMHSA grants will help inform which and for whom AOT can be most effective, to help avoid poor outcomes for this vulnerable population.

Treatment Beds versus Jail Beds

The national survey of senior law enforcement officials finding that increased service calls is due to an inability to keep persons with mental illness hospitalized long enough to achieve clinical stability reflects the current reality that the number of psychiatric beds is grossly inadequate to serve the population's needs. Experts estimate a need for a minimum of one publicly funded acute psychiatric bed for every 2,000 people for hospitalization for individuals with serious psychiatric disorders; according to the most recent national data from the American Hospital Association's Annual Survey of Hospitals, there is currently one acute publicly funded

psychiatric bed for every 5,053 people nationwide.[72] The number of long-term publicly funded hospital beds that remain for patients who are so ill they have become involved in the criminal justice setting after being charged with a felony crime has fallen to fewer than 12 publicly funded beds per 100,000 population in the United States, the lowest level since these data have been tracked.[73] It has also resulted in inmates in psychiatric crisis in jail settings waiting weeks and months for transfer to a long-term publicly funded state hospital bed to receive necessary treatment. The shortage of long-term publicly funded beds has led to unacceptably lengthy delays for competency restoration services. The United States District Court in the state of Washington ruled that a delay of more than seven days between a finding of incompetency to stand trial and the commencement of competency restoration services is unconstitutional.[74] Several other states, including Oregon, Louisiana, Pennsylvania, Alabama, and Colorado, have been successfully sued over this issue and face court orders, settlement agreements, or consent decrees. The shortage of publicly funded psychiatric beds in both acute community and long-term settings make increasing the use of diversion strategies that reduce hospital and criminal justice recidivism critical.[75]

California, despite being among the wealthiest states in the country, falls well below the national average with only one public psychiatric bed for every 5,856 people, significantly lower than the nation's average of one bed for every 4,959 people.[72] This shortage of public acute psychiatric beds creates crisis situations in California's cities. To illustrate, San Francisco's total number of psychiatric beds (acute, nonacute, private pay, and uninsured) is 153. With a population of 837,442, San Francisco has one bed for every 5,473 and is at a deficit of 266 acute psychiatric beds to meet minimum quality standards for its size.[74] In 2018, 50,400 mental health-related 911 calls were made to dispatchers in San Francisco, an average of 4,200 each month. In response to the calls for service, police officers responded and contacted the mentally ill person in most cases (66%) which led to detainment for an involuntary psychiatric assessment (64%). A small but significant fraction of calls for service (3%) led to criminal charges being filed. When a person commits a misdemeanor crime and suffers from mental illness, officers have limited options for diverting people out of the criminal justice system because of overcrowding in the one devoted psychiatric emergency room at San Francisco's County hospital and the lack of acute psychiatric beds to admit involuntarily detained persons for further treatment.

Consequently, even though San Francisco's County Jail population has declined in recent years, those with mental illness remain over-represented.[76] Between 35% and 40% of San Francisco County Jail inmates receive care from behavioral health care services and 17% receive treatment for a serious mental illness. Providing mental health care in correctional institutions is challenging; the settings are fundamentally punitive environments where control and security are the top priority. There is extensive research that demonstrates that persons with mental illness are harmed, not helped, by incarceration.[77] When incarcerated, they are likely to engage in self-harm behaviors,[78] incur disciplinary infractions which can lead to placement in solitary confinement,[79] be targets of use of force by correctional officers, and are victimized by other prisoners.[80,81] These persons are released into the community without adequate follow-up into programs suited to their needs and in some cases, are released without needed medications. Negative experiences in the jail environment and the failure to provide for community re-entry with ongoing psychiatric services worsens the likelihood of a return into substance abuse, homelessness, and criminal recidivism.

The San Francisco Budget and Legislative Analyst's Office on Jail Population, Costs, and Alternatives reported that the jail houses 240 inmates with serious mental illness who would benefit from psychiatric beds appropriate to their needs rather than incarceration.[74] A Behavioral Health Justice Center which provides mental health services designed to interrupt the cycle has been proposed to break the cycle of homelessness, addiction, and criminal recidivism for the persons with severe mental illness population involved in the criminal justice system. The center is based on a system of interconnected programs that creates a continuum of mental health care treatment options for individuals with mental illness in the justice system specifically designed to prevent recidivism. The proposed Behavioral Health Justice Center is similar in design to Miami's Mental Health Diversion Facility (MHDF) which is scheduled to open in 2020.[82] The MHDF is designed to be part of a larger continuum of services for people with mental illness in the criminal justice

system in Dade County, Florida. The MHDF will provide a continuum of care, ranging from intensive treatment in the crisis-stabilization unit on the second floor (to which some will be involuntarily committed), to dental and primary care, basketball in the gym, and employment training in the culinary arts. In terms of bed count, three levels will be available: 40 beds for the crisis-stabilization unit, 120 for short-term residential treatment (stays of about 90 days), and 48 for the residential-treatment facility (180-day stays). The MHDF will further expand upon the efforts of Judge Steve Leifman whose Eleventh Judicial Circuit Criminal Mental Health Project (CMHP), which includes pre-arrest and post-arrest mental health diversion programs, and has dramatically reduced recidivism rates for people involved. Since implementation, recidivism rates for people accused of misdemeanors dropped from 75% to 20%, and people accused of felonies have a recidivism rate of only 6%.[76]

In early 2019, the Los Angeles County Board of Supervisors made a decision that represents a "paradigm shift" in the treatment of inmates and efforts to seek alternatives to incarceration.[83] Supervisors voted down a 2.2-billion proposal to build a Consolidated Correctional Treatment Facility to replace the dilapidated Central Jail, which was built in 1963. Instead, the money will be used to fund construction of a Mental Health Treatment Center comprised of series of smaller mental health centers rather than a single, large hospital. The new complex would offer inmates re-entry programs, supportive housing, community-based services, and other alternatives. The Los Angeles County Department of Health Services would oversee the new facility, rather than the Sheriff's Department, which currently manages all jail operations. The Mental Health Treatment Center would house a greater number of persons with mental illness than are currently housed in all the County hospitals combined. The plan marks a landmark shift in philosophy toward the care of inmates and recognizes the reality of the current jail population: inmates who have medical or mental illness now make up an estimated 70% of people held in the county jail system and they need treatment services to successfully break free from the criminal justice system.

Conclusion

Measurement of the benefit effects of CIT, and co-responding teams, is an expectedly challenging endeavor, yet one we are obliged to undertake given patient wellbeing, officer wellbeing, and use of huge swaths of public money related to the intersection of these three realms. Co-responding is a natural progression of professional collaboration between police and expert mental health professionals. Both police and mental health professionals carry analogous duties that involve deeply intimate and intrusive interactions with mental health patients: police use degrees of force, and psychiatric medical professionals use degrees of restraint. These teams both take on responsibility for public safety. Both have the legal power to limit another human's freedom to move about as that human wishes. Both ask deeply personal questions of individuals who are at an inherent disadvantage by being in a position of losing ordinary control from a social level to bodily and mental levels. Both teams work in fractured systems that carry risk for harm to the professional – an issue especially marked for police – and in which these teams witness very ill patients struggle in for up to decades. Police and expert mental health professionals share much common ground, from the field to the emergency department, and, so far, co-responding teams appear to help patients and may also bode well for multiplying the beneficial effects of the efforts of mental health experts and police. The entire goal of this work is to help patients and mitigate their languishing in ineffective care. Progress is being made, but there are still many improvements needed.

Whether or not officers are CIT trained, psychiatric emergency service units and emergency rooms in medical hospitals are frequently the de facto endpoint for police who are managing acute mental health patient calls. Once an officer hands off a psychiatrically acute patient in an emergency department, the duty of the police in response to a psychiatric call has been completed, and the patient is then in a setting ostensibly designed for his or her psychiatric needs.

When police arrive at an emergency room with a detained patient on an involuntary hold, three parties are directly involved: the patient, the emergency room staff, and the police officers. Each of these parties is in a position of being outside their usual element. The patients are outside their usual element by having some of their rights taken away and facing various configurations of police and psychiatric professionals. The police are out of their element by being in a medical environment. And finally, the emergency room staff are out of their element by now being partnered with police during an often lengthy hand-off process, when an acute patient is in custody on the unit. Police and psychiatric professionals in the emergency room usually are not formally trained to work together, despite the need. Although this broad problem warrants being addressed, the implementation of CIT does create configurations of police and mental health professionals, proximal to the emergency room setting, that may improve outcomes for patients and lead to better safety for police and mental health responders.[84]

From the Memphis Model in 1988 to current CIT-related mental health skills training, there are numerous national efforts to optimize police expertise regarding mental health signs and symptoms, and reduce the risk of harm. Co-responding police/mental health programs, in the form of mobile response, shows benefits through the combined expertise of these professionals. Co-responding teams are finding success in a variety of measures: aborting crises-related harm, linkage to more effective follow-up care, better follow-up adherence, diversion from the criminal justice system, lower admissions, increased mental health acumen among officers, cost savings, and a more sophisticated perception of persons with mental illness by officers.[85]

To be clear, the police portion of co-responding teams appears to be moving toward better optimization with use of CIT. CIT training helps police, while working with dispatch, to identify when CRTs are indicated. In one study, officers involved in co-responding teams reported a sense of better understanding of mental illness and improved collaboration in the field. Police shared the frustration of their mental health colleagues when needed mental health resources were not available in the community they both serve.[85] Outcome reviews have shown that, compared to police emergency contacts, the use of co-responding teams increased the number of 911 calls identified as warranting a mental health response. Co-responding teams are more successful at linking individuals to mental health services who had not received care previously, facilitate greater engagement in outpatient care after the emergency contact, and spend less time on-scene compared to police only contacts. Finally, patients who have received services from a co-responding team express that they have been heard, received meaningful advice, and feel a decreased sense of isolation.

Acknowledgments

The authors wish to thank Randall Hagar, Director of Government Affairs at the California Psychiatric Association for his long-standing dedication toward improving care for persons with serious mental illness in California and his ongoing efforts to expand services under Intercept 0.

Disclosure

The authors have nothing to disclose.

References

1. Dunn T, Dempsey C. Agitation in field settings: emergency medical services providers and law enforcement. In: Zeller SL, Nordstrom KD, Wilson MP, eds. *Diagnosis and Management of Agitation.* New York, NY: Cambridge University Press; 2017.

2. Treatment Advocacy Center. Emergency hospitalization for evaluation: assisted psychiatric treatment standards by state. www.treatmentadvocacycenter.org/storage/doc uments/Emergency%5FHospitalization%5Ffor%5FEvalu ation.pdf (accessed June 2020).

3. Counsel of State Governments – Justice Center. Stepping up initiative. https://csgjusticecenter.org/me ntal-health/county~improvement-project/stepping-up/pdf (accessed February 2019).

4. Reuland M, Draper L, Norton B. Improving responses to people with mental illness: tailoring law enforcement initiatives to individual jurisdictions. Bureau of Justice Assistance, Council of State Governments Justice Center; 2010. www.bja.gov/Publ ications/CSG_LE_Tailoring.pdf (accessed June 2020).

5. Dupont R, Major Cochran S, Pillsbury S. Crisis Intervention Team Core Elements. The University of Memphis, School of Urban Affairs and Public Policy, Department of Criminology and Criminal Justice, CIT Center; 2007. http://cit.memphis.edu/pdf/CoreEleme nts.pdf (accessed June 2020).

6. Bakeman R, Broussard B, D'Orio B, Watson CW. Police officers' volunteering for (rather than being assigned to) Crisis Intervention Team (CIT) training: evidence for a beneficial self-selection effect. *Behav Sci Law.* 2017; **35**(5–6): 470–479.

7. Compton MT, Bakeman R, Broussard B, et al. The police-based crisis intervention team (CIT) model: I. Effects on officers' knowledge, attitudes, and skills. *Psychiatr Serv.* 2014; **65**(4): 517–522.

8. van den Brink RH, Broer J, Tholen AJ, et al. Role of the police in linking individuals experiencing mental health crises with mental health services. *BMC Psychiatry.* 2012; **12**: 171.

9. El-Mallakh PL, Kiran K, El-Mallakh RS. Costs and savings associated with implementation of a police crisis intervention team. *South Med J.* 2014; **107**(6): 391–395.

10. Compton MT, Demir Neubert BN, Broussard B, et al. Use of force preferences and perceived effectiveness of actions among Crisis Intervention Team (CIT) police officers and non-CIT officers in an escalating psychiatric crisis involving a subject with schizophrenia. *Schizophr Bull.* 2011; **37**(4): 737–745.

11. Compton MT, Broussard B, Reed TA, et al. Survey of police chiefs and sheriffs and of police officers about CIT programs. *Psychiatr Serv.* 2015; **66**(7): 760–763.

12. Demir B, Broussard B, Goulding SM, et al. Beliefs about causes of schizophrenia among police officers before and after crisis intervention team training. *Community Ment Health J.* 2009; **45**(5): 385–392.

13. Silverstone PH, Krameddine YI, DeMarco D, et al. A novel approach to training police officers to interact with individuals who may have a psychiatric disorder. *J Am Acad Psychiatry Law.* 2013; **41**(3): 344–355.

14. Krameddine YI, DeMarco D, Hassel R, et al. A novel training program for police officers that improves interactions with mentally ill individuals and is cost-effective. *Front Psychiatry.* 2013; **4**: 9.

15. Gur OM. Persons with mental illness in the criminal justice system: police interventions to prevent violence and criminalization. *J Police Crisis Negot.* 2010; **10**(1–2): 220–240.

16. Dempsey C. Beating mental illness: crisis intervention team training and law enforcement response trends. *South Calif Interdiscip Law J.* 2017; **26**(2): 323–340.

17. Lamanna D, Shapiro GK, Kirst M, et al. Co-responding police-mental health programmes: service user experiences and outcomes in a large urban centre. *Int J Ment Health Nurs.* 2018; **27**(2): 891–900.

18. Kisely S, Campbell LA, Peddle S, et al. A controlled before-and-after evaluation of a mobile crisis partnership between mental health and police services in Nova Scotia. *Can J Psychiatry.* 2010; **55**(10): 662–668.

19. Lee SJ, Thomas P, Doulis C, et al. Outcomes achieved by and police and clinician perspectives on a joint police officer and mental health clinician mobile response unit. *Int J Ment Health Nurs.* 2015; **24**(6): 538–546.

20. McKenna B, Furness T, Oakes J, et al. Police and mental health clinician partnership in response to mental health crisis: a qualitative study. *Int J Ment Health Nurs.* 2015; **24**(5): 386–393.

21. Evangelista E, Lee S, Gallagher A, et al. Crisis averted: how consumers experienced a police and clinical early

response (PACER) unit responding to a mental health crisis. *Int J Ment Health Nurs.* 2016; **25**(4): 367–376.

22. Lopez H. *A Descriptive Study of LAPD's Co-Response Model for Individuals with Mental Illness.* Long Beach, CA: ProQuest School of Social Work, University of California; 2016. www.equitasproject.org/wp-content /uploads/2017/06/Lopez-Thesis-on-Co-responder-model.pdf (accessed June 2020).

23. Policy Research Associates, SAMHSA's Gains Center for Behavioral Health and Justice Transformation. Developing a comprehensive plan for mental health and criminal justice collaboration: the Sequential Intercept Model. www.prainc.com/wp-content/uploa ds/2015/10/SIMBrochure.pdf (accessed June 2020).

24. Policy Research Associates. The Sequential Intercept Model: advancing community-based solutions for justice-involved people with mental and substance use disorders. www.prainc.com/wp-content/uploads/ 2017/08/SIM-Brochure-Redesign0824.pdf (accessed June 2020).

25. Los Angeles Police Department, Los Angeles Department of Mental Health. Community mental health resource guide. www.equitasproject.org/wp-content/uploads/2017/06/LAPDTriFoldFinal-2-15-17-updated.pdf (accessed February 2019).

26. National Alliance on Mental Illness, Glendale Chapter. Guidelines for effective communication with 911 dispatch. http://namiglendale.org/dealing-with-911/ (accessed June 2020).

27. Houston Police Department, Mental Health Division. Emergency guide. www.houstoncit.org/emergency-guide/ (accessed June 2020).

28. National Alliance on Mental Illness, Dallas Chapter. 911 Checklist. www.namidallas.org/uploads/2/2/4/3/224331 50/911_checklist_2015.pdf (accessed February 2019).

29. Houston Police Department, Mental Health Division. Crisis call diversion. www.houstoncit.org/ccd/ (accessed June 2020).

30. The Counsel of State Governments, Justice Center. "What If," to Real Results: US Police Departments Explore Innovative, Collaborative Ways to Address Growing Mental Health Crisis. https://csgjusticecen ter.org/mental-health/posts/from-what-if-to-real-results-u-s-police-departments-explore-innovative-collaborative-ways-to-address-growing-mental-health-crisis/pdf. (accessed February 2019).

31. Bernstein M. Next year a 9-1-1 mental health emergency call won't automatically bring a Portland cop. *The Oregonian.* 2011. www.oregonlive.com/portland/index .ssf/2011/12/next_year_a_911_call_from_a_me.html (accessed June 2020).

32. White Bird Clinic. CAHOOTS (Crisis Assistance Helping Out On The Streets). https://whitebirdclinic .org/services/cahoots/ (accessed June 2020).

33. Los Angeles Police Department. Barricaded suspects. *Training Bulletin, Volume XLV, Issue 4.* December 2016. https://recordsrequest.lacity.org/do cuments/748737 (accessed June 2020).

34. Wogan JB, Cournoyer C. How police chiefs plan to avoid "lawful but awful" shootings, governing the states and localities. *Governing.* February 2, 2016. w ww.governing.com/topics/public-justice-safety/gov-police-chiefs-shootings.html (accessed June 2020).

35. Biasotti MA. The Impact of Mental Illness on Law Enforcement Resources. Naval Postgraduate School Center for Homeland Defense and Security; 2011. w ww.treatmentadvocacycenter.org/storage/docu ments/The_%20Impact_of_Mental_Illness_on_Law_ Enforcement_Resources.pdf (accessed March 2019).

36. Sevy S, Nathanson K, Visweswaraiah H, et al. The relationship between insight and symptoms in schizophrenia. *Compr Psychiatry.* 2004; **45**(1): 16–19.

37. Dell'Osso L, Pini S, Cassano GB, et al. Insight into illness in patients with mania, mixed mania, bipolar depression and major depression with psychotic features. *Bipolar Disord.* 2002; **4**(5): 315–322.

38. Pini S, Cassano GB, Dell'Osso L, et al. Insight into illness in schizophrenia, schizoaffective disorder, and mood disorders with psychotic features. *Am J Psychiatry.* 2001; **158**(1): 122–125.

39. Amador XF, Flaum M, Andreasen NC, et al. Awareness of illness in schizophrenia and schizoaffective and mood disorders. *Arch Gen Psychiatry.* 1994; **51**(10): 826–836.

40. Fennig S, Everett E, Bromet EJ, et al. Insight in first-admission psychotic patients. *Schizophr Res.* 1996; **22**(3): 257–263.

41. Arango C, Amador X. Lessons learned about poor insight. *Schizophr Bull.* 2011; **37**(1): 27–28.

42. Misdrahi D, Tessier A, Swendsen J, et al. Determination of adherence profiles in schizophrenia using self-reported adherence: results from the FACE-SZ dataset. *J Clin Psychiatry.* 2016; **77**(9): e1130–e1136.

43. Hui CLM, Poon VWY, Ko WT, et al. Risk factors for antipsychotic medication non-adherence behaviors and attitudes in adult-onset psychosis. *Schizophr Res.* 2016; **174**(1–3): 144–149.

44. Czobor P, Van Dorn RA, Citrome L, et al. Treatment adherence in schizophrenia: a patient-level meta-analysis of combined CATIE and EUFEST studies. *Eur Neuropsychopharmacol.* 2015; **25**(8): 1158–1166.

45. Myers N, Bhatty S, Broussard B, et al. Clinical correlates of initial treatment disengagement in first-episode psychosis. *Clin Schizophr Relat Psychoses.* 2017; **11**(2): 95–102.

46. Levin JB, Seifi N, Cassidy KA, et al. Comparing medication attitudes and reasons for medication nonadherence among three disparate groups of individuals with serious mental illness. *J Nerv Ment Dis*. 2014; **202**(11): 769–773.

47. Brain C, Allerby K, Sameby B, et al. Drug attitude and other predictors of medication adherence in schizophrenia: 12 months of electronic monitoring (MEMS®) in the Swedish COAST-study. *Eur Neuropsychopharmacol*. 2013; **23**(12): 1754–1762.

48. Compton MT, Gordon TL, Goulding SM, et al. Patient-level predictors and clinical correlates of duration of untreated psychosis among hospitalized first-episode patients. *J Clin Psychiatry*. 2011; **72**(2): 225–232.

49. Hill M, Crumlish N, Whitty P, et al. Nonadherence to medication four years after a first episode of psychosis and associated risk factors. *Psychiatr Serv*. 2010; **61**(2): 189–192.

50. Pijnenborg GH, Timmerman ME, Derks EM, et al. Differential effects of antipsychotic drugs on insight in first episode schizophrenia: data from the European First-Episode Schizophrenia Trial (EUFEST). *Eur Neuropsychopharmacol*. 2011; **25**(6): 808–816.

51. Kim JH, Ann JH, Lee J. Insight change and its relationship to subjective well-being during acute atypical antipsychotic treatment in schizophrenia. *J Clin Pharm Ther*. 2011; **36**(6): 687–694.

52. Wiffen BD, Rabinowitz J, Fleischhacker WW, et al. Insight: demographic differences and associations with one-year outcome in schizophrenia and schizoaffective disorder. *Clin Schizophr Relat Psychoses*. 2010; **4**(3): 169–175.

53. Treatment Advocacy Center. A background paper from the Office of Research & Public Affairs: serious mental illness and anosognosia; 2016. www .treatmentadvocacycenter.org/key-issues/anosogno sia/3628-serious-mental-illness-and-anosognosia (accessed June 2020).

54. Treatment Advocacy Center. A background paper from the Office of Research & Public Affairs: anosognosia, non-treatment, and violent behavior; 2016. www.treatmentadvocacycenter.org/key-issues/ anosognosia/3636-anosognosia-non-treatment-and-violent-behavior (accessed June 2020).

55. Tsai G, Quanbeck CD. Assisted outpatient treatment and outpatient commitment. In: Rosner R, Scott C, eds. *Principles and Practice of Forensic Psychiatry, 3rd edn*. Boca Raton, FL: CRC Press; 2017: 131–144.

56. Swartz MS, Swanson JW, Steadman HJ, Robbins PC, Monahan J. New York State assisted outpatient treatment program evaluation. New York State Assisted Outpatient Treatment Program Evaluation,

Duke University School of Medicine; 2009. https://o mh.ny.gov/omhweb/resources/publications/aot_pro gram_evaluation/report.pdf (accessed June 2020).

57. Swartz MS, Swanson J, Hiday V, et al. A randomized controlled trial of outpatient commitment in North Carolina. *Psychiatr Serv*. 2001; **52**(3): 325–329.

58. Treatment Advocacy Center. What is AOT? www .treatmentadvocacycenter.org/storage/documents/ao t-one-pager.pdf (accessed June 2020).

59. Treatment Advocacy Center. A background paper from the Office of Research & Public Affairs: the role of Assisted Outpatient Treatment in reducing violence. www.treatmentadvocacycenter.org/evi dence-and-research/learn-more-about/3634-the-role -of-assisted-outpatient-treatment-in-reducing-violence (accessed June 2020).

60. Swartz M, Swanson J, Wagner H, et al. Can involuntary outpatient commitment reduce hospital recidivism?: findings from a randomized trial with severely mentally ill individuals. *Am J Psychiatry*. 1999; **156**(12): 1968–1975.

61. Swanson J, Swartz M, Elbogen E, et al. Effects of involuntary outpatient commitment on subjective quality of life in persons with severe mental illness. *Behav Sci Law*. 2003; **21**(4): 473–491.

62. Wagner H, Swartz M, Swanson J, et al. Does involuntary outpatient commitment lead to more intensive treatment? *Psychol Public Policy Law*. 2003; **9**(1–2): 145–158.

63. Van Dorn R, Swanson J, Swartz M, et al. Continuing medication and hospitalization outcomes after assisted outpatient treatment in New York. *Psychiatr Serv*. 2010; **61**(10): 982–987.

64. Swanson J, Van Dorn R, Swartz M, et al. The cost of assisted outpatient treatment: can it save states money? *Am J Psychiatry*. 2013; **170**(12): 1423–1432.

65. Swartz M, Swanson J. Economic grand rounds: can states implement involuntary outpatient commitment within existing state budgets? *Psychiatr Serv*. 2013; **64**(1): 7–9.

66. Treatment Advocacy Center. A Promising Start: Results from a California Survey Assessing the Use of Laura's Law. 2019. www.treatmentadvocacycenter.org/a-promis ing-start (accessed June 2020).

67. Cripps SN, Swartz MS. Update on assisted outpatient treatment. *Curr Psychiatry Rep*. 2018; **20**(12): 112.

68. Munetz MR, Ritter C, Teller JLS, et al. Association between hospitalization and delivery of assisted outpatient treatmentwith and without assertive community treatment. *Psychiatr Serv*. 2019; **70**(9): 833–836.

69. National Institute of Justice, Office of Justice Programs. Program profile: Assisted Outpatient

Treatment. www.crimesolutions.gov/ProgramDetails .aspx?ID=228 (accessed June 2020).

70. Substance Abuse and Mental Health Services Administration. Assisted outpatient treatment grant program for individuals with serious mental illness [grant announcement]. 2016. www.samhsa.gov/gran ts/grant-announcements/sm-16-011 (accessed June 2020).

71. Meldrum ML, Kelly EL, Calderon R, et al. Implementation status of assisted outpatient treatment programs: a national survey. *Psychiatr Serv.* 2016; **67**(6): 630–635.

72. California Hospital Association. California psychiatric bed annual report. www.calhospital.org/ PsychBedData.pdf (accessed March 2019).

73. Treatment Advocacy Center. Going, going, gone: trends and consequences of eliminating state psychiatric beds, 2016. www .treatmentadvocacycenter.org/storage/documents/go ing-going-gone.pdf (accessed June 2020).

74. Disability Rights Washington. AB v DSHS (Trueblood): reforming Washington's forensic mental health system. www.disabilityrightswa.org/ca ses/trueblood/ (accessed June 2020).

75. Treatment Advocacy Center. Competency restoration versus psychiatric treatment. www .treatmentadvocacycenter.org/fixing-the-system/fea tures-and-news/4126-the-distinction-between-com petency-restoration-and-psychiatric-treatment (accessed June 2020).

76. Haney C, Johnson JK, Lacey K, Romano M. Justice that heals: promoting behavioral health, safeguarding the public, and ending our overreliance on jails. https://sfdi strictattorney.org/sites/default/files/Document/BHJC% 20Concept%20Paper_Final_0.pdf (accessed June 2020).

77. Bewley MT, Morgan RD. A national survey of mental health services available to offenders with mental illness: who is doing what? *Law Hum Behav.* 2011; **35** (5): 351–363.

78. Kaba F, Lewis A, Glowa-Kollisch S, et al. Solitary confinement and risk of self-harm among jail inmates. *Am J Public Health.* 2014; **104**(3): 442–447.

79. Lamb HR, Weinberger LE. Understanding and treating offenders with serious mental illness in public sector mental health. *Behav Sci Law.* 2017; **35**(4): 303–318.

80. Blitz CL, Wolff N, Shi J. Physical victimization in prison: the role of mental illness. *Int J Law Psychiatry.* 2008; **31**(5): 385–393.

81. Wolff N, Blitz CL, Shi J. Rates of sexual victimization in prison for inmates with and without mental disorders. *Psychiatr Serv.* 2007; **58**(8): 1087–1094.

82. Eide S. Keeping the mentally ill out of jail: an innovative Miami-Dade program shows the way. *City Journal.* Autumn, 2018. www.city-journal.org/miami-dade-criminal-mental-health-project (accessed June 2020).

83. Lau M. In landmark move, L.A. County will replace Men's Central Jail with mental health hospital for inmates. *Los Angeles Times.* February 13, 2019. www .latimes.com/local/lanow/la-me-jail-construction-20 190212-story.html (accessed June 2020).

84. Kubiak S, Comartin E, Milanovic E, et al. Countywide implementation of crisis intervention teams: multiple methods, measures and sustained outcomes. *Behav Sci Law.* 2017; **35**(5–6): 456–469.

85. Shapiro GK, Cusi A, Kirst M, et al. Co-responding police-mental health programs: a review. *Adm Policy Mental Health.* 2015; **42**(6): 606–620.

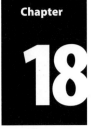

Chapter

18

Dopamine Antagonist Antipsychotics in Diverted Forensic Populations

Michael A. Cummings, George J. Proctor, and Ai-Li W. Arias

Introduction

In community settings, the principle barriers to independent living, stable relationships, and gainful employment arise from the negative and cognitive symptom domains of schizophrenia spectrum disorders.[1,2] In contrast, the positive symptoms of psychosis often are the gateway (e.g. via persecutory delusion associated with anger) to arrest and criminalization for the mentally ill.[3,4] Since the clinical discovery of chlorpromazine in 1952, dopamine antagonism in the mesolimbic dopamine circuit has been central to treating the positive symptoms of psychosis.[5,6] The hyperactivity of the mesolimbic circuit and the normalizing effects of the dopamine antagonist antipsychotics are illustrated in Figure 18.1.

In this review, we seek to understand the roles of dopamine antagonist antipsychotics, including the use of long-acting or depot formulations and plasma concentrations, in controlling the positive symptoms of psychosis, thereby supporting decriminalization of those suffering from psychotic disorders.[7]

Principle Text

The French pharmaceutical firm, Rhône-Poulenc, began exploring polycyclic antihistamine compounds in 1933. This led to the approval and clinical introduction of diphenhydramine in 1946. Promethazine, a phenothiazine derivative, was approved the following year. Although this compound produced sedation, decreased motor activity, and indifference

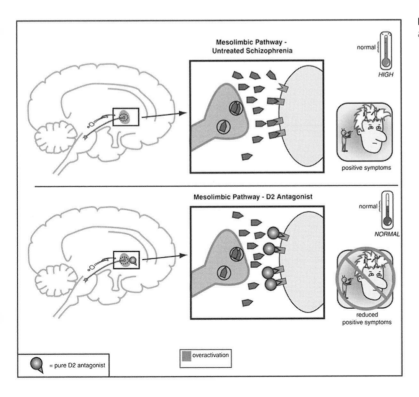

Figure 18.1 Mesolimbic pathway and D$_2$ antagonists.

to stimulation in rats, it had much more limited effects in humans.

In 1948, a French surgeon named Pierre Huguenard began using a combination of promethazine and pethidine (a.k.a. meperidine), an opioid, as pre-operative medications to calm and sedate patients. Henry Laborit, another French surgeon, subsequently proposed to Rhône-Poulenc that a more effective replacement for promethazine be sought. Consequently in December 1950, the chemist Paul Charpentier produced various compounds related to promethazine, including RP-4560 or chlorpromazine.

Chlorpromazine appeared to be the most promising compound because of its lesser peripheral effects. Chlorpromazine was distributed for testing in humans between April and August 1951. In this context, Henry Laborit tested chlorpromazine at the Val-de-Grâce Military Hospital in Paris. Dr. Laborit found the drug effective, as it produced a state akin to artificial hibernation. In fact, Dr. Laborit became such a proponent of chlorpromazine that it became colloquially known as "Laborit's drug."

Nevertheless, chlorpromazine's use as a pre-operative drug was cut short by its propensity to induce orthostatic hypotension and syncope via antagonism at α-adrenergic receptors. Despite this failure, a French psychiatrist named Pierre Deniker had been aware of chlorpromazine and was interested in using it to calm psychotic and manic patients at St. Anne's Hospital in Paris. Dr. Deniker's application of chlorpromazine to psychiatric patients was supported by Professor Jean Delay, who was the superintendent of St. Anne's during that time. Treatment with chlorpromazine proved more successful than Dr. Deniker and Dr. Delay had hoped. It reduced positive psychotic symptoms such as delusional ideation and hallucinations. Additionally, it calmed agitated and regressed behaviors while promoting emotional stability. Consequently, the success of chlorpromazine in psychiatry was likened to the discovery of antibiotics with respect to medical importance. Chlorpromazine's achievement led to the development of first-generation antipsychotics, several of which continue to be used clinically today (see Table 18.1).[8]

Clozapine, the first second-generation antipsychotic, was synthesized by Schmuts and

Table 18.1 First-generation dopamine antagonists

Medication generic name	Chemical group	Comments
Acepromazine	Phenothiazine	Used primarily in veterinary medicine
Benperidol	Butyrophenone	
Bromperidol	Butyrophenone	
Carpipramine	Tricyclic	
Chlorpromazine	Phenothiazine	First antipsychotic
Chlorprothixene	Thiothixene	
Clocapramine	Tricyclic	
Clopenthixol	Thiothixene	
Clorotepine	Tricyclic	
Clotiapine	Tricyclic	
Compazine	Phenothiazine	Used as antiemetic
Cyamemazine	Phenothiazine	
Dixyrazine	Phenothiazine	
Droperidol	Butyrophenone	Used primarily for anesthesia
Flupentixol	Thioxanthene	
Fluphenazine	Phenothiazine	Available as long-acting injectable
Fluspirilene	Diphenylbutylpiperidine	
Haloperidol	Butyrophenone	Available as long-acting injectable
Levomepromazine	Phenothiazine	

Table 18.1 (cont.)

Medication generic name	Chemical group	Comments
Loxapine	Tricyclic	Available as nasal spray
Mesoridazine	Phenothiazine	Discontinued
Molindone	Other	Discontinued
Moperone	Butyrophenone	Discontinued
Mosapramine	Tricyclic	
Pearlapine	Tricyclic	
Penfluridol	Diphenylbutylpiperidine	
Perazine	Phenothiazine	
Pericyazine	Phenothiazine	
Perphenazine	Phenothiazine	
Pimozide	Diphenylbutylpiperidine	Prone to QT prolongation
Pipamperone	Butyrophenone	Discontinued
Pipotiazine	Phenothiazine	
Prochlorperazine	Phenothiazine	
Promazine	Phenothiazine	Discontinued
Promethazine	Phenothiazine	Antipsychotic precursor
Prothipendyl	Phenothiazine	
Sulpiride	Benzamide	
Sultopride	Benzamide	
Thioproperazine	Phenothiazine	Available in Canada only among English-speaking countries
Thioridazine	Phenothiazine	Discontinued
Thiothixene	Thioxanthene	
Timiperone	Butyrophenone	
Trifluoperazine	Phenothiazine	
Triflupromazine	Phenothiazine	Discontinued
Veralipride	Benzamide	
Zuclopenthixol	Thioxanthene	

Notes: Derived from the U.S. and E.U. Pharmacopeias (www.USP.ORG and www.EDQM.EU)
Bold indicates those medications in common use in the United States.

Eichenberger in 1958. It has since become the gold standard for the management of treatment-resistant schizophrenia and pointed to pathological mechanisms in schizophrenia spectrum disorders beyond dysregulation of dopamine (i.e. glutamate hypoactivity and, perhaps, muscarinic hypoactivity).[9] The success of clozapine and its difficult adverse effect profile ignited substantial research in pursuit of antipsychotics that would be as effective as clozapine but with an improved safety profile.[10] This plethora of research resulted in the synthesis and approval of several second-generation dopamine antagonists (see Table 18.2).[11]

Mechanisms

Despite various chemical subtypes, a wide range of potencies at dopamine D_2 receptors, and important differences in side-effect profiles based on affinities for and actions at other receptors (i.e. adrenergic, histamine, acetylcholine, serotonin receptors, etc.), all of the dopamine antagonist antipsychotics share a principle mechanism for exerting their antipsychotic effects, namely, induction of depolarization blockade at the dopamine neurons that give rise to the mesolimbic dopamine pathway.[12] For the first-generation antipsychotics, this depolarization blockade

Table 18.2 Second-generation dopamine antagonists

Medication generic name	Chemical group	Comments
Amisulpride	Benzamide	
Asenapine	Tricyclic	Available as orally dissolving tablet only
Blonanserin	Other	
Iloperidone	Benzisoxazole/ benzisothiazole	
Lurasidone	Benzisoxazole/ benzisothiazole	Effective for bipolar depression
Melperone	Butyrophenone	
Nemonapride	Benzamide	
Olanzapine	Tricyclic	Modest glutamate modulation at high plasma concentrations (>120 ng/ml)
Paliperidone	Benzisoxazole/ benzisothiazole	Available in controlled release and long-acting injectable formulations
Perospirone	Benzisoxazole/ benzisothiazole	
Quetiapine	Tricyclic	Metabolite effective for bipolar depression
Remoxipride	Benzamide	
Risperidone	Benzisoxazole/ benzisothiazole	Available in long-acting injectable formulation
Sertindole	Other	
Ziprasidone	Benzisoxazole/ benzisothiazole	
Zotepine	Tricyclic	

Notes: Derived from the U.S. and E.U. Pharmacopeias (www.USP.ORG and www.EDQM.EU)

Bold indicates commonly in use in the U.S.

accounted for circa 92% to 93% of antipsychotic efficacy for these drugs.[13] Among the second-generation antipsychotics, dopamine antagonism and depolarization blockade remains the likely principle mechanism of action, although some (e.g. olanzapine) may exert modest antipsychotic effects via the modulation of glutamate signal transduction.[14] In this context, clozapine is unique in that it likely provides little, if any, of its antipsychotic efficacy via direct effects on dopamine signaling, instead more likely acting via robust modulation of glutamate.[15] Thus, the first step in treating positive psychotic symptoms is to provide the patient with an adequate exposure to the initial chosen dopamine antagonist antipsychotic for an adequate amount of time.

Antipsychotic Trials

A recent consensus paper identified the parameters of an adequate antipsychotic trial as a trial of at least six weeks duration and a dose of at least 600 mg chlorpromazine equivalents. A duration of four months was given for long-acting injectable (LAI) antipsychotics. Because medication adherence is often poor, this paper held a single antipsychotic plasma concentration measurement to be a minimal standard, while a more optimal standard was held to be two plasma concentration measurements separated by at least two weeks without prior notification of the patient. A further important principle of adequate antipsychotic trials is pursuit of the trial until one of three endpoints is achieved: improvement of psychotic signs and symptoms; emergence of intolerable adverse effects that cannot be managed via reasonable interventions; or, a point of futility is reached, for example, saturation of D_2 dopamine receptors or flattening of the drug's receptor occupancy curve.[16]

Importantly, failure to achieve a 20% to 30% reduction in psychotic symptoms in response to two or more adequate dopamine antagonist trials indicates that the patient is treatment-resistant; that is, the patient exhibits a pharmacodynamic failure in response to adequate dopamine antagonism. Additionally, such treatment resistance portends a poor probability of response to most antipsychotic agents. Most first- and second-generation antipsychotic medications show a response rate of 0% to 5% among such patients, while high plasma concentration olanzapine (120–200 ng/ml) produces a response rate of about 7%.[17] Moreover, data suggest for treatment-resistant schizophrenic patients that responsiveness to even clozapine begins to decline at about 2.8 years of treatment-resistant status.[18] The low probability of response to antipsychotics other than clozapine combined with data indicating a response-decay curve to even clozapine after 2.8 years among treatment-resistant schizophrenia spectrum disordered patients argues strongly in favor of clozapine treatment as soon as strictly defined treatment resistance is identified. That is, further time should not be wasted in pursuing treatments with a low probability of success, thereby diminishing even the superior efficacy of clozapine in patients who are pharmacodynamic failures with respect to dopamine antagonism.[19,20]

In the context of treatment-resistant schizophrenia, it is also worth noting that although there are a number of augmentation strategies ranging from antipsychotic polypharmacy to addition of medications from additional classes, the effect sizes of these strategies have been described as small or modest.[21] Exceptions to this analysis include augmentation with mood stabilizers in schizophrenic patients exhibiting early acute psychomotor agitation or in patients exhibiting a mood component or bipolar diathesis.[22–24] It is also worth noting that dopamine partial agonist antipsychotics may be more effective for the negative and cognitive symptom domains of schizophrenia spectrum disorders than the positive symptom domain.[25–27]

The second route to treatment failure for the dopamine antagonists is pharmacokinetic. In general, data have suggested that for the dopamine antagonists, optimal antipsychotic response occurs when dopamine D_2 and D_3 receptor occupancies are roughly in the 60% to 80% range.[28] This is why assuring adequate receptor occupancy for an adequate period of time is critical to providing an adequate dopamine antagonist trial.[14] In this context, it is worth noting that plasma concentrations of the antipsychotics correlate much more tightly

Table 18.3 Optimal plasma concentration ranges for selected dopamine antagonist antipsychotics

Antipsychotic	Optimal trough plasma concentration range
Fluphenazine	0.8–2.0 ng/ml in most patients
	2.0–4.0 ng/ml in more ill patients
Haloperidol	5.0–20.0 ng/ml in most patients
	20.0–30.0 ng/ml in more ill patients
Olanzapine	40–120 ng/ml in most patients
	120–200 ng/ml in more ill patients
Paliperidone	28–112 ng/ml
Perphenazine	0.8–4.0 ng/ml

Note: Derived from the California Department of State Hospitals Psychotropic Medication Policy, Chapter 41, Appendix – Therapeutic Plasma Concentrations for Antipsychotics and Mood Stabilizers (2019).

with relevant receptor occupancies than the prescribed dose.[29] Numerous factors can affect the relationship between dose and plasma concentration, including adherence, absorption, distribution, catabolism, and elimination.[30] Hence, measuring antipsychotic plasma concentrations provides a much more precise and accurate means to assuring adequate receptor occupancy. (Please see the companion article in this volume entitled, "Monitoring and Improving Antipsychotic Adherence in Outpatient Forensic Diversion Programs," by Meyer, J.M.)

Optimal plasma concentration ranges for selected dopamine antagonist antipsychotics are shown in Table 18.3.[22,31]

Measuring plasma antipsychotic concentrations can be useful in various clinical circumstances ranging from benchmarking an optimal clinical response to assessing poor or extensive metabolism or investigating the clinical decompensation of a previously stable patient.[32]

While patient factors such as drug absorption, distribution, catabolism, and elimination play important roles in determining antipsychotic efficacy, they often pale in importance when compared with medication adherence.[33] This is especially true in forensic settings, where medication diversion often becomes an added challenge.[34] The use of LAI antipsychotics provides the most reliable means to address issues of nonadherence or diversion.[35] Because decriminalizing a portion of the

Table 18.4 LAI dopamine antagonist antipsychotic initiation

LAI antipsychotic	Comments on initiation
Fluphenazine	For each 10 mg of oral fluphenazine per day, prescribe 25 mg of fluphenazine decanoate I.M. q week times three and then continue for every 2 weeks at 12.5 mg to a maximum of 100 mg as guided by plasma concentration measurements. Optimal for most patients is 0.8–2.0 ng/ml. Some more treatment-resistant patients may require plasma concentrations of 2.0–4.0 ng/ml. Note that fluphenazine decanoate exhibits both an immediate and delayed release from its vehicle, requiring initial reduction or discontinuation of oral dosing in some individuals to avoid post-injection emergence of neurologic adverse effects.
Haloperidol	Because haloperidol decanoate has little immediate release phase, a loading dose strategy is required to avoid a need for prolonged co-administration of an oral antipsychotic. That is, administration at a fixed dose would require 3–5 months to reach steady state. Give 100–300 mg I.M. q 1-week times two to three doses. For each 100 mg used in loading, the average steady-state plasma concentration is 7.75 ng/ml. Measurement of a plasma concentration before the third loading dose will assist in determining whether the third loading dose is needed. Measurement of a plasma concentration shortly before the first maintenance dose will be helpful in fine tuning ongoing dosing. Optimal for most patients is 5–20 ng/ml. A few more treatment-resistant patients may require plasma concentrations of 20–30 ng/ml. Adverse neurological effects become more frequent at plasma concentrations >20 ng/ml. Maintenance dosing should begin 14 days after the last loading injection. For maintenance, give on average 100 mg q 4 weeks per 20 mg of the prior oral haloperidol daily dose. If the maintenance dose exceeds 300 mg, then divide the dose and administer every 14 days, as the maximum injectable volume is 3 ml.
Olanzapine	LAI olanzapine is available in 150, 210, 300, and 405 mg doses. Oral equivalents have not been established. There is no need for oral cross-over or loading. Note, however, that a circa 0.1% risk of delirium, obtundation, and coma follows each dose. Direct nursing observation is required for a minimum of 3 h following each injection.
Paliperidone	Give an initial dose of 234 mg followed by a second initiation dose of 156 mg after 1 week. Initial doses should be deltoid. Maintenance doses may be deltoid or gluteal. The modal maintenance dose is 117 mg q 4 weeks, with a dose range of 39–234 mg. A dose of 234 mg per month produces 9-hydroxy-risperidone plasma concentrations comparable to 4–5 mg of oral risperidone per day (risperidone + 9-hydroxy-risperidone). Oral risperidone or paliperidone is not required after the initiation phase. Paliperidone palmitate extended-release (Invega Trinza®) is restricted to patients who have received effective and stable treatment with paliperidone palmitate (Invega Sustenna®) for a minimum of 4 months. At the time the next dose of paliperidone palmitate would be due, give the equivalent dose of paliperidone palmitate extended-release (Invega Trinza®)
Risperidone	Initiate depot risperidone (Consta®) at 25–50 mg. q 2 weeks, while continuing oral risperidone treatment. After 3 weeks have passed since the initial injection, taper and discontinue oral risperidone treatment. Each 25 mg of LAI risperidone produces plasma concentrations of risperidone + 9-hydroxy-risperidone comparable to 2 to 3 mg of oral risperidone. Risperidone also is available in a subcutaneous formulation (Perseris®) which can be given in abdominal subcutaneous injections of 90 mg (0.6 ml) or 120 mg (0.8 ml), achieving plasma concentrations comparable to 3 or 4 mg of oral risperidone, respectively, at about 1 week, obviating the need for oral cross-over. Injections of this formulation are monthly.

Notes: Derived from the California Department of State Hospitals Psychotropic Medication Policy, Chapter 09, Depot Antipsychotics (2019). Also derived from package inserts for olanzapine (Zyprexa Relprevv®), paliperidone (Invega Sustenna® and Invega Trinza®), and risperidone (Risperdal Consta®), as well as references 40, 41, 42, and 43. Web sites: www.DrugInserts.COM/lib/rx/meds/Zyprexa-Relprevv-1. www.InvegaSustenna.COM; www.InvegaTrinza.COM; and www.DrugInserts.COM/lib/rx/meds/Risperdal-Consta-1.

arrested mentally ill population would involve release to community settings, assurance of continued treatment becomes a critical requirement for the success of any such program.[36] Additionally, it is worth noting that LAI antipsychotics have been associated with decreased rates of violence and criminality when compared with their oral counterparts.[37] In fact, the benefits of LAI antipsychotics are such that they produce an approximately 30% reduction in mortality risk when compared with the same antipsychotics prescribed in oral formulations in schizophrenia spectrum disordered patients.[38]

Unfortunately, LAI antipsychotics are infrequently used and thus are less familiar.[39] In particular, clinicians may be unfamiliar with strategies for initiating LAI antipsychotic treatment or transitioning from oral to depot formulations of dopamine antagonist antipsychotics.[40–43] Initiation/transition strategies are summarized in Table 18.4.

Conclusions

While negative and cognitive psychotic symptoms are major barriers to successful social functioning and employment in the community at large, it is more often positive psychotic symptoms that result in behaviors that lead to arrest and criminalization. Dopamine antagonist antipsychotics provide the cornerstone of treatment for positive psychotic symptoms and may provide an effective means to divert the mentally ill from the path of criminalization and incarceration. Critical to their success, however, are antipsychotic trials of therapeutic dose/plasma concentration for an adequate period of time. Moreover, such medication trials should be pursued to one of three endpoints: (1) successful improvement of psychotic signs and symptoms; (2) emergence of intolerable adverse effects that do not respond to reasonable interventions; or (3) arrival at a point of futility (e.g. saturation of D_2 dopamine receptors or flattening of the medication's receptor occupancy curve).

In those patients who have pharmacodynamic failures of two adequate trials of first- or second-generation dopamine antagonist antipsychotics, a trial of clozapine should be pursued vigorously. This is true because other antipsychotics, with or without augmentation, are unlikely to produce an adequate response in patients with strictly defined treatment-resistant schizophrenia. Moreover, some data indicate that even clozapine's efficacy in this context begins to fade after treatment resistance has been present for 2.8 years. Thus, our treatment-resistant schizophrenia patients would be better served if we clinicians do not waste time pursuing multiple antipsychotic trials or seemingly endless augmentation trials which are not likely to be successful.

With respect to pharmacokinetic failures, it should be emphasized that plasma concentrations are a much better means to assess antipsychotic trial adequacy than medication dose. In this context, it must be acknowledged that the failure of medication adherence is a major cause of pharmacokinetic failure. In short, if the medication does not make it into the patient, then there is no hope for an adequate antipsychotic response. Moreover, the issue of adherence is especially important to decriminalization of the mentally ill, as such individuals would return to the community as an inherent goal of decriminalization. To date, the only formulations of the antipsychotics that we clinicians can be certain are reliably making it into the patient on an ongoing basis are the LAI antipsychotics. In fact, data indicate that these formulations produce superior antipsychotic responses and even reduce mortality when compared with their oral counterparts. They are nevertheless underutilized, often being thought of as medications "of last resort." Instead, the available data support that the LAI antipsychotics should be one of our most frequently used tools, especially in forensic populations.

Disclosure

Dr. Cummings, Dr. Proctor, and Dr. Arias declare that they have nothing to disclose.

References

1. Grove TB, Tso IF, Chun J, et al. Negative affect predicts social functioning across schizophrenia and bipolar disorder: findings from an integrated data analysis. *Psychiatry Res.* 2016; **243**: 198–206.

2. Kaneko K. Negative symptoms and cognitive impairments in schizophrenia: two key symptoms negatively influencing social functioning. *Yonago Acta Med.* 2018; **61**(2): 91–102.

3. Ullrich S, Keers R, Coid JW. Delusions, anger, and serious violence: new findings from the MacArthur violence risk assessment study. *Schizophr Bull.* 2014; **40**(5): 1174–1181.

4. Fazel S, Zetterqvist J, Larsson H, Langstrom N, Lichtenstein P. Antipsychotics, mood stabilisers, and risk of violent crime. *Lancet.* 2014; **384**(9949): 1206–1214.

5. Urs NM, Peterson SM, Caron MG. New concepts in dopamine D2 receptor biased signaling and implications for schizophrenia therapy. *Biol Psychiatry.* 2017; **81**(1): 78–85.

6. Howes OD, McCutcheon R, Owen MJ, Murray RM. The role of genes, stress, and dopamine in the development of schizophrenia. *Biol Psychiatry.* 2017; **81**(1): 9–20.

7. Rotter M, Carr WA. Targeting criminal recidivism in mentally ill offenders: structured clinical approaches. *Community Ment Health* J. 2011; **47**(6): 723–726.

8. Lopez-Munoz F, Alamo C, Cuenca E, et al. History of the discovery and clinical introduction of chlorpromazine. *Ann Clin Psychiatry.* 2005; **17**(3): 113–135.

9. Melkersson K, Lewitt M, Hall K. Higher serum concentrations of tyrosine and glutamate in schizophrenia patients treated with clozapine, compared to in those treated with conventional

antipsychotics. *Neuro Endocrinol Lett.* 2015; **36**(5): 465–480.

10. Crilly J. The history of clozapine and its emergence in the US market: a review and analysis. *Hist Psychiatry.* 2007; **18**(1): 39–60.

11. Shen WW. A history of antipsychotic drug development. *Compr Psychiatry.* 1999; **40**(6): 407–414.

12. Grace AA. The depolarization block hypothesis of neuroleptic action: implications for the etiology and treatment of schizophrenia. *J Neural Transm Suppl.* 1992; **36**: 91–131.

13. Miyamoto S, Duncan GE, Marx CE, Lieberman JA. Treatments for schizophrenia: a critical review of pharmacology and mechanisms of action of antipsychotic drugs. *Mol Psychiatry.* 2005; **10**(1): 79–104.

14. Howes O, McCutcheon R, Stone J. Glutamate and dopamine in schizophrenia: an update for the 21st century. *J Psychopharmacol.* 2015; **29**(2): 97–115.

15. Veerman SR, Schulte PF, de Haan L. The glutamate hypothesis: a pathogenic pathway from which pharmacological interventions have emerged. *Pharmacopsychiatry* 2014; **47**(4–5): 121–130.

16. Howes OD, McCutcheon R, Agid O, et al. Treatment-resistant schizophrenia: treatment response and resistance in psychosis (TRRIP) working group consensus guidelines on diagnosis and terminology. *Am J Psychiatry.* 2017; **174**(3): 216–229.

17. Stroup TS, Gerhard T, Crystal S, Huang C, Olfson M. Comparative effectiveness of clozapine and standard antipsychotic treatment in adults with schizophrenia. *Am J Psychiatry.* 2016; **173**(2): 166–173.

18. Yoshimura B, Yada Y, So R, Takaki M, Yamada N. The critical treatment window of clozapine in treatment-resistant schizophrenia: secondary analysis of an observational study. *Psychiatry Res.* 2017; **250**: 65–70.

19. Kerwin R. When should clozapine be initiated in schizophrenia?: some arguments for and against earlier use of clozapine. *CNS Drugs.* 2007; **21**(4): 267–278.

20. Doyle R, Behan C, O'Keeffe D, et al. Clozapine use in a cohort of first-episode psychosis. *J Clin Psychopharmacol.* 2017; **37**(5): 512–517.

21. Galling B, Roldan A, Hagi K, et al. Antipsychotic augmentation vs. monotherapy in schizophrenia: systematic review, meta-analysis and meta-regression analysis. *World Psychiatry.* 2017; **16**(1): 77–89.

22. Stahl SM, Morrissette DA, Cummings M, et al. California state hospital violence assessment and treatment (Cal-VAT) guideline. *CNS Spectr.* 2014; **19** (5): 449–465.

23. Fond G, Boyer L, Favez M, et al. Medication and aggressiveness in real-world schizophrenia: results from the FACE-SZ dataset. *Psychopharmacology.* 2016; **233**(4): 571–578.

24. Garriga M, Pacchiarotti I, Kasper S, et al. Assessment and management of agitation in psychiatry: expert consensus. *World J Biol Psychiatry.* 2016; **17**(2): 86–128.

25. Mossaheb N, Kaufmann RM. Role of aripiprazole in treatment-resistant schizophrenia. *Neuropsychiatr Dis Treat.* 2012; **8**: 235–244.

26. Veerman SRT, Schulte PFJ, de Haan L. Treatment for negative symptoms in schizophrenia: a comprehensive review. *Drugs.* 2017; **77**(13): 1423–1459.

27. Stahl SM. Drugs for psychosis and mood: unique actions at D3, D2, and D1 dopamine receptor subtypes. *CNS Spectr.* 2017; **22**(5): 375–384.

28. Wulff S, Pinborg LH, Svarer C, et al. Striatal D(2/3) binding potential values in drug-naive first-episode schizophrenia patients correlate with treatment outcome. *Schizophr Bull.* 2015; **41**(5): 1143–1152.

29. Urban AE, Cubala WJ. Therapeutic drug monitoring of atypical antipsychotics. *Psychiatr Pol.* 2017; **51**(6): 1059–1077.

30. Fan J, de Lannoy IA. Pharmacokinetics. *Biochem Pharmacol.* 2014; **87**(1): 93–120.

31. Meyer JM, Cummings MA, Proctor G, Stahl SM. Psychopharmacology of persistent violence and aggression. *Psychiatr Clin North Am.* 2016; **39**(4): 541–556.

32. Dahl SG. Plasma level monitoring of antipsychotic drugs: clinical utility. *Clin Pharmacokinet.* 1986; **11**(1): 36–61.

33. Tharani AJ, Farooq S, Saleem F, Naveed A. Compliance to antipsychotic medication: a challenge for client, family and health care providers. *J Pak Med Assoc.* 2013; **63**(4): 516–518.

34. Pilkinton PD, Pilkinton JC. Prescribing in prison: minimizing psychotropic drug diversion in correctional practice. *J Correct Health Care.* 2014; **20**(2): 95–104.

35. Marcus SC, Zummo J, Pettit AR, Stoddard J, Doshi JA. Antipsychotic adherence and rehospitalization in schizophrenia patients receiving oral versus long-acting injectable antipsychotics following hospital discharge. *J Manag Care Spec Pharm.* 2015; **21**(9): 754–768.

36. McGuire AB, Bond GR. Critical elements of the crisis intervention team model of jail diversion: an expert survey. *Behav Sci Law.* 2011; **29**(1): 81–94.

37. Mohr P, Knytl P, Vorackova V, Bravermanova A, Melicher T. Long-acting injectable antipsychotics for prevention and management of violent behaviour in psychotic patients. *Int J Clin Pract*. 2017; **71**(9): e12997.

38. Taipale H, Mittendorfer-Rutz E, Alexanderson K, et al. Antipsychotics and mortality in a nationwide cohort of 29,823 patients with schizophrenia. *Schizophr Res*. 2017; **197**: 274–280.

39. Iyer S, Banks N, Roy MA, et al. A qualitative study of experiences with and perceptions regarding long-acting injectable antipsychotics: part II-physician perspectives. *Can J Psychiatry*. 2013; **58**(5 Suppl 1): 23s–29s.

40. Siragusa S, Saadabadi A. Fluphenazine. In: *StatPearls*. Treasure Island (FL): StatPearls Publishing LLC; 2018.

41. Quraishi S, David A. Depot haloperidol decanoate for schizophrenia. *Cochrane Database Syst Rev*. 2000; **1999**(2): CD001361.

42. Park EJ, Amatya S, Kim MS, et al. Long-acting injectable formulations of antipsychotic drugs for the treatment of schizophrenia. *Arch Pharm Res*. 2013; **36**(6): 651–659.

43. Citrome L. Sustained-release risperidone via subcutaneous injection: a systematic review of RBP-7000 (PERSERIS™) for the treatment of schizophrenia. *Clin Schizophr Relat Psychoses*. 2018; **12**(3): 130–141.

Monitoring and Improving Antipsychotic Adherence in Outpatient Forensic Diversion Programs

Jonathan M. Meyer

Introduction

California has the largest population of mentally ill defendants nationwide, and on June 27, 2018, the governor signed into law Assembly Bill 1810 that offered every county the opportunity to establish diversion program procedures (Section 15), and opened program access to all mental health diagnoses excluding antisocial personality disorder, borderline personality disorder, and pedophilia.[1] This measure thus reflects the increasing nationwide interest in channeling seriously mentally ill individuals away from traditional legal processes into pre-trial diversion programs.[2] On an individual level the goal is to provide treatment for mental health conditions, decrease the legal burden and consequences of arrest, and facilitate integration with community support structures. Despite the expense of jail diversion, a fiscal benefit is realized immediately through reduced costs of custodial care, especially for defendants deemed incompetent to stand trial who may have faced lengthy detours through jail and state hospital competency restoration programs.[3] The longer-term fiscal benefit is derived from those who successfully complete mental health court treatment, as diversion program completers experience fewer post-treatment arrests and days incarcerated.[4,5]

While the use of community-based resources allows appropriate diversion clients to be managed as outpatients, provision of care outside controlled settings (e.g. jail and hospital) presents a set of challenges for monitoring treatment fidelity. Schizophrenia patients benefit from mental health court participation, and schizophrenia spectrum disorders remain the core group targeted by many diversion programs across the nation.[6] For schizophrenia spectrum disorders antipsychotic medication is the foundation of treatment, and medication nonadherence not only increases illness relapse risk but is also associated with higher recidivism rates in forensic patients. Among a cohort of 63 prison parolees with a schizophrenia diagnosis previously found not guilty by reason of insanity, poor adherence to treatment increased the odds of reoffense by 10-fold (OR = 10.42; $p = 0.001$).[7] Importantly, in a large ($n = 11,462$) Canadian study of offenders with schizophrenia and a mean follow-up of 10 years, lower antipsychotic adherence levels were significantly associated with increased adjusted risk ratios (ARR) of violent (ARR = 1.58; 95% CI = 1.46–1.71) and nonviolent (ARR = 1.41; 95% CI = 1.33–1.50) offenses compared to those with high adherence rates ($\geq$ 80%).[8] Although jail diversion programs must provide a comprehensive array of services, including supported housing, case management, substance use treatment, and appropriate rehabilitative options (i.e. cognitive, psychosocial, vocational), maintenance of participant psychiatric stability is key to the successful completion of mental health court dictates. Because antipsychotic nonadherence looms as one of the biggest factors in psychiatric relapse and recidivism, measures to track and mitigate nonadherence must be incorporated into the treatment protocols of all diversion programs.[9] The purpose of this focused review is to provide a description of how evidence-based strategies, including pill counts, plasma antipsychotic levels, and long-acting injectable (LAI) antipsychotics, can be implemented in outpatient diversion programs with the goal of minimizing risks of treatment failure related to inadequate antipsychotic treatment.

Pill Counts to Track Nonadherence in Schizophrenia Patients

Although the cause may be lack of insight, cognitive dysfunction, or other aspects of the disorder (e.g. substance use and homelessness), antipsychotic nonadherence is exceedingly common among schizophrenia

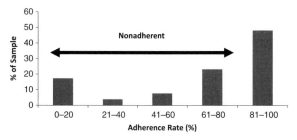

Figure 19.1 Four-week MEMSCap data on 52 outpatients with schizophrenia.[12]

patients.[10] Whether the adherence metric is pill count, medication possession ratio, or plasma antipsychotic levels, an estimated 50% of schizophrenia patients are nonadherent with antipsychotic therapy.[10] Even for schizophrenia patients knowingly enrolled in studies employing specially designed Medication Event Monitoring System electronic chips (MEMSCap) to record each pill bottle opening,[11] adherence rates (by pill count) remain low. One MEMSCap study (*n* = 52) found that only 48% of schizophrenia patients took 80% of their doses over four weeks, with 17.3% of patients taking ≤ 20% of their antipsychotic[12] (Figure 19.1). Employing 70% as the adherence threshold, another MEMSCap study noted a nonadherence rate of 57% among a group of chronic schizophrenia spectrum patients (*n* = 61).[13] The latter study also illustrates the concept that patients and clinicians are poor judges of the extent of nonadherence: the patient self-report of nonadherence was 5%, and the physician estimate of nonadherence was only 7%.[13] These MEMSCaps studies illustrate several important concepts: pill count is an excellent measure of adherence for patients on oral medication; plasma antipsychotic levels are not as well correlated with adherence as are pill counts; pill counts and plasma levels are superior to clinician estimates of adherence.[11,14] As will be discussed later, the additional value provided by plasma antipsychotic levels rests in allowing one to differentiate nonresponders due to inadequate drug levels from those who are treatment-resistant.[15]

For patients who respond to an antipsychotic that is available as an LAI, conversion to the depot formulation is appropriate and can be guided by manufacturer recommendations, and a recent review paper is dedicated to this topic.[16] Unfortunately, most antipsychotics and the commonly used first-line mood stabilizers lithium and divalproex are available only in oral forms. The use of pill counts can rapidly identify poor oral medication adherence and permit interventions to avert the psychiatric and forensic consequences. Diversion programs typically have measures to assure that patients have a supply of oral psychiatric medication, so refill records are of less importance than in other outpatient programs. However, the fact that a patient has refilled a medication is not a guarantee that the medication is ingested, a fact borne out by numerous studies.[17,18] Pill counts are thus a critical tool for ensuring oral medication adherence. As diversion patients typically meet with a staff member every week, weekly pill counts are an appropriate interval, with the exact day of the week varying (if possible) to avert pill dumping by higher-functioning patients when the assessment day is pre-assigned. As diversion enrollees transition to more independent living situations and also demonstrate the ability to self-monitor, the frequency of pill counts can decrease.

Use of Long-Acting Injectable Antipsychotics

Despite the best efforts of diversion program staff, many patients will struggle with oral medication adherence, thus necessitating conversion to an LAI formulation. Moreover, diversion enrollees often have a historical pattern of oral medication nonadherence when not in supervised treatment, so instituting an LAI prior to exiting the diversion program is appropriate to forestall symptomatic relapse and recidivism.[2] That schizophrenia patients with criminal justice contact have high rates of treatment nonadherence served as the basis for a pragmatically informed randomized trial of usual oral medications versus an LAI (paliperidone palmitate) in adult schizophrenia patients who had been in custody within the prior two years.[19] The primary endpoint was time to treatment failure over 15 months defined by one of many outcomes: arrest or incarceration; psychiatric hospitalization; increased psychiatric services to prevent hospitalization; treatment discontinuation or supplementation due to inadequate efficacy, safety, or tolerability; completed suicide. Among the 444 subjects included in the final analysis, paliperidone palmitate was associated with a significant delay in time to first treatment failure compared to oral antipsychotics (hazard ratio 1.43; 95% CI, 1.09–1.88; *p* = 0.011). Treatment failure rates in the LAI and oral cohorts over 15 months were 39.8% and 53.7%, respectively, with arrest and psychiatric hospitalization the most common reasons for treatment failure (21.2% versus 29.4% and 8.0% versus 11.9%, respectively).[20] The superiority of an LAI versus comparable oral antipsychotics seen in that trial parallels conclusions from meta-analyses of other randomized and controlled study designs.[21]

Table 19.1 provides basic kinetic details on the LAI antipsychotics available in the USA as of January 2019. Although there are 10 separate agents listed, these fall into four broad groups: the first-generation antipsychotics (FGAs) (haloperidol or fluphenazine decanoate), risperidone or its metabolite

paliperidone (Consta®, Perseris®, Invega Sustenna®, Invega Trinza®), aripiprazole (Abilify Maintena®, Aristada®, Aristada Initio®), and olanzapine (Replrevv®). Detailed information on the use of these LAI antipsychotics and unique safety issues with olanzapine pamoate (Relprevv®) can be found in recent reviews.[16,26] While some patients will refuse an LAI, and others might not respond to or tolerate the available LAI options, successful conversion to an LAI vastly simplifies concerns about antipsychotic nonadherence. The failure of a patient to be seen at the prearranged time for the injection immediately alerts

Table 19.1 Kinetic properties of depot antipsychotics available in the United States[16,22,23]

Drug	Vehicle	Dosage	Tmax	$T_{1/2}$ multiple dosing	Able to be loaded
Fluphenazine decanoate	Sesame oil	12.5–100 mg/2 wks	0.3–1.5 days	14 days	Yes
Haloperidol decanoate	Sesame oil	25–400 mg/4 wks	3–9 days	21 days	Yes
Risperidone subcutaneous (Perseris®)	Water	90–120 mg/4 wks	4–6 h (1st peak) ~ 8 days (2nd peak)	9–11 days	Not needed
Risperidone microspheres (Risperdal Consta®)	Water	12.5–50 mg/2 wks	21 days	3–6 days	No (21–28 days oral overlap)
Paliperidone palmitate (Invega Sustenna®)	Water	39–234 mg/4 wks	13 days	25–49 days	Yes
Paliperidone palmitate (3 mo) (Invega Trinza®)*	Water	273–819 mg/12 wks	84–95 days (deltoid) 118–139 days (gluteal)	30–33 days	No
Olanzapine pamoate (Zyprexa Relprevv®)**	Water	150–300 mg/2 wks 300–405 mg/4 wks	7 days	30 days	Yes
Aripiprazole monohydrate (Abilify Maintena®)	Water	300–400 mg/4 wks	6.5–7.1 days	29.9–46.5 days	No (14 days oral overlap)
Aripiprazole lauroxil (Aristada®)***	Water	441 mg, 662 mg, 882 mg/4 wks 882 mg/6 wks 1064 mg/8 wks	41 days (single dose)[24] 24.4–35.2 days (repeated dosing)[25]	53.9–57.2 days	No (Start with ALNCD 675 mg IM+30 mg oral OR 21 days oral overlap)
Aripiprazole lauroxil nanocrystal (Aristada Initio)****	Water	675 mg once	27 days (range: 16 to 35 days)	15–18 days (single dose)	—

* Only for those on paliperidone palmitate monthly for four months. Cannot be converted from oral medication.

** See US FDA bulletin: (www.fda.gov/Drugs/DrugSafety/ucm356971.htm).

*** 21 days oral overlap unless starting with aripiprazole lauroxil nanocrystal + single 30 mg oral dose.

**** Aripiprazole lauroxil nanocrystal (ALNCD) is only used for initiation of treatment with aripiprazole lauroxil, or for resumption of treatment. It is always administered together with the clinician determined dose of aripiprazole lauroxil, although the latter can be given up to 10 days after the aripiprazole lauroxil nanocrystal injection.

clinical staff that something is amiss. Unlike oral medications, the long half-lives of LAI preparations also provide a cushion of time to locate the patient before antipsychotic plasma levels become subtherapeutic.[21]

The choice of an LAI is dependent on patterns of response and tolerability during prior antipsychotic exposure. Use of FGA LAIs is necessary for patients who require higher levels of dopamine D_2 antagonism than that provided by second-generation antipsychotics (SGAs); however, for those who are sensitive to D_2 antagonism, risperidone/paliperidone and aripiprazole are better choices. Risperidone and paliperidone have a risk for hyperprolactinemia which exceeds that for any other antipsychotic, including FGAs and aripiprazole, but risperidone and paliperidone also have lower risk for parkinsonism, akathisia, and dystonia than an FGA.[27] Aripiprazole and the FGAs are the LAIs with the lowest weight-gain risk and therefore might be preferable for patients at higher risk for weight gain due to younger age or nonwhite race/ethnicity.[28]

Monitoring Plasma Antipsychotic Levels to Track Adherence and Optimize Antipsychotic Response

In certain circumstances there might be a suspicion of pill dumping by patients on oral antipsychotics, so plasma antipsychotic levels can be used to monitor adherence.[11] As noted later, fluctuations of more than 30% in trough plasma levels are usually indicative of adherence issues, assuming that levels are obtained at approximately the same time after the last dose and that no new medications have been introduced to influence antipsychotic kinetics.[14] The other important use of plasma antipsychotic levels is to guide dosing adjustments, especially in nonresponders. Even when adherence is assured on the basis of regular pill counts or use of an LAI formulation, there is extensive interindividual variation in antipsychotic metabolism, and a wide range of antipsychotic levels at which patients respond.[16] When adherence is removed from the equation, inadequate response can only be due to one of two issues: subtherapeutic plasma antipsychotic levels (due to underdosing or kinetic interactions) or treatment resistance.[29] Before deciding that an adherent patient who failed two or more antipsychotics is treatment-resistant, subtherapeutic antipsychotic levels must be ruled out. In

a British study of 99 outpatients deemed to have treatment-resistant schizophrenia and in need of a clozapine trial, 35% had subtherapeutic antipsychotic levels, 34% of which (n = 12) were undetectable.[29]

Basic Principles for Obtaining Plasma Antipsychotic Levels

Table 19.2 outlines the important issues in obtaining plasma antipsychotic levels. For oral medication in particular, consistency in the time since last dose is critical to interpreting changes in levels over time. Table 19.3 provides estimated trough plasma levels for antipsychotics and commonly used LAI formulations. A single data point can be difficult to interpret, so when levels are unexpectedly high or low based on a given dose a repeat level must be ordered. How one reacts to a high plasma level will depend on the clinical scenario as described in Table 19.2. Embedded in the discussion of response to high plasma antipsychotic levels is the reality that there is no agreed-upon maximum level for antipsychotics, a fact reflected in the significant disparity between laboratory reference ranges (Table 19.4). The following section on managing antipsychotic nonresponse provides a nuanced discussion of the concepts that should underlie the use of plasma antipsychotic levels to pursue efficacy in nonresponders.

Use of Plasma Levels to Track Adherence

Long-acting injectable antipsychotics are designed to have long half-lives and, with repeated dosing at the prescribed interval, should exhibit limited month-to-month variation in trough plasma levels.[26] During the first year of treatment there may be an upward trend in plasma antipsychotic levels beyond that predicted by kinetic parameters, and this is related to the systemic delivery of the antipsychotic from its depot reserve, resulting in a greater fraction of medication available for redistribution into tissues.[49] As the tissue compartment becomes saturated, plasma levels will increase, so antipsychotic levels should be monitored every 2–3 months during the first year of treatment, and dosing adjustments made as necessary.

Assuming that an oral antipsychotic is taken daily and the plasma level is obtained as a 12-h trough (±2 h), there should be less than 30% variation between determinations.[14] Variations ≥ 50% are typically due to nonadherence but may reflect the

Table 19.2 How to obtain and respond to plasma antipsychotic levels[30]

Timing	Oral antipsychotics: The standard is a 12 h trough, although variation by ± 2 h is acceptable and should not meaningfully influence results. Antipsychotics should ideally be administered as a single bedtime dose. For those on twice daily dosing, the morning dose must be held until the level is drawn. If there is doubt about the latter, repeat the level.
	Depot antipsychotics: The standard is to obtain a trough level on the morning of the next injection or up to 3 days prior.
Expected variation	Oral antipsychotics: Up to 30% for 12 h trough levels. Marked trough plasma level fluctuations (>50%) on the same dose indicate nonadherence.
	Depot antipsychotics: Limited variation in trough levels at steady state.
Response to low plasma levels	Oral antipsychotics: When there are no prior plasma levels for a patient on oral antipsychotics and the value is more than 50% below that predicted for the dose (Table 19.3), nonadherence is the likely culprit. A repeat level will be instructive. Marked plasma level fluctuations (>50%) on the same dose indicate nonadherence, while consistent levels (especially with multiple data points) with limited fluctuation may indicate absorption or drug metabolism issues.
	Depot antipsychotics: Levels below that expected for the dose are indicative of drug metabolism issues.
Response to high plasma levels	The first rule of thumb is patient safety as determined by clinical evaluation. When no prior levels are available, many clinicians become alarmed when very high levels are returned from the laboratory and reflexively reduce doses without first determining whether the level fits the clinical picture. Most patients with very high plasma concentrations typically exhibit adverse effects consistent with the level. Moreover, as noted in Table 19.4, there is wide variation in what laboratories refer to as a "high" antipsychotic levels. Before any actions are taken, a few steps need to be performed.
	(a) The patient must be evaluated in person.
	(b) For those on divided daily oral doses, an attempt must be made to determine if the level was a true trough, or if a morning dose was inadvertently given prior to the blood draw.
	(c) When there are adverse effects, the next oral dose can be held and modest dose reduction is preferable to discontinuation (e.g. 25%). For depot medications, the time to next injection should be delayed until the adverse effects have abated.
	(d) When there is a complete absence of adverse effects, this must be noted in the record as the reason for not changing the dose immediately, and for ordering a repeat level. Occasional patients will be encountered who both tolerate and respond to high antipsychotic plasma levels beyond what the local laboratory recommends (see Tables 19.5 and 19.6). If the level is above the point of futility, slow dose reduction (e.g. 10% per month) is necessary to prevent rebound psychosis.[31,32]

addition of an inhibitor or inducer that has altered the antipsychotic kinetics. A common example is the 50% drop in plasma clozapine levels seen in patients who resume smoking.[30] If no inhibitors or inducers have been added, nonadherence is the issue and it needs to be addressed by the combination of pill counts and repeat plasma levels to confirm that the patient is ingesting the medication and not discarding it. Although plasma antipsychotic levels may not return from the laboratory for as long as two weeks, repeated determinations will establish a range of expected levels when the patient is adherent.

Use of Antipsychotic Plasma Levels to Manage Nonresponse

With respect to oral antipsychotic treatment, meta-analyses of numerous clinical trials have shown that minimal response to a given dose after two weeks portends low likelihood of response to that dose at week 6.[50] For patients who fail to respond meaningfully to a given oral antipsychotic dose after two weeks, further dose escalation is indicated in the absence of limiting adverse effects. The time frame for dosing adjustments is markedly different for LAI antipsychotics and depends on the half-life of the agent. In general, antipsychotic titration should be terminated only for one of three reasons: (a) intolerable adverse effects, (b) marked improvement, and (c) plasma levels that indicate low likelihood of further improvement (i.e. levels are at the point of futility).[31] Despite the known dose correlations (Table 19.3), even adherent patients or those on LAI antipsychotics may have surprisingly low plasma levels due to genetic variations that make the individual an ultrarapid metabolizer for specific cytochrome P450 enzymes.[31] Determination of the antipsychotic level is the only means to distinguish those who are kinetic failures (as manifested by sub-therapeutic plasma levels) and those who are treatment-resistant and in need of clozapine.[29]

Table 19.3 Predicted steady-state trough plasma levels by dose for select antipsychotics

Oral medications	Relationships and supporting data
Aripiprazole	Concentration (ng/ml) = 12 × oral dose (mg/d)[33] 20 mg/d -> 230 ± 193 ng/ml
Clozapine	• 40 year old male, 80 kg, clozapine/norclozapine ratio of 1.32 Concentration (ng/ml) = 1.08 × oral dose (mg/d) (nonsmokers) Concentration (ng/ml) = 0.67 × oral dose (mg/d) (smokers) 325 mg -> 350 ng/ml[34] (nonsmokers) 525 mg -> 350 ng/ml[34] (smokers) • 40 year old female, 70 kg, clozapine/norclozapine ratio of 1.32 Concentration (ng/ml) = 1.32 × oral dose (mg/d) (nonsmokers) Concentration (ng/ml) = 0.80 oral dose (mg/d) (smokers) 265 mg -> 350 ng/ml[34] (nonsmokers) 435 mg -> 350 ng/ml[34] (smokers)
Haloperidol	Concentration (ng/ml) = 0.78 × oral dose (mg/d) 10 mg/d -> 7.79 ± 4.79 ng/ml[35]
Fluphenazine	Concentration (ng/ml) = 0.08 × oral dose (mg/d) (nonsmokers) Concentration (ng/ml) = 0.04 × oral dose (mg/d) (smokers) 22.9 mg -> 1.83 ± 0.94 ng/ml[36] (nonsmokers) 20.4 mg -> 0.89 ± 0.43 ng/ml[36] (smokers)
Olanzapine	Concentration (ng/ml) = 2.00 × oral dose (mg/d) (nonsmokers) Concentration (ng/ml) = 1.43 × oral dose (mg/d) (smokers) 10 mg -> 20 ng/ml[37] (nonsmokers) 14 mg -> 20 ng/ml[38] (smokers)
Paliperidone	Concentration (ng/ml) = 4.09 × oral dose (mg/d) (adult sample, n=221)[39] Concentration (ng/ml) = 2.59 × oral dose (mg/d) (Korean sample, n=100)[39]
Perphenazine	Concentration (ng/ml) = 0.08 × oral dose (mg/d) (2D6 PM)[40] Concentration (ng/ml) = 0.04 × oral dose (mg/d) (2D6 EM)
Risperidone + 9-OH Risp (active moiety)	Active Moiety Concentration (ng/ml) = 7.00 × oral dose (mg/d)[41] Risp/9-OH Risp Ratio: 0.2 (range 0.1–0.3)[42]
LAI Medications	**Relationships and Supporting Data**
Aripiprazole lauroxil	882 mg/month: 219 ng/ml[24]
Aripiprazole monohydrate	400 mg/month: 212 ng/ml[43]
Fluphenazine decanoate	25 mg/2 weeks: 1.27 ng/ml[44]
Haloperidol decanoate	100 mg/month: 2.94 ± 0.33 ng/ml (52 week data)[45]
Paliperidone palmitate (monthly)	Monthly dose (mg) × 0.1645 (ng/ml)[46]
Risperidone microspheres	50 mg/2 weeks: 32.2 ± 18.0 ng/ml (52 week data)[47]
Risperidone subcutaneous	90 mg/month = 3 mg oral risperidone = 21 ng/ml[48] 120 mg/month = 4 mg oral risperidone = 28 ng/ml[48]

Abbreviations: EM = extensive metabolizer; PM = poor metabolizers.

While there is limited agreement on the high end of the therapeutic range, most laboratories present a narrow range of values that represent the therapeutic threshold for antipsychotic therapy. Table 19.5 presents working definitions of therapeutic threshold, tolerability threshold, and point of futility to help guide treatment decisions, and evidence-based values derived from the literature are noted in Table 19.6.[31] In inadequate responders without adverse effects, the plasma antipsychotic level is important in deciding whether the minimum response threshold has been met.

Having a value at or slightly above the response threshold is no guarantee of response as the patient may need a plasma level at the high end of the range, but it does serve as a useful initial target for nonresponders with levels below the threshold.[51] As the titration proceeds to higher plasma levels in search of greater efficacy, most patients will not be able to tolerate levels above the tolerability threshold; however, for those who do, there is little clinical value in exceeding the point of futility beyond which response rates are close to zero.[31] As laboratories present a wide range of values for the

Table 19.4 Variations in laboratory plasma antipsychotic reference ranges

| | Therapeutic range (ng/ml)* | | | | | | | |
| | ARUP | | LabCorp | | Mayo Clinic | | Quest | |
Analyte	Lower	Upper	Lower	Upper	Lower	Upper	Lower	Upper
Fluphenazine	0.5	2.0	1.0	10.0	1.0	10.0	Not provided	
Haloperidol**	5.0	20.0	1.0	10.0	5.0	16.0	5.0	15.0
Olanzapine	20.0	80.0	10.0	80.0	10.0	80.0	5.0	75.0
Clozapine***	Not well established		Not provided		Therapeutic range > 350 ng/ml		See below	

* Sites accessed January 15, 2019:

ARUP Laboratories: https://www.aruplab.com

LabCorp: https://www.labcorp.com/test-menu/search

Mayo Clinic Laboratories: https://www.mayomedicallaboratories.com

Quest: http://www.questdiagnostics.com/testcenter/TestDetail.action

(866-697-8378; for Cloz: 800-421-4449 x5440; for Flu: 866-522-6649)

** ARUP reports that the toxic haloperidol level is > 42.0 ng/ml

LabCorp reports a potentially toxic haloperidol level is > 50.0 ng/ml

Mayo provides the following text: "A therapeutic window exists for haloperidol; patients who respond at serum concentrations between 5 and 16 ng/mL show no additional improvement at concentrations >16 to 20 ng/mL. Some patients may respond at concentrations < 5 ng/mL, and others may require concentrations significantly > 20 ng/mL before an adequate response is attained."

*** ARUP reports that the toxic clozapine level is ≥ 1500 ng/ml

Quest reports a level range only for norclozapine: 25–400 ng/ml. Patient reports contain the following referring to the plasma clozapine level: "The therapeutic response begins to appear at 100 mcg/L. Refractory schizophrenia appears to require a therapeutic concentration of at least 350 mcg/L (trough, at steady state). Toxic range: > 1000 mcg/L." [NB: mcg/L = ng/mL].

Table 19.5 Concepts for use of plasma antipsychotic levels

Therapeutic threshold	The plasma level below which likelihood of response is low (but not zero). Example: in a clinical trial of haloperidol, response rate for levels < 2 ng/ml was 9% compared to 73% for levels 5–12 ng/ml.[51]
Tolerability threshold	The plasma level at which 80% of patients have intolerable adverse effects. Example: in a clinical trial of fluphenazine, 80% of subjects with a plasma level of 2.72 ng/ml manifested intolerable adverse effects.[51]
Point of futility	Some schizophrenia may not develop parkinsonism, akathisia, dystonia, or other dose limiting adverse effects despite doses that significantly exceed the tolerability threshold. Example: based on clinical trials data and clinical experience, the chances of responding to a plasma fluphenazine level > 4.0 ng/ml is virtually nil, yet plasma levels as high as 16 ng/ml have been reported in the literature.[31,52]

upper end of their reference range (or in some instances no value at all), the point of futility should serve as an evidence-based marker that the clinician can aim for, assuming tolerability, but once reached serves as the defining point to terminate that antipsychotic trial.

Conclusions

Diversion programs offer an opportunity for patients to receive treatment for their psychiatric illness along with the possibility of having a criminal charge dismissed. The successful completion of diversion programs is associated with decreased recidivism rates, but when patients are treated outside of controlled settings medication nonadherence potentially undermines any gains made through diversion program participation. Nonadherence is the norm among patients with schizophrenia and starts at the time of initial diagnosis; moreover, those with a history of criminal contact comprise an enriched pool of treatment nonadherent patients necessitating the use of

Table 19.6 Response, tolerability, and futility thresholds for select antipsychotics

	Response threshold (ng/ml)	Tolerability threshold (ng/ml)	Point of futility (ng/ml)
Haloperidol	3–5	18–20	30
Fluphenazine	0.8–1.0	2.7–2.8	4.0
Clozapine	350	800–1000	>1000
Risperidone + 9-OH Risperidone	??	??	112
Olanzapine	23.2	176	200

strategies to track antipsychotic therapy in all diversion enrollees. The use of LAI antipsychotics removes issues that surround oral medication non-adherence and should be considered for most diversion patients. When oral antipsychotic therapy is required (e.g. treatment-resistant patients on clozapine), pill counts are highly correlated with medication adherence and must be implemented. While less familiar to many clinicians, antipsychotic plasma levels represent a useful tool to track medication adherence, and, importantly, to prevent treatment failures from subtherapeutic plasma levels. Through a combination of multiple tools, the odds of psychiatric stability increase, and with it the likelihood of diversion program completion.

Disclosures

Dr. Meyer reports having received speaking or advising fees from Acadia Pharmaceuticals, Alkermes, Allergan, Intra-Cellular Therapies, Janssen Pharmaceutica, Merck, Neurocrine, Otsuka America, Inc., Sunovion Pharmaceuticals, and Teva Pharmaceutical Industries.

References

1. California Assembly Bill 1810. Pretrial Diversion, Section 15. 2018.

2. Case B, Steadman HJ, Dupuis SA, et al. Who succeeds in jail diversion programs for persons with mental illness?: a multi-site study. *Behav Sci Law*. 2009; 27(5): 661–674.

3. Renner M, Newark C, Bartos BJ, et al. Length of stay for 25, 791 California patients found incompetent to stand trial. *J Forensic Leg Med*. 2017; 51: 22–26.

4. Steadman HJ, Redlich A, Callahan L, et al. Effect of mental health courts on arrests and jail days: a multisite study. *Arch Gen Psychiatry*. 2011; 68(2): 167–172.

5. Gill KJ, Murphy AA. Jail diversion for persons with serious mental illness coordinated by a prosecutor's office. *Biomed Res Int*. 2017; 2017: 7917616.

6. Comartin E, Kubiak SP, Ray B, et al. Short- and long-term outcomes of mental health court participants by psychiatric diagnosis. *Psychiatr Serv*. 2015; 66(9): 923–929.

7. Oueslati B, Fekih-Romdhane F, Mrabet A, et al. Correlates of offense recidivism in patients with schizophrenia. *Int J Law Psychiatry*. 2018; 58: 178–183.

8. Rezansoff SN, Moniruzzaman A, Fazel S, et al. Adherence to antipsychotic medication and criminal recidivism in a Canadian provincial offender population. *Schizophr Bull*. 2017; 43(5): 1002–1010.

9. Lamberti JS. Understanding and preventing criminal recidivism among adults with psychotic disorders. *Psychiatr Serv*. 2007; 58(6): 773–781.

10. Dufort A, Zipursky RB. Understanding and managing treatment adherence in schizophrenia. *Clin Schizophr Relat Psychoses*. 2019. Jan 3. doi:10.3371/CSRP.ADRZ.121218. [Epub ahead of print]

11. Brain C, Sameby B, Allerby K, et al. Twelve months of electronic monitoring (MEMS) in the Swedish COAST-study: a comparison of methods for the measurement of adherence in schizophrenia. *Eur Neuropsychopharmacol*. 2014; 24(2): 215–222.

12. Remington G, Teo C, Mann S, et al. Examining levels of antipsychotic adherence to better understand nonadherence. *J Clin Psychopharmacol*. 2013; 33(2): 261–263.

13. Byerly MJ, Thompson A, Carmody T, et al. Validity of electronically monitored medication adherence and conventional adherence measures in schizophrenia. *Psychiatr Serv*. 2007; 58(6): 844–847.

14. Velligan DI, Wang M, Diamond P, et al. Relationships among subjective and objective measures of adherence to oral antipsychotic medications. *Psychiatr Serv*. 2007; 58(9): 1187–1192.

15. McCutcheon R, Beck K, Bloomfield MA, et al. Treatment-resistant or resistant to treatment?:

antipsychotic plasma levels in patients with poorly controlled psychotic symptoms. *J Psychopharmacol.* 2015; **29**(8): 892–897.

16. Meyer JM. Converting oral to long acting injectable antipsychotics: a guide for the perplexed. *CNS Spectr.* 2017; **22**(S1): 14–28.

17. Velligan DI, Lam YW, Glahn DC, et al. Defining and assessing adherence to oral antipsychotics: a review of the literature. *Schizophr Bull.* 2006; **32**(4): 724–742.

18. Xu DR, Gong W, Gloyd S, et al. Measuring adherence to antipsychotic medications for schizophrenia: concordance and validity among a community sample in rural China. *Schizophr Res.* 2018; **201**: 307–314.

19. Alphs L, Mao L, Rodriguez SC, et al. Design and rationale of the Paliperidone Palmitate Research in Demonstrating Effectiveness (PRIDE) study: a novel comparative trial of once-monthly paliperidone palmitate versus daily oral antipsychotic treatment for delaying time to treatment failure in persons with schizophrenia. *J Clin Psychiatry.* 2014; **75**(12): 1388–1393.

20. Alphs L, Benson C, Cheshire-Kinney K, et al. Real-world outcomes of paliperidone palmitate compared to daily oral antipsychotic therapy in schizophrenia: a randomized, open-label, review board-blinded 15-month study. *J Clin Psychiatry.* 2015; **76**(5): 554–561.

21. Kishimoto T, Hagi K, Nitta M, et al. Effectiveness of long-acting injectable vs oral antipsychotics in patients with schizophrenia: a meta-analysis of prospective and retrospective cohort studies. *Schizophr Bull.* 2018; **44**(3): 603–619.

22. Alkermes Inc. *Aristada Initio Package Insert.* Walltham MA: Alkermes Inc.; 2018.

23. Indivior Inc. *Perseris Package Insert.* North Chesterfield, VA: Indivior Inc.; 2018.

24. Hard ML, Mills RJ, Sadler BM, et al. Aripiprazole lauroxil: pharmacokinetic profile of this long-acting injectable antipsychotic in persons with schizophrenia. *J Clin Psychopharmacol.* 2017; **37**(3): 289–295.

25. Hard ML, Mills RJ, Sadler BM, et al. Pharmacokinetic profile of a 2-month dose regimen of aripiprazole lauroxil: a phase I study and a population pharmacokinetic model. *CNS Drugs.* 2017; **31**(7): 617–624.

26. Meyer JM. Understanding depot antipsychotics: an illustrated guide to kinetics. *CNS Spectr.* 2013; (18 Suppl 1): 55–68.

27. Leucht S, Cipriani A, Spineli L, et al. Comparative efficacy and tolerability of 15 antipsychotic drugs in schizophrenia: a multiple-treatments meta-analysis. *Lancet.* 2013; **382**(9896): 951–962.

28. Meyer JM, Rosenblatt LC, Kim E, et al. The moderating impact of ethnicity on metabolic outcomes during treatment with olanzapine and aripiprazole in patients with schizophrenia. *J Clin Psychiatry.* 2009; **70**(3): 318–325.

29. McCutcheon R, Beck K, D'Ambrosio E, et al. Antipsychotic plasma levels in the assessment of poor treatment response in schizophrenia. *Acta Psychiatr Scand.* 2017; **137**(1): 39–46.

30. Meyer JM, Stahl SM. *The Clozapine Handbook.* Cambridge, UK: Cambridge University Press; 2019.

31. Meyer JM. A rational approach to employing high plasma levels of antipsychotics for violence associated with schizophrenia: case vignettes. *CNS Spectr.* 2014; **19**(5): 432–438.

32. Iyo M, Tadokoro S, Kanahara N, et al. Optimal extent of dopamine D2 receptor occupancy by antipsychotics for treatment of dopamine supersensitivity psychosis and late-onset psychosis. *J Clin Psychopharmacol.* 2013; **33**(3): 398–404.

33. Sparshatt A, Taylor D, Patel MX, et al. A systematic review of aripiprazole – dose, plasma concentration, receptor occupancy, and response: implications for therapeutic drug monitoring. *J Clin Psychiatry.* 2010; **71**(11): 1447–1556.

34. Rostami-Hodjegan A, Amin AM, Spencer EP, et al. Influence of dose, cigarette smoking, age, sex, and metabolic activity on plasma clozapine concentrations: a predictive model and nomograms to aid clozapine dose adjustment and to assess compliance in individual patients. *J Clin Psychopharmacol.* 2004; **24**(1): 70–78.

35. Wei FC, Jann MW, Lin HN, et al. A practical loading dose method for converting schizophrenic patients from oral to depot haloperidol therapy. *J Clin Psychiatry.* 1996; **57**(7): 298–302.

36. Ereshefsky L, Jann MW, Saklad SR, et al. Effects of smoking on fluphenazine clearance in psychiatric inpatients. *Biol Psychiatry.* 1985; **20**(3): 329–332.

37. Bishara D, Olofinjana O, Sparshatt A, et al. Olanzapine: a systematic review and meta-regression of the relationships between dose, plasma concentration, receptor occupancy, and response. *J Clin Psychopharmacol.* 2013; **33**(3): 329–335.

38. Haslemo T, Eikeseth PH, Tanum L, et al. The effect of variable cigarette consumption on the interaction with clozapine and olanzapine. *Eur J Clin Pharmacol.* 2006; **62**(12): 1049–1053.

39. Schoretsanitis G, Spina E, Hiemke C, et al. A systematic review and combined analysis of therapeutic drug monitoring studies for oral paliperidone. *Expert Rev Clin Pharmacol*. 2018; **11**(6): 625–639.

40. Linnet K, Wiborg O. Steady-state serum concentrations of the neuroleptic perphenazine in relation to CYP2D6 genetic polymorphism. *Clin Pharmacol Ther*. 1996; **60**(1): 41–47.

41. de Leon J, Sandson NB, Cozza KL. A preliminary attempt to personalize risperidone dosing using drug-drug interactions and genetics: part II. *Psychosomatics*. 2008; **49**(4): 347–361.

42. de Leon J, Wynn G, Sandson NB. The pharmacokinetics of paliperidone versus risperidone. *Psychosomatics*. 2010; **51**(1): 80–88.

43. Mallikaarjun S, Kane JM, Bricmont P, et al. Pharmacokinetics, tolerability and safety of aripiprazole once-monthly in adult schizophrenia: an open-label, parallel-arm, multiple-dose study. *Schizophr Res*. 2013; **150**(1): 281–288.

44. Marder SR, Midha KK, Van Putten T, et al. Plasma levels of fluphenazine in patients receiving fluphenazine decanoate. Relationship to clinical response. *Br J Psychiatry*. 1991; **158**: 658–665.

45. Jann MW, Wei FC, Lin HN, et al. Haloperidol and reduced haloperidol plasma concentrations after a loading dose regimen with haloperidol decanoate. *Prog Neuropsychopharmacol Biol Psychiatry*. 1996; **20**(1): 73–86.

46. Schoretsanitis G, Spina E, Hiemke C, et al. A systematic review and combined analysis of therapeutic drug monitoring studies for long- acting paliperidone. *Expert Rev Clin Pharmacol*. 2018; **11**(12): 1237–1253.

47. Fleischhacker WW, Eerdekens M, Karcher K, et al. Treatment of schizophrenia with long-acting injectable risperidone: a 12-month open-label trial of the first long-acting second-generation antipsychotic. *J Clin Psychiatry*. 2003; **64**(10): 1250–1257.

48. Ivaturi V, Gopalakrishnan M, Gobburu JVS, et al. Exposure-response analysis after subcutaneous administration of RBP-7000, a once-a-month long-acting Atrigel formulation of risperidone. *Br J Clin Pharmacol*. 2017; **83**(7): 1476–1498.

49. Ereshefsky L, Mascarenas CA. Comparison of the effects of different routes of antipsychotic administration on pharmacokinetics and pharmacodynamics. *J Clin Psychiatry*. 2003; **64**(Suppl 16): 161B–1623.

50. Samara MT, Leucht C, Leeflang MM, et al. E arly improvement as a predictor of later response to antipsychotics in schizophrenia: a diagnostic test review. *Am J Psychiatry*. 2015; **172**(7): 617–629.

51. Midha KK, Hubbard JW, Marder SR, et al. Impact of clinical pharmacokinetics on neuroleptic therapy in patients with schizophrenia. *J Psychiatry Neurosci*. 1994; **19**(4): 254–264.

52. Nyberg S, Dencker SJ, Malm U, et al. D(2)- and 5-HT(2) receptor occupancy in high-dose neuroleptic-treated patients. *Int J Neuropsychopharmacol*. 1998; **1**(2):95–101.

Pharmacological Treatment of Violence in Schizophrenia

Martin T. Strassnig, Vanessa Nascimento, Elizabeth Deckler, and Philip D. Harvey

Clinical Implications

- Most patients with schizophrenia, save for a small minority, are not chronically aggressive or violent.
- Known predictors of violence include patients with co-morbid substance use disorders (SUDs) and nonadherence with prescribed treatments, those with co-morbid personality disorders, and those with frequent relapses/arrests/civil commitments.
- Among the few modifiable risk factors for violent behavior in patients with schizophrenia is treatment with antipsychotics.
- Aside from clozapine, it appears that treatment with long-acting injectable (LAI) medications is superior to oral antipsychotic in terms of violence prevention. Moreover, LAI facilitate the successful implementation of functional skills training in people with schizophrenia. For the high-risk recidivist target population, better life skills have the potential to also reduce risk for contact with the legal system, including an improved ability to live independently in supported environments and interact appropriately with others.
- High-risk patients who are resistant to treatment with other antipsychotics should receive treatment with clozapine due to its direct positive effects on impulsive violence, along with a reduction in co-morbid risk factors such as SUDs.

Acute treatment of schizophrenia patients is often triggered by attempting to thwart aggression or violence in an inpatient hospital setting. Administration of oral or injectable antipsychotics to acutely agitated patients, perhaps in conjunction with a benzodiazepine, can lead to rapid de-escalation. Short-acting intramuscular formulations of atypical antipsychotics are now available, perhaps with better tolerability compared to the short-acting intramuscular formulation of haloperidol.

New alternative formulations that avoid injections including inhalation and sublingual administration have also become available, further adding to the therapeutic options for calming down acutely agitated patients.[1] In contrast, the treatment of chronic aggression and violence can be a more vexing problem in clinical and community settings, including successful transitioning to an outpatient setting and successful residence in the community.[2] Most patients with schizophrenia are not chronically aggressive or violent; among patients with schizophrenia, there is a small increase in violence and violent offending on average compared to general population standards in the USA and Europe.[3,4] However, much of the excess risk appears to be mediated by substance abuse co-morbidity. Unfortunately, the small subgroup of patients who commit violent acts under certain circumstances are frequently the focus of intense media scrutiny, negatively affecting the public perception of the entire population of schizophrenia patients.[5] This contributes to the stigma associated with mental illness, which is considered to be the most significant obstacle to the development of mental health services.[6] In fact, patients with psychosis are more likely to be victims rather than perpetrators of violence.[7]

Aggression and violence are often used interchangeably although in a strict sense, they are two slightly different concepts albeit located along the same continuum: aggression usually involves threatening behavior, whereas violence goes a step further, and adds an act of furtherance, involving physical harm to others. For the purpose of our review, we will include both aggression and violence towards others, while also acknowledging that aggression and violence are multifactorially and dynamically determined. Moreover, there is often a systematic bias in studying violence in schizophrenia, with many samples examining patients who are involuntarily committed to inpatient facilities or who are undomiciled and receive no mental health treatment, while also abusing substances. Because involuntary commitment criteria often require that the patient has already engaged in threatening or otherwise dangerous behaviors, only the patients already likely to commit violent acts or those who have expressed such an intent are being studied in most inpatient samples. Similarly, outpatient studies are often either retrospective studies of violent acts or include only patients civilly committed in outpatient settings, with the same selection bias applicable.

Known predictors of violence include patients with co-morbid substance use disorders (SUDs) and nonadherence with prescribed treatments, those with co-morbid personality disorders, and those with a history of violence, frequent relapses/hospitalizations/arrests/and/or commitments.[8] Lifelong antisocial behavior often predated by childhood conduct disorder is a risk factor as well.[4] Comprehensive earlier studies from the New York State Mental Health System, and later the California State Hospital System have delineated three types of violence that are common among patients with schizophrenia: psychosis-driven, impulsive (for example, due to fear, anger, provocation), and predatory.[9,10] Viewed from a caregiver perspective, the burden of dealing with aggression and violence falls on family members, clinical care staff, roommates, law enforcement, and staffs of emergency rooms and jails, adding a dynamic element that can be either helpful or detrimental, depending on how the interaction is perceived by the aggressor. Effective management of violence thus requires consideration of these risk factors and circumstances as they interact with the type of violence encountered, in addition to pharmacological treatment, as reviewed below.

Because a large proportion of violent patients end up in jail, a variety of jail diversion programs has been implemented in the USA and Europe, among other countries, to reduce their presence in the criminal justice system. Although they vary in their structure and procedures and operate from different juncture points within the criminal justice process, all jail diversion programs have at their core the idea that persons with severe mental illness should be redirected to mental health services rather than the penal system.[11] Moreover, linking the mentally ill accused and offenders to community-based treatment services shifts the locus of intervention to community-based mental health treatment, reducing jail time while

better serving the mental health needs of these patients. However, patients in these programs do not typically receive court-ordered medications and many of the co-morbidities that are associated with future violence risk (e.g. substance use, antisocial PD, violence history) limit their effectiveness for future violence prevention.

Antipsychotics, Impulsive Aggression and Violence in Schizophrenia

Among the few modifiable risk factors for violent behavior in patients with schizophrenia is the success of treatment with antipsychotic medication.[2,12] Psychosis-driven aggression and violence can be addressed with treatment of the underlying psychosis. As such, standard treatment algorithms apply including those recommended for otherwise treatment-resistant patients.[13] Clozapine is the preferred treatment for resistant psychosis, but remains largely underutilized. Impulsive aggression, the most common form of aggression in schizophrenia patients, does appear to respond well to clozapine also. For example, clozapine has been shown to reduce aggression, hostility, and violent behavior,[14] coinciding with empirical observations that patients with schizophrenia who take clozapine are less likely to engage in physical and verbal aggression[15,16] and are less likely to require restraints and seclusion in hospital settings.[17] In other words, along with its effects on otherwise treatment-resistant psychotic symptoms, clozapine may have direct antiviolence effects, such as its demonstrated effects on suicidal behaviors,[18] and moreover, possible direct effects on smoking and substance abuse as well, addressing key independent risk factors for violence, further reducing risk.[19] If so, clozapine may effectively address several domains involved in the generation of violence including psychosis-driven and impulsive violence while reducing a major co-morbid risk factor (SUDs), a possibility we aim to examine in our review as well.

Finally, in a subset of recidivist offenders, lasting treatment adherence is oftentimes difficult to achieve. In these patients, there have been efforts to augment adherence, including through the use of long-acting injectable (LAI) antipsychotics and other, non-pharmacological interventions that aim to reduce other, dynamic risk factors for violence. Since there is little evidence that LAI medications are effective in patients who are treatment-resistant to oral medications, we will review the databases separately as most people with schizophrenia treated with clozapine are in fact treatment-resistant regardless of their level of violence, substance abuse or smoking status.

Treatment Adherence and the Use of LAI Antipsychotics for Violence Prevention

Poor treatment adherence is common in the schizophrenia population; rates of nonadherence have been found to be as high as 50–75%.[20] Although nonadherence to medical treatment is often this common in general medical conditions, the consequences of nonadherence in schizophrenia are more immediate than, say, the consequence of nonadherence to blood pressure or lipid lowering medications. Factors associated with poor adherence to antipsychotic medication include the patient's insight into illness, homelessness, family support, and the efficacy, side effects, and cost of medication.[21] Poor treatment adherence is of particular concern in patients with co-morbid substance use and those with prior involvement with the legal system, which are also risk factors for violence. Nonadherence often becomes a precursor to frequent symptom exacerbations, including increased propensity for violent behaviors. Certain predictors of violence are found in higher rates among patients with schizophrenia compared to the general population; these predictors include low socioeconomic status, unemployment, alcohol abuse, and antisocial personality disorder.[22] The relationship between poor adherence and violence in patients with schizophrenia has been demonstrated. Proper treatment with antipsychotics reduces violence by decreasing positive symptoms of schizophrenia, whereas nonadherence to antipsychotics is associated with higher rates among violence.

Patients with schizophrenia who are nonadherent are faced with multiple repercussions outside of recidivism. Risk of relapse is 3.7 times greater in patients with schizophrenia who are nonadherent in comparison to patients who are adherent. Moreover, nonadherence predisposes patients to a higher risk of psychiatric rehospitalization, emergency room visits, substance abuse or relapse to substance use, attempted suicide,[21] and being the victim of a crime.[23] With every psychotic episode, patients with schizophrenia suffer from a worsened disease state and further deterioration of social functioning, including evidence of structural brain changes associated with relapse and retreatment.[24] Consequently, it is imperative to consider relapse prevention as a treatment target in the management of schizophrenia.

Long-Acting Injectable (LAI) Antipsychotics

LAI antipsychotics assure delivery of therapeutic levels of medications over several weeks, and with more recent LAI formulations for up to three months, essentially eliminating the need for daily oral medication administration. Although the primary indication for LAI use is poor treatment adherence, less than one-fifth of patients with schizophrenia receive their medication in the form of an LAI.[23] Despite the persistent stigma that follows LAIs and the unsubstantiated and antiquated notion that LAIs cause more adverse effects than oral antipsychotic medications (OAPs), it has been found that LAIs and OAPs do not differ significantly regarding adverse effects.[20] Additionally, adherence remains a barrier to efficacious treatment in patients with schizophrenia who are treated with OAPs. One-third of patients on OAPs are poorly adherent to their medication.[23]

There is a limited number of retrospective studies and prospective trials that suggest LAI may have clinical benefit in schizophrenia patients with high risk of violent behavior. One study by Arango et al. reported that patients with schizophrenia who were considered violent had significantly fewer violent episodes after treatment with LAI medications compared to those treated with OAPs.[22] Moreover, LAIs can effectively reduce the severity of hostility, aggression, and frequency of violent incidents. When patients are adherent to their treatment, LAIs reduce both violent and nonviolent offending behaviors.[25]

Additionally, LAIs have been found to be superior to oral antipsychotics in reducing violent behavior in patients with schizophrenia both with and without co-morbid substance abuse.[25] Substance abuse is highly prevalent among patients with schizophrenia. Studies show that 47% of patients with schizophrenia have lifetime co-morbid substance abuse and 27% have current substance abuse.[26] Nearly 50% of patients with schizophrenia report substance abuse prior to their first episode of schizophrenia.[27] While schizophrenia is a risk factor for violence, substance abuse, regardless if accompanied by a co-morbid diagnosis or not, is known to increase the risk of violence.[26] Therefore, the ability of LAI to treat patients with co-morbid substance abuse makes it an even more desirable treatment option. LAIs may also benefit patients in early-phase or first-episode schizophrenia,[23] possibly improving long-term outcome.

Although systematic bias is often present in studies examining violence in schizophrenia, the Paliperidone Palmitate Research in Demonstrating Effectiveness (PRIDE) study was designed to reflect real-world management of patients with schizophrenia and is therefore worth discussing.[28] The PRIDE study was a 15-month, randomized, prospective study of adult patients with a history of incarceration in addition to a DSM-IV diagnosis of schizophrenia conducted between May 2010 and December 2013. The authors hypothesized that existing clinical trials comparing LAI and oral antipsychotics generated inconclusive results due to failure to enroll individuals representative of patients with schizophrenia in real-world settings. The authors of the PRIDE study note that by failing to enroll patients with complex co-morbidities and histories, the factors which complicate management of schizophrenia such as co-morbid substance abuse, unemployment, and unstable living conditions remain unaccounted for. By creating broader criteria for PRIDE study participants, the authors hoped to produce study results with greater generalizability in comparison to previous studies. Efforts were made to recruit participants who would normally be excluded from trials, such as patients from homeless shelters, soup kitchens, and jail-release or diversion programs. Furthermore, participants were not excluded for a history of substance abuse, although individuals with history of intravenous drug abuse within three months of screening or with an opiate dependence disorder were excluded. Additionally, the study allowed for substantial flexibility in terms of treatment decisions and analyzed clinically relevant endpoints with an explanatory approach, which resulted in an overall pragmatic study design.

Participants were randomly assigned to treatment with one of the seven reviewed oral antipsychotics or with a monthly long-acting injection of paliperidone palmitate. The primary endpoint was time to first treatment failure, defined as either arrest/incarceration, psychiatric hospitalization, suicidal behavior, discontinuation of antipsychotic treatment or supplementation with an additional antipsychotic due to inadequate efficacy, or a necessary increase in psychiatric services to prevent impending psychiatric hospitalization.

The results of the PRIDE study demonstrated that once-monthly treatment with paliperidone palmitate was more effective in delaying treatment failure than treatment with daily oral antipsychotics. In terms of adherence, 95.2% of patients in the paliperidone palmitate group has a medication possession ratio (MPR) greater than 80%, whereas merely 24.3% of patients in the oral antipsychotic group were found to have an MPR greater than 80%. In summary, the PRIDE study results indicate that medication choice may improve outcomes for patients with schizophrenia who are at risk for treatment failure.

In the PRIDE study, 40% of the paliperidone palmitate patients and 54% of the oral antipsychotic patients had a treatment failure event. However, the time to first failure was 416 days in the paliperidone group and 226 in the oral medication group. Twenty-one percent of the paliperidone group and 29% of the oral treatment group had an arrest, with the time to the first arrest being found to be considerably different: median time to arrest in the paliperidone group was over 450 days, with the time to arrest for the oral medication group being 274 days. Thus, there is considerable evidence that LAI treatment provides extensive protection against hospitalization and arrest even in cases with lengthy histories of multiple arrests and hospitalizations. This head-to-head randomized trial provides quite convincing evidence of efficacy for relapse and arrest reduction.

Additional Benefits of LAI Medications

Many people with schizophrenia who have a history of recidivist violence have other schizophrenia-related co-morbidities. These include deficits in the abilities to everyday functioning skills. While functional skills deficits are most strongly related to negative symptoms and cognitive deficits,[29] there is emerging evidence that clinical stability induced by LAI treatment is also correlated with improvements in everyday functioning. In the most recent example, Fu et al.[30] reported that long-term treatment with LAI medications led to persistent benefits in everyday functioning indexed with a targeted clinical rating scale, particularly when compared to patients receiving placebo treatment. These results are similar to results of previous studies that have suggested gains in everyday functioning with successful LAI treatment,[31] reductions in risk for homelessness,[32] and improvement in outcomes in first episode samples.[33] Thus, treatment with LAI medications seems to facilitate other interventions aimed at improving functional outcomes in people with schizophrenia. For the high-risk recidivist population, improvement in life skills might also reduce risk of contact with the legal system, due to increases in the ability to live independently in supported environments and interact more proficiently with others.

Who Should Not Receive LAI Treatment?

Although there are very few indications that LAI actually lead to more side effects than oral medications, there is also no evidence that patients who are treatment-resistant to oral medication in trials with adequate adherence would receive any additional benefits from LAI. Thus, a pre-qualification for using LAI treatment is demonstrated adequate response to oral formulations of the same medications. For patients who are treatment-resistant to antipsychotic medication and by extension, to LAI, there is only one effective treatment for treatment resistance, and that is clozapine. In the sections below, we will describe the use of clozapine as a violence reduction treatment and evaluate which subset of patients would benefit the most from clozapine.

Clozapine for Violence

Clozapine is among the most unique pharmacological treatments for severe mental illness. It is the only treatment approved for treatment resistance and suicidal behavior in schizophrenia, and has also been extensively researched for its effects on co-morbid smoking and SUDs, the latter being a major risk factor for violence. As noted above, psychotic symptoms, either due to nonresponse or treatment discontinuation in otherwise treatment-responsive patients, can be drivers of violence. Clozapine may have a direct effect on violence reduction, in line with its known suicide risk reduction, or indirectly, due to a reduction in psychotic symptoms and SUDs in otherwise nonresponsive patients.

In our literature review, we examined prospective studies and other evidence (case series, and retrospective studies). We divided the prospective studies we reviewed into randomized and nonrandomized trials.

Randomized Controlled Trials

A randomized double-blind controlled trial involving 101 patients, with aggression as the target symptom, was performed with participants who were inpatients of the research ward at a hospital.[34] Compared to olanzapine and haloperidol, clozapine had the best antiaggressive effect in the trial, as indexed by reductions in the primary outcomes scale, the Barratt Impulsiveness Scale. The researchers in the study stated their belief that reduced aggressiveness was a direct result of effects of clozapine on impulsivity and depression, with clozapine's serotonergic action likely playing a role.

A 12-week prospective, randomized, double-blind trial involving 100 inpatients diagnosed with schizophrenia targeted aggression measured with the Modified Overt Aggression Scale (MOAS).[35] Inpatients were randomized to either haloperidol, olanzapine, or clozapine in equal numbers. The study found that there was no significant difference in the response to psychotic symptoms across the three medications, although both olanzapine and clozapine were more effective than haloperidol at reducing aggressiveness. Similar results were found in a randomized, double-blind trial focusing on 110 inpatients with either schizophrenia or schizoaffective disorder.[36] The study compared clozapine, olanzapine, and haloperidol in their antiviolence effect on these patients, and also used the MOAS as the outcomes. This study found that clozapine was superior to haloperidol and olanzapine in its antiaggressive effect, while the antipsychotic effect of the three drugs was equal. These findings again suggest an anti-impulsive aggression effect of clozapine that is independent of its antipsychotic effect.

A prospective, double-blinded, and randomized trial looked at the effectiveness of clozapine, olanzapine, haloperidol, and risperidone on treating hostility in 157 patients with schizophrenia or schizoaffective disorder.[37] The study participants were inpatients at state psychiatric hospitals either in New York or North Carolina. The patients were intended to receive a target daily dose of 500 mg of clozapine. The study determined that clozapine decreased aggressiveness in patients compared to the other treatments with minimal differences in antipsychotic efficacy.

In a secondary analysis from the first phase of the CATIE schizophrenia trial, patients were randomized to one of the four atypical antipsychotics, other than clozapine, or a typical agent.[38] Although violence was reduced for the entire sample, there were no differences between the groups in rates of reduction, with rates of violence being minimal at baseline (19%) compared to other studies. This study highlights the fact that most randomized trials do not suggest that atypical medications other than clozapine have significant potential to reduce violence.

Overall, the results from these studies suggest there may be a direct antiaggressive effect of clozapine operative when compared to other typical and atypical antipsychotic medications, independent of symptom reductions.

Other Evidence (Nonrandomized Trials and Case Series)

Three nonrandomized, prospective studies examined the effect of clozapine on violence reduction and clozapine treatments were suggested to be protective against future aggressive behavior[39,40] and fewer restraint episodes in the hospital.[41] One large, nonrandomized observational study in 675 participants with either schizophrenia or bipolar disorder, with patients recruited from homeless shelters, jails, hospitals, and the streets, did not find enough evidence to determine if clozapine decreased violence in this population, but it asserted that not enough patients with schizophrenia are prescribed clozapine in order to make an accurate conclusion.[42]

A nonrandomized, prospective study of 20 children examined clozapine's impact on aggression in adolescents. The study participants were treatment-resistant schizophrenia inpatients at a child psychiatric center, and all were treated with clozapine.[43] The number and frequency of emergency injectable medication events, emergency oral medication events, and/or seclusions were assessed for each of the patients both before and after clozapine treatment, with the incidence of these events drastically decreasing after the administration of clozapine. In addition, administration of clozapine also allowed patients to be discharged to less restrictive environments more expediently.

Several case series were similar in that they all produced results that demonstrated clozapine's effectiveness for violence reduction.[44–46]

We also identified a number of large-scale retrospective studies relevant to this review. All of these studies concluded that treatment with clozapine resulted in a measurable decrease in aggressiveness, violence, and/or hostility in the study participants.[16,47–51]

In summary, clozapine appears to be beneficial in reducing aggressiveness in patients suffering from schizophrenia and schizoaffective disorder. Compared to other antipsychotics, several studies demonstrate that clozapine's antiaggressive effects are superior to those of haloperidol, olanzapine, and risperidone and both dependent and independent of its antipsychotic effects. Finally, even in the presence of co-morbidities such as intellectual disability and antisocial tendencies, clozapine was effective. These data indicate that clozapine should be considered as a treatment for violence in any patient who manifests continued violence, hostility, or aggression after other treatments, regardless of psychosis.

Outpatient Civil Commitment

A fundamental conflict exists between individual autonomy and the need for treatment of people suffering from severe mental illness, inclusive of potentially violent patients.[52] This challenge is magnified when aggression and violence are involved. Given that the common consequence of violence to patient perpetrators is incarceration, often for lengthy terms, there is a clear argument that outpatient commitment (OPC), applied fairly, has benefits to both patients and society as a whole.

Under US Civil Law, OPC orders, issued by a judge, mandate people with serious mental illness (SMI) to adhere to outpatient treatment in order to prevent recidivism and improve outcomes. According to recent data, at least 46 states and the District of Columbia had commitment statutes permitting some form of OPC,[53] with inconsistent implementation, evaluation, and funding across states. The first such program was implemented in North Carolina in 1983, a "preventive" form of OPC used as the model for OPC laws implemented in other states, often named for murder victims who were killed by people with severe mental illness, such as "Kendra's Law" in New York or "Laura's Law" in California. Involuntary administration of medication is usually explicitly prohibited under the authority of OPC and, if indicated, requires separate legal authority and procedures for administration of involuntary medication. The patient may be sent to a hospital for evaluation if needed, depending on state law.

The ethics and effectiveness of OPC orders continue to be debated.[54] Major limitations that have led to unclear evidence include difficulties in conducting and interpreting trials, the definition and measurement of violence, comparing outcomes across different health systems nationally, working with a frequently uncooperative and risky population, small sample sizes, and selection bias. What is often missing in the debate, however, is the above-mentioned restriction on administering compulsory medication. This appears to be a major limitation to programs designed to facilitate treatment in people whose reason for placement under involuntary treatment orders is often triggered by nonadherence to medication.

Among the United States' civil commitment programs, the program in New York had the most solid funding and implementation, allowing for adequate outcome evaluation, compared to other states. NY patients under OPC orders did appear to have improved outcomes, in contrast to results from a recent meta-analysis utilizing international data: 58 among the noted results were reduced hospitalization and length of stay, higher rates of receiving psychotropic medication prescriptions and intensive case management services, and greater engagement in outpatient treatment with resultant decreased safety-risk, a 17% reduction in offenses, 11% in initial-victimizations, and 22% for repeat-perpetrations.[55] Another, similar study pointed out that community treatment order (CTO)-initiated rehospitalization was associated with a 13% reduced initial-perpetration risk, a 17% reduced initial-victimization risk, and a 22% reduced repeat-victimization risk.[56]

Recommendations

The treatment of chronic aggression and violence in schizophrenia involves assessment of interdependent risk factors including the type of aggression (psychosis-driven, impulsive, or predatory), co-morbidities (SUDs), antisocial behavior, and environmental factors. Antipsychotics are not effective for predatory violence. Psychosis-driven violence is likely the most easily accessible type of violence encountered, and follows the same treatment algorithm as for partially/unresponsive patients, eventually oftentimes involving LAIs or clozapine. Aside from clozapine, it appears that treatment with LAI medications is superior to oral antipsychotic in terms of violence prevention.

Moreover, LAI facilitate the successful implementation of functional skills training in people with schizophrenia. For the high-risk recidivist target population, better life skills have the potential to also reduce risk for contact with the legal system, including an improved ability to live independently in supported environments and interact appropriately with others. High-risk patients who are resistant to treatment with other antipsychotics should receive treatment with clozapine.

Impulsive violence appears to respond well to clozapine also, due to its direct positive effects on impulsive violence, along with a reduction in co-morbid risk factors such as SUDs. Moreover, the direct antiviolence effect of clozapine lends itself particularly well to treating violent offenders. CTOs should be stringently implemented and if needed, hospitalization is initiated so that these treatments can be safely introduced, or restarted.

Treatment Algorithm

In patients with a history of nonadherence and a history of violent acts during relapses, a trial of LAI seems to be a reasonable first step. As treatment nonresponse and the need for clozapine is determined on the basis of 12 weeks of treatment or less, a rapid decision regarding treatment response, within three one-month injection cycles, can be made. For individuals who are involuntarily committed, LAI treatment also reduces the need for monitoring for surreptitious nonadherence to medication. In cases where adherence to oral medication can be ascertained, the benefits of LAI to oral medications of the same type/class are not proven.

In cases with history of treatment resistance, clozapine treatment appears indicated in any cases and certain for any cases with a history of violence. As noted above, violence may be reduced even in the presence of clozapine nonresponse for psychotic symptoms. Thus, for individuals who do manifest clear treatment response but are not intolerant, clozapine as an antiviolence treatment seems viable.

Finally, as noted elsewhere in this issue (Chapter 21), cognitive, social cognitive, and functional skills training appears to have violence reduction potential on its own. As these interventions have optimal efficacy in patients with greater clinical stability, concurrent optimized antipsychotic treatment would seem critical, regardless of whether the treatment was LAI or clozapine.

Acknowledgments

The authors completed all work on this paper.

Disclosures

In the last three years, Dr. Harvey has received consulting fees or travel reimbursements from Akili, Alkermes, Allergan, Biogen, Boehringer Ingelheim, Forum Pharma, Genentech (Roche Pharma), Intra-Cellular Therapies, Jazz Pharma, Lundbeck Pharma, Minerva Pharma, Otsuka America (Otsuka Digital Health), Sanofi Pharma, Sunovion Pharma, Takeda Pharma, and Teva. This consultation work was on phase 2 or 3 drug development and is not related to the content of this paper. Dr. Strassnig has served as a consultant to Bracket. This consultation work was on phase 3 drug development and is not related to the content of this paper. Ms. Nascimento has nothing to disclose. Ms. Deckler has nothing to disclose.

References

1. Citrome L, Volavka J. The psychopharmacology of violence: making sensible decisions. *CNS Spectr.* 2014; **19**(5): 411–418.

2. Meyer JM, Cummings MA, Proctor G, et al. Psychopharmacology of persistent violence and aggression. *Psychiatr Clin North Am.* 2016; **39**(4): 541–556.

3. Fazel S, Gulati G, Linsell L, et al. Schizophrenia and violence: systematic review and meta-analysis. *PLoS Med.* 2009; **6**(8): e1000120.

4. Witt K, van Dorn R, Fazel S. Risk factors for violence in psychosis: systematic review and meta-regression analysis of 110 studies. *PLoS One.* 2013; **8**(2): e55942.

5. Sariaslan A, Lichtenstein P, Larsson H, et al. Triggers for violent criminality in patients with psychotic disorders. *JAMA Psychiatry.* 2016; **73**(8): 796–803.

6. Torrey EF. Stigma and violence: isn't it time to connect the dots? *Schizophr Bull.* 2011; **37**(5): 892–896.

7. Bhavsar V, Bhugra D. Violence towards people with mental illness: assessment, risk factors, and management. *Psychiatry Clin Neurosci.* 2018; **72**(11): 811–820.

8. Walsh E, Buchanan A, Fahy T. Violence and schizophrenia: examining the evidence. *Br J Psychiatry.* 2002; **180**: 490–495.

9. Nolan KA, Volavka J, Czobor P, et al. Aggression and psychopathology in treatment-resistant inpatients with schizophrenia and schizoaffective disorder. *J Psychiatr Res.* 2005; **39**(1): 109–115.

10. Quanbeck CD, McDermott BE, Lam J, et al. Categorization of aggressive acts committed by chronically assaultive state hospital patients. *Psychiatr Serv.* 2007; **58**(4): 521–528.

11. Sirotich F. The criminal justice outcomes of jail diversion programs for persons with mental illness: a review of the evidence. *J Am Acad Psychiatry Law.* 2009; **37**(4): 461–472.

12. Volavka J, Van Dorn RA, Citrome L, et al. Hostility in schizophrenia: an integrated analysis of the combined Clinical Antipsychotic Trials of Intervention Effectiveness (CATIE) and the European First Episode Schizophrenia Trial (EUFEST) studies. *Eur Psychiatry.* 2016; **31**: 13–19.

13. Morrissette DA, Stahl SM. Treating the violent patient with psychosis or impulsivity utilizing antipsychotic poly pharmacy and high-dose mono therapy. *CNS Spectr.* 2014; **19**: 439–448.

14. Patchan K, Vyas G, Hackman AL, et al. Clozapine in reducing aggression and violence in forensic populations. *Psychiatr Q.* 2018; **89**(1): 157–168.

15. Ratey JJ, Leveroni C, Kilmer D, et al. The effects of clozapine on severely aggressive psychiatric inpatients in a state hospital. *J Clin Psychiatry.* 1993; **54**(6): 219–223.

16. Rabinowitz J, Avnon M, Rosenberg V. Effect of clozapine on physical and verbal aggression. *Schizophr Res.* 1996; **22**(3): 249–255.

17. Chiles JA, Davidson P, McBride D. Effects of clozapine on use of seclusion and restraint at a state hospital. *Hosp Community Psychiatry.* 1994; **45**(3): 269–271.

18. Sinyor M, Remington G. Is psychiatry ignoring suicide?: the case for clozapine. *J Clin Psychopharmacol.* 2012; **32**(3): 307–308.

19. Brunette MF, Drake RE, Xie H, et al. Clozapine use and relapses of substance use disorder among patients with co-occurring schizophrenia and substance use disorders. *Schizophr Bull.* 2006; **32**(4): 637–643.

20. Misawa F, Kishimoto T, Hagi K, et al. Safety and tolerability of long acting injectable versus oral antipsychotics: a meta-analysis of randomized controlled studies comparing the same antipsychotics. *Schizophr Res.* 2016; **176**(2–3): 220–230.

21. Khan AY, Salaria S, Ovais M, et al. Depot antipsychotics: where do we stand? *Ann Clin Psychiatry.* 2016; **28**(4): 289–298.

22. Arango C, Bombin I, Gonzalez-Salvador T, et al. Randomised clinical trial comparing oral versus depot formulations of zuclopenthixol in patients with schizophrenia and previous violence. *Eur Psychiatry.* 2006; **21**(1): 34–40.

23. Correll CU, Citrome L, Haddad PM, et al. The use of long-acting injectable antipsychotics in schizophrenia: evaluating the evidence. *J Clin Psychiatry.* 2016; **77**(Suppl 3): 1–24.

24. Rezansoff SN, Moniruzzaman A, Fazel S, et al. Adherence to antipsychotic medication and criminal recidivism in a Canadian provincial offender population. *Schizophr Bull.* 2017; **43**(5): 1002–1010.

25. Lynn Starr H, Bermak J, Mao L, et al. Comparison of long-acting and oral antipsychotic treatment effects in patients with schizophrenia, comorbid substance abuse, and a history of recent incarceration: an exploratory analysis of the PRIDE study. *Schizophr Res.* 2018; **194**: 39–46.

26. Iozzino L, Ferrari C, Large M, et al. Prevalence and risk factors of violence by psychiatric acute inpatients: a systematic review and meta-analysis. *PLoS One.* 2015; **10**(6): e0128536.

27. Trudeau KJ, Burtner J, Villapiano AJ, et al. Burden of schizophrenia or psychosis-related symptoms in adults undergoing substance abuse evaluation. *J Nerv Ment Dis.* 2018; **206**(7): 528–536.

28. Alphs L, Benson C, Cheshire-Kinney K, et al. Real-world outcomes of paliperidone palmitate compared to daily oral antipsychotic therapy in schizophrenia: a randomized, open-label, review board-blinded 15-month study. *J Clin Psychiatry.* 2015; **76**(5): 554–561.

29. Strassnig M, Bowie C, Pinkham AE, et al. Which levels of cognitive impairments and negative symptoms are related to functional deficits in schizophrenia? *J Psychiatr Res.* 2018; **104**: 124–129.

30. Fu DJ, Turkoz I, Walling D, et al. Paliperidone palmitate once-monthly maintains improvement in functioning domains of the personal and social performance scale compared with placebo in subjects with schizoaffective disorder. *Schizophr Res.* 2018; **192**: 185–193.

31. Montemagni C, Frieri T, Rocca P. Second-generation long-acting injectable antipsychotics in schizophrenia: patient functioning and quality of life. *Neuropsychiatr Dis Treat.* 2016; **12**: 917–929.

32. Sajatovic M, Ramirez LF, Fuentes-Casiano E, et al. A 6-month prospective trial of a personalized behavioral intervention + long acting injectable antipsychotic in individuals with schizophrenia at risk of treatment non adherence and homelessness. *J Clin Psychopharmacol.* 2017; **37**(6): 702–707.

33. Medrano S, Abdel-Baki A, Stip E, et al. Three-year naturalistic study on early use of long-acting injectable antipsychotics in first episode psychosis. *Psychopharmacol Bull.* 2018; **48**(4): 25–61.

34. Krakowski MI, Czobor P. Depression and impulsivity as pathways to violence: implications for antiaggressive treatment. *Schizophr Bull.* 2014; **40**(4): 886–894.

35. Krakowski MI, Czobor P, Citrome L, et al. Atypical antipsychotic agents in the treatment of violent patients with schizophrenia and schizoaffective disorder. *Arch Gen Psychiatry.* 2006; **63**(6): 622–629.

36. Krakowski M, Czobor P, Citrome L. Weight gain, metabolic parameters, and the impact of race in aggressive inpatients randomized to double-blind clozapine, olanzapine or haloperidol. *Schizophr Res.* 2009; **110**(1–3): 95–102.

37. Citrome L, Volavka J, Czobor P, et al. Effects of clozapine, olanzapine, risperidone, and haloperidol on hostility among patients with schizophrenia. *Psychiatr Serv.* 2001; **52**(11): 1510–1514.

38. Swanson JW, Swartz MS, Van Dorn RA, et al. Comparison of antipsychotic medication effects on reducing violence in people with schizophrenia. *Br J Psychiatry.* 2008; **193**(1): 37–43.

39. Hodgins S, Riaz M. Violence and phases of illness: differential risk and predictors. *Eur Psychiatry.* 2011; **26**(8): 518–524.

40. Swanson JW, Swartz MS, Elbogen EB. Effectiveness of atypical antipsychotic medications in reducing violent behavior among persons with schizophrenia in community-based treatment. *Schizophr Bull.* 2004; **30**(1): 3–20.

41. Chengappa KN, Vasile J, Levine J, et al. Clozapine: its impact on aggressive behavior among patients in a state psychiatric hospital. *Schizophr Res.* 2002; **53** (1–2): 1–6.

42. Fond G, Boyer L, Boucekine M, et al. Illness and drug modifiable factors associated with violent behavior in homeless people with severe mental illness: results from the French Housing First (FHF) program. *Prog Neuropsychopharmacol Biol Psychiatry.* 2019; **90**: 92–96.

43. Kranzler H, Roofeh D, Gerbino-Rosen G, et al. Clozapine: its impact on aggressive behavior among children and adolescents with schizophrenia. *J Am Acad Child Adolesc Psychiatry.* 2005; **44**(1): 55–63.

44. Chalasani L, Kant R, Chengappa KN. Clozapine impact on clinical outcomes and aggression in severely ill adolescents with childhood-onset schizophrenia. *Can J Psychiatry.* 2001; **46**(10): 965–968.

45. Cohen SA, Underwood MT. The use of clozapine in a mentally retarded and aggressive population. *J Clin Psychiatry.* 1994; **55**(10): 440–444.

46. Hotham JE, Simpson PJ, Brooman-White RS, et al. Augmentation of clozapine with amisulpride: an effective therapeutic strategy for violent treatment-resistant schizophrenia patients in a UK high security hospital. *CNS Spectr.* 2014; **19**(5): 403–410.

47. Ifteni P, Szalontay AS, Teodorescu A. Reducing restraint with clozapine in involuntarily admitted patients with schizophrenia. *Am J Ther.* 2017; **24**(22): 222–226.

48. Volavka J. The effects of clozapine on aggression and substance abuse in schizophrenic patients. *J Clin Psychiatry.* 1999; **60**: 43–46.

49. Balbuena L, Mela M, Wong S, et al. Does clozapine promote employability and reduce offending among mentally disordered offenders? *Can J Psychiatry.* 2010; **55**(1): 50–56.

50. Kraus JE, Sheitman BB. Clozapine reduces violent behavior in heterogeneous diagnostic groups. *J Neuropsychiatry Clin Neurosci.* 2005; **17**(1): 36–44.

51. Kelly DL, Conley RR, Feldman S, et al. Adjunct divalproex or lithium to clozapine in treatment-resistant schizophrenia. *Psychiatr Q.* 2006; **77**(1): 81–95.

52. Kisely SR, Campbell LA. Compulsory community and involuntary outpatient treatment for people with severe mental disorders. *Schizophr Bull.* 2015; **41**(3): 542–543.

53. Swartz MS, Bhattacharya S, Robertson AG, et al. Involuntary outpatient commitment and the elusive pursuit of violence prevention. *Can J Psychiatry.* 2017; **62**(2): 102–108.

54. Barnett P, Matthews H, Lloyd-Evans B, et al. Compulsory community treatment to reduce readmission to hospital and increase engagement with community care in people with mental illness: a systematic review and meta-analysis. *Lancet Psychiatry.* 2018; **5**(12): 1013–1022.

55. Swartz MS, Wilder CM, Swanson JW, et al. Assessing outcomes for consumers in New York's assisted outpatient treatment program. *Psychiatr Serv.* 2010; **61**(10): 976–981.

56. Segal SP, Rimes L, Hayes SL. The utility of outpatient commitment: reduced-risks of victimization and crime perpetration. *Eur Psychiatry.* 2019; **56**: 97–104.

Chapter

21

Neurocognition and Social Cognition Training as Treatments for Violence and Aggression in People with Severe Mental Illness

Mackenzie T. Jones and Philip D. Harvey

Introduction

There is a wide-ranging belief that people with severe mental illnesses (SMI) are violent or dangerous. Most patients with schizophrenia are not chronically aggressive or violent; among patients with schizophrenia, there is a small increase in violence and violent offending on average compared with general population standards in the USA and Europe.[1,2] However, violence on the part of people with SMI has several features that differentiate it from violence in the general population. First, it is less likely to be motivated by financial reasons. Second, it can be unpredictable and directed toward strangers. Not being financially motivated, it is more challenging for the general public to avoid. While few people would walk alone in a dark and deserted part of a large city, most people in general would not feel like they need to avoid standing on a subway platform. However, most people who push strangers off subway platforms, leading to fatal injuries, have mental illness and generally have no connection with the people that they attack.[3] In fact, in 20 of 20 cases with available background information reviewed by Martell and Dietz, the offenders and the victims did not know each other, and the offenders were psychotic.[3]

Despite the fact that random violence can occur with people with SMI, during the period that was surveyed in the study, 1977–1991, there were at least 1,600 and up to 2,605 murders per year in New York when this survey was conducted.[4] Thus, 20 out of approximately 30,000 murders were attributable to random subway platform pushing. As a result, although the offenses were striking, random, and terrifying, these are extremely uncommon. This still does not reduce the sensationalism of violence in the media and resulting stigmatization.[5]

Most victims of aggressive behavior on the part of people with SMI are family members, fellow patients, and mental health professionals who are injured while attempting to treat members of the SMI group. So, much like violence in general, most violence in people with SMI stays within the patient's social network and needs to be viewed accordingly. The most common cases of violence in SMI are violent acts directed at people with whom the patient is very familiar. This may not be different from the general population, wherein physical abuse of family members is very common, and the majority of homicides are still committed by people who know the people that they kill. For example, among male homicide victims, only 29% were killed by someone they did not know, and assaults were committed by someone known to the victim in 64% of cases as well.[6]

Aggressive and violent behavior, including both verbal and physical aggression, have considerable adverse consequences for people with SMI. For example, most state hospital beds in America are occupied by forensically committed people with SMI. In California, for example, there are five state hospitals where no more than 10% of the residents are nonforensic cases.[7] Even for state hospital patients who are not committed, aggression and violence are the primary reason for long hospital stays. For example, White et al.[8] reported on the reasons that prevented discharge from a state hospital during a period of aggressive downsizing. Out of a total of 894 patients considered for discharge, only 27% could be discharged, with the primary reasons preventing discharge, in order of importance, being impulsivity, hostility, excitement, and uncooperativeness. Cognitive performance, hallucinations, and negative symptoms did not predict the likelihood of discharge, although delusions did. As a result, several of the features of individuals with specific treatment-resistant symptoms, despite pharmacological therapies, prevent discharges even when the hospital management is highly motivated to empty the hospital. Considering that verbal aggression is also a barrier to successful discharge from long-term care, actual physical violence is not required to prevent discharge to less restrictive settings.[9]

Determinants of Aggression and Violence

There are several potential causes of violent behavior on the part of people with SMI, based on correlational studies. These include intellectual, cognitive, and social-cognitive deficits, psychopathic/antisocial traits, skills deficits, substance abuse, and specific psychotic features. Each of these potential causes will be briefly addressed before we discuss potential treatments that target these symptoms.

Cognitive Impairments

Although cognitive impairments are common in SMI and are clearly correlated with many elements of disability, the research on cognitive impairment as a determinant of violence has yielded some highly specific findings. Although people with SMI do not commonly manifest co-morbid intellectual disability (ID), the research on violence in SMI, particularly among state hospital patients, suggests that this is more common in violent patients.[10] Global cognitive performance deficits are commonly found to be associated with risk for violence, although the patterns of specific cognitive impairments, however, are somewhat inconsistently associated. For example, Ahmed et al.[11] found an overall difference between violent and nonviolent state hospital inpatients on the MATRICS Consensus Cognitive Battery, but only working memory and verbal learning were subscales significantly worse in aggressive patients. In contrast, Serper et al.[12] found that impairments in executive functioning predicted increased violence during acute admissions, and Krakowski and Czobor[13] found more executive functioning impairments in lower aggression cases.

Social-Cognitive Deficits

There are several different domains of social cognition, including understanding the mental states of others,

recognizing emotions, and making attributions for the reasons that others act the way that they do.[14] These elements of social cognition diverge in their functional importance. Understanding mental states and recognizing emotions appear to be related to impairments in everyday social functioning, while attributions fail to predict these types of disability.[15] However, attribution style predicts the presence of paranoid ideation, which, particularly when delusional in severity, is associated with unprovoked attacks on others.[16] Thus, attributional style may contribute to a belief that others are mistreating you, leading to attempts to contravene and reduce threats. In fact, a recent study suggested a direct impact of social-cognitive deficits on violent behavior, while neurocognition's effects were mediated through social-cognitive functioning and deficits in everyday functioning.[17]

Antisocial Traits

Scores on the Psychopathy Checklist (PCL) have been compared across aggressive and nonaggressive patients with SMI. The results are quite consistent, in that PCL scores were the best predictor of community violence on the part of people with SMI in the MacArthur risk assessment study.[18] A series of studies of hospitalized inpatients have generated similar findings. For example, Krakowski and Czobor[13] found that PCL scores were the best predictor of high levels of aggression, and Volavka[19] reviewed the research literature and suggested that psychopathic traits were responsible for more violent assaults in patient units compared with psychotic symptoms.

Skills Deficits

Skills deficits in schizophrenia include reduced ability to perform everyday social and functionally skilled acts.[20] These deficits can lead to considerable frustration because tasks that are easily completed by others are challenging, time-consuming, and poorly performed. Further, social skill deficits can also lead to problems in interacting with others, which can interact with negative attributions and lead to negative interactions. As noted above, deficits in real-world functioning were found to be associated with violent acts.[17] Further evidence for this argument is provided by Martinez Martin et al.,[21] who found that impairments in the ability to perform everyday activities and social competencies were associated with increased aggressive behavior.

Specific Psychotic Symptoms

Both paranoid delusions and command hallucinations have been found to be associated with violent acts.[22,23] The relationship between these symptoms and violence is face-valid, in that it is easy to understand why an individual could become violent upon hearing voices directing him/her to engage in violent acts. However, in addition to paranoia and hallucinations, lack of insight is clearly required. If the individual were aware that the voices or ideas constituted a psychotic symptom, they would be considerably less likely to act on them.[24]

Substance Abuse

Violence in nonhospitalized people with SMI is more common in individuals with concurrent substance abuse.[25] Abuse of several different drugs is common in schizophrenia and is estimated to have a prevalence as high as 50%.[26] The most commonly abused substances are alcohol, cannabis, and cocaine. Individuals with co-morbid schizophrenia and substance abuse are found to have the highest rates of violent behavior;[27] so reducing substance abuse might have a beneficial effect.[28]

Interventions Targeting Cognitive and Social-Cognitive Deficits

As the treatments for psychosis as a violence reduction strategy are presented elsewhere in this special issue, we will focus on the treatment of cognitive and social-cognitive deficits and their potential for violence reduction. Further, there have been several treatment efforts targeting cognition that have been applied to substance abuse in dual diagnosis populations. Pharmacological treatments aimed at cognition and social cognition have been disappointing,[29,30] and so herein we focus on computerized cognitive training (CCT) and computerized social-cognitive training (CSCT). An overview of the CCT and CSCT evaluation studies that we discuss is presented in Table 21.1.

Training Interventions Aimed at Cognition and Social Cognition

Despite the failures of pharmacological interventions for cognition and social cognition in schizophrenia, there are very encouraging results from computerized training interventions. The ultimate aim of cognitive interventions for patients with schizophrenia is to improve social and everyday functioning. To evaluate such interventions, it is important to investigate multiple levels of efficacy, including near transfer of skills to improved performance on similar nontrained tasks, far transfer of skills to improved performance on more demanding tasks, and generalizable, or environmental, transfer of skills to improved real-world everyday functioning. While there has been debate over the efficacy of CCT due to overstated commercial claims,[31,32] several meta-analyses of CCT efficacy have found that it has small-to-moderate effect sizes.[33,34] The largest meta-analysis to date encompassing 40 independent studies involving 2,104 participants showed that CCT provides small-to-moderate benefits in generalizable cognitive domains, particularly within relatively stable patients in both inpatient and outpatient settings.[34] Further concurrent psychosocial interventions were found to lead to functional gains.

Since social-cognitive deficits are separable from neuropsychological deficits[35] and social cognition has been found to predict social functioning better than other neurocognitive domains in patients with schizophrenia,[36,37] social cognition and interaction training (SCIT)[38] and CSCT have also been developed in recent years following the success of CCT in the treatment of cognitive impairment and resultant functional deficits in SMI. Combs et al. developed SCIT, which is a group intervention based upon a manual whose content a group must progress through at its own pace in weekly 1-h sessions.[38] It includes a combination of psychoeducation, drill-and-repeat skill practice, strategy games, heuristic rehearsal, and homework assignments in which participants are encouraged to practice with a family member or acquaintance outside of the group. The results suggested modest benefits in improving social functioning and negative symptoms, but not in the realm of social cognition. This was slightly surprising because SCIT was expected to have downstream effects on functioning and symptoms through improvement in social cognition. It was also demonstrated that greater dosages of SCIT might lead to greater outcomes. Later, larger-scale studies have confirmed the efficacy of the training and again suggested that dose effects are important.[39]

Considering that a greater dosage leads to better outcomes and the fact that the SCIT program requires a trained clinician team, long treatment durations,

Table 21.1 Results of cognitive and social cognitive training on violence and determinants of violence

Study	Sample size	Population (inpatient/ outpatient)	Training CCT, social cognition, combined	Outcomes measures 1. Cognition and social cognition 2. Clinical 3. Violence and related factors (functioning, substance abuse)
Combs et al.[38]	Total SCZ N = 28 1. CSCT (18) 2. Control (10)	Inpatient (forensic)	SCIT	1. Cognition and social cognition performance-based measures 2. PANSS 3. Observed incidents of aggression
Roberts et al.[39]	Total SCZ N = 66 1. CSCT (SCIT) (33) 2. TAU (33)	Outpatient	CSCT	1. Cognition and social cognition, performance-based measures and rating scales 2. PANSS 3. None
Nahum et al.[40]	Total CSCT (34) 1. SCZ N = 17 2. HC N = 17	Outpatient	CSCT	1. Cognition and social cognition performance-based measures 2. None 3. None
Lindenmayer et al.[42]	Total SCZ N = 59 1. CCT + CSCT (32) 2. CCT (CR) alone (27)	55 inpatients 4 outpatients	Combined vs. CCT	1. Cognition and social cognition performance-based measures 2. PANSS 3. PSP
Lindenmayer et al.[43]	Total SCZ N = 78 1. CCT + CSCT (39) 2. CCT (CR) alone (39)	Inpatient and outpatient	Combined	1. Cognition and social cognition performance-based measures 2. PANSS 3. PSP
Fisher et al.[44]	Total SCZ N = 111 1. CCT+CSCT (57) 2. CCT alone (54)	Outpatients	Combined	1. Cognition and social cognition performance-based measures 2. PANSS 3. None
Sacks et al.[45]	Total SCZ N = 19	Outpatients	Combined	1. Cognition and social cognition performance-based measures 2. PANSS 3. None
Russell et al.[46]	Total SCZ N = 40 1. CSCT (26) 2. Control (14) O	Outpatients	CSCT	1. Cognition and social cognition performance-based measures 2. SAPS/SANS/BDI 3. None
Eack et al.[48] Feasibility	Total SCZ N = 31 1. CCT (CET) (22) 2. TAU (9)	Outpatient substance misusers	Combined	1. Cognition and social cognition performance-based measures 2. BPRS/Wing Negative Symptom Scale/ Raskin Depression Rating Scale/COVI 3. GAS; timeline follow-back interview for substance use
Eack et al.[49] Outcomes	Total SCZ N = 31 1. CCT (CET) (22) 2. TAU (9)	Outpatient substance misusers	Combined	1. MCCB/MSCEIT 2. None 3. Timeline follow-back interview for substance use/Addiction Severity Index
Cullen et al.[51] Violence and antisocial behavior outcomes	Total N = 84 (69 SCZ 15 other) 1. CCT (R&R) (44) 2. TAU (40)	Inpatient (forensic)	CCT	1. None 2. PANSS/HCR-20/DUDIT 3. MacArthur Community Violence Instrument verbal aggression/drug or alcohol use/leave violations
Cullen et al.[52] Social-cognitive outcomes	Total MDO N = 84 (69 SCZ) 1. CCT (44) 2. TAU (40)	Inpatient (forensic)	CCT	1. Social cognition performance-based measures 2. PANSS/HCR-20 3. Crime Pics II/NAS

Table 21.1 (cont.)

Study	Sample size	Population (inpatient/outpatient)	Training CCT, social cognition, combined	Outcomes measures 1. Cognition and social cognition 2. Clinical 3. Violence and related factors (functioning, substance abuse)
Ahmed et al.[53]	Total SCZ N = 78 1. CCT (CR) (42) 2. Control (36)	Inpatient	CCT	1. Cognition performance-based measures 2. PANSS 3. OAS
Kumar et al.[54]	Total SCZ N = 16 1. CCT (8) 2. TAU (8)	Inpatient	CCT	1. None 2. PANSS 3. PANSS Hostility Item
Ussorio et al.[55]	Total SCZ N = 56 1. Short duration of untreated psychosis (28) 2. Long duration of untreated psychosis (28)	Outpatient	CCT	1. Cognition and social cognition performance-based measures 2. PANSS/BPRS 3. PSP

and organized patient groups, there are limits to the practicality of applying these treatments in clinical settings. To address this, Nahum et al. evaluated the feasibility of SocialVille, an online program designed to treat social cognition deficits in patients with schizophrenia by specifically targeting the domains of affect perception, social cue perception, theory of mind, and self-referential processing, through 19 computerized exercises.[40] While the design of the experiment prevented any claims of efficacy, it did conclude that CSCT would be feasible in this patient population and may help with some of the practicality limits facing SCT.

With the established success of CCT on cognition, the success of SCT on both social cognition and neurocognition, and the confirmed feasibility of CSCT, programs were eventually developed to augment cognitive training with SCT. Kurtz et al. performed a meta-analysis to investigate the effects of SCT programs alone, as well as combined cognitive training and SCT on social cognition and functioning.[41] The meta-analysis found that SCT demonstrated improvement in the social cognition domains of facial affect recognition and theory of mind, but no improvements were seen in attributional style or social perception.[41] Most significantly, the meta-analysis found that moderate-to-large effects on improvement were confirmed by observer-rated measures of functioning for both inpatients and outpatients, suggesting that SCT provides benefits to patients that are generalizable to their overall functioning. They did not find any changes in patients' positive or negative symptoms or any relationship between dosage and increased effects.

While Kurtz et al. investigated the effects of multiple types of programs, they did not investigate whether SCT in isolation or in combination with cognitive remediation (CR) had differential effects on social or neurocognition. Lindenmayer et al.,[42] however, did examine whether CR alone had a different effect on social cognition from CR combined with CSCT. A program originally developed for autism spectrum patients – Mind Reading: An Interactive Guide to Emotions – was used as CSCT intervention, while COGPACK was used as CR intervention. The study found that combined CR and CSCT resulted in greater improvement than CR alone in measures of social cognition, social functioning, and neurocognition. Since CR alone did, however, still contribute to some improvements on its own, the results suggest that improved neurocognition may be a necessary prerequisite for improved social-cognitive ability in treatment, but not sufficient to account for all potential improvement. The design of the study did not include a CSCT-only group, so no conclusions could be made on whether CSCT alone would have been sufficient to obtain improvements in social cognition. However, the combined CR and CSCT program did have a unique impact on generalization of social functioning skills, whereas CR alone did not.

In a replication of these findings in a separate sample of patients, Lindenmayer et al. reported that combined CCT and CSCT led to greater gains in social cognition and neurocognition.[43] Further, the combined intervention led to the greatest gains in everyday functioning, indexed by work performance. A similar study by Fisher et al. evaluated targeted cognitive training, specifically auditory and visual processing training, and CSCT compared with targeted cognitive training alone.[44] These authors did not find that a combined intervention demonstrated significantly more improvement in most domains of cognition and functioning, although they did find that combined training resulted in greater improvements in reward processing, specifically increased consummatory and anticipatory pleasure, which have been linked to motivated and goal-directed behavior, as well as prosody identification. This was significant because of past findings suggesting that the relationship between social cognition and social functioning is mediated by the level of motivation, with more support for the theory that poor social-cognitive abilities impeded motivation, leading to poor functioning.

Another study by Sacks et al. looked at a similar combination of auditory cognitive training and CSCT and found that the training resulted in significant gains in neurocognition, certain domains of social cognition (emotion identification, social perception, and self-referential source memory), as well as a decrease in positive symptoms.[45] They were also able to show that the effects of CSCT were generalized to more complex social-cognitive abilities outside of what was targeted during training, where other studies failed to demonstrate the generalization of skills.[46,47] This study showed that a cost-effective, efficient, and scalable combined CCT and CSCT program could improve generalizable cognition skills and reduce positive symptoms in patients with schizophrenia.

With results demonstrating the ability of cognitive training and SCT to reduce positive symptoms, but mixed results with regard to other symptoms and overall real-world functioning, studies also began to investigate the feasibility of cognitive training and SCT for more specific groups of patients with schizophrenia, specifically substance abusers. Eack et al. looked at whether cognitive enhancement therapy (CET) could improve cognitive impairments in patients with schizophrenia who misuse substances.[48] The study found mixed results regarding feasibility and efficacy of the training in the patient population due to difficulty engaging and retaining participants. In many cases, this was due to positive symptom instability leading to a withdrawal from the study and ambivalence from the patients toward additional treatment approaches. Even with considerable attrition, intent-to-treat analyses demonstrated that CET resulted in significant improvements in neurocognitive, social-cognitive, and functional outcomes. Thus, the study demonstrated that cognitive remediation can be feasibly applied to substance-using patients with schizophrenia. Another report by Eack et al. published additional results from the same study that included the substance use trajectories for patients with schizophrenia who received CET compared with those who received usual care.[49] Patients receiving CET demonstrated significantly greater and faster reductions in alcohol use that were associated with cognitive improvements in processing speed, visual learning, and problem-solving. And, while patients only demonstrated greater, faster reductions in alcohol use and not cannabis use, cognitive improvements were associated with overall less likelihood of alcohol and cannabis use over the 18-month trial. This is highly relevant to the issue of violence, wherein substance abuse is consistently associated with violent acts on the part of people with schizophrenia as described above.

Cognitive and Social-Cognitive Training and Violence Reduction

As noted above, violence can be associated with deficits in everyday functional and social skills, which may be the end product of cognitive impairments or ID. Social-cognitive impairment appears to be directly associated with violent behavior, and substance abuse coupled with SMI is associated with the highest risk of violent behavior. Thus, the studies reviewed above suggest that both CCT and CSCT improve, directly or indirectly, some of the major risk factors for violent behavior. There is currently a gap in therapeutic resources designed to adequately address the frequency and severity of violent behaviors in patients with schizophrenia. Given the success of CR and SCT programs at improving neurocognition and social cognition, these programs could directly reduce violence and aggression in patients with schizophrenia.

Several studies have directly examined the impact of training in social-cognitive and neurocognitive abilities and their impacts on violent behavior as an outcome variable. These have included studies of neurocognitive and social-cognitive interventions alone, and in combination. These have also used quite wide-ranging patient populations, including those specifically selected for being incarcerated. Darmedru et al. performed the first systematic review to investigate whether CR and SCT are effective in managing violent and aggressive behaviors.[50] They identified 11 relevant studies: 2 investigated nonspecific cognitive remediation interventions, 2 investigated SCIT, 5 investigated reasoning and rehabilitation (R&R) or revised reasoning and rehabilitation, and the final 2 investigated metacognitive training (MCT). All 11 studies showed reduced violence and aggression in various ways, including reduced violent thinking and behavior, reduced physical and violent assaults, and reduced disruptive and aggressive behaviors. The effects were seen in both inpatient and outpatient settings at both early and later stages of disease.

A series of studies by Cullen et al. presented detailed results on both social-cognitive outcomes as well as violent and antisocial outcomes in offenders with SMI at a forensic hospital.[51,52] The social-cognitive outcomes demonstrated moderate improvements in impulsive/carelessness style subscale of the SPSI (Social Problem Solving Inventory), the avoidant style subscale of the SPSI, and small improvements in the total SPSI score.[52] When analyzing the impacts on behavior, the R&R group showed significant reduction in verbal aggression and leave violations compared with the control group following treatment, with reduced verbal aggression being maintained during the 12-month follow-up, though the reduction did not sustain statistical significance.[51]

Ahmed et al. evaluated the benefits of a nonspecific cognitive remediation program within a mixed sample of forensic and mental health patients at a state hospital.[53] The study looked at neurocognition and psychotic symptoms as primary outcomes and functional capacity, experiential recovery, and aggression as secondary outcomes.[53] Those who completed CR showed improvements in the attention, working memory, verbal learning, and overall cognitive functioning domains of neurocognition.[53] Furthermore, the cognitive remediation group demonstrated greater reductions in verbal and physical aggression compared with the control group.[53]

There were no statistically significant differences in WASI IQs between forensic and mental health

patients in Ahmed et al.'s study, although forensic patients had IQs that were five points lower and they also had one fewer year of education (approximately nine years) than standard mental health patients. Interestingly, forensic participants did show greater deficits in working memory and verbal learning relative to mental health patients, as well as increased verbal, object, self, and physical aggression at baseline. The fact that the group with reduced working memory and verbal learning at baseline also had increased aggression at baseline, in addition to the findings that improved working memory and verbal learning skills accompanied reduced aggression following a CR program, further supports the concept that CR reduces aggression through its effects on cognition. It was not possible to further examine whether there were improvements in everyday functioning, because the entire sample was hospitalized at a state psychiatric facility.

The SCIT intervention that reported on changes in aggression was also administered to forensic inpatients.[54] The intervention demonstrated improvements in social cognition, improvements in self-reported social relationships, and fewer aggressive incidents. All changes were independent of clinical symptoms over time, supporting the effectiveness of SCIT as well as the generalization of SCIT to the patients' behaviors. However, the experiment was not a randomized controlled trial, and participants were recruited based on their interest in SCIT, so that motivation or insight may have impacted external validity.

MCT targets active positive symptoms, particularly delusions, as a variant of cognitive behavioral therapy. While studies have shown an improvement in total PSP (Personal and Social Performance scale), which includes a subscale on disturbing and aggressive behaviors, neither of the studies looked specifically at reductions in violence or aggression.[54,55] This appears to be a promising area for future work.

What Are the Mechanisms That Lead to Violence Reduction Following Social-Cognitive and Neurocognitive Training?

Cognitive and social-cognitive training has been shown to reduce violence in schizophrenia patients across multiple environments, including forensic settings. While some cognitive training focuses on problem-solving, some of the other most effective cognitive training strategies improve multitasking, which likely makes the world easier to manage and less confusing for patients. This is probably particularly important for patients with ID who may be more easily overwhelmed with managing concurrent demands. In addition to reducing violence, SCT does also improve social-cognitive functioning. Cognitive training has been shown to augment progress in SCT, producing faster social-cognitive gains, faster cognitive gains, and greater functional gains. Thus, the effect of SCT on violence reduction appears to be direct, with improvements in violence related to the extent of improvement in social cognition.

So, there are several substrates of possible treatment related reductions in violence.

- Improving neurocognition can lead to reduced stress in functional domains.
- Specific neurocognitive improvements (e.g. impulsivity, problem-solving) can be directly related to reductions in impulsive aggressive actions.
- Improving social-cognitive abilities can lead to direct reductions in aggression based on interpersonal suspiciousness.
- Neurocognitive improvements in areas such as problem-solving can lead to reduced substance abuse.

There are some remaining issues to be addressed. For example, the studies to date have not defined treatment response for violence reduction in terms of criterion-referenced outcomes, nor examined the rates of treatment response for violence reduction. Thus, at this time we cannot specify the number needed to treat in order to estimate the likelihood of an individual with schizophrenia manifesting a good response to neurocognitive or social-cognitive treatment. Further, the predictors of treatment response are as yet undefined, and we do not know, for example, whether there are some factors, such as antisocial tendencies or elements of substance abuse, that would preclude a beneficial response to treatment if these are present. Antisocial tendencies do not seem to be particularly responsive to prior treatments. A final concern is whether treatment programs should be tailored to individual social cognition or neurocognitive domains or whether structured curriculum based interventions are preferable. Some studies targeting other outcomes, such as employment, have found that combined treatments with a social and neurocognitive focus have greater benefits.[42]

Conclusion

The current state of research suggests that combined intervention programs targeting neurocognitive, social cognitive, and everyday functional skills lead to the best outcomes for traditional rehabilitation targets such as work. Similarly, it appears likely that a broad-spectrum approach, combining CCT, CSCT, and skills-based approaches targeting social and everyday functional skills, would have the greatest potential for violence reduction. Additionally, as CCT and CSCT are easily delivered on computers and to groups of patients, these approaches have the potential to be highly cost-effective, especially when the cost of incarceration is considered in comparison to the use of these treatments.

Disclosures

Ms. Jones has nothing to disclose. Dr. Harvey reports personal fees from Alkermes, personal fees from Allergan, personal fees from Akili, personal fees from Boehringer-Ingelheim, personal fees from Forum Pharma, personal fees from Genentech, personal fees from Intra-Cellular Therapies, personal fees from Jazz Pharma, personal fees from Lundbeck, personal fees from Minerva, personal fees from Otsuka, personal fees from Sanofi, grants and personal fees from Takeda, personal fees from Teva, other from Verasci, outside the submitted work.

References

1. Fazel S, Gulati G, Linsell L, et al. Schizophrenia and violence: systematic review and meta-analysis. *PLoS Med.* 2009; **6**(8): e1000120.

2. Witt K, van Dorn R, Fazel S. Risk factors for violence in psychosis: systematic review and meta-regression analysis of 110 studies. *PLoS One.* 2013; **8**(2): e55942.

3. Martell DA, Dietz PE. Mentally disordered offenders who push or attempt to push victims onto subway tracks in New York City. *Arch Gen Psychiatry.* 1992; **49**(6): 472–475.

4. The Disaster Center. New York Crime Rates 1960–2016. www.disastercenter.com/crime/nycrime.htm (accessed June 2020).

5. Torrey EF. Stigma and violence: isn't it time to connect the dots? *Schizophr Bull.* 2011; **37**(5): 892–896.

6. McQuade KM. Victim-offender relationship. In: Albanese JS, ed. *The Encyclopedia of Criminology and Criminal Justice*. Hoboken, NJ: Blackwell Publishing Ltd; 2014.

7. California Department of State Hospitals. Welcome. www.dsh.ca.gov/about_Us/ (accessed June 2020).

8. White L, Parrella M, McCrystal-Simon J, et al. Characteristics of elderly psychiatric patients retained in a state hospital during downsizing: a prospective study with replication. *Int J Geriatr Psychiatry*. 1997; **12**(4): 474–480.

9. Bowie CR, Moriarty PJ, Harvey PD, et al. Aggression in elderly schizophrenia patients: a comparison of nursing home and state hospital residents. *J Neuropsychiatry Clin Neurosci*. 2001; **13**(3): 357–366.

10. Puri BK, Richardson AJ, Higgins CJ, et al. Reduction in IQ in patients with schizophrenia who have seriously and dangerously violently offended. *Schizophr Res*. 2002; **53**(3): 267–268.

11. Ahmed AO, Richardson J, Buckner A, et al. Do cognitive deficits predict negative emotionality and aggression in schizophrenia? *Psychiatry Res*. 2018; **259**: 350–357.

12. Serper M, Beech DR, Harvey PD, Dill C. Neuropsychological and symptom predictors of aggression on the psychiatric inpatient service. *J Clin Exp Neuropsychol*. 2008; **30**(6): 700–709.

13. Krakowski MI, Czobor P. Proneness to aggression and its inhibition in schizophrenia: interconnections between personality traits, cognitive function and emotional processing. *Schizophr Res*. 2017; **184**: 82–87.

14. Pinkham AE, Penn DL, Green MF, et al. The social cognition psychometric evaluation study: results of the expert survey and RAND panel. *Schizophr Bull*. 2014; **40**(4): 813–823.

15. Pinkham AE, Penn DL, Green MF, et al. Social cognition psychometric evaluation: results of the initial psychometric study. *Schizophr Bull*. 2016; **42** (2): 494–504.

16. Pinkham AE, Harvey PD, Penn DL. Paranoid individuals with schizophrenia show greater social cognitive bias and worse social functioning than non-paranoid individuals with schizophrenia. *Schizophr Res Cogn*. 2016; **3**: 33–38.

17. O'Reilly K, Donohoe G, Coyle C, et al. Prospective cohort study of the relationship between neuro-cognition, social cognition and violence in forensic patients with schizophrenia and schizoaffective disorder. *BMC Psychiatry*. 2015; **15**: 155.

18. Skeem L, Mulvey EP. Psychopathy and community violence among civil psychiatric patients: results from the MacArthur Violence Risk Assessment Study. *J Consult Clin Psychol*. 2001; **69**: 358–374.

19. Volavka J. Violence in schizophrenia and bipolar disorder. *Psychiatr Danub*. 2013; **25**(1): 24–33.

20. Harvey PD, Velligan DI, Bellack AS. Performance-based measures of functional skills: usefulness in clinical treatment studies. *Schizophr Bull*. 2007; **33**(5): 1138–1148.

21. Martinez-Martin N, Fraguas D, Garcia-Portilla MP, et al. Self-perceived needs are related to violent behavior among schizophrenia outpatients. *J Nerv Ment Dis*. 2011; **199**(9): 666–671.

22. Keers R, Ullrich S, Destavola BL, et al. Association of violence with emergence of persecutory delusions in untreated schizophrenia. *Am J Psychiatry*. 2014; **171** (3): 332–339.

23. Shawyer F, Mackinnon A, Farhall J, et al. Acting on harmful command hallucinations in psychotic disorders: an integrative approach. *J Nerv Ment Dis*. 2008; **196**(5): 390–398.

24. Ekinci O, Ekinci A. Association between insight, cognitive insight, positive symptoms and violence in patients with schizophrenia. *Nord J Psychiatry*. 2013; **67**(2): 116–123.

25. Haddock G, Eisner E, Davies G, et al. Psychotic symptoms, self-harm and violence in individuals with schizophrenia and substance misuse problems. *Schizophr Res*. 2013; **151**(1–3): 215–220.

26. Hunt GE, Large MM, Cleary M, et al. Prevalence of comorbid substance use in schizophrenia spectrum disorders in community and clinical settings, 1990–2017: systematic review and meta-analysis. *Drug Alcohol Depend*. 2018; **191**: 234–258.

27. Van Dorn R, Volavka J, Johnson N. Mental disorder and violence: is there a relationship beyond substance use? *Soc Psychiatry Psychiatr Epidemiol*. 2012; **47**: 487–503.

28. Ntounas P, Katsouli A, Efstathiou V, et al. Comparative study of aggression – dangerousness on patients with paranoid schizophrenia: focus on demographic data, PANSS, drug use and aggressiveness. *Int J Law Psychiatry*. 2018; **60**: 1–11.

29. Keefe RS, Buchanan RW, Marder SR, et al. Clinical trials of potential cognitive-enhancing drugs in schizophrenia: what have we learned so far? *Schizophr Bull*. 2013; **39**(2): 417–435.

30. Bradley ER, Woolley JD. Oxytocin effects in schizophrenia: reconciling mixed findings and moving forward. *Neurosci Biobehav Rev*. 2017; **80**: 36–56.

31. Simons DJ, Boot WR, Charness N, et al. Do "brain-training" programs work? *Psychol Sci Public Interest*. 2016; **17**(3): 103–186.

32. Harvey PD, McGurk SR, Mahncke H, et al. Controversies in computerized cognitive training. *Biol Psychiatry Cogn Neurosci Neuroimaging.* 2018; **3** (11): 907–915.

33. McGurk SR, Twamley EW, Sitzer DI, et al. A meta-analysis of cognitive remediation in schizophrenia. *Am J Psychiatry.* 2007; **164**(12): 1791–1802.

34. Wykes T, Huddy V, Cellard C, et al. A meta-analysis of cognitive remediation for schizophrenia: methodology and effect sizes. *Am J Psychiatry.* 2011; **168**(5): 472–485.

35. Harvey PD, Penn D. Social cognition: the key factor predicting social outcome in people with schizophrenia? *Psychiatry (Edgmont).* 2010; **7**(2): 41–44.

36. Brekke JS, Hoe M, Long J, et al. How neurocognition and social cognition influence functional change during community-based psychosocial rehabilitation for individuals with schizophrenia. *Schizophr Bull.* 2007; **33**(5): 1247–1256.

37. Fett AK, Viechtbauer W, Dominguez MD, et al. The relationship between neurocognition and social cognition with functional outcomes in schizophrenia: a meta-analysis. *Neurosci Biobehav Rev.* 2011; **35**(3): 573–588.

38. Combs DR, Adams SD, Penn DL, et al. Social Cognition and Interaction Training (SCIT) for inpatients with schizophrenia spectrum disorders: preliminary findings. *Schizophr Res.* 2007; **91**(1–3): 112–116.

39. Roberts DL, Combs DR, Willoughby M, et al. A randomized, controlled trial of Social Cognition and Interaction Training (SCIT) for outpatients with schizophrenia spectrum disorders. *Br J Clin Psychol.* 2014; **53**(3): 281–298.

40. Nahum M, Fisher M, Loewy R, et al. A novel, online social cognitive training program for young adults with schizophrenia: a pilot study. *Schizophr Res Cogn.* 2014; **1**(1): e11–e19.

41. Kurtz MM, Richardson CL. Social cognitive training for schizophrenia: a meta-analytic investigation of controlled research. *Schizophr Bull.* 2012; **38**(5): 1092–1104.

42. Lindenmayer JP, McGurk SR, Khan A, et al. Improving social cognition in schizophrenia: a pilot intervention combining computerized social cognition training with cognitive remediation. *Schizophr Bull.* 2013; **39**(3): 507–517.

43. Lindenmayer JP, Khan A, McGurk SR, et al. Does social cognition training augment response to computer-assisted cognitive remediation for schizophrenia? *Schizophr Res.* 2018; **201**: 180–186.

44. Fisher M, Nahum M, Howard E, et al. Supplementing intensive targeted computerized cognitive training with social cognitive exercises for people with schizophrenia: an interim report. *Psychiatr Rehab J.* 2017; **40**(1): 21–32.

45. Sacks S, Fisher M, Garrett C, et al. Combining computerized social cognitive training with neuroplasticity-based auditory training in schizophrenia. *Clin Schizophr Rel Psychoses.* 2013; **7** (2): 78–86.

46. Russell TA, Green MJ, Simpson I, et al. Remediation of facial emotion perception in schizophrenia: concomitant changes in visual attention. *Schizophr Res.* 2008; **103**(1–3): 248–256.

47. Penn DL, Roberts DL, Combs D, et al. Best practices: the development of the Social Cognition and Interaction Training program for schizophrenia spectrum disorders. *Psychiatr Serv.* 2007; **58**(4): 449–451.

48. Eack SM, Hogarty SS, Greenwald DP, et al. Cognitive Enhancement Therapy in substance misusing schizophrenia: results of an 18-month feasibility trial. *Schizophr Res.* 2015; **161**(2–3): 478–483.

49. Eack SM, Hogarty SS, Bangalore SS, et al. Patterns of substance use during cognitive enhancement therapy: an 18-month randomized feasibility study. *J Dual Diag.* 2016; **12**(1): 74–82.

50. Darmedru C, Demily C, Franck N. Cognitive remediation and social cognitive training for violence in schizophrenia: a systematic review. *Psychiatry Res.* 2017; **251**: 266–274.

51. Cullen AE, Clarke AY, Kuipers E, et al. A multisite randomized trial of a cognitive skills program for male mentally disordered offenders: violence and antisocial behavior outcomes. *J Consult Clinical Psychol.* 2012; **80**(6): 1114–1120.

52. Cullen AE, Clarke AY, Kuipers E, et al. A multi-site randomized controlled trial of a cognitive skills programme for male mentally disordered offenders: social-cognitive outcomes. *Psychol Med.* 2012; **42**(3): 557–569.

53. Ahmed AO, Hunter KM, Goodrum NM, et al. A randomized study of cognitive remediation for forensic and mental health patients with schizophrenia. *J Psychiatr Res.* 2015; **68**: 8–18.

54. Kumar D, Zia Ul Haq M, Dubey I, et al. Effect of meta-cognitive training in the reduction of positive symptoms in schizophrenia. *Eur J Psychother Couns.* 2010; **12**(2): 149–158.

55. Ussorio D, Giusti L, Wittekind CE, et al. Metacognitive training for young subjects (MCT young version) in the early stages of psychosis: is the duration of untreated psychosis a limiting factor? *Psychol Psychother.* 2016; **89**(1): 50–65.

Examining Violence Among Not Guilty by Reason of Insanity State Hospital Inpatients Across Multiple Time Points: The Roles of Criminogenic Risk Factors and Psychiatric Symptoms

Darci Delgado, Sean M. Mitchell, Robert D. Morgan, and Faith Scanlon

Introduction

Institutional violence and associated risk factors within state hospitals have largely remained unexamined in the literature in spite of high violence prevalence rates: almost one-third (31.4%) of state hospital inpatients will engage in a violent assault during their hospitalization course.[1] This dearth of research is particularly true for state hospital inpatients adjudicated not guilty by reason of insanity (NGRI). An NGRI status indicates that an individual has been evaluated and deemed guilty of a criminal act but, due to mental disease or defect, was incapable of either knowing or understanding the nature of their act or was incapable of distinguishing between right and wrong at the time of their crime.[2] Unfortunately, the majority of research examining violence and associated risk factors has been conducted among state hospital inpatients upon release into the community.[3,4] Such research provides little insight into violence that occurs within the walls of the hospital and jeopardizes the safety of the patients and staff. Existing research also has not focused specifically on NGRI inpatients, but rather state hospital inpatients broadly. This is problematic because preliminary research demonstrated that the rates of violence toward other patients and staff were higher among NGRI inpatients than patients committed as incompetent to stand trial.[1] To further expand this scant literature, the current study aimed to evaluate both psychiatric symptoms and criminogenic risk (i.e. risk factors that, when present, increase an individual's risk of engaging in criminal activity and/or violence) as they relate to institutional violence over time during NGRI inpatients' hospitalization.

Narrow research has been conducted on psychiatric symptoms and criminogenic risk factors that may contribute to institutional violence risk among NGRI inpatients. Particularly concerning is that research examining violence among NGRI inpatients[5] has largely focused on psychiatric symptoms while neglecting criminogenic risk factors.[6,7] Given that an NGRI commitment status indicates a nexus between criminal behavior and mental illness, research examining traditional criminal risk factors for violence, in conjunction with psychiatric symptoms, may elucidate important treatment targets for NGRI inpatients and enhance institutional safety.

The relationship between severe mental illness and violence is complex.[8] A recent meta-analysis indicated that approximately one in five community psychiatric inpatients engaged in violent behavior during their hospitalization.[9] This study also found that among other factors (e.g. being male, history of violence, and alcohol abuse diagnosis), schizophrenia was linked to institutional violence.[9] Similarly, in another sample of community psychiatric inpatients, schizophrenia was associated with increased risk of institutional assault.[10] Furthermore, in a forensic state hospital sample, 82% of which were NGRI inpatients, both impulsivity and psychiatric symptoms, as measured by the Brief Psychiatric Rating Scale, were associated with greater violence.[5] Moreover, based on a literature review and synthesis of qualitative features of violent prisoners, those with a severe mental illness diagnosis (schizophrenia or other psychotic disorder, bipolar disorder, or major depression) and active psychiatric symptoms (psychotic symptoms, confusion, or depression) were more likely to engage in institutional violence than those without these characteristics.[11] Taken together, this research suggests a link between severe mental illness and violence risk among psychiatric inpatients and individuals who are criminally engaged. However, these studies did not take another body of literature into consideration when examining violence – namely the role of criminogenic risk factors. It was long assumed that criminal justice involvement for individuals with mental illness was due to untreated mental illness;[12] however, in the past 15 years, it has been recognized that criminogenic risk significantly contributes to criminal justice involvement to a greater degree than does psychopathology.[13,14]

Research has identified eight central criminogenic risk factors including: antisocial personality, antisocial attitudes, antisocial peers, substance abuse, history of antisocial behavior, relationship/familial problems, vocational difficulties, and lack of leisure activities.[15] There is concordance between these criminogenic risk factors and factors that have been associated with institutional violence within forensic settings. For example, a recent meta-analysis examined individual factors that differentiate violent versus nonviolent psychiatric inpatients across a variety of inpatient settings, including a community acute psychiatric hospital, a forensic hospital, and veterans inpatient psychiatric units.[16] This study found multiple risk factors that increased probability of violence, two of which could be considered related to criminogenic risk factors: a history of violence and a history of substance abuse.[16] Additionally, a diagnosis of schizophrenia was most strongly associated with increased inpatient violence compared to all other diagnoses. Other studies have indicated that antisocial behavior, criminality, and impulsivity were associated with institutional violence in forensic psychiatric hospitals and correctional settings.[17,18] In sum, these studies indicate that independently, psychiatric symptoms and criminogenic risk factors may be important predictors for violence among individuals with psychiatric symptoms and criminal justice involvement. As such, these factors may also confer greater risk for violent behavior among NGRI inpatients, which is the focus of the current study.

Given the multifaceted relation between mental illness, criminogenic risk, and violence, the current study sought to provide clarity on this topic in a sample of NGRI state hospital inpatients – a high-risk and understudied group. Because NGRI patients are at the crossroads of mental illness and criminality, the current study examined associations between psychiatric symptoms, criminal risk factors,

and future institutional violence. As an exploratory aim, we provided updated rates of violence among NGRI inpatients, as well as descriptions of patient characteristics. First, we hypothesized that NGRI inpatients who engaged in institutional violence during the six-month follow-up period would report more severe psychiatric symptoms at the time of assessment compared to NGRI inpatients who did not engage in institutional violence during the follow-up period when controlling for previous violence. Second, we hypothesized that NGRI patients who engaged in institutional violence during the six-month follow-up period would report higher criminogenic risk at the time of assessment than people who did not engage in institutional violence during the follow-up period when controlling for previous violence.

Methods

Participants

Participants consisted of 164 male (82%), 33 female (16.5%), and 3 transgender (1.5%) forensic mental health inpatients adjudicated NGRI and hospitalized under California Penal Code 1026 in the California Department of State Hospitals (DSH). Participants had a mean age of 44.57 years (SD = 12.55), and were predominantly Caucasian (n = 74, 37%) and African-American (n = 39, 19.5%); however, other racial groups were represented, including American Indian/Native American (n = 7, 3.5%), and Asian (n = 11, 5.5%). Additionally, 25 (12.5%) participants were Hispanic. Data on racial and ethnic identity were missing for one participant. Most participants were single or non-partnered (n = 146, 73%), whereas the remainder were married/partnered (n = 18, 9%), divorced or separated (n = 29, 14.5%), or widowed (n = 6, 3%). The majority of participants identified as heterosexual (n = 159, 79.5%). The average years of education were 12.72 (SD = 2.34).

Participants were hospitalized for an average of 7.21 years (SD = 6.47). Many participants reported previous misdemeanor (n = 138, 69%; n = 3 missing data) or felony convictions (n = 131, 65.5%; n = 5 missing data). Participants' primary psychiatric diagnosis was identified from their medical files and included schizophrenia (n = 84, 42%), schizoaffective disorder (n = 65, 32.5%), bipolar I (n = 21, 10.5%), and major depressive disorder (n = 6, 3%). The remaining 11% of participants (n = 22) had another disorder, including substance use disorder, delusional disorder, pedophilic disorder, or unspecified psychotic disorder. Two individuals (1%) had a primary diagnosis of antisocial personality disorder.

Overall, demographics of the participants appear to generally reflect the composition of the total NGRI patient population of these facilities. Point-in-time administrative census data at the time of data collection found that the NGRI inpatients include 85.4% males and 14.6% females while the mean age of NGRI inpatients was 49.7 years (SD =13.2). The overall NGRI inpatient population at these institutions had a higher average length of hospitalization when compared to the research sample (hospital-wide mean = 9.88 years; SD = 8.29 versus sample mean = 7.21 years; SD = 6.47). The percentages of the total hospital NGRI population's primary diagnoses appear similar to the percentages of the research sample's diagnoses: schizophrenia (51.5%); schizoaffective disorder (30.2%); bipolar disorder (7.1%); major depressive disorder (2.8%); and other diagnoses including substance abuse disorder, personality disorder, and delusional disorder (8.3%). Administrative data were not available for other demographic categories including ethnicity, partnership status, or mean years of education.

Measures

The Demographics and History Questionnaire

The Demographics and History Questionnaire is a self-report questionnaire developed for this study to obtain information on participants' demographics (e.g. age, race, gender), criminal history, and psychiatric history.

The Self-Appraisal Questionnaire

The Self-Appraisal Questionnaire (SAQ)[19] is a 72-item true/false self-report measure of criminogenic risk factors that is commonly used in clinical and research settings to assess criminal risk. The SAQ produces a total score and seven subscale scores (i.e., Alcohol and Drug Abuse, Anger, Antisocial Associates, Antisocial Personality Disorder, Conduct Problems, Criminal History, and Criminal Tendencies). This measure has evidenced adequate internal consistency (Cronbach's alpha ranging from 0.69 to 0.88),[20,21] and concurrent and predictive validity for assessing recidivism.[22] High SAQ total scores are associated with significantly higher rates of violent offenses and institutional infractions, as well as a greater frequency of previous offenses and arrests,[20] reconviction,[21] and reincarceration.[22] For

the purposes of the current study, only the SAQ total score (Cronbach's alpha = 0.89) was used as a general indicator of criminogenic risk.

The Brief Symptom Inventory

The Brief Symptom Inventory (BSI)[23] is a 53-item self-report measure assessing psychiatric symptom distress during the past week. Participants respond to the BSI items with a five-point Likert-type response option (ranging from 0 = *not at all* to 4 = *extremely*[24]). Nine symptom dimension scores (e.g. somatization, depression, anxiety), and three global indices (i.e. General Severity Index [GSI], Positive Symptom Total, Positive Symptom Distress Index) can be calculated from the BSI, with higher scores indicating greater psychiatric symptoms and distress. The nine BSI dimensions have shown strong convergent validity with the SCL-90-R (alpha ≥ 0.92).[23] The GSI produces an overall score from the average of all the participant's responses;[23] for this reason, the GSI was used in the current study (Cronbach's alpha = 0.96). The GSI has shown strong test–retest reliability (alpha = 0.90)[23] and internal consistency (Cronbach's alpha = 0.97).[24]

The Measure of Criminal Attitudes and Associates

The Measure of Criminal Attitudes and Associates (MCAA) is a self-report measure of participants' number of criminal associates (Part A) and participants' criminal attitudes (Part B).[25] Part A assesses the participants' number of and contact with criminal associates to produce a Criminal Friend Index. Higher scores on this index indicate more involvement with criminal associates and are correlated with total number of convictions (Pearson's $r = 0.36$) and incarcerations (Pearson's $r = 0.44$).[26] Part B is comprised of 46 items assessing criminal attitudes with agree/disagree response options. Part B produces four criminal attitudes subscale scores including Attitudes toward Entitlement, Attitudes toward Associates, Attitudes toward Violence, and Antisocial Intent. For the current study, the Criminal Friends Index, Attitudes toward Violence (Cronbach's alpha = 0.83), and the Antisocial Intent (Cronbach's alpha = 0.75) subscales were used. We did not use the Attitudes toward Entitlement (Cronbach's alpha = 0.64) or Attitudes toward Associates (Cronbach's alpha = 0.63) scales due to low reliability values.

Institutional Violence

Institutional violence data were collected from a review of administrative data (special incident reports) electronically captured as part of general operations at each state hospital facility. Violence included aggressive acts toward staff or another patient in which an act of hitting, pushing, kicking, spitting, gassing, or similar acts are directed to cause potential or actual injury. Verbal aggression was not included. Violence toward staff or other patients during six months before and six months after completion of the self-report questionnaires listed above was recorded. These data were coded separately for violence before (i.e. previous institutional violence) and after (follow-up institutional violence) the self-report assessments where 0 = no violence and 1 = violence. See Table 22.2 for a breakdown of the violence data.

Procedure

Prior to the initiation of this study, all procedures were approved by the Texas Tech University and the California Committee for the Protection of Human Subjects, two institutional review boards for the protection of human subjects. Potential participants consisted of all NGRI forensic mental health patients from two secure hospitals within the DSH. As all study materials were in English, only English speaking/reading patients were eligible for participation. Patients received a general announcement that a study was in progress and all NGRI patients were afforded an opportunity to express interest in the study. Potential participants that expressed interest in the study met individually with a member of the research team and were informed of the nature and purpose of the study and consented to participate. Potential participants who were unable to provide consent or declined participation were excused to return to their regularly scheduled activities. Patients consenting to participate were administered the San Diego Quick Assessment of Reading Ability,[27] a brief reading level screening test. Those who scored a reading level below sixth grade were excluded from the remainder of the study. Those scoring a sixth grade or higher reading level were provided a manila envelope containing the measures in counter-balanced order. Participants were instructed to complete the measures without including identifying information (e.g. name, patient number), and they were not compensated for their participation. Overall, 237 NGRI inpatients were approached to participate in this study. Of these individuals, 18 declined participation (7.6% refusal rate). Of the remaining 219 individuals

that agreed to learn about the study, 12 did not meet the eligibility requirement (e.g. reading level), resulting in 207 total consented participants.

Data Analysis Plan

Statistical Package for the Social Sciences (SPSS) version 25 was used to conduct all analyses. Frequency analyses were used to explore the institutional violence data. One-way analysis of covariance (ANCOVA) and multivariate analysis of covariance (MANCOVA) were used to test the hypotheses that NGRI inpatients who engaged in institutional violence during the six-month follow-up period would report more severe psychiatric symptoms and higher criminogenic risk at the time of assessment compared to NGRI inpatients who did not engage in institutional violence during the follow-up period. Follow-up institutional violence was dichotomized into 1 = violence and 0 = no violence, which was used as the independent variable. ANCOVA was used to test mean differences in the BSI GSI scores, SAQ total scores, and the MCAA Criminal Friends Index scores between the follow-up violence groups after controlling for previous institutional violence (dichotomized into 1 = violence and 0 = no violence). Similarly, MANCOVA was used to test differences in the linear combination of the MCAA Attitudes toward Violence scores and the MCAA Antisocial Intent scores between follow-up violence groups after controlling for previous institutional violence.

To better clinically contextualize the results, receiver operating characteristic (ROC) curve analyses were conducted, and a preliminary clinical cutoff score is provided for analyses that indicated significant mean differences between the follow-up violence groups on the criminal risk or psychiatric severity distress measures. The ROC curve analyses were conducted bivariately (i.e. one predictor and one criterion variable) given that is how these assessments would likely be used in clinical settings.

Results

Data Screening and Preparation

Missing data were imputed using expectation maximization, given that only 3.11% of the data were missing and missingness was completely at random (Little's Missing Completely at Random Test; χ^2[21,047, N = 204] = 15,285.28, p >0.999).[28] Four participants were missing violence information from their chart;

therefore, they were excluded from the analyses. We identified univariate outliers, which were considered as variable scores that were greater than ±3.29 SD from the mean. All univariate outliers were winsorized and retained in the dataset for the analyses.[28] Multivariate outliers were identified using Mahalanobis Distance, but there were no multivariate outliers. Furthermore, the dependent variable distributions were assessed for normality. The SAQ total score was not significantly skewed. The BSI GSI, MCAA Criminal Friends Index, MCAA Antisocial Intent, and MCAA Attitudes toward Violence distributions were significantly positively skewed; therefore, a square root transformation (i.e. sqrt) was performed, which best normalized the distributions.[28]

Preliminary Analyses

Covariates were considered if they were significantly different between the two groups: those with follow-up institutional violence and those without. There were no significant difference between the groups on age ($F[1,175] = 0.001$, $p = 0.979$), years of education ($F[1,175] = 0.03$, $p = 0.871$), race/ethnicity ($\chi^2[5, N = 200] = 2.36$, $p = 0.757$), gender ($\chi^2[2, N = 200] = 2.41$, $p = 0.300$), or sexual orientation ($\chi^2[4, N = 200] = 3.31$, $p = 0.508$). Therefore, no demographic variables were included as covariates in the analyses. Previous institutional violence was significantly associated with follow-up institutional violence ($\chi^2[1, N = 200] = 23.91$, $p < 0.001$); therefore, previous institutional violence was

used as a covariate in the analyses. This is consistent with previous literature that indicates that previous violence is a strong predictor of future violence.[29] Therefore, we are testing if psychiatric symptom severity and criminal risk differ between the follow-up institutional violence groups, beyond what is accounted for by a strong, known predictor (previous violence). See Table 22.1 for bivariate correlations and descriptive statistics for the variables included in the analyses.

Exploratory analyses

As seen in Table 22.2, 94.6% of those who were not previously violent were also not violent at follow-up. Additionally, 33.3% of those who were previously violent were also violent at follow-up. These data indicate that the majority of those who were and were not previously violent will go on to be nonviolent.

Primary analyses

Using ANCOVA, differences in the BSI GSI (sqrt) scores were tested between follow-up institutional violence groups after adjusting for previous institutional violence. Levene's Test indicated that error variances were not significantly different between the follow-up violence groups ($F[1,198] = 0.30$, $p = 0.587$), which is congruent with the assumption of ANCOVA. After adjusting for previous institutional violence ($F[1,197] = 2.55$, $p = 0.112$, $\eta_p^2 = 0.01$, observed power = 0.36), the mean difference between the follow-up institutional violence groups on the BSI GSI (sqrt) was not

Table 22.1 Bivariate correlations

	1	2	3	4	5	6
1. Previous violence	–					
2. Follow-up violence	0.35**	–				
3. SAQ total	0.21**	0.21**	–			
4. BSI GSI (sqrt)	0.14*	0.11	0.33**	–		
5. MCAA Criminal Friends Index (sqrt)	08	0.08	0.35**	0.05	–	
6. MCAA Violence (sqrt)	0.21**	0.19**	0.40**	0.27**	0.18**	–
7. MCAA Intent (sqrt)	0.05	0.11	0.44**	0.26**	0.19**	0.51**

Abbreviations: BSI GSI, Brief Symptom Inventory Global Severity Index score; MCAA Index, Measure of Criminal Attitudes and Associates Criminal Friends Index score; MCAA Intent, Measure of Criminal Attitudes and Associates Criminal Intent score; MCAA Violence, Measure of Criminal Attitudes and Associates Attitudes toward Violence score; SAQ total, Self-Appraisal Questionnaire total score; sqrt, the variable was square root transformed.

*$p < 0.05$.

**$p < 0.01$.

Table 22.2 Contingency table of the number of participants who were previously violent and who were violent at follow-up

		Previous violence (n)		
		No	Yes	Total
Follow-up violence (n)	No	158	22	180
	Yes	9	11	20
	Total (n)	167	33	200

Table 22.3 Means and standard deviations of the dependent variables for those who were and were not violent at follow-up

	Follow-up violence		No follow-up violence	
	M	SD	M	SD
SAQ total*	29.18	9.59	21.76	10.38
BSI GSI (sqrt)	0.85	0.36	0.72	0.38
MCAA Criminal Friends Index (sqrt)	2.50	1.80	2.01	1.88
MCAA Violence (sqrt)	1.79	1.00	1.19	0.93
MCAA Intent (sqrt)	1.61	0.83	1.29	0.85

Abbreviations: BSI GSI, Brief Symptom Inventory Global Severity Index score; MCAA Index, Measure of Criminal Attitudes and Associates Criminal Friends Index score; MCAA Intent, Measure of Criminal Attitudes and Associates Criminal Intent score; MCAA Violence, Measure of Criminal Attitudes and Associates Attitudes toward Violence score; SAQ Total, Self-Appraisal Questionnaire total score; sqrt, the variable was square root transformed.

*Significant (p<0.05) mean difference after adjusting for previous institutional violence.

significant ($F[1,197] = 0.78$, $p = 0.378$, $\eta_p^2 = 0.00$, observed power = 0.14), indicating that psychiatric symptom distress was not associated with institutional violence at follow-up after considering participants' previous institutional violence. See Table 22.3 for means and standard deviations.

Differences in the SAQ total scores were tested between follow-up institutional violence groups after adjusting for previous institutional violence. Levene's Test indicated that error variances were not significantly different between the follow-up institutional violence groups ($F[1,198] = 0.95$, $p = 0.332$). After adjusting for previous institutional violence ($F[1,197] = 4.63$, $p = 0.032$, $\eta_p^2 = 0.02$, observed power = 0.57), the mean difference between the follow-up institutional violence groups on the SAQ total score was significant ($F[1,197] = 4.62$, $p = 0.033$, $\eta_p^2 = 0.02$, observed power = 0.57). See Table 22.3 for means and standard deviations. That is, participants with higher SAQ total scores were statistically significantly more likely to engage in future institutional violence after accounting for their previous violent behaviors during hospitalization.

Although risk assessment is beyond the scope of this study, given the significant relation between SAQ total scores and institutional violence, we decided to conduct a supplemental analysis to provide additional clinical context to the findings. Specifically, bivariate ROC curve analyses demonstrated that the SAQ total score was significantly associated with follow-up violence (OR = 1.07, $p = 0.004$), and yielded an area under the curve (AUC) statistic of 0.71 (where an AUC of 0.50 would indicate chance-level prediction of follow-up violence). Youden's J Index was calculated to identify the SAQ total score that places equal emphasis on high sensitivity and specificity (i.e. the SAQ total score that had best balance between the highest true positive rate [sensitivity] and the lowest false positive rate [1-specificity] when predicting follow-up institutional violence). A *preliminary* SAQ total cutoff score of 23 produced the best balance between sensitivity (0.75) and specificity (0.61). In other words, a score of 23 has

a 75% chance of correctly identifying someone with future institutional violence; however, a score of 23 has a 39% (1-specificity) chance of falsely identifying that an individual will engage in future institutional violence. Therefore, an individual scoring over a 23 on the SAQ total score may be more likely to engage in later institutional violence; however, the false positive rate should be strongly considered, and the SAQ total score should not be used as a sole measure to assess the potential for future institutional violence.

Differences in the MCAA Criminal Friends Index (sqrt) scores were tested between follow-up violence groups after adjusting for previous violence. Levene's Test indicated that errors variances were not significantly different between the follow-up violence groups ($F[1,198] = 1.24$, $p = 0.267$). After adjusting for previous violence ($F[1,197] = 0.66$, $p = 0.418$, $\eta_p^2 = 0.00$, observed power = 0.13), the mean difference between the follow-up violence groups on the MCAA Criminal Friends Index (sqrt) was not significant ($F[1,197] = 0.57$, $p = 0.451$, $\eta_p^2 = 0.00$, observed power = 0.12). This finding indicated that associating with criminal friends was not related to institutional violence at follow-up after accounting for previous institutional violence. See Table 22.3 for means and standard deviations.

Lastly, using MANCOVA, differences in the MCAA Attitudes toward Violence (sqrt) scores and the MCAA Criminal Intent (sqrt) scores were tested between follow-up violence groups after adjusting for previous violence. Homogeneity of covariance matrices was tested using Box's M Test, which was not significant (Box's $M = 0.58$, $F[3,13\ 296.09] = 0.19$, $p = 0.905$). After adjusting for previous violence (Wilk's $\Lambda = 0.97$, $F[2, 196] = 3.24$, $p = 0.041$, $\eta_p^2 = 0.03$, observed power = 0.61), there was no significant difference in the linear combination of these MCAA (sqrt) variables (Wilk's $\Lambda = 0.98$, $F[2,196] = 1.76$, $p = 0.174$, $\eta_p^2 = 0.02$, observed power = 0.37). These results indicate that attitudes toward violence and criminal intent were not significantly associated with follow-up institutional violence after adjusting for previous institutional violence. See Table 22.3 for means and standard deviations.

Discussion

The current study aimed to test differences in assessments of psychiatric symptom severity and criminogenic risk factors between NGRI state hospital inpatients who engaged in intuitional violence six months following the assessments and NGRI inpatients who did not engage in violence during the follow-up period when controlling for previous violence. Specifically, we hypothesized NGRI inpatients who engaged in institutional violence during the six-month follow-up period would report more severe psychiatric symptoms and higher criminogenic risk at the time of assessment compared to NGRI inpatients who did not engage in institutional violence during the follow-up period. We also provided an exploratory description of patterns in institutional violence and preliminary cutoff scores for criminogenic risk assessments that were significantly associated with follow-up institutional violence.

Our study elucidated patterns in institutional violence among NGRI inpatients. Data indicated that 16.5% and 10% of this sample of NGRI inpatients engaged in institutional violence toward other patients or staff in the six months prior to and six months following the self-report assessments, respectively. Additionally, most patients who were not previously violent did not go on to be violent during the follow-up period; only 33.3% of those who were previously violent also engaged in violence during the follow-up period. Given the sample's modest average length of hospitalization (7.21 years, SD = 6.47), these exploratory results indicated violence prevalence rates that are lower than the overall forensic inpatient violence rate of 31.4% found in previous studies.[1] However, considering the sample's length of hospitalization at the time of the study, this prevalence rate is consistent with general findings that an individual's risk of violence is highest

upon and soon after admission, and then decreases over the course of hospitalization.[30] These exploratory results aid in the provision of general rates of violence for those in this stage of their hospitalization and treatment.

The results in the current study also partially supported our hypotheses. That is, one of our assessments of criminogenic risk (the SAQ total score) was significantly higher among NGRI inpatients who engaged in institutional violence during the follow-up period compared to those who did not, after controlling for previous institutional violence. However, our findings did not support significant differences between the follow-up institutional violence groups on specific aspects of criminogenic risk – specifically our measures of criminal attitudes (MCAA Attitudes toward Violence and the MCAA Criminal Intent) and criminal associates (MCAA Criminal Friends Index) after controlling for previous institutional violence. Similarly, there were no significant differences between the follow-up institutional violence groups on our assessment of psychiatric symptoms distress severity (the BSI GSI scores) after controlling for previous institutional violence. Although research has indicated that psychiatric symptoms are significantly associated with violence among other psychiatric patients, including inpatients,[6,7] our results do not support this association among NGRI inpatients after considering their previous violence. Perhaps NGRI state hospital inpatients – particularly in our sample – are more psychiatrically stabilized given their length of hospitalization compared to participants in previous studies that may include acute inpatients in other settings.[9,10] This finding suggests that solely treating psychiatric symptoms may not be sufficient for reducing institutional violence among NGRI inpatients. Furthermore, when predicting violence, it is advisable to integrate comprehensive risk assessments in the assessment process (e.g. at admission) rather than focusing on specific aspects of problematic behavior (e.g. antisocial cognitions).

Traditional forensic state hospital treatment has focused on psychopharmacological interventions targeting active psychiatric symptoms.[31] The results from this study are best understood in the consideration of what treatment needs remain *after* mental health symptoms are ameliorated. This cohort of NGRI inpatients, in an intermediate stage of treatment, is no longer committing violence due to acute symptomatology but instead due to residual, untreated criminogenic risk. These findings are consistent with previous research indicating that criminogenic factors, more so than psychiatric symptoms, increase risk for violence,[13,17,18] and parallel recent findings in the correctional literature whereby justice-involved individuals with mental illness are at greater risk for criminal recidivism due to criminogenic factors than mental health functioning.[32,33]

Implications for Policy and Practice

Regarding the assessment implications of our findings, we conducted exploratory analyses to further contextualize the significant difference in SAQ total scores between the follow-up institutional violence groups. Results indicated that a *preliminary* SAQ total cutoff score of 23 maximized the sensitivity and specificity of the prediction of institutional violence six months later. More specifically, a score of 23 demonstrated a 75% chance of correctly identifying someone with future institutional violence; however, there was also a 39% chance of falsely identifying that an individual will engage in future institutional violence. We discourage clinicians from using the SAQ total score (or comparable risk assessment measure) as a sole measure of NGRI inpatients' potential for future violence. Instead, it is important to synthesize risk predictions with other violence risk assessments (e.g., Violence Risk Screening – 10 [V-RISK-10],[34] Historical-Clinical-Risk Management-20, Version 3,[35] Short Term Assessment of Risk and Treatability[36]) and objective data (e.g. previously recorded violence) to best understand how to conceptualize the patient's potential for violence, others' safety, and the best treatment for the patient. Furthermore, replication of cutoff scores for predicting institutional violence using the SAQ or other risk measures is necessary; however, our results provide the first step toward evidence-based guidelines for using risk predictions to guide treatment efforts at reducing institutional violence among NGRI inpatients.

Clinical utility of risk assessments should not be limited to pre-release assessments, but should also be used as an important treatment-planning tool with NGRI inpatients who are at an intermediate stage of their treatment pathway and inpatient hospitalization. Some of the major hurdles to an NGRI inpatient's successful release from a state hospital include institutional rule violations and violence. These results show that criminogenic risk factors play a key role in violence, thereby greatly influencing eventual treatment success. By assessing criminogenic risk, a clinician would identify treatment targets – that is, substance abuse, criminal thinking, or anger management – as a focus of treatment. Importantly, holistically integrating criminogenic risk in treatment of mental illness may result in the even greater treatment success.[37–39] Leveraging treatments that target these criminogenic needs could be a beneficial addition to the traditional psychiatric symptom-focused approach to treatment of NGRI inpatients.

Limitations and Future Directions

This study is not without limitations. First, we assessed criminogenic risk and psychiatric symptom severity at one time point and our follow-up violence records from the six months following our self-report assessments. Therefore, our study could not detect potentially important short-term changes in psychiatric symptoms or criminal risk that could impact violence, as indicated in previous studies.[40] This could possibly explain some of our nonsignificant findings. Additionally, participants were in the DSH system, and they were required to have at least a sixth grade English reading level and demonstrate the capability for informed consent to participate. Our sample was also largely male and had been hospitalized for several years. Therefore, these findings may not generalize to other state hospital systems, NGRI inpatients with greater demographic heterogeneity, or those who do not meet our inclusion criteria. In addition, these findings may not generalize to patients who are earlier in their hospitalization course. Given the participants' length of hospitalization, our participants were likely more psychiatrically stabilized than more recently admitted patients; therefore, they may not have been experiencing as severe psychiatric distress measured by the BSI. It is possible that newer patients who are less psychiatrically stabilized would demonstrate a different relation between their psychiatric symptoms and future violence. Furthermore, our study used self-report measures as our primary predictors, which are subject to recall bias and false reporting. Alternative measures of psychiatric symptom distress and criminal risk should be considered. Although we had data on institution violence reported in the patients' hospital records, which provided objective violence data, it is possible that there was institutional violence that was not observed by staff or that was not recorded, which could impact the effect sizes of our results. Similarly, the observed power statistics (i.e. the probability of detecting an effect if there is one) for our analyses were low, especially for nonsignificant results; however, it should be noted that the effect sizes for nonsignificant results were also very small (e.g. $\eta_p^2 = 0.01$). Thus, a very large sample would be necessary to detect such small effect sizes, which would likely lack clinical meaning. Nevertheless, the low power in the current study could have produced a false negative finding. Therefore, further replication of our work is warranted.

Future directions for this line of research are considerable. Examination of the interplay between psychiatric symptoms and criminogenic risk factors in the prediction of institutional violence amongst other commitment types (mentally disordered offender, incompetent to stand trial, etc.) could aid in the generalizability of the current study's results across all forensic state hospital inpatients. Additionally, future examination of different stages of hospitalization (i.e. recent admission versus intermediate hospitalization versus approaching discharge to community) could help identify the most suitable window of time to target criminogenic risk treatment. Future research should also consider more intensive longitudinal research designs that allow for a more fine-grained examination of risk factors for violence among NGRI inpatients overtime. Finally, replication of the use of the SAQ, an efficient self-report measure of criminogenic risk, as a predictive measure of inpatient violence in NGRI inpatients could represent a next step in establishing evidence-based guidelines for assessing this population's violence risk.

Conclusion

Targeting the treatment of criminogenic risk factors, in addition to psychiatric symptoms, is an important and necessary facet of providing evidence-based care to the NGRI inpatient population. In this sample, criminogenic risk, and not psychiatric symptoms, was predictive of six months of post-assessment institutional violence, when controlling for previous violence. A holistic approach of examining both psychiatric and criminogenic risk factors throughout the course of hospitalization will facilitate a greater understanding of pertinent violence risk factors, but also help pave the way for a treatment plan that adequately captures all domains of factors to help an individual succeed in both a forensic state hospital and, eventually, in the community.

Acknowledgments

Part of the work of Sean M. Mitchell was supported by a grant from the National Institute of Mental Health (S.M.M., T32 MH020061).

Disclosure

The authors declare no conflict of interest.

References

1. Broderick C, Azizian A, Kornbluh R, Warburton K. Prevalence of physical violence in a forensic psychiatric hospital system during 2011–2013: patient assaults, staff assaults, and repeatedly violent patients. *CNS Spectr.* 2015; **20**(3): 319–330.

2. §CA Penal Code 1026.

3. Vitacco MJ, Balduzzi E, Rideout K, Banfe S, Britton J. Reconsidering risk assessment with insanity acquittees. *Law Hum Behav.* 2018; **42**(5): 403.

4. Almeida F, Moreira D, Moura H, Mota V. Psychiatric monitoring of not guilty by reason of insanity outpatients. *J Forensic Leg Med.* 2016; **38**: 58–63.

5. McDermott BE, Edens JF, Quanbeck CD, Busse D, Scott CL. Examining the role of static and dynamic risk factors in the prediction of inpatient violence: variable- and person-focused analyses. *Law Hum Behav.* 2008; **32**(4): 325–338.

6. Grevatt M, Thomas-Peter B, Hughes G. Violence, mental disorder and risk assessment: can structured clinical assessments predict the short-term risk of inpatient violence? *J Forens Psychiatry Psychol.* 2004; **15**(2): 278–292.

7. Ross D, Hart S, Webster C. *Aggression in Psychiatric Patients: Using the HCR-20 to Assess Risk for Violence in Hospital and in the Community.* Port Coquitlam, Canada: Riverview Hospital; 1998.

8. Douglas KS, Guy LS, Hart SD. Psychosis as a risk factor for violence to others: a meta-analysis. *Psychol Bull.* 2009; **135**(5): 679.

9. Iozzino L, Ferrari C, Large M, Nielssen O, De Girolamo G. Prevalence and risk factors of violence by psychiatric acute inpatients: a systematic review and meta-analysis. *PLoS One.* 2015; **10**(6): e0128536.

10. Flannery RB, Wyshak G, Tecce JJ, Flannery GJ. Characteristics of American assaultive psychiatric patients: review of published findings, 2000–2012. *Psychiatr Q.* 2014; **85**(3): 319–328.

11. Schenk AM, Fremouw WJ. Individual characteristics related to prison violence: a critical review of the literature. *Aggress Violent Behav.* 2012; **17**(5): 430–442.

12. Morgan RD, Flora DB, Kroner DG, et al. Treating offenders with mental illness: a research synthesis. *Law Hum Behav.* 2012; **36**(1): 37.

13. Skeem JL, Steadman HJ, Manchak SM. Applicability of the risk-need-responsivity model to persons with mental illness involved in the criminal justice system. *Psychiatr Serv.* 2015; **66**(9): 916–922.

14. Draine J, Salzer MS, Culhane DP, Hadley TR. Role of social disadvantage in crime, joblessness, and homelessness among persons with serious mental illness. *Psychiatr Serv.* 2002; **53**(5): 565–573.

15. Andrews DAB. *The Psychology of Criminal Conduct, 5th edn.* Cincinnati, OH: Anderson Publishing Company; 2010.

16. Dack C, Ross J, Papadopoulos C, Stewart D, Bowers L. A review and meta-analysis of the patient factors associated with psychiatric inpatient aggression. *Acta Psychiatr Scand.* 2013; **127**(4): 255–268.

17. Walters GD. Predicting institutional adjustment and recidivism with the psychopathy checklist factor scores: a meta-analysis. *Law Hum Behav.* 2003; **27**(5): 541–558.

18. Douglas KS, Strand S, Belfrage H, Fransson G, Levander S. Reliability and validity evaluation of the Psychopathy Checklist: Screening Version (PCL: SV) in Swedish correctional and forensic psychiatric samples. *Assessment.* 2005; **12**(2): 145–161.

19. Loza W. Self-Appraisal Questionnaire (SAQ): a tool for assessing violent and non-violent recidivism. In: *Handbook of Recidivism Risk/Needs Assessment Tools.* Hoboken, NJ: Wiley; 2018: 165.

20. Loza W, Conley M, Warren B. Concurrent cross-validation of the Self-Appraisal Questionnaire: a tool for assessing violent and nonviolent recidivism and institutional adjustment on a sample of North Carolina offenders. *Int J Offender Ther Comp Criminol.* 2004; **48**(1): 85–95.

21. Mitchell O, Caudy MS, MacKenzie DL. A reanalysis of the Self Appraisal Questionnaire: psychometric properties and predictive validity. *Int J Offender Ther Comp Criminol.* 2013; **57**(4): 445–459.

22. Loza W, Neo LH, Shahinfar A, Loza-Fanous A. Cross-validation of the Self-Appraisal Questionnaire: a tool for assessing violent and nonviolent recidivism with female offenders. *Int J Offender Ther Comp Criminol.* 2005; **49**(5): 547–560.

23. Derogatis LR, Melisaratos N. The brief symptom inventory: an introductory report. *Psychol Med.* 1983; **13**(3): 595–605.

24. Derogatis LR. *BSI Brief Symptom Inventory. Administration, Scoring, and Procedures Manual.* Minneapolis, MN: National Computer Systems (NCS); 1993.

25. Mills JF, Kroner DG. Measures of criminal attitudes and associates: user guide. Unpublished instrument and user guide; 1999.

26. Mills JF, Kroner DG, Forth AE. Measures of Criminal Attitudes and Associates (MCAA) development, factor structure, reliability, and validity. *Assessment.* 2002; **9**(3): 240–253.

27. LaPray M, Ross H. San Diego quick assessment. *J Reading.* 1969; **12**: 305–307.

28. Tabachnick BG, Fidell LS. *Using Multivariate Statistics, 6th edn.* Boston, MA: Pearson; 2013.

29. Lussier P, Verdun-Jones S, Deslauriers-Varin N, Nicholls T, Brink J. Chronic violent patients in an inpatient psychiatric hospital: prevalence, description, and identification. *Crim Justice Behav.* 2010; **37**(1): 5–29.

30. Broderick C. Violence report: DSH violence 2010–2017. Sacramento, CA: Department of State Hospitals; 2019.

31. Warburton K. The new mission of forensic mental health systems: managing violence as a medical syndrome in an environment that balances treatment and safety. *CNS Spectr.* 2014; **19**(5): 368–373.

32. Morgan RD, Fisher WH, Duan N, Mandracchia JT, Murray D. Prevalence of criminal thinking among state prison inmates with serious mental illness. *Law Hum Behav.* 2010; **34**(4): 324–336.

33. Skeem JL, Winter E, Kennealy PJ, Louden JE, Tatar I, Joseph R. Offenders with mental illness have criminogenic needs, too: toward recidivism reduction. *Law Hum Behav.* 2014;**38**(3):212.

34. Bjørkly S, Hartvig P, Heggen F-A, Brauer H, Moger T. Development of a brief screen for violence risk (V-RISK-10) in acute and general psychiatry: an introduction with emphasis on findings from a naturalistic test of interrater reliability. *Eur Psychiatry.* 2009;**24**(6):388–394.

35. Douglas KS, Hart SD, Webster CD, Belfrage H. HCR-20V3: Assessing Risk for Violence: User Guide. British Columbia, Canada: Simon Fraser University; 2013.

36. Webster C, Martin M, Brink J, Nicholls T, Desmarais S. Manual for the Short-Term Assessment of Risk and Treatability (START; Version 1.1). Coquitlam, Canada: British Columbia Mental Health & Addiction Services; 2009.

37. Morgan RD, Kroner D, Mills JF. A Treatment Manual for Justice Involved Persons with Mental Illness: Changing Lives and Changing Outcomes: Abingdon, UK: Routledge; 2017.

38. Morgan RD, Kroner DG, Mills JF, Bauer RL, Serna C. Treating justice involved persons with mental illness: preliminary evaluation of a comprehensive treatment program. *Crim Justice Behav.* 2014;**41**(7):902–916.

39. Gaspar M, Brown L, Ramler T, et al. Therapeutic outcomes of changing lives and changing outcomes for male and female justice involved persons with mental illness. *Crim Justice Behav.* 2019: 0093854819879743.

40. Skeem JL, Schubert C, Odgers C, Mulvey EP, Gardner W, Lidz C. Psychiatric symptoms and community violence among high-risk

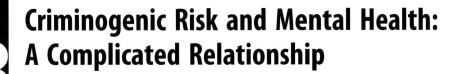

Chapter 23

Criminogenic Risk and Mental Health: A Complicated Relationship

Robert D. Morgan, Faith Scanlon, and Stephanie A. Van Horn

Criminogenic Risk and Mental Health: A Complicated Relationship

The relationship between criminogenic risk and mental illness in justice-involved persons with mental illness (PMI) is complex and poorly understood. As previously noted,[1] the general public is misinformed on the nature of this relationship, erroneously believing that mental illness causes violence and crime. This perception is compounded by news reports immediately speculating about mental illness in response to sensationalized criminal acts such as mass shootings, as well as in popular and social media. Of greater concern, however, is when clinicians, administrators, and policymakers are also misinformed. Criminal risk includes static (e.g. age, gender) and dynamic (e.g. antisocial attitudes, substance misuse) factors that place an individual at greater risk of involvement in crime. Criminogenic risk, on the other hand, refers to dynamic risk factors that directly contribute to criminal behavior and therefore need to be a focus of intervention (e.g. need to reduce antisocial attitudes, need to reduce substance misuse). Known criminogenic risk factors provide treatment targets for professional service providers and decision- and policymakers aiming to reduce crime.

Criminogenic risk is well understood in correctional settings and often guides the nature of rehabilitative services.[2] Criminogenic risk is less understood in mental health circles, however, and even when working with justice-involved PMI, mental health professionals often remain uninformed on the necessity of including criminogenic risk factors in mental health treatments. In fact, mental health professionals working with incarcerated PMI have historically emphasized mental health recovery (e.g. reduce symptomatology, medication management) over, and at times to the exclusion of, criminogenic risk.[3,4] This is particularly problematic given evidence that targeting criminogenic risk

reduces criminal involvement, including for PMI (see[5] for a thorough review). Notably, it is the first author's experience that when consulting with mental health professionals in correctional and forensic settings, there remains a belief that PMI are involved in the criminal justice system due to lack of adequate mental health care, and that mental illness is the primary culprit when it comes to these individuals' criminal behavior. However, research data clearly refute this position such that this naivety and lack of understanding of criminogenic risk is inexcusable.

Researchers have clearly demonstrated the link of criminal risk with criminal outcomes for PMI. In fact, a body of literature now supports the conclusion that mental illness is not the driving force behind PMI's criminal justice involvement, but that criminogenic risk (dynamic risk factors commonly associated with criminal activity) is likely the primary cause of crime, similar to criminal justice populations that do not have mental illness (see for example[6–8]). In other words, it is now well understood that the relationship of mental illness to crime is weak and that other factors, including criminogenic factors, better account for crime.[9] Most compelling in this line of investigation were the results of a meta-analysis showing that traditional criminogenic risk factors (e.g. antisocial attitudes, antisocial associates, substance misuse) were better predictors of criminal justice involvement (i.e. recidivism) than were traditional clinical (i.e. mental health) factors for justice-involved PMI.[10] In fact, results demonstrated that the variables that best predicted recidivism for PMI were essentially the same as the variables that predicted recidivism for offenders without mental illness. Specifically, this body of research demonstrates that justice-involved PMI exhibit criminal risk factors similarly to nonmentally ill criminal justice populations across a variety of criminal justice settings and populations, including prison inmates,[11–13] young jail inmates,[14] forensic psychiatric patients[15] and justice-involved PMI hospitalized in acute inpatient psychiatric units.[15,16] Nevertheless, the traditional approach of targeting psychiatric stabilization remains the predominant service model used for justice-involved PMI[17] without concomitant services targeting their criminal risk or criminalness. Thus, it is not surprising that traditional psychiatric services have had limited impact on criminal justice outcomes.[18] To be effective, services for justice-involved PMI must address the co-occurring issues of mental illness and criminal risk.[7,11,18]

Although it is clear that criminogenic risk places PMI at risk for criminal justice involvement, we still do not know the nature of this criminogenic–mental illness relationship. Importantly, then, we also do not know how this relationship impacts treatment needs, and of ultimate concern, what this relationship means in terms of individual and societal outcomes. Bartholomew and Morgan[1] proposed that "mental illness and criminalness feed each other in a continuous loop" (p. 5) as depicted in Figure 23.1. If Figure 23.1 accurately reflects the relationship between mental illness and criminalness, there would be a complex directionality such that mental illness and criminalness are independent (untreated mental illness results in increased psychiatric recidivism and untreated criminalness results in increased criminal recidivism), but also multidirectional such that untreated mental illness results in increased

criminal risk, and vice versa. In this latter relationship, for example, a PMI experiencing decompensation in terms of mental health functioning (e.g. increased symptomatology) will experience reciprocal decompensation in their cognitive and behavioral controls that allow them to manage their criminal risk.

From the Risk-Need-Responsivity (RNR) model, the criminalness-mental illness relationship, as depicted in Figure 23.1, suggests that mental illness may be a responsivity factor for crime, but of equal importance is that criminalness may be a responsivity issue for mental health functioning. The nature of this relationship and the conceptualization of mental illness and criminalness as risk or responsivity factors will, in our opinion, guide the next wave of research. Such research will have practical implications beyond our understanding of this relation with the potential to significantly alter how we approach the issue of mental illness across the criminal justice landscape, and similarly, how we address criminal justice involvement across the mental health landscape. Even as we write this narrative discussing both criminal justice and mental health systems – structured as separate entities in the United States – we recognize that such research may help break the artificial silos that now exist, which put justice-involved PMI in a criminal justice or mental health system vacuum.

Applying the Model of Co-Morbid Mental Illness and Criminalness in Mental Health Settings

Although criminalness is typically considered in the context of corrections, it is relevant in community mental health settings as well. For example, in a sample of 79 men and 63 women in an acute inpatient psychiatric unit, more than half (n = 74, 52.1%) endorsed previously being convicted of a crime (misdemeanor and/or felony).[15] This finding is consistent with the rate of criminal justice involvement in a similar sample of psychiatric inpatients from another acute inpatient psychiatric unit where among 61 patients (32 male, 29 female), 55.7% (n = 34) reported they had been convicted of a crime.[19] Compared to inpatient samples, the prevalence of prior convictions in outpatient mental health care samples appears to be a little less, with one study showing a prevalence of about 36%.[20]

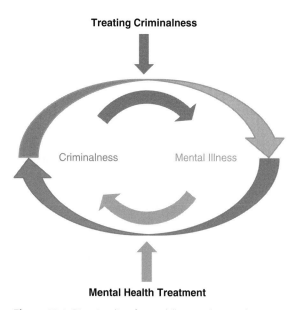

Treating Criminalness

Criminalness   Mental Illness

Mental Health Treatment

Figure 23.1 Directionality of mental illness and criminalness.

Beyond the prevalence of criminal justice involvement in mental health samples, there is a need to further examine the nature of the mental illness-criminalness relation in community-based psychiatric patients. One important variable linked to criminalness is antisocial attitudes, which are attitudes or dispositions that violate the social norm, including criminal and defiant behavior. Antisocial attitudes or cognitions are considered a primary risk factor for predicting crime. In fact, antisocial cognition is one of the "Central Eight,"[5] which consists of the strongest empirically validated criminal risk factors. Importantly for purposes of this discussion, antisocial attitudes are prevalent in justice-involved persons with and without mental illness alike.[11] Thus, this provides an important variable from which to explore the nature of the mental illness-criminalness relationship.

Among a cross-sectional sample of 61 inpatients mentioned above, scores on the Psychological Inventory of Criminal Thinking Styles[21] (PICTS) General Criminal Thinking scale, an overall self-report measure of criminal thinking, was significantly associated with a number of the self-reported Millon Clinical Multiaxial Inventory-III[22] (MCMI) scales of psychiatric syndromes, including the clusters of clinical syndromes scale (Anxiety, Somatoform, Bipolar, Dysthymic, Alcohol, Drug, and Post-Traumatic Stress disorder scales; $n = 61$, $\beta = 0.513$, $p < 0.001$, $R^2_{adj} = 0.251$), severe clinical syndromes scale (Thought Disorder, Major Depression, and Delusional Disorder scales; adjusting for sex, $n = 61$, $\beta = 0.442$, $p < 0.001$, $R^2_{adj} = 0.208$), Borderline scale (adjusting for sex, $n = 60$, $\beta = 0.477$, $p < 0.001$, $R^2_{adj} = 0.244$), Antisocial scale (adjusting for relationship status, $n = 49$, $\beta = 0.732$, $p < 0.001$, $R^2_{adj} = 0.517$), and an average of the combined raw MCMI scales which was used as a holistic measure of mental health symptomology ($n = 61$, $\beta = 0.604$, $p < 0.001$, $R^2_{adj} = 0.354$).[19] Furthermore, the General Criminal Thinking scale scores accounted for 20.8% to 51.7% of the variance in these MCMI scales. This suggests that the relation between criminal thinking and mental health symptomology is an appreciable one for justice-involved PMI, and that criminal thinking may be contributing to a variety of psychiatric symptoms, thereby interfering with mental health treatment. It should be noted, however, that due to the cross-sectional nature of this data, it is not feasible to make causal or temporal conclusions regarding the relationship of these constructs.

Although criminal thinking, as measured by the PICTS, was a significant predictor of symptoms associated with mental illness, criminal risk was not statistically significantly associated with self-reported length of psychiatric hospitalization (a behavioral indicator of the patients' mental health functioning) in a subsample of this clinical population. Specifically, neither the PICTS General Criminal Thinking scale ($n = 19$, $\beta = 0.071$, $p = 0.773$, $R^2_{adj} = -0.054$), nor the Criminal Sentiments Scale-Modified[23] (CSSM) Total Score ($n = 16$, $\beta = 0.068$, $p = 0.803$, $R^2_{adj} = -0.066$) was statistically significantly associated with current length of hospitalization in the psychiatric facility. In other words, antisocial cognitions were related to psychiatric symptoms, but not length of hospital stay. This finding suggests that criminalness is a responsivity factor for mental illness given the obtained relationship with psychiatric symptomatology, but not for psychiatric recovery as criminalness was not predictive of length of hospitalization. Given these are correlational findings from cross-sectional data, more research is needed to explore the nature of these relationships, including temporality and causation.

We further examined the mental illness-criminalness relationship by studying the relationship between psychiatric functioning and institutional misconduct. Specifically, we assessed the extent to which severe psychiatric symptomology (i.e. mania and thought disorders), criminal attitudes, and the interaction between the two were related to both violent and nonviolent disciplinary infractions among an incarcerated population ($n = 265$). Among violent infractions, main effects of gender ($\beta = 2.49$, $p = <0.0001$), criminal attitudes ($\beta = 0.02$, $p = <0.0001$), symptoms of mania ($\beta = 0.05$, $p = 0.001$), and thought disorder ($\beta = -0.04$, $p = 0.01$) were noted. A model that included all possible interactions between mania, thought disorder, and criminal attitudes was also examined. None of the interactions were significant; however, all previously mentioned main effects remained significantly related to violent misconduct. When looking at nonviolent infractions, gender ($\beta = 1.52$, $p < 0.0001$) and criminal attitudes ($\beta = 0.01$, $p = 0.04$) were statistically significant contributors to the model; however, the practical significance of criminal attitudes was negligible. Neither mania ($p = 0.70$) nor thought disorder ($p = 0.37$) was significantly related to nonviolent infractions.[24] Results from this study again suggest that criminalness and mental illness play a role in disruptive behavior. Furthermore, given that mental illness and criminal attitudes were not related to nonviolent infractions, it is possible that as the behavior becomes more antisocial, both mental illness and criminalness factors should be addressed.[24] As this was a retrospective study, conclusions regarding the causal nature of these relationships cannot be drawn; however, the results support the hypothesis that criminalness is a responsivity factor when addressing mental health concerns.

Collectively if these findings are supported by further research, they suggest that criminalness is a vital, albeit overlooked factor in the treatment of PMI in community mental health settings – many of whom have a history of criminal justice involvement. Furthermore, these findings highlight that criminogenic risk is not only important for criminal risk outcomes, but that it is also entangled in mental health treatment, making psychiatric symptoms more problematic (i.e. criminalness is a responsivity issue for PMI). In other words, the presence of criminalness (a broader concept than criminogenic risk) can negatively impact not only an individual's psychiatric symptoms, but also motivation, commitment, and sustained efforts toward recovery. For example, a PMI high in antisocial attitudes may find self-medication for symptom management more convenient with more pleasurable psychoactive effects (and fewer negative side effects) than working through the complexities and bureaucracy of the community mental health system to receive their psychotropic medications. Therefore, in order to improve outcomes in justice-involved PMI, it is essential to attend to criminogenic risk not only in criminal justice settings (e.g. corrections), but also in both forensic and nonforensic psychiatric settings. Given the conclusion that mental illness and criminalness have an interactive and reciprocal relationship, these results and the resulting model (Figure 23.1) have significant treatment implications; however, it is first relevant to discuss the assessment of criminalness broadly, but also specifically as it pertains to psychiatric patients.

Using Risk Assessments to Inform Psychiatric Treatment Planning

Risk assessments serve multiple purposes when providing services to criminal justice-involved persons, with the most common being to inform

security and release decisions. Initially, risk classification was based on clinical judgments (e.g. "gut feelings") that were primarily informed by unstructured interviews with the justice-involved individual. Overall, these judgments of risk lacked accuracy, and better methods were needed.[25,26] The second generation of risk assessments improved upon its predecessor by including structured assessments; however, they were not theoretically informed and mainly assessed for risk factors that were static and unchangeable (e.g. prior criminal history, type of offense).[27] Although this generation of assessments improved upon the first generation, they were only marginally useful in predicting future criminal behavior given their focus on unchangeable risks.[5] The third generation of risk assessments continued to implement structured assessments but expanded to include dynamic risk factors that could be addressed in an attempt to improve risk estimates. Finally, the fourth generation of risk assessment has attempted to address the difficulty of translating the information gleaned from these assessments to appropriate use for classification and treatment by incorporating elements of case management.[5]

Although the use of risk assessment instruments has increased exponentially over the last decade, there remains considerable debate regarding how to most effectively communicate their results.[28] One of the more contentious topics centers around whether actuarial (i.e. statistical method of estimating risk using risk factors with known probabilities) or structured professional judgment (SPJ) instruments (i.e. incorporates actuarial information but estimate of risk is at the discretion of the assessor) yield more accurate predictions; however, an exploration of the current issues surrounding violence risk assessment called attention to two key misunderstandings in this debate.[28] First, the assessment of risk is a process and the administration of one actuarial instrument cannot be considered a stand-alone risk assessment.[28] Second, people, not instruments, make decisions regarding risk and a risk assessment that does not address all known risk factors, whether through actuarial or SPJ methods, is neither comprehensive nor sufficient.[28]

There are other notable issues regarding the communication of risk assessment results. Some risk assessment results are communicated in "categories" of risk (i.e. high, moderate, low); however, studies have shown that clinicians' interpretation of these terms vary widely.[28] Other risk assessment results are communicated in terms of an individual's likelihood of reoffending. Studies have shown that individuals, including highly educated professionals and clinicians, tend to neglect base rate information when making individual predictions whether the information is presented categorically or probabilistically.[29,30] Furthermore, some research has found that inclusion of risk relevant information in narrative form can lead clinicians to overestimate risk, despite this information having been included in the estimated probability of reoffense.[31] Collectively then, the accuracy of risk assessments means little if the results are not communicated clearly, interpreted accurately,[28] and effectively used to inform treatment for justice-involved PMI in both criminal justice and mental health settings.

A variety of measures are available for the prediction of risk. The Level of Service Inventory-Revised (LSI-R) is the most commonly used risk assessment worldwide with over one million official administrations in the year 2010 alone.[32] A summary of the meta-analytic studies of the LSI-R indicated that its average predictive criterion validity for predicting general recidivism is 0.36, and 0.25 for predicting violent recidivism.[27] Other research has indicated LSI-R scores are also predictive of halfway house success, parole success, self-reported criminal activity (as opposed to new arrests or convictions), and institutional misconduct.[33] The LSI-R and its fourth-generation revision, the Level of Service/Case Management Inventory (LS/CMI), have been shown to be predictive of reoffending in a wide range of justice-involved persons, including those with severe mental illness[34] and drug offenses.[35]

A large-scale meta-analysis of other commonly used risk assessments found overall moderate predictive validity for violent recidivism for the Historical, Clinical and Risk Management Violence Risk Assessment Scheme (HCR-20; $r = 0.25$), the Psychopathy Checklist-Revised (PCL-R; $r = 0.24$), and the Violence Risk Appraisal Guide (VRAG; $r = 0.27$).[36] Some differences among these measures were noted in terms of predicting institutional violence, with the HCR-20 evidencing the strongest predictive validity ($r = 0.31$) and the PCL-R evidencing the weakest ($r = 0.15$).[36] An examination of violence prediction in a sample of psychiatrically institutionalized justice-involved persons also found that the HCR-20

and PCL-R were significant predictors of both verbal and physical aggression.[37] Interestingly, findings also indicated the Brief Psychiatric Rating Scale evidenced a strong relationship with physical and verbal aggression in this population.[37]

Clearly, risk assessments can provide invaluable information pertaining to security and release decisions; however, information regarding risk should also be used to guide treatment.[38] Measures that include an examination of dynamic risk factors can inform treatment planning by helping clinicians understand important issues to address in treatment that will ultimately reduce risk and subsequently improve public safety.

The LS/CMI[33] is an excellent example of a theoretically driven risk assessment instrument that can function both as a tool to inform decision-makers regarding risk of reoffense, and as a tool to ensure that the intensity and targets of treatment are appropriate. Research has continually shown that the individuals who need the most intensive services are those with a higher probability of reoffending.[31,38,39] Even more importantly, research has also shown that providing intensive services to low-risk individuals can increase their risk of reoffending.[38] The LS/CMI functions as a risk assessment tool by examining an individual's risk on each of the Central Eight risk factors and providing a total score that is associated with a risk category (i.e. low, moderate, high). It functions as a treatment planning tool when clinicians use the information learned about criminogenic risk to prioritize treatment goals. For example, an individual with high scores on the antisocial attitudes and employment subscales would best be served by cognitive behavioral therapy to address criminal thinking, as well as vocational training and assistance with job placement.

Another theoretically grounded, comprehensive risk assessment instrument that was designed to address treatment needs is the Violence Risk Scale (VRS).[40] The VRS assesses 6 static and 20 dynamic risk factors and includes an assessment of the individual's treatment readiness on each dynamic risk factor, as indicated by their stage of change (for an in-depth discussion, see Reference[41]). The inclusion of treatment readiness allows the clinician to choose appropriate interventions for an individual's readiness to change, and when used multiple times during treatment also allows the VRS to function as a measure of treatment progress.[40] The VRS evidences good predictive validity, with area under the curve values ranging from 0.73 ($p < 0.001$) for any reoffense at one-year follow-up, to 0.74 ($p < 0.001$) for any reoffense at three-year follow-up.[40]

Although several risk assessments can be used to inform treatment planning to address criminal risk factors, there is no widely available assessment that addresses both criminogenic and psychiatric risk simultaneously. Currently, treatment providers must use a battery of assessments to identify the co-occurring needs of justice-involved PMI. The Services Matching Instrument[42] (SMI) is being developed to meet this need. The SMI is intended as an integrated, theoretically grounded treatment planning tool designed to identify empirically identified risk factors for both criminal (e.g. criminal history, criminal associates) and psychiatric recidivism (e.g. psychiatric symptomology, social support). A preliminary examination of the psychometric properties of the SMI suggests the measure evidences good test retest reliability ($r = 0.78$ to 0.91), concurrent validity ($r = 0.41$ to 0.67), and internal consistency ($r = 0.77$ to 0.94),[43] with additional evaluation of the measures psychometric properties in progress.

The assessment of risk has evolved significantly in the last several decades and can be an invaluable tool in improving public safety; however, risk assessment instruments are underutilized in terms of improving criminal rehabilitation. Unfortunately, these instruments fail to capture how mental illness may affect the presentation of criminogenic risk factors, and vice versa. More work is needed to develop measures that integrate these needs for the growing population of justice involved PMI, and to examine the efficacy and accuracy of how risk is interpreted by clinicians and communicated to decision-makers. In addition, more research is needed to better understand the interaction of criminalness and severity of mental illness symptomology such that treatment needs can be more fully conceptualized and prioritized.

Treating Criminalness and Mental Illness

The lead author has written about treating justice-involved PMI and the necessity of targeting mental illness and criminalness as co-occurring problems;[4,11,44] however, these discussions have not fully captured the complexity of the criminalness-mental illness relationship. It is easy to think of criminalness and mental illness as univariate constructs with both impacting unique outcomes of interest (criminalness impacting criminal recidivism and mental illness impacting psychiatric recidivism) and we often develop treatments accordingly. For example, recent efforts to modify cognitive behavioral therapy programs aimed at reducing criminal risk (e.g. *Moral Reconation Therapy*[45]) to also address issues of mental illness[46] are done in this vein. But simply adding mental health-focused treatment strategies or interventions to programs designed to treat criminalness, and vice versa, does not account for the complexity of the criminalness-mental illness relationship and risks missing the treatment mark.

It is commonly understood in health and behavioral health circles that the more problem areas introduced into an individual's life (e.g. mental illness, criminalness, substance abuse, physical disability), the more problematic (and typically negative) the outcomes.[47] There are many examples of this in educational, medical, psychiatric, and criminal justice literatures, but one example highlights this concern specifically for justice-involved PMI.

Research examining barriers to employment has demonstrated that a criminal record[48–50] and mental illness[51–53] are significant barriers to employment. Stigma is a serious concern when it comes to employment for those involved in the justice system (see Reference[50] for a thorough review); however, most concerning for justice-involved PMI is that these barriers are compounded when both mental illness and criminal history are present. In other words, employers appear least likely to hire individuals with both a criminal record and mental illness, compared to those with just a criminal record or PMI who are not justice-involved;[54,55] multiple areas of concern result in poorer outcomes.

Given these findings across a range of disciplines, it is not surprising to find suggestions for treating co-occurring disorders in a unified treatment protocol (see for example[56]) or a combined/interdisciplinary approach (see Reference[57]). It was in this vein that *Changing Lives and Changing Outcomes*[58] (*CLCO*[1]) was developed. *CLCO* is a comprehensive program systematically developed to meet the unique treatment

---

[1] Disclaimer that the first author of this paper is also the first author of this commercially available program; however, the authors of CLCO do not accept royalties on this program and all proceeds support student research.

needs of individuals with co-occurring mental health and criminogenic concerns. The aim of this program is not to cure mental illness or criminalness, but rather to maximize adaptive behaviors to optimize functioning while reducing psychiatric relapse and criminal reoffending. Although *CLCO* is rooted in cognitive behavioral theory, with a significant psychoeducational component outlined in a comprehensive and structured treatment manual, the uniqueness of the program is in the *integration* of best mental health practices and best correctional rehabilitation practices throughout the therapeutic modules. In other words, consistent with Figure 23.1, the aim of *CLCO* is to treat not only the unique features of mental illness and the unique criminogenic needs of justice-involved PMI, but to also treat these problems as integrated, with complex ties to both criminal justice and mental health outcomes of interest. For example, one of the *CLCO* modules entitled "Mental Illness and Criminalness Awareness" is not limited to understanding mental illness. Rather, it also incorporates awareness of one's criminal proclivity and how problems in one area (i.e. mental illness or criminalness) can increase problems in the other domain. Similarly, the Medication Adherence module not only emphasizes the role of psychotropic medication in recovery from mental illness, but also as a responsible life choice that is consistent with achieving one's prosocial life goals (i.e. a better choice in regard to criminal justice outcomes than, for example, "self-medicating" with illicit substances).

We use *CLCO* not as an example of the best treatment program available for justice-involved PMI, but rather as an example of how treatments – regardless of one's treatment of choice – need to integrate treatments of mental health and criminogenic risk in treatment work with justice-involved PMI. As the research summarized in this paper demonstrates, this means going beyond merely adding a mental health focus to an already effective correctional program (e.g. *Thinking for a Change, Moral Reconation Therapy*). Instead, the field should aim to develop and incorporate treatments that are meaningfully integrated, to better meet the need of, address, and account for the complex, interwoven relation of mental illness and criminalness in correctional and psychiatric settings alike.

Although these treatment recommendations historically have stronger ties in criminal justice settings, these recommendations are also reflective of changes needed in forensic and nonforensic psychiatric settings. In forensic settings, for example, treatments for competency restoration and insanity should not be limited to psychiatric recovery. This may appear less relevant in the legal context of competency to stand trial, where the emphasis is typically on abatement of symptoms that impact one's ability to factually and rationally understand proceedings or to assist in one's defense. Although criminal risk is not predictive of competency restoration outcomes,[59] as Gowensmith and colleagues[60] alluded, failure to integrate a holistic perspective that includes an individual's criminogenic risk presents a missed opportunity. Although competency may be restored with a univariate focus on mental health functioning, sustained competency, further psychiatric recovery efforts, and reduced criminal and psychiatric recidivism outcomes are possibly missed. In nonforensic settings, it is common to encounter a significant number of patients with justice involvement (i.e. approximately 50% of patients) such that psychiatric recovery (see for example, *Illness Management and Recovery*[61]) needs to also account for the criminalness-mental illness relationship. At the very least, it appears that criminalness is a responsivity factor for mental illness. Therefore, given the impact of criminogenic risk factors on psychiatric symptomatology, recovery efforts that do not account for criminogenic risk will fall short of treatment goals.

Conclusion

Over the last several decades, researchers, policymakers, and clinicians alike have developed a growing appreciation for the complex and nuanced relationship between mental illness and crime. As a result, there have been significant clinical advances in the management of justice-involved PMI, such that it is no longer acceptable to ignore the co-occurring mental health and criminogenic needs of this high-risk population, be it in terms of assessment or treatment. In order to maintain this momentum, researchers must continue to examine the nature of the mental illness-criminalness relationship, how it may affect treatment needs, and of ultimate concern, how treatment of these co-occurring needs contributes to both psychiatric and criminal justice outcomes. In the meantime, policymakers, criminal justice administrators, and clinicians alike must address what we already know about the complexity of this issue, and develop holistic, wraparound policies and clinical strategies to assist justice-involved PMI to achieve improved quality of life, prolonged psychiatric recovery, and improved public safety. A multidisciplinary effort to recognize and address this reciprocal relationship will be required if we have any hope of achieving these goals.

Acknowledgment

The authors wish to thank Dr. Jeremy Mills for his comments on a previous draft of this manuscript.

Disclosures

Robert Morgan, Faith Scanlon, and Stephanie Van Horn do not have any disclosures.

References

1. Bartholomew NR, Morgan RD. Comorbid mental illness and criminalness implications for housing and treatment. *CNS Spectr*. 2015; **20**(3): 231–240.

2. Bonta J, Andrews DA. Risk-need-responsivity model for offender assessment and rehabilitation. *Rehabilitation*. 2007; **6**(1): 1–22.

3. Bewley MT, Morgan RD. A national survey of mental health services available to offenders with mental illness: who is doing what? *Law Hum Behav*. 2011; **35**(5): 351–363.

4. Morgan RD, Flora DB, Kroner DG, et al. Treating offenders with mental illness: a research synthesis. *Law Hum Behav*. 2012; **36**(1): 37–50.

5. Bonta J, Andrews DA. *The Psychology of Criminal Conduct*. New York, NY: Routledge; 2016.

6. Ditton PM. *Mental Health and Treatment of Inmates and Probationers*. Washington, DC: US Department of Justice, Bureau of Justice Statistics; 1999.

7. Draine J, Salzer MS, Culhane DP, Hadley TR. Role of social disadvantage in crime, joblessness, and homelessness among persons with serious mental illness. *Psychiatr Serv*. 2002; **53**(5): 565–573.

8. Fisher WH, Silver E, Wolff N. Beyond criminalization: toward a criminologically informed framework for mental health policy and services research. *Adm Policy Ment Health*. 2006; **33**(5): 544–557.

9. Skeem JL, Winter E, Kennealy PJ, et al. Offenders with mental illness have criminogenic needs, too: toward recidivism reduction. *Law Hum Behav*. 2014; **38**(3): 212.

10. Bonta J, Law M, Hanson K. The prediction of criminal and violent recidivism among mentally disordered offenders: a meta-analysis. *Psychol Bull*. 1998; **123**(2): 123.

11. Morgan RD, Fisher WH, Duan N, Mandracchia JT, Murray D. Prevalence of criminal thinking among state prison inmates with serious mental illness. *Law Hum Behav*. 2010; **34**(4): 324–336.

12. Wolff N, Morgan RD, Shi, J. Comparative analysis of attitudes and emotions among inmates: does mental illness matter? *Crim Justice Behav*. 2013; **40**(10): 1092–1108.

13. Wolff N, Morgan RD, Shi J, Fisher W, Huening J. Comparative analysis of thinking styles and emotional states of male and female inmates with and without mental disorders. *Psychiatr Serv*. 2011; **62**: 1485–1493.

14. Wilson AB, Farkas K, Ishler K, et al. Criminal thinking styles among people with serious mental illness in jail. *Law Hum Behav*. 2014; **38**(6): 592–601.

15. Bolaños AD, Mitchell SM, Morgan RD, et al. A comparison of criminogenic risk factors between psychiatric inpatients with and without criminal justice involvement (in preparation).

16. Gross NR, Morgan RD. Understanding persons with mental illness who are and are not criminal justice involved: a comparison of criminal thinking and psychiatric symptoms. *Law Hum Behav*. 2013; **37**(3): 175–186.

17. Skeem JL, Manchak S, Peterson JK. Correctional policy for offenders with mental illness. *Law Hum Behav*. 2011; **35**(2): 110–126.

18. Hodgins S, Muller-Isberner R, Freese R, et al. A comparison of general adult and forensic patients with schizophrenia living in the community. *Int J Forensic Ment Health*. 2007; **6**(1): 63–75.

19. Scanlon F, Morgan RD, Mitchell SM, et al. Community mental health settings and the criminal justice systems: The institutions of justice-involved persons with mental illness (in preparation).

20. Theriot MT, Dulmus CN, Sowers KM, et al. Factors relating to self identification among bullying victims. *Child Youth Serv Rev*. 2005; **27**(9): 979–994.

21. Walters GD. The psychological inventory of criminal thinking styles: part II. Identifying simulated response sets. *Crim Justice Behav*. 1995; **22**(4): 437–445.

22. Millon T, Millon C, Davis RD, et al. *Millon Clinical Multiaxial Inventory-III (MCMI-III): Manual*. Minneapolis, MN: Pearson/PsychCorp; 2009.

23. Shields IW, Simourd DJ. Predicting predatory behavior in a population of incarcerated young offenders. *Crim Justice Behav*. 1991; **18**(2): 180–194.

24. Van Horn SA, Morgan RD, Grabowski KE. Examining the relationship between criminalness, mental illness and institutional misconduct (in preparation).

25. Dawes RM, Faust D, Meehl PE. Clinical versus actuarial judgment. *Science*. 1989; **243**: 1668–1674.

26. Monahan J. *Predicting Violent Behavior: An Assessment of Clinical Techniques*. Thousand Oaks, CA: Sage Publications; 1981.

27. Andrews DA, Bonta J, Wormith JS. The recent past and near future of risk and/or need assessment. *Crime Delinq*. 2006; **52**(1): 7–27.

28. Mills JF. Violence risk assessment: a brief review, current issues, and future directions. *Can Psychol*. 2017; **58**(1): 40–49.

29. Mills JF, Kroner DG. The effect of base-rate information on the perception of risk for re-offence. *Am J Forensic Psychol*. 2006; **24**: 45–56.

30. Walters GD, Kroner DG, DeMatteo D, Locklair BR. The impact of base rate utilization and clinical experience on the accuracy of judgments made with the HCR-20. *J Forensic Psychol Pract*. 2014; **14**(4): 288–301.

31. Hilton NZ, Harris GT, Rawson K, Beach CA. Communicating violence risk information to forensic decision makers. *Crim Justice Behav*. 2005; **32**(1): 97–116.

32. Wormith JS. The legacy of DA Andrews in the field of criminal justice: how theory and research can change policy and practice. *Int J Forensic Ment Health*. 2011; **10**(2): 78–82.

33. Andrews DA, Bonta J, Wormith JS. *The Level of Service/Case Management Inventory (LS/CMI)*. Toronto, Ontario: Multi-Health Systems; 2004.

34. Ferguson AM, Ogloff JR, Thomson L. Predicting recidivism by mentally disordered offenders using the LSI-R: SV. *Crim Justice Behav*. 2009; **36**(1): 5–20.

35. Kelly CE, Welsh WN. The predictive validity of the Level of Service Inventory—Revised for drug-involved offenders. *Crim Justice Behav*. 2008; **35**(7): 819–831.

36. Campbell MA, French S, Gendreau P. The prediction of violence in adult offenders: a meta-analytic comparison of instruments and methods of assessment. *Crim Justice Behav*. 2009; **36**(6): 567–590.

37. Gray NS, Hill C, McGleish A, et al. Prediction of violence and self-harm in mentally disordered offenders: a prospective study of the efficacy of HCR-20, PCL-R, and psychiatric symptomatology. *J Consult Clin Psychol*. 2003; **71**(3): 443.

38. Andrews DA, Dowden C. Risk principle of case classification in correctional treatment: a meta-analytic investigation. *Int J Offender Ther Comp Criminol*. 2006; **50**(1): 88–100.

39. Lowenkamp CT, Latessa EJ, Holsinger AM. The risk principle in action: what have we learned from 13,676 offenders and 97 correctional programs? *Crime Delinq*. 2006; **52**(1): 77–93.

40. Wong SC, Gordon A. The validity and reliability of the Violence Risk Scale: a treatment-friendly violence risk assessment tool. *Psychol Public Policy Law*. 2006; **12**(3): 279.

41. Prochaska JO, DiClemente CC. *The Transtheoretical Approach: Crossing Traditional Boundaries of Therapy*. Homewood, IL: Dow Jones-Irwin; 1984.

42. Morgan RD, Kroner DG, Mills JF, Olafsson BN. The Services Matching Instrument. Unpublished assessment.

43. Olafsson BN, Morgan RD, Kroner DG. The services matching instrument: development, reliability and preliminary validity (in preparation).

44. Morgan RD, Kroner DG, Mills JF, Batastini AB. Treating criminal offenders. In: Weiner IB, Otto RK, eds. *Handbook of Forensic Psychology, 4th edn*. Hoboken, NJ: John Wiley & Sons; 2013: 795–838.

45. Little GL, Robinson KD. Moral reconation therapy: a systematic step-by-step treatment system for treatment-resistant clients. *Psychol Rep*. 1988; **62**: 135–151.

46. Rotter M, Carr WA. Targeting criminal recidivism in mentally ill offenders: structured clinical approaches. *Community Ment Health J*. 2011; **47**(6): 723–726.

47. Goodell S, Druss BG, Walker ER, Mat M. *Mental Disorders and Medical Comorbidity*. Cambridge, MA: The Synthesis Project, MIT; 2011.

48. Holzer HJ, Raphael S, Stoll MA. How willing are employers to hire ex-offenders? *Focus*. 2004; **23**(2): 40–43.

49. Petersilia J. Prisoner re entry: public safety and reintegration challenges. *Prison J*. 2001; **81**(3): 360–375.

50. Varghese FP, Hardin EE, Bauer RL, Morgan RD. Attitudes toward hiring offenders: the roles of criminal history, job qualifications, and race. *Int J Offender Ther Comp Criminol*. 2009; **54**(5): 769–782.

51. Corrigan P. How stigma interferes with mental health care. *Am Psychol*. 2004; **59**(7): 614.

52. Alexander L, Link B. The impact of contact on stigmatizing attitudes toward people with mental illness. *J Ment Health*. 2003; **12**(3): 271–289.

53. Overton SL, Medina SL. The stigma of mental illness. *J Couns Dev*. 2008; **86**(2): 143–151.

54. Batastini AB, Bolanos AD, Morgan RD. Attitudes toward hiring applicants with mental illness and criminal justice involvement: the impact of education and experience. *Int J Law Psychiatry*. 2014; **37**(5): 524–533.

55. Graffam J, Shinkfield AJ, Hardcastle L. The perceived employability of ex-prisoners and offenders. *Int J Offender Ther Comp Criminol.* 2008; **52**(6): 673–685.

56. Allen LB, McHugh RK, Barlow DH. Emotional disorders: a unified protocol. In: Barlow DH, ed. *Clinical Handbook of Psychological Disorders: A Step-by-Step Treatment Manual.* New York, NY: Guilford Press; 2008: 216–249.

57. Aaronson CJ, Katzman GP, Gorman JM. Combination pharmacotherapy and psychotherapy for the treatment of major depression and anxiety disorders. In: Nathan PE, Gorman JM, eds. *A Guide to Treatments that Work*, 3rd edn. New York, NY: Oxford University Press; 2007.

58. Morgan RD, Kroner D, Mills JF. *A Treatment Manual for Justice Involved Persons with Mental Illness:* *Changing Lives and Changing Outcomes.* New York, NY: Routledge; 2018.

59. Colwell LH, Gianesini J. Demographic, criminogenic, and psychiatric factors that predict competency restoration. *J Am Acad Psychiatry Law.* 2011; **39**(3): 297–306.

60. Gowensmith WN, Frost LE, Speelman DW, Therson DW. Lookin' for beds in all the wrong places: outpatient competency restoration as a promising approach to modern challenges. *Psychol Public Policy Law.* 2016; **22**(3): 293–305.

61. Gingerich S, Mueser KT. *Illness Management and Recovery Implementation Resource Kit.* Rockville, MD: Substance Abuse and Mental Health Services Administration, Center for Mental Health Services; 2004.

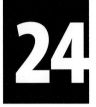
Implementation of a Specialized Treatment Program to Reduce Violence in a Forensic Population

Susan Velasquez, Andrea Bauchowitz, David Pyo, and Megan Pollock

Changing Trends in Forensic Populations

The California Department of State Hospitals (DSH) manages the psychiatric care of almost 7,000 patients admitted to any of its five hospitals. Over 90% of these patients have forensic commitments, meaning they have been charged with, or convicted of, a crime. Treating patients with mental illness and criminal behavior reflects a general trend within state psychiatric facilities.[1,2] An increase in physical violence towards staff and patients has been attributed to this mandate to care for patients with both severe mental illness and criminal backgrounds.[1,3,4] Addressing violence is a pressing need within state hospital systems, as a safe treatment environment is essential to the delivery of effective care.

Treating psychiatric symptoms alone has not been effective in reducing violence associated with severe mental illness.[5] Furthermore, treating patients without considering their violent behaviors is apt to complicate their timely discharge into the community. In addition to symptoms of severe mental illness, criminogenic risk factors perpetuate criminal thinking and behavior.[6] These risk factors include, but are not limited to, association with antisocial peers, antisocial attitudes, substance abuse, poor family relations, and difficulties with employment. Research demonstrates that addressing the criminogenic as well as mental health needs of justice-involved patients significantly improves outcomes in terms of criminal behaviors and psychiatric symptoms.[5] Traditionally, criminogenic risks were addressed in correctional treatment settings and the generalizability to other settings is recently being explored in detail.[7] A study of the DSH patient population revealed that criminogenic risk clearly exists in many state psychiatric hospital patients.[8] These findings expose a necessary paradigm shift in treatment planning within state psychiatric facilities.

Historically, state psychiatric hospitals were tasked with providing humane psychosocial care for persons diagnosed with severe mental illness, a mindset and practice remaining predominant today. Traditionally, addressing violence risk was not routinely implemented in treatment planning. Given the current and growing forensic patient population, outdated practices to address violent behaviors for the wellbeing of patients and staff must be amended.

A key struggle in these efforts is lack of continuum of care in the state psychiatric system.

Considering a Continuum of Care

Andrews and Bonta's Risk-Need-Responsivity Model (RNR) outlines a system to address criminogenic risk.[9] The overarching principles of the RNR model are to deliver treatments based on an empirically solid theory (i.e. cognitive and social learning theories) in a humane manner considering idiothetic factors. The Risk aspect of the model suggests that those at highest risk for violence receive more frequent and intense treatment. The Needs aspect highlights that these treatments ought to target the specific risk factors that are associated with criminal behavior. Lastly, the Responsivity aspect emphasizes the importance that these treatments are targeted to the individuals' cognitive skills, learning style, and motivation.

Those at highest risk for violence require a higher level of care, including more intensive treatment dosing with a physical plant outlay that promotes safety of staff and patients. Treatment is only effective when safety needs are addressed; accordingly, a structured and secure environment is necessary for the provision of effective treatment to those at highest risk for violence. Towards this goal, DSH leadership envisioned an enhanced treatment program (ETP) to provide an additional level of care for patients at greatest risk for violence. Within this program, criminogenic risk is considered for each patient referral and treatment decisions are guided by violence risk factors. Through this novel approach to treatment, DSH aims to create a center of excellence, delivering care in a setting that balances safety and treatment of severely mentally ill patients at highest risk for violence.

Environmental Security: Past, Present, and Future

The juxtaposition of how to efficaciously treat persons diagnosed with serious psychiatric illness who engage in aggressive behaviors "transcends boundaries of time, place, age, diagnostic and criminal justice status."[10] The deinstitutionalization movement from the Community Mental Health Act of 1963 resulted in an increasingly forensic psychiatric population in state hospital settings. The role of state hospitals has become one of managing populations deemed inappropriate for other settings[2]. Most patients admitted to state hospitals have a history of physical aggression, thus creating an unsafe work environment. In recent years, violence rates have notably increased in state hospital settings both for forensically and civilly committed patients.[1] Front-line staff, such as psychiatric technicians and nurses, are at heightened risk given their frequent contact with patients. Paralleling this trend, physical violence committed by DSH patients is increasing. In 2016, 1,528 physical assaults on staff occurred and 1,308 physical assaults were attempted. In 2017, these rates rose to 1,650 attempted physical assaults and 1,644 incidents where contact on staff occurred.[4] Given the rising violence, it became imperative that DSH leadership investigate national and international approaches to treating the most violent patients.

A critical first step was to research other practices to understand treatment approaches for violent patients requiring the highest security. From this a key take-home message was creating treatment units with single bedrooms some with their own bathrooms. Recent research revealed single bedrooms with private bathrooms may be the single most important design intervention for reducing stress and aggression on psychiatric wards.[11] Substantial research in correctional settings and community mental health housing found residing in dormitories reliably correlates with reduced privacy, higher crowding stress, more aggressive behaviors, illness complaints, and social withdrawal.[11]

Psychiatric facilities typically have dorm-style housing due to the high volume of patients. The only way to remove a dangerous patient from others is via seclusion or restraints. Common safety protocols for imminent dangerousness is use of seclusion and restraints. Without such safety procedures, violence increases, and treatment progress deteriorates.[12,13] This is clearly documented in one of the most comprehensive and successful inpatient programs for chronic institutionalized psychiatric patients conducted by Paul and Lentz (1977).[14] Paul and Lentz developed a rigorous social learning inpatient program leading to significant reductions in aggression.[12,13] Within this program, seclusion was used as a standard safety protocol for imminent dangerousness for violence when needed for a maximum of 48 hours of seclusion. Over two years, the program exhibited a reduction from 30 assaults to 10 assaults per week. An unexpected state mandate reduced the established allotment of 48 hours of seclusion to a maximum of two hours. In the following two years, assaults skyrocketed in this program from 10 per week to 75 assaults per week.[13]

Research demonstrates that security is necessary to create an environment that allows for therapeutic work to happen.[15] The ETP arose aligning with the RNR's key principle of treating patients at highest risk for violence with the highest dosages of care. The construction of the ETP has been thoughtfully designed to have low social and spatial density, meaning all patients will have their own bedroom and increased square footage in common areas with good line of sight including cameras. Patients will have daily access to outdoor spaces. The ETP staff can lock patient room doors when clinically indicated based on dangerousness. Given the high volume of unpredictable physical violence, the ability to lock doors based on each patient's risk of violence will greatly reduce the need for use of restraints and seclusion. The ETP has specialized door portals and a no-contact treatment room which includes a windowed-divider and two separate entrances. This allows for safe delivery of therapeutic intervention to even the most dangerous patients. This unique feature employs a fresh approach to maintain needed physical environmental safety with reduced use of seclusion and restraints. The use of seclusion and restraints can lead to a reactive management of violence as legally patients can only be placed in seclusion or restraints when exhibiting imminent dangerousness. The option of locked door status based on individual violence risk factors affords a preventative approach to violence. The ETP will continue to review and use environmental design in programming to create a safe atmosphere to deliver evidence-based practices to the most challenging patients.

From Idea to Implementation

The process of developing an ETP from a theoretical idea to a sustainable program involved the communication, strategic planning, and execution of the vision of this program. As aforementioned, a recognition of a needed paradigm shift is needed to adequately treat patients at the highest risk for violence. This recognition led to taking the vision of providing care for patients at highest risk of violence into an action plan.

The first step was to secure the support of involved stakeholders. One of the first stakeholder groups enlisted was the labor unions. Due to the increased employee violence the labor unions were keenly aware of the need for a structured and secure treatment environment in which their members could work without the fear of violence. The support of the labor unions was key in securing the sponsorship of a California legislator in the writing and passing of legislation (Enhanced Treatment Programs, Assembly Bill No. 1340[16]). This process was arduous and took bold leadership from within DSH, labor unions, and other California State legislators. It was this assembly bill that secured funding for the structural changes needed on the ETP units and allowed the use of locked doors based on clinical indicators for highest risk of violence, initiating a preventative approach to violence beyond just the criteria of imminent dangerousness. Furthermore, the ETP was funded for staffing at an enhanced level compared to the standard treatment environment.

Following passage of the legislation, clinical and administrative employees of DSH were enlisted for support. Psychiatric technicians and registered nurses were overwhelmingly the most supportive. These employees are routinely exposed to violence on the units and welcomed the development of a space where they could safely treat highly dangerous patients. The support of DSH staff was utilized in the formation of numerous workgroups to identify key tasks needed for the successful implementation of the ETP. These tasks included: the development of a forensic focused treatment plan, selecting evidence-based treatment modalities, writing of policies, development of unit operational procedures, and development and

execution of an extensive training for ETP staff. Utilizing DSH staff in the planning of the ETP was paramount in the successful implementation of the program vision.

Violence Risk Informed Treatment Planning

The next stage of development was to create a specific treatment framework to tackle the need of reducing violence in our forensic population. Current scientific literature indicates the initial phase of informed treatment includes implementation of a comprehensive violence risk assessment that determines the typology of aggression and violence risk factors.[1,6,17] There is a longstanding trend in the field of violence risk assessment focusing on identifying dynamic violence risk factors as theoretically they are amenable to change (e.g. via treatment), and can reduce violence potential if altered.[18–20] Recent research has provided evidence for the categorization of aggression perpetrated within psychiatric facilities into three types based on motivation and etiology (psychotic, impulsive, and organized), and the need to target treatments based on these categories.[21,22] In order to determine typology and identify dynamic risk factors for the ETP, structured professional judgment (SPJ) instruments including the Historical Clinical Risk Management 20 Version 3 (HCR20v3[23]), Short-Term Assessment of Risk and Treatability (START[24]), and Hare Psychopathy Checklist-Revised (PCL-R[25]) were selected. These instruments have garnered empirical support for their use in the justice-involved and forensic populations in determining typology and dynamic risk factors with regards to violence prediction and treatment planning.[26–28]

Final considerations regarding the implementation of a comprehensive risk assessment within the ETP included the bifurcation of treatment provider and violence risk assessor and the need for repeated assessment of violence risk.[17,29] Given the myriad issues that arise when treatment providers are tasked with forensic evaluations of their patients, the Forensic Needs Assessment Team (FNAT) was developed to serve as independent evaluators providing risk assessments on a repeated schedule.[1,16,30]

Treatment to Address Violence Risk

Research indicates that consideration of psychosocial treatments, modalities, and theories that elicit the greatest probability for producing change and reducing violence be considered following the assessment of violence risk.[31] However, there is currently a dearth of interventions specifically to reduce violence with the mentally ill population. Much of the scientific literature focuses on criminal recidivism more broadly with justice-involved persons, and only a few investigating interventions specifically targeting violence recidivism in persons with serious mental illness (SMI).[6,7,13] Theoretical modalities and associated interventions with empirical support for their use with either the SMI or justice-involved population were therefore considered. We also considered how these interventions would address the typology of violence and dynamic risk factors identified in the comprehensive risk assessment. These included the RNR treatment model and numerous interventions that fall within the cognitive-behavioral and social-learning theory principles.[6,13] Other frameworks of treatment, including Positive Psychology, Trauma Informed Care (TIC), and Motivational Interviewing (MI), were considered given their utility in treating aspects related to violence (e.g. trauma, substance abuse) and compatibility with RNR principles (e.g. responsivity, attitudes towards treatment). These frameworks of treatment were part of the trending zeitgeist with various pilot programs demonstrating promising outcomes in the DSH system. Table 24.1 illustrates the relationship between typology of violence and treatments provided in the ETP.

Research indicates that treatment programs and interventions adherent to the principles of RNR are the most effective on recidivism outcomes.[6,7,32] Given the strength of support found in the literature, interventions selected for the ETP were ones that were consistent with RNR principles. Some of the major interventions

selected for the ETP included Changing Lives Changing Outcomes (CLCO[33]), CBT for Psychosis (CBT-P[34]), Dialectical Behavioral Therapy (DBT[35]), and restorative- and social cognition-based cognitive rehabilitation interventions. These include Social Cognition and Interaction Training (SCIT[36]) and BrainHQ which is a computer-based cognitive restoration treatment program with strong empirical support.[37]

The CLCO model is purported to be a treatment intended for use with persons involved in the criminal justice system and concurrently diagnosed with a mental illness.[33] The model integrates best practices in both social learning and cognitive behavioral theories with the goals of enhancing quality of life, improving mental health status, and reducing criminal and psychiatric recidivism. Although the fact that CLCO is relatively new in the field, there is promising data to support its use in producing positive outcomes for justice-involved mentally ill persons.[38]

Unlike CLCO, the other RNR-consistent treatments listed have not been specifically designed for persons in the criminal justice system. These treatments have historically been used to treat mentally ill persons and are theoretically tied to various dynamic risk factors and types of aggression. However, they have only recently garnered support for their use in forensic populations.[13,31] DBT was originally developed to treat parasuicidal behaviors in women diagnosed with borderline personality disorder. A meta-analysis of existing research also illustrated the efficacy of DBT in reducing physical aggression among persons with histories of violence and violent offending.[39] CBT-P was originally developed for persons experiencing symptoms of psychosis. One study of CBT-P on persons in treatment (both inpatient and outpatient) with histories of violence demonstrated promising findings in the reduction of violence.[40] Cognitive rehabilitation has been utilized to treat neurocognitive and neurodevelopmental disorders to increase functioning. In a study of cognitive rehabilitation in forensic patients, O'Reilly and colleagues[41] supported the use of cognitive rehabilitation interventions to improve several cognitive functions and reduce risk (e.g. moved to lower security unit). Persons with schizophrenia often display social deficits.[42] Social skills training (SST) for schizophrenia is a well-established evidence-based treatment for social dysfunctions.[43] Improved social functioning often leads to better interpersonal relationships, which may help reduce a person's aggressive behaviors.

Table 24.1 Typologies of violence and treatment modalities in the ETP

Typology of violence	Treatment	Modality
Organized	CLCO	RNR
	Positive Psychology	Positive Psychology
Psychotic	CBT-P	RNR
	SST	RNR
Impulsive	DBT	RNR
	Cognitive rehabilitation	RNR
	Sensory modulation	TIC
	MI	Substance abuse

Also included in the ETP are interventions demonstrating merit in reducing violence in this population but without clear theoretical connections to the RNR model. These interventions (TIC, MI, Positive Psychology) are not necessarily adversarial to the RNR model, and in many ways align with those principles. Substance abuse disorders have been indicated as having the strongest relationship to violence, in general.[1] MI has traditionally been used to treat substance use disorders and to enhance motivation for internal change, including behavioral change.[44]

As the primary goal of the ETP is to promote behavioral change (i.e. reduce violence), it stands to reason that MI would be included especially when considering the support for its use in justice-involved populations.[45] Behavior modification generally requires replacing maladaptive behaviors with more adaptive ones. Positive Psychology attempts to foster the development of novel behaviors and potentially replace antisocial behaviors with pro-social ones.[46] Trauma has been identified as a violence risk factor and appears conceptually related to the impulsive typology of aggression.[47] In this study, persons who were exposed to early victimization, had childhood conduct problems, and were diagnosed with a schizophrenia spectrum disorder, were more likely to engage in violent behaviors as adults.

Data Collection of Clinical Outcomes

The final step of developing the ETP was to include a methodology for data collection of clinical outcomes in order to evaluate its effectiveness in reducing violence.[1] Some of the variables to be collected include incidence of violence, as well as its typology and severity. Collecting these data allows for a systematic approach to evaluate the effectiveness of not only an individual treatment plan, but the broader treatment program.

Conclusion

Treatment of forensic patients who are at the highest risk of perpetuating violence requires an innovative model for adequate assessment and treatment of this population (Table 24.2). Working with stakeholders across state entities provided DSH the opportunity to design and implement an innovative treatment program to address the changing safety, security, and treatment needs in a state psychiatric facility. This unique treatment program seeks to reduce the

Table 24.2 ETP model of treating violence in forensic facilities

Environmental security	Single room with bathroom
	Intensive milieu locked door enhanced staffing
Violence risk assessment	Independent forensic evaluation Quarterly assessment
Treatment based on risk factors	CLCO CBT-P DBT MI Positive Psychology SCIT Brain HQ TIC SST
Data collection	Outcome data Incidences of aggression, severity, type

perpetration of violence within a forensic population, allowing for a safer environment for residents and staff members while simultaneously increasing the efficacy of treatments. Extensive data collection is essential to evaluating outcomes in terms of the program's effectiveness. Some questions pertaining to the nature of pathologies of referred patients, their specific treatment needs, and the response to treatment remain and will be addressed in future publications.

Disclosure

Dr. Velasquez, Dr. Bauchowitz, Dr. Pyo, and Dr. Pollock have no conflicts of interest to disclose.

References

1. Warburton K. The new mission of forensic mental health systems: managing violence as a medical syndrome in an environment that balances treatment and safety. *CNS Spectr.* 2014; **19**: 368–373.

2. Fisher W, Geller, JL, Pandiani, JA. The changing role of the state psychiatric hospital. *Health Affairs.* 2009; **28** (3): 676–684.

3. Bader S, Evans, SE, Welsh, E. Aggression among psychiatric inpatients: the relationship between time, place, victims, and severity ratings. *J Am Psychiatr Nurses Assoc.* 2014; **20**(3): 179–186.

4. Broderick C. Violence report: DSH violence 2010–2017. California Department of State Hospitals; 2019: 265.

5. Morgan R, Flora DB, Kroner DG, et al. Treating offenders with mental illness: a research synthesis. *Law Hum Behav.* 2012; **36**(1): 37–50.

6. Andrews D. The risk-need-responsivity (RNR) model of correctional assessment and treatment. In: Dvoskin J, Skeem, JL, Novaco, RW, Douglas, KS, eds. *Using Social Science to Reduce Violent Offending.* New York: Oxford University Press; 2012: 127–156.

7. Skeem J, Steadman HJ, Manchak SM. Applicability of the risk-need-responsivity model to persons with mental illness involved in the criminal justice system. *Psychiatr Serv.* 2015; **66**: 916–922.

8. Delgado D, Mitchell SM, Morgan RD, Scanlon, F. Examining violence among not guilty by reason of insanity state hospital inpatients across multiple timepoints: the roles of criminogenic risk factors and psychiatric symptoms. Manuscript submitted for publication. 2019

9. Andrews D, Bonta J, Hoge RD. Classification for effective rehabilitation: rediscovering psychology. *Crim Justice Behav.* 1990; **17**(1): 19–52.

10. Sugarman P, Dickens G. The evolution of secure and forensic mental healthcare. In: Sugarman P, Dickens GL, Picchioni MM, eds. *Handbook of Secure Care.* London: RCPsych Publications; 2015.

11. Ulrich R, Bogren L, Gardiner SK, Lundin S. Psychiatric ward design can reduce aggressive behavior. *J Environ Psychol.* 2018; **57**: 53–66.

12. Glynn S, Mueser KT. Social learning for chronic mental inpatients. *Schizophr Bull.* 1986; **12**(4): 648–668.

13. Douglas KS, Nicholls TL, Brink J. Interventions for the reduction of violence by persons with serious mental illness. In: Kleespies PM, ed. *The Oxford Handbook of Behavioral Emergencies and Crises.* New York: Oxford University Press; 2016: 466–488.

14. Paul G, Lentz R. *Psychosocial Treatment of Chronic Mental Patients: Milieu versus Social-Learning Programs.* Cambridge, MA: Harvard University Press; 1977.

15. Crichton J. Defining high, medium, and low security in forensic mental healthcare: the development of the matric of security in Scotland. *J Forens Psychiatry Psychol.* 2009; **20**(3): 333–353.

16. Achadjian K. Assembly Bill No. 1340. Enhanced Treatment Programs. 2014.

17. Douglas K, Skeem JL. Violence risk assessment: getting specific about being dynamic. *Psychol Public Policy Law.* 2005; **11**(3): 347–383.

18. Dvoskin J, Heilbrun K. Risk assessment and release decision-making: toward resolving the great debate. *J Am Acad Psychiatry Law.* 2001; **29**: 6–10.

19. Kraemer H, Kazdin AE, Offord DR, et al. Coming to terms with the terms of risk. *Arch Gen Psychiatry.* 1997; **54**: 337–343.

20. De Vries Robbe M, De Vogel V, Douglas KS, Nijman HLI. Changes in dynamic risk and protective factors for violence during inpatient forensic psychiatric treatment: predicting reductions in post discharge community recidivism. *Law Hum Behav.* 2015; **39**(1): 53–56.

21. Quanbeck C. Forensic psychiatric aspects of inpatient violence. *Psychiatr Clin North Am.* 2006; **29**: 743–760.

22. Stahl S, Morrissette DA, Cummings M, et al. California State Hospital Assessment and Treatment (Cal-VAT) guidelines. *CNS Spectr.* 2014; **19**: 4490465.

23. Douglas K, Hart SD, Webster CD, Belfrage H. *HCR-20V3: Professional guidelines for evaluating risk of violence.* Mental Health, Law, and Policy Institute, Simon Fraser University; 2013.

24. Webster C, Nicholls TL, Martin ML, Desmarais SL, Brink J. Short-Term Assessment of Risk and Treatability (START): the case for a new violence risk structured professional judgment scheme. *Behav Sci Law.* 2006; **24**: 757–766.

25. Hare R. *The Hare Psychopathy Checklist-Revised, 2nd edn.* Toronto, Canada: Multi-Health Systems; 2003.

26. Penney S, Marshall LA, Simpson AIF. The assessment of dynamic risk among forensic psychiatric patients transitioning to the community. *Law Hum Behav.* 2016; **40**: 374–386.

27. Hogan N, Olver ME. Assessing risk for aggression in forensic psychiatric inpatients: an examination of five measures. *Law Hum Behav.* 2016; **40**(3): 233–243.

28. Hogan N, Olver ME. Static and dynamic assessment of violence risk among discharged forensic patients. *Crim Justice Behav.* 2019; **47**(7): 923–938.

29. Watt K, Storey JE, Hart D. Violence risk identification, assessment and management practices in inpatient psychiatry. *J Threat Assess Management.* 2018; **5**(3): 155–172.

30. Greenberg S, Shuman DA. Irreconcilable conflict between therapeutic and forensic roles. *Prof Psychol Res Pr.* 1997; **28**(1): 50–57.

31. Douglas K, Nicholls TL, Brink J. Reducing the risk of violence among people with serious mental illess: a critical analysis of treatment approaches. In: Kleespies P, ed. *Behavioral Emergencies: An Evidence-Based Resource for Evaluating and Managing Risk of Suicide, Violence, and Victimization.* Washington, DC: American Psychological Association; 2009.

32. Viljoen J, Cochrane DM, Jonnson MR. Do risk assessment tools help manage and reduce risk of

violence and reoffending?: a systematic review. *Law Hum Behav.* 2018; **42**(3): 181–214.

33. Morgan R, Kroner DG, Mills JF. *A Treatment Manual for Justice Involved Persons with Mental Illness.* New York: Routledge; 2018.

34. Kingdon D, Turkington D. *Cognitive Therapy of Schizophrenia.* New York: Guilford Press; 2005.

35. Linehan M. *Cognitive-Behavioral Treatment of Borderline Personality Disorder.* New York: Guilford Press; 1993.

36. Roberts D, Penn D, Combs D. *Social Cognition and Interaction Training (SCIT).* New York: Oxford University Press; 2016.

37. Shah T, Weinborn M, Verdile G, Sohrabi H, Martins R. Enhancing cognitive functioning in healthy older adults: a systematic review of the clinical significance of commercially available computerized cognitive training in preventing cognitive decline. *Neuropsychol Rev.* 2017; **27**(1): 62–80.

38. Morgan R, Kroner DG, Mills JF, Bauer R, Serna C. Treating justice involved persons with mental illness: preliminary evaluation of a comprehensive treatment program. *Crim Justice Behav.* 2014; **41**: 902–916.

39. Frazier S, Vela J. Dialectical behavior therapy for the treatment of anger and aggressive behaviors: a review. *Aggress Violent Behav.* 2014; **19**(2): 156–163.

40. Haddock G, Barrowclough C, Shaw JJ, et al. Cognitive-behavioural therapy v. social activity therapy for people with psychosis and a history of

violence: randomised controlled trial. *Br J Psychiatry.* 2009; **194**: 152–157.

41. O'Reilly K, Donohoe G, O'Sullivan D, et al. A randomized controlled trial of cognitive remediation for a national cohort of forensic patients with schizophrenia or schizoaffective disorder. *BMC Psychiatry.* 2019; **19**: 27.

42. Kern R, Glynn SM, Horan WP, Marder SR. Psychosocial treatments to promote functional recovery in schizophrenia. *Schizophr Bull.* 2009; **35**(2): 347–361.

43. Bellack A, Mueser KT, Gingerich S, Agresta J. *Social Skills Training for Schizophrenia: A Step-by-Step Guide.* New York: The Guilford Press; 2004.

44. Miller W, Rollnick S. *Motivational Interviewing: Helping People Change, 3rd edn.* New York: Guilford Press; 2013.

45. Ginsburg J, Mann RE, Rotgers F, Weekes JR. Motivational interviewing with criminal justice populations. In: Miller W, Rollnick SR, eds. *Motivational Interviewing: Preparing People for Change.* New York: Guilford Press; 2002: 333–346.

46. Barlett M, Desteno D. Gratitude and prosocial behavior: helping when it costs you. *Psychol Sci.* 2006; **17**(4): 319–324.

47. Swanson J, Van Dorn RA, Swartz MS, et al. Alternative pathways to violence in persons with schizophrenia: the role of childhood antisocial behavior problems. *Law Hum Behav.* 2008; **32**: 228–240.

From Trauma-Blind to Trauma-Informed: Rethinking Criminalization and the Role of Trauma in Persons with Serious Mental Illness

Helga Thordarson and Tiffany Rector

Introduction

This article explores how wide-ranging effects of exposure to psychological trauma in mentally ill individuals continue to be largely overlooked, contributing to poor outcomes and a flood of mentally ill individuals into the court system and correctional care. Even in state hospitals and community mental health settings, the consequences of trauma often go unrecognized and untreated in highly vulnerable individuals. The authors posit that a trauma-informed lens is needed to move "trauma-blind" systems forward to more enlightened, evidence-based care and treatment. The traditional criminalization hypothesis refers to the funneling of serious mental illness (SMI) individuals into the criminal justice system as a result of deinstitutionalization and inadequate community mental health resources. This article explores how expanding notions about criminalization that identify factors beyond SMI still miss the mark by underestimating or omitting the role of trauma. Chronic under-recognition of trauma-related disorders contributes to misattributions about the cause and meaning of behaviors that pose common management problems in prisons, state hospitals, conditional release and community-based mental health programs, homeless shelters, and communities. A trauma-informed perspective offers insight for care providers (and individuals) seeking to understand acts of aggression, self-injury, high risk medical refusals, impulsivity, substance abuse, medication nonadherence, rule-breaking, and heightened reactivity to perceived disrespect, shaming, coercion, and power differentials. The authors encourage providers to take a new look at clients who demonstrate these behaviors with the view that for many SMI individuals, these responses do not represent treatment resistance or reckless risk-taking, but rather, *complex, adaptive behaviors that arise from traumatic life histories.*

While trauma-informed care (TIC) is not the answer to all problems, it offers a more effective and compassionate approach to challenges facing SMI individuals and the systems that treat them. TIC fosters awareness of the lifelong effects of psychological trauma, shifting the clinical question from "What's wrong with you?" to "What happened to you?" In trauma-informed systems, the impact of trauma is recognized at all levels and proactive policies and procedures are employed to mitigate harm and reduce retraumatization. TIC is associated with improved mental health outcomes, patient satisfaction, and significant reductions in violence, sexually risky behavior, substance abuse, containment-related injuries, seclusion and restraint, and use of sedative hypnotics in acute inpatient settings.[1–3]

TIC is a national standard promoted by public health agencies across the U.S. and beyond. Leaders in mental health care increasingly view trauma-informed perspectives as critical, and this paper serves as a call to action. TIC offers a roadmap for organizational change that supports safer environments for patients, inmates, and staff. A crucial first step is increasing awareness of trauma prevalence and impact among SMI individuals.

Trauma Prevalence

Life histories replete with trauma are the norm for individuals involved with mental health services and the criminal justice system. Per the Substance Abuse and Mental Health Services Administration (SAMHSA), trauma is "an almost universal experience among people who use public mental health, substance abuse and social services, as well as people who are justice-involved or homeless."[4] Studies affirm that nearly all individuals treated in inpatient and forensic psychiatric settings are survivors of trauma, with reported lifetime prevalence rates of 98% in a mixed group of in/outpatients with SMI and 100% in male forensic inpatients – with 75% of the latter endorsing exposure in childhood.[5,6] SMI mental health patients are also far more likely than the general population to be victims of trauma or violence in the previous year.[7] High levels of trauma exposure and mental illness are found in correctional settings as well. Per the Treatment Advocacy Center, "Los Angeles County Jail, Chicago's Cook County Jail, or New York's Riker's Island Jail each hold more mentally ill inmates than any remaining psychiatric hospital in the United States" and overall, more SMI individuals reside in jails and prisons than in psychiatric facilities; the Center estimates that 15% of prisoners and 20% of inmates in jails are seriously mentally ill.[8] Other studies report higher rates of SMI in incarcerated persons; in Iowa, almost half (48%) of prisoners were diagnosed with a mental disorder and 29% were diagnosed with SMI.[9] Despite the almost universal presence of traumatic life histories in SMI individuals, studies consistently demonstrate gross, systemic under-recognition of trauma-related disorders.

Trauma and Related Disorders Often Go Unrecognized

A significant number of SMI individuals warrant a concurrent diagnosis of post-traumatic stress disorder (PTSD), but few individuals are diagnosed. In a multisite study, 43% of SMI patients met criteria for PTSD upon evaluation, but only 2% were identified as such; a follow-up study found a 35% rate of PTSD in SMI patients.[5,10] In a community mental health setting 33% of patients with SMI met criteria for PTSD, but only 4% were identified.[11] A review conducted in a large forensic state hospital found that only 1.4% of patients were diagnosed with PTSD.[12] A systematic review of 34 articles determined that PTSD is a common co-morbid condition, with most studies reporting prevalence ranging from 20% to 30% with schizophrenia and higher co-morbidity (40%) with concurrent substance abuse.[13] A comprehensive review covering 30 years of data and 33 studies concluded that the mean prevalence rate for PTSD in the context of SMI was 30%.[14] Prevalence of "complex" PTSD (arising from prolonged, early, repeated traumatic experiences that are interpersonal in nature) was 31% in a sample of patients diagnosed

with borderline personality disorder.[15] Trauma exposure is also elevated in adults with intellectual disability[16] and varies with socioeconomic status, poverty, gender, sexual orientation, and other demographic factors.[1]

Accurate diagnosis of PTSD in the presence of SMI can be challenging. Severe trauma symptoms may be misinterpreted as evidence of personality or psychotic disorder, and dissociation can be difficult to differentiate from psychosis.[17] Flashbacks and hypervigilance may be interpreted as congruent with symptoms of paranoia or schizophrenia rather than concurrent PTSD.[13,14] Other reasons for low diagnostic rates include a widespread belief that SMI individuals are unreliable historians, despite studies demonstrating accurate self-report of traumatic events even in the presence of active psychiatric symptoms.[18,19] In cases where co-occurring PTSD is wholly unrecognized, effective clinical management and compassionate care prove challenging.

The Impact of Trauma

Childhood trauma is powerfully associated with serious issues that are routinely encountered in treating mentally ill patients and inmates, including leading causes of physical illness and mortality, psychiatric illness, substance abuse, and risk-taking behaviors in adulthood. The landmark Adverse Childhood Experiences (ACE) study (conducted by Kaiser Permanente in partnership with the Centers for Disease Control) queried 17,000 people and found that the number of traumatic events in a person's early life is robustly correlated with subsequent heart, liver, and lung disease, smoking, obesity, sexually transmitted diseases, substance use, depression, suicidal behavior, hallucinations, and other life problems.[20] The authors note that our earliest experiences are "not lost, but, like a child's footprints in wet cement, are often life-long" and that unrecognized and untreated trauma represent a costly public health problem. Other studies reveal that early exposure to trauma results in alterations in brain structure and function including, but not limited to, changes in the sensory system and hippocampus, increased activity in the amygdala, decreased activity in the prefrontal cortex, enlarged ventricles, decreased gray matter, and neurochemical changes such as increased dopamine and decreased serotonin.[21–23]

While specific causal pathways are not yet fully understood, a growing body of research reveals a relationship between early trauma and later violence and criminality. A study associated with the ongoing ACE project found early childhood trauma was associated with aggression and adult criminality in male offenders.[24] The authors note that the powerful effects of trauma are too often ignored in treatments addressing criminality and that interventions that do not attempt "to heal these neurobiological wounds are destined to fail." In a study of nearly 4,000 imprisoned males, those with histories of childhood physical or sexual abuse reported more substance abuse, symptoms of depression and anxiety, and interpersonal problems arising from difficulties with self-regulation and aggression.[25] A recent meta-analysis indicated that individuals with psychosis and histories of maltreatment in childhood were twice as likely to be violent as SMI patients lacking that history.[26] Trauma also exacerbates expression of co-morbid conditions: in patients with schizophrenia, PTSD is associated with increased suicidality, severity of positive symptoms, neurocognitive impairment, lower levels of functioning, and poor quality of life.[13] Exposure to early trauma has also been connected to repeated self-injurious behavior in adulthood,[27] emotional dysregulation, and increased irritability.[28]

Unrecognized Trauma Leads to Poor Outcomes

A pervasive lack of understanding about symptoms and adaptive behaviors common to SMI trauma survivors increases risk of poor outcomes, negative encounters with staff, and unwanted contact with the criminal justice system. A core tenet of TIC is that *all behavior has purpose and meaning*. An individual who erupts aggressively in the medication line upon being touched without warning may have an early life history that makes sense of a seemingly "unprovoked" outburst. Similarly, there may be a discoverable, reality-based rationale at work when an individual repeatedly refuses her gynecological appointments despite a history of cervical cancer. Authors of the landmark ACE study note that too frequently providers focus narrowly on the presenting problem "which is often only the marker for the real problem which lies buried in time, concealed by patient shame, secrecy, and sometimes amnesia – and frequent clinician discomfort."[20] Without

a trauma-informed lens and abiding curiosity, patients may well appear irrational, pathological, reckless, or resistant. TIC teaches us that patterns of behavior that appear unhealthy or destructive may represent the best available "solution" to an even worse problem facing that individual. Uninformed responses that disregard the challenges and needs of traumatized individuals may result in disengagement, inadequate treatment, or contribute to increased reactivity, aggression, and instability.[29] All of this sets the stage for a revolving door between the streets, community, state hospital, and correctional settings.

The Criminalization Hypothesis and Trauma

The most common conceptualization of the criminalization hypothesis is that persons with SMI are disproportionately represented in the criminal justice system because untreated psychiatric symptoms bring them into contact with law enforcement, and that rerouting them to appropriate mental health treatment is the solution. To that end, concerted efforts have been made over the past 20 years to provide community-based alternatives such as jail diversion programs, problem-solving courts, specialized probation and parole caseloads, and forensic mental health services emphasizing psychiatric rehabilitation.[30,31] The Sequential Intercept Model has served as a framework for identifying points of intervention that might "prevent individuals from entering or penetrating deeper into the criminal justice system."[32] The primary goal of these "first generation" interventions was to ensure individuals with SMI were properly linked with needed mental health services, and often involved pre-booking and post-booking diversion, Forensic Assertive Community Treatment (FACT), and Forensic Intensive Case Management (FICM).[29,31,33] However, a growing body of literature suggests the standard criminalization hypothesis does not wholly account for the large number of SMI in the criminal justice system, and that purely untreated mental illness only accounts for 5–10% of those individuals.[34–36]

One study of post-booking jail diversion found only 8% of crimes to be related to mental illness, while 26% were related to substance abuse; which led researchers to call for an expanded view of criminalization that includes other criminal risk factors inherent to the environments of SMI individuals such as poverty, homelessness, employment instability, and substance abuse.[36,37] A 2010 study of released prisoners revealed that 7% of crimes were linked to psychosis or survival behaviors resulting from socioeconomic disadvantage (respectively classified as "psychotic" and "disadvantaged"); however, the largest group (90% of mentally ill, 68% of non-mentally ill) were classified as "reactive" and found to have the highest likelihood of further criminal justice involvement. Group members were characterized by hostility, disinhibition, and "emotionally motivated responses to perceived provocation." Among the mentally ill reactive group, substance abuse was determined to be a motivating factor in the majority of offenses. Based upon findings, the researchers called for additional attention to be paid to the same criminogenic risk factors shared by offenders without mental illness.[35] In both studies, raters determined motivating behavior based on review of police reports and interviews with offenders; however, the methodologies used did not account for the fact that many traumatized individuals, particularly those who are untreated, lack sufficient insight to recognize or verbalize the full range of motivations/impulses behind their behavior. Furthermore, both studies failed to recognize the integral role trauma can play in substance abuse, hostility, disinhibition, and emotional reactivity.

Trauma: The Missing Piece

We suggest that criminalization occurs in an ongoing manner, not only at the time of first law enforcement contact, but well into the custodial and treatment phases. While SMI and/or other factors might lead individuals to be incarcerated or judicially committed to treatment, the story doesn't end there. Once in the criminal justice system, trauma-based behaviors are often misinterpreted and wrongly attributed to purely criminogenic factors, leading to improper or inadequate treatment interventions, power struggles with staff, and ultimately retraumatization. In some cases, the stigma associated with certain types of criminal behavior, and those who commit it, may also play a role in staff insensitivity and inadequate attention to complex treatment needs.[38] While some acknowledge the role trauma can play in SMI entering the system,[39] we would argue that many seeking to expand the criminalization hypothesis still overlook the role trauma plays in *continued* criminalization of this population once incarcerated or remanded to care.

Additionally, trauma *may underlie other risk factors* contributing to criminalization. For example, both illicit drug use and homelessness are strongly connected to traumatic life histories. The ACE study strikingly revealed a powerful, dose-dependent relationship between early traumatic experiences and later intravenous drug use, noting a 4,600% greater likelihood of heroin or methamphetamine use (via injection) in males with an ACE score of six versus males with scores of zero.[20] The SHIFT study found trauma to be one of two factors predicting long-term housing instability.[40] Still, much of the research reconceptualizing criminalization appears to be siloed from concurrent literature on the impact of trauma. This disconnect continues to be a barrier to developing comprehensive, multifaceted approaches that reduce SMI involvement in the criminal justice system.

Some researchers have begun to incorporate trauma into broader models, and we urge others to explore this topic more fully. One suggested second generation approach is the "person-place framework," which calls for targeted interventions for mental illness, criminogenic risk, and other risk factors arising from social and environmental disadvantages commonly experienced by SMI persons, such as addiction and trauma exposure.[31] Others suggest the Risk-Need-Responsivity (RNR) Model[41] should be updated to reflect current research indicating reactivity, impulsivity, and need for excitement can actually be trauma responses rather than indicators of antisocial personality.[42] One researcher recommends treatment planning that addresses both criminogenic risk and responsivity factors – like trauma – "that can create barriers to positive outcomes."[29] The common theme in evolving research is that services aimed at mental illness alone may only be partially effective;[29,33,37,43] therefore, it is incumbent upon all of us in the mental health and criminal justice systems to regroup and evolve beyond the strategies employed over the last two decades.

We propose a comprehensive expanded view of the criminalization hypothesis that recognizes the *interplay and overlap of all factors* available in current research. Identified factors contributing to criminalization of SMI include: untreated mental illness, substance abuse, social and environmental factors, criminogenic risk, and unrecognized/untreated trauma (See Figure 25.1 – original visual representation of an "Expanded model of the criminalization hypothesis.")

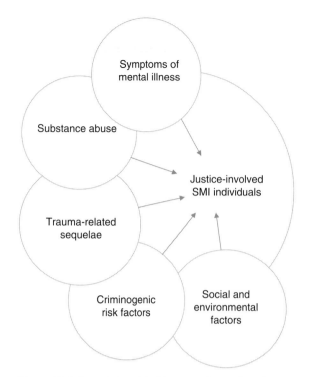

Figure 25.1 Expanded model of the criminalization hypothesis.

How Trauma-Informed Principles Can Help

Trauma-informed systems offer the possibility of improved outcomes in multiple areas; however, trauma can only be healed within systems that are not retraumatizing. Every member of an organization, from those who serve as first point of contact to executive leadership, must understand the impact trauma has on an individual's development, and common behaviors traumatized individuals exhibit.[44] It is important for service providers to recognize that these behaviors are not always characterological, but may have developed over time as adaptive strategies for coping with the impact of trauma.[45] This understanding can translate into more sensitive responses throughout the service delivery process. A hallmark of trauma-informed care is that each interaction is made with the intention of contributing to recovery and reducing the likelihood of retraumatization.[44]

It is also important to understand how one's environment – within criminal justice or mental health settings – can be further traumatizing. Lack of control, hopelessness over circumstances, necessary security protocols, and exposure to institutional

TEN IMPLEMENTATION DOMAINS

1. Governance and Leadership
2. Policy
3. Physical Environment
4. Engagement and Involvement
5. Cross Sector Collaboration
6. Screening, Assessment, Treatment Services
7. Training and Workforce Development
8. Progress Monitoring and Quality Assurance
9. Financing
10. Evaluation

Figure 25.2 Expanded model of the criminalization hypothesis.

violence can trigger traumatized individuals who already experience significant anxiety, hypervigilance, and irritability.[29] Even the traumatizing effect of a person's own committing offense warrants further attention.[6] The vicarious trauma of staff can also lead to an unhealthy workforce, and institutional trauma that fosters reactivity and "management by crisis."[46] Transparency, flexibility, communication, and compassion at all levels can go a long way toward increasing physical and psychological safety for staff and those they serve.

Some mental health and correctional staff may perceive trauma-informed interventions as ineffective or even dangerous; however, quite to the contrary, they assist in the development of prosocial coping skills, safer and more peaceful milieus with fewer incidents, and improved staff morale.[46] Staff across mental health and correctional settings should be trained to recognize signs and symptoms of trauma-reactivity, employ trauma-informed de-escalation techniques, create more trauma-informed physical environments whenever possible, and provide appropriate referral to trauma-specific treatments.

SAMHSA offers organizations a guide for implementing trauma-informed care across multiple domains, including not only workforce training and provision of trauma-specific services, but areas such as physical environment, leadership, and policy. (See Figure 25.2 – public domain image of SAMHSA's "Ten Implementation Domains."[47])

Clinical and Policy Implications

Given the high prevalence of trauma within the SMI population, universal trauma precautions should be employed in agencies that serve them.[6,29] In other words, policies and procedures should reflect the assumption that every individual has a trauma history. Cross-sector training on trauma, its impact, and its behavioral expression can begin to change the hearts and minds of staff within mental health and criminal justice systems. A shift in system culture can then pave the way for changes that minimize environmental stressors, and encourage appropriate referral/linkage to evidence-based trauma-specific assessment and treatment. Trauma should be meaningfully integrated into risk management and viewed as a "universal component" of violence risk assessment.[48] Trauma-informed case formulations can guide treatment planning and trauma-focused interventions that have been identified as safe and effective with SMI patients.[49] Exploring individuals' support systems may offer valuable information that can assist with such formulations.[29]

With regard to program/research design and evaluation, consumers should be integrated whenever possible to ensure the wisdom of those with "lived experience" serves as a guide for change. Further, the principles of trauma-informed care must be operationalized in terms of specific activities and competencies that can be evaluated and replicated.[42] A distinction should be made between mental health and public safety outcomes when selecting interventions. Program reviews over recent years show few instances where criminal justice and mental health outcomes were considered in tandem;[31] however, this must change through appropriate cross-sector collaboration that also integrates community re-entry, conditional release, and other community supervision entities. Some communities have found Sequential Intercept Mapping workshops to be useful tools for collaboration between systems, education about available services and resources, and identification of service gaps.[29]

We urge systems to work together toward the following goals:

- Build cultures that embody TIC principles and practice relationship-based care and curiosity. Change culture first, then implement trauma-specific services.
- Integrate trauma as a core component of violence risk assessment and incident/risk management (utilize trauma-informed case formulations).
- Implement sensitive trauma screening and assessment practices, and evidence-based treatments, including, but not limited to sensory modulation and somatosensory therapies, Cognitive Behavioral Therapy (CBT), and Eye Movement Desensitization and Reprocessing (EMDR).
- Address staff trauma to support healthier milieus and authentic, engaged, relationship-based care with SMI individuals.
- Engage in cross-sector training and collaboration, identify desired mental health and criminal justice outcomes, and develop an integrated plan for measurement and evaluation.

Conclusion

Over recent years, concerted efforts have been made by mental health and criminal justice systems to reduce criminalization of the mentally ill, yet large numbers of SMI persons continue to fill jails, prisons, and state hospitals. Only with an expanded view of the multiple interconnected factors that contribute to criminalized SMI can systems begin to work together to address this complex social issue. To paraphrase Maya Angelou, *now that we know better, we can do better*. Acknowledging the powerful role of trauma is an important step toward healing, increased resilience, and mutual understanding. Building trauma-responsive organizations will enhance safety and bring renewed sense of purpose, meaning, and connection for individuals and the providers who serve them.

Acknowledgments

The authors would like to thank the many dedicated trauma champions working to foster positive change, kindness, and clinical curiosity in the California Department of State Hospitals.

Funding

Helga Thordarson has no research, consulting, or other funding sources to report.

Tiffany Rector has no research, consulting, or other funding sources to report.

Disclosures

Helga Thordarson has nothing to disclose.

Tiffany Rector has nothing to disclose.

References

1. Center for Substance Abuse Treatment (US). *Trauma Informed Care in Behavioral Health Services. Treatment Improved Protocol (TIP) Series, No. 57.* Rockville, MD: Substance Abuse and Mental Health Services Administration; 2014.

2. Muskett C. Trauma-informed care in inpatient mental health settings: a review of the literature. *Int J Ment Health Nurs.* 2013; **23**(1): 51–59.

3. Riemer D. Creating sanctuary: reducing violence in a maximum security forensic psychiatric hospital unit. *Forensic Nurses.* 2009; **15**(1): 302.

4. Substance Abuse and Mental Health Services Administration. Creating a Trauma-Informed Criminal Justice System for Women: Why and How. www.nasmhpd.org/sites/default/files/Women%20in%20Corrections%20TIC%20SR(2).pdf (accessed June 2020).

5. Mueser KT, Goodman LB, Trumbetta SL, et al. Trauma and posttraumatic stress disorder in severe mental illness. *J Consult Clin Psychol.* 1998; **66**(3): 493–499.

6. McKenna G, Jackson N, Browne C. Trauma history in a high secure male forensic inpatient population. *Int J Law Psychiatry.* 2019; **66**: 101475.

7. Khalifeh H, Oram S, Osborn D, Howard LM, Johnson S. Recent physical and sexual violence against adults with severe mental illness: a systematic review and metaanalysis. *Int Rev Psychiatry.* 2016; **28**(5): 433–451.

8. Treatment Advocacy Center. Serious mental illness prevalence in jails and prisons. 2016. www.treatmentadvocacycenter.org/evidence-and-research/learn-more-about/3695 (accessed June 2020).

9. Al-Rousan T, Rubenstein L, Sieleni B, Deol H, Wallace RB. Inside the nation's largest mental health institution: a prevalence study in a state prison system. *BMC Public Health.* 2017; **17**(1): 342.

10. Mueser KT, Salyers MP, Rosenberg SD, et al. Interpersonal trauma and posttraumatic stress disorder in patients with severe mental illness: demographic, clinical, and health correlates. *Schizophr Bull.* 2004; **30**(1): 45–57.

11. Howgego IM, Owen C, Meldrum L, et al. Posttraumatic stress disorder: an exploratory study examining rates of trauma and PTSD and its effects on client outcomes in community mental health. *BMC Psychiatry.* 2005; **5**: 21.

12. Alexander A, Welsh E, Glassmire DM. Underdiagnosing posttraumatic stress disorder in a state hospital. *J Forensic Psychol Pract.* 2016; **16**(5): 448–459.

13. Seow LSE, Ong C, Mahesh MV, et al. A systematic review on comorbid posttraumatic stress disorder in schizophrenia. *Schizophr Res.* 2016; **176**(2–3): 441–451.

14. Mauritz MW, Goossens PJJ, Draijer N, van Achterberg T. Prevalence of interpersonal trauma exposure and trauma-related disorders in severe mental illness. *Eur J Psychotraumatol.* 2013; **4**.

15. Ford JD, Fournier D. Psychological trauma and post-traumatic stress disorder among women in community mental health aftercare following psychiatric intensive care. *J Psychiatr Intensive Care.* 2007; **3**(1): 27–34.

16. Wigham S, Emerson E. Trauma and life events in adults with intellectual disability. *Curr Dev Disord Rep.* 2015; **2**: 93–99.

17. Lysaker P, LaRocco V. The prevalence and correlates of trauma-related symptoms in schizophrenia spectrum disorder. *Compr Psychiatry.* 2008; **49**: 330–334.

18. Grubaugh AL, Zinzow HM, Paul L, Egede LE, Frueh BC. Trauma exposure and posttraumatic stress disorder in adults with severe mental illness: a critical review. *Clin Psychol Rev.* 2011; **31**: 883–899.

19. Fisher HL, Craig TK, Fearon P, et al. Reliability and comparability of psychosis patients' retrospective reports of childhood abuse. *Schizophr Bull.* 2009; **37** (3): 546–553.

20. Felitti VJ, Anda RF. The relationship of adverse childhood experiences to adult health, well-being, social function, and healthcare. In: Lanius R, Vermetten E, Pain C, eds. *The Impact of Early Life Trauma on Health and Disease; The Hidden Epidemic.* New York: Cambridge University Press; 2010: 77–87.

21. Dannlowski U, Struhrmann A, Beutelmann V, et al. Limbic scars: long-term consequences of childhood maltreatment revealed by functional and structural magnetic resonance imaging. *Biol Psychiatry.* 2012; **71**: 286–293.

22. Ford JD. Neurobiological and developmental research: clinical implications. In: Courtois CA, Ford JD, eds. *Treating Complex Traumatic Stress Disorders: An Evidence-Based Guide.* New York: Guilford Press; 2009: 31–58.

23. Read J, Fosse R, Moskowitz A, Perry B. The traumagenic neurodevelopmental model of psychosis revisited. *Neuropsychiatry.* 2014; (4): 65–79.

24. Reavis JA, Looman J, Franco KA, Rojas B. Adverse childhood experiences and adult criminality: how long must we live before we possess our own lives? *Perm J.* 2013; **17**(2): 44–48.

25. Wolff N, Shi J. Childhood and adult trauma experiences of incarcerated persons and their

relationship to adult behavioral health problems and treatment. *Int J Environ Res Public Health*. 2012; **9**: 1908–1926.

26. Green K, Browne K, Chou S. The relationship between childhood maltreatment and violence to others in individuals with psychosis: a systematic review and meta-analysis. *Trauma Violence Abuse*. 2019; **20**(3): 358–373.

27. Cleare S, Wetherall K, Clark A, et al. Adverse childhood experiences and hospital-treated self-harm. *Int J Environ Res Public Health*. 2018; **15**: 1235.

28. Bielas H, Barra S, Skrivanek C, et al. The associations of cumulative adverse childhood experiences and irritability with mental disorders in detained male adolescent offenders. *Child Adolesc Psychiatry Ment Health*. 2016; **10**: 34.

29. Pinals DA. Crime, violence, and behavioral health: collaborative community strategies for risk mitigation. *CNS Spectr*. 2015; **20**: 241–249.

30. DeMatteo D, LaDuke C, Locklair BR, Heilbrun K. Community-based alternatives for justice-involved individuals with severe mental illness: diversion, problem-solving courts, and reentry. *J Crim Justice*. 2013; **41**: 64–71.

31. Epperson MW, Wolff N, Morgan RD, et al. Envisioning the next generation of behavioral health and criminal justice interventions. *Int J Law Psychiatry*. 2014; **37**(5): 427–438.

32. Munetz MR, Griffin PA. Use of the sequential intercept model as an approach to decriminalization of people with serious mental illness. *Psychiatr Serv*. 2006; **57**(4): 544–549.

33. Wolff N, Frueh C, Juening J, et al. Practice informs the next generation of behavioral health and criminal justice interventions. *Int J Law Psychiatry*. 2013; **36**(1): 1–10.

34. Skeem JL, Manchak S, Peterson JK. Correctional policy for offenders with mental illness: creating a new paradigm for recidivism reduction. *Law Hum Behav*. 2011; **35**: 110–126.

35. Peterson J, Skeem JL, Hart E, Vidal S, Keith F. Analyzing offense patterns as a function of mental illness to test the criminalization hypothesis. *Psychiatr Serv*. 2010; **61**(12): 1217–1222.

36. Junginger J, Claypoole K, Laygo R, Crisanti A. Effects of serious mental illness and substance abuse on criminal offenses. *Psychiatr Serv*. 2006; **57**(6): 879–882.

37. Draine J, Salzer MS, Culhane DP, Hadley TR. Role of social disadvantage in crime, joblessness, and homelessness among persons with serious mental illness. *Psychiatr Serv*. 2002; **53**(5): 565–573.

38. Wiechelt SA, Shdaimah CS. Trauma and substance abuse among women in prostitution: implications for a specialized diversion program. *J Forensic Soc Work*. 2011; **1**(2): 159–184.

39. Pinals DA, Felthous AR. Introduction to this double issue: jail diversion and collaboration across the justice continuum. *Behav Sci Law*. 2017; **35**: 375–379.

40. Hayes MA, Zonneville M, Bassuk E. The SHIFT (Service and Housing Interventions for Families in Transition) study: final report. American Institutes for Research; 2010. https://www.air.org/resource/service-and-housing-interventions-families-transition-shift-study-final-report (accessed June 2020).

41. Bonta J, Andrews DA. Risk-need-responsivity model for offender assessment and rehabilitation (User Report 2007–06). Public Safety Canada; 2007.

42. Leitch L. Action steps using ACEs and trauma-informed care: a resilience model. *Health Justice*. 2017; **5**(1): 1–10.

43. Fisher WH, Silver E, Wolff N. Beyond criminalization: toward a criminologically informed framework for mental health policy and services research. *Adm Policy Ment Health*. 2006; **33**(5): 544–557.

44. Elliott DE, Bjelajac P, Fallot RD, Markoff LS, Reed BG. Trauma-informed or trauma-denied: principles and implementation of trauma-informed services for women. *J Community Psychol*. 2005; **33** (4): 461–477.

45. Stainbrook K, Penney D, Elwyn L. The opportunities and challenges of multi-site evaluations: lessons from the jail diversion and trauma recovery national cross-site evaluation. *Eval Program Plann*. 2015; **50**: 26–35.

46. Miller NA, Najavits LM. Creating trauma-informed correctional care: a balance of goals and environment. *Eur J Psychotraumatol*. 2012; **3**(1): 17246.

47. Substance Abuse and Mental Health Services Administration. *SAMHSA's Concept of Trauma and Guidance for a Trauma-Informed Approach. HHS Publication No. (SMA) 14–4884*. Rockville, MD: Substance Abuse and Mental Health Services Administration; 2014.

48. Horowitz D, Guyer M, Sanders K. Psychological approaches to violence and aggression: contextually anchored and trauma-informed interventions. *CNS Spectr*. 2015; **20**: 190–199.

49. Swan S, Keen N, Reynolds N, Onwumere J. Psychological interventions for posttraumatic stress symptoms in psychosis: a systematic review of outcomes. *Front Psychol*. 2017; **8**: 341.

The Indistinguishables: Determining Appropriate Environments for Justice-Involved Individuals

Sean E. Evans and Shannon M. Bader

Perhaps one of the most outstanding weaknesses of contemporary psychological theory is the relative neglect of the environment by many of the most influential theoretical viewpoints.

Isidor Chein, The Environment as a Determinant of Behavior[1]

Introduction

History may not repeat itself, but there seem to be reverberating themes. One such theme is the challenge of "how" and "where" to manage people who behave in dangerous, scary, or unacceptable ways. Throughout time, these individuals have been placed in institutional settings or facilities; the names of which often belied the philosophical approach popular at the time. Reform schools and correctional institutions were providing discipline, instruction, and behavioral guidance while asylums and sanatoriums were places of rest and recovery. In the 1840s, Dorothea Dix began to argue that individuals with mental illness were distinct from criminals and should not be housed in jails or prison.[2] Her descriptions of inhumane treatment within jail settings resulted in the establishment of state psychiatric hospitals around the country. Now, after nearly 200 years of advancements in medicine, penological research, psychological treatments, and public policies, the question of "how" and "where" to best manage people remains unanswered. Modern day jail diversion programs and mental health courts continue to promote Dix's perspective that mentally ill individuals should be provided appropriate treatment, not languish in jail or prison. However, this ideal has not become a reality. The living conditions and medical treatment for people with mental illness within facilities remain a primary public policy issue for the American Civil Liberties Union and the National Alliance on Mental Illness with large class action lawsuits occurring each year. Similarly, the Department of Justice continues to order jails and prisons into receivership for inadequate care. Dix's proposition was a simple one. Criminals and antisocial individuals should be housed and safely contained in jails and prisons but individuals with mental illness should be admitted to hospitals for treatment. Unfortunately, the question of "how" and "where" remains because the reality of people who behave in dangerous, scary, or unacceptable ways is much more complex. We argue that there is a population of individuals not so clearly criminal or mentally ill (see Figure 26.1). Furthermore, individuals in this indistinguishable group can be incorrectly placed either at a correctional institution or psychiatric facility and experience possible harm, poorer outcomes, and potential for further misclassification.

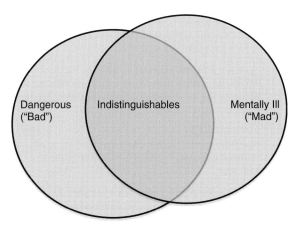

Figure 26.1 The criminalization of mental illness – the "bad" versus "mad" dichotomy.

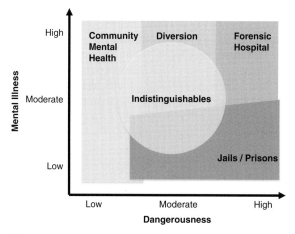

Figure 26.2 Decriminalizing mental illness – a dimensional model.

The Sorting Hat

In the *Harry Potter*[3] book series, the Sorting Hat magically determines which college or house at the wizard school each new student should be assigned. Once the Sorting Hat is placed on the students' head, it can hear their thoughts and then makes a determination about their appropriate placement within minutes or even seconds. According to the books, the hat makes very few errors. When examining individuals entering the criminal justice system, there is no such magical sorting mechanism available. Instead of wizard houses, the classification is whether the person is dangerous or mentally ill. Indeed, the initial options for classification are whether the person is "bad" or "mad." Often, the police officers first called to the scene of a disturbance or crime are forced to immediately determine whether the subject is dangerous, mentally ill, or under the influence of an intoxicant. Based on their training and initial impressions, the police officers then determine if it is necessary to ticket or arrest the person, take them to jail, or transport them to a local hospital for treatment. Each of these actions requires presumptions about whether the person is dangerous and requires containment or is ill and needs treatment. These assessments occur very quickly and often with little to no background information.

Although some people are easily identifiable as dangerous while others undoubtedly require immediate mental health care, there is a population of individuals that are not so clearly sorted. These indistinguishables encompass a wide range of presentations. Some may have a mild mental illness that is typically well managed but currently exacerbated by substance abuse; others may have no mental illness but are unexpectedly acting aggressive or bizarre; while another may appear belligerent and socially inappropriate but not necessarily violent or even mentally ill. Indeed, the kinds of indistinguishables are innumerable. For this reason, *the simple distinction between either dangerous or mentally ill is incomplete.* Not all individuals with a diagnosis of a mental illness require inpatient treatment. Similarly, not all individuals who have engaged in illegal behaviors require incarceration to ensure community safety. The binary distinction between dangerousness and mental illness ignores the dimensional nature of these constructs (see Figure 26.2). Dorothea Dix would likely agree that only the most dangerous require incarceration and only the severely mentally ill require hospitalization. People demonstrating both significant mental illness and dangerous behaviors are appropriate for inpatient forensic treatment but those with less serious illness can remain in community settings.

Even with this more nuanced view that incorporates spectrums of dangerousness and mental illness, the indistinguishables remain. Where is the appropriate placement for an individual stabilized on antipsychotic medication but continuing to act aggressively? What about the patient who intermittently decompensates and then sets fires? We propose that inappropriate placement into the incorrect facility, treatment location, or security rating can result in poorer clinical outcomes, longer lengths of stay, and violence.

From Deinstitutionalization to Transinstitutionalization

In 1939, the British psychiatrist Lionel S. Penrose observed that the availability of psychiatric beds for the mentally ill reduced the incidence of crime and therefore decreased the number of people in prison.[4] This inverse relationship between the proportion of people in psychiatric hospitals and prisons became known as the Penrose hypothesis.[4–7] Empirical support for the Penrose hypothesis continues to be debated; however, the basic premise that individuals are categorized as "mad" (mentally ill) or "bad" (criminal) remains a ubiquitous part of our social ecologies.

Since Penrose's observation, two significant trends have taken place in the United States. First, as a result of the *deinstitutionalization* movement, there are fewer psychiatric beds available to serve the growing number of mentally ill individuals. Coinciding with the advent of psychotropic medications in the 1950s, psychiatric hospitals began releasing patients with the promise that these patients could receive more humane and effective treatment in the community. In 1955, for instance, there were 559,000 state hospital beds for a population of 164 million people; however, only 40 years later that number dropped to 72,000 state hospital beds for a population of 250 million.[8]

The second trend is the exponential increase in incarceration rates and prisons. Since the early 1970s, the United States has witnessed an unprecedented increase in the total number of incarcerated individuals.[9] The total number of people incarcerated between 1980 and its peak in 2008 rose from 501,836 to 2.3 million in the United States.[10] When adjusting for population, the rates of incarceration from 1980 to 2008 rose from 310 inmates per 100,000 adults to 1,000 inmates per 100,000 adults.[10] To provide a global comparison, the United States has more persons in jail and prison than what is reported in China (approximately 1.6 million inmates) and Brazil (approximately 673,000 inmates).[10]

The *transinstitutionalization* trends have resulted in blending of individuals with the full range of mental illness and the full range of dangerousness at prisons, jails, forensic hospitals, and psychiatric hospitals. In other words, a patient at a forensic hospital may show the identical pattern of illness severity and dangerousness as a prison inmate. The only distinction may be how they were originally sorted. Importantly, research suggests that there can be critical consequences when an indistinguishable does not have both the mental health services and containment they need.

Mental Illness in Prison and Jails

Penological research over the last decades has argued that for some inmates, prison and jail can create new symptoms and exacerbate pre-existing symptoms of mental illness. Solitary confinement and entire super-max facilities that utilize isolation as a key method to deter violence, contraband trading, or escape have received the most attention.[11] Now called extended control units or ECUs, these units typically have inmates locked into a single cell with no windows 22 to 23 hours per day. The inmates in ECUs have limited access to exercise, work, religious services, or rehabilitation programs. The amount of interaction between staff and inmates varies from facility to facility with some being characterized as total deprivation of human contact.[12] Research on these populations has demonstrated that some ECU inmates have psychosis that quickly resolves when they are transferred to a less

restrictive area of the prison and that many develop "SHU Syndrome."[13] First coined in 1983, SHU Syndrome was characterized by severe confusion, mutism, hallucinations, hyper-responsivity to any stimuli, and delusional beliefs that include persecutory thoughts or ideas of reference among inmates with no history of mental illness.[14,15] During two high profile court cases, *Madrid v. Gomez*[16] and *Jones 'El v. Berge,*[17] the courts concluded that ECU prison housing "is known to cause severe psychiatric morbidity, disability, suffering and mortality" and required screening procedures to ensure that inmates with existing diagnoses of schizophrenia spectrum disorders, past suicidality, or intellectual disabilities could not be sent to the ECU because the risk of exacerbating their symptoms was too high.

The creation or exacerbation of mental illness in this type of extreme prison setting may not be surprising but additional research suggests that some general population inmates also experience an increase in their psychiatric symptoms. A recent report[18] suggested that about 14% of state and federal prisoners and 26% of jail inmates reported experiences that met the threshold for "serious psychological distress" (SPD). Moreover, about 37% of prisoners and 44% of jail inmates had been informed by a mental health professional that they have a mental disorder.[18] Of those prisoners with a mental disorder, major depressive disorder was the most common disorder (24% for prisoners and 30% for jail inmates), with bipolar disorder the second most common (17% and 25% respectively). When compared to the standardized adult population of the United States (5%), three times as many prisoners met the threshold for SPD (14%). Jail inmates were five times more likely to meet the threshold of SPD (26%) than the adult general population. Female prisoners and jail inmates were even more likely to meet the threshold for SPD than males.[18] These findings suggest that the environment of the prison or jail setting may be disproportionately detrimental to some inmates more than others. It is possible that this group of inmates would experience fewer psychiatric symptoms, require less medication, and have better community re-entry if they had been in a nonprison setting such as a diversion program or forensic hospital.

Violence in Psychiatric Hospitals

With shifts in the law that now require dangerousness (and not the need for treatment alone) as the primary legal criteria for involuntary treatment, more civilly committed patients are being admitted to state hospitals with an increased risk for violence. For example, an analysis of patients within the California Department of State Hospitals (DSH) found that civilly committed patients engaged in more acts of physical violence towards staff and other patients than forensically committed patients.[19] Research on the rate of inpatient aggression varies considerably in the literature, which is likely due to how violence is defined, measured, and documented;[20] however, approximately 20%–40% of psychiatric inpatients exhibit violent behaviors while in hospital settings.[21] Notably, patients within inpatient psychiatric settings have higher rates of violence than individuals with mental illness living in the community.[22,23] In sum, these large studies highlight that patients needing mental health treatment may also simultaneously need containment and security to manage their dangerousness.

A host of patient factors, including severe and chronic psychiatric symptomatology, cognitive impairment, personality disorders, impulsivity, criminal justice system involvement, and trauma histories, play a significant role in violent inpatient behaviors among psychiatric patients. Additionally, research into the relationship between situational and environmental factors and inpatient aggression have suggested that the physical environment, crowding, ward organization, hospital management style, institutional responses to violence, staff mixture, staff training, patient population, uninvolved psychiatric leadership, as well as temporal and location factors can all influence the frequency and severity of aggression within psychiatric hospitals.[24-28] Studies have shown that violent patients can evoke anger and fear in staff members leading to team splitting and treatment disagreements,[29] staff members becoming passive and engaging in scapegoating,[30] and experiencing strong negative feelings (countertransference) towards patients.[31] Based on this literature, patients who are psychiatrically stable and continue to be violent towards staff might create even stronger reactions in staff and significantly undermine the therapeutic milieu that the inpatient psychiatric unit is attempting to facilitate. Indeed, the psychiatric and forensic hospitals intended for treatment may not incorporate the necessary safety and security measures inherent to prison settings.

Solutions: The Appropriate Environment for Indistinguishables

This research highlights that many individuals are likely incorrectly sorted into facilities that do not match their dangerousness or mental health needs. Our current binary system of "mad" versus "bad" does not allow for full assessment of the indistinguishable to determine their ideal placement. There are some model programs and research findings that suggest solutions to this dichotomy. First, we propose that settings designed to fulfill dual needs, both containment and mental health milieu treatment, may be the most apt placement for the indistinguishables.

The indistinguishables require admission to a facility appropriate for their both their psychiatric and security needs. Jails, prisons, and forensic hospitals must be prepared for individuals across the entire spectrum of mental illness and dangerousness. Marrying the necessary security measures with a treatment focus can improve the outcomes of a larger range of inmates and patients, reducing the possibility of SHU syndrome or violence. Indeed, human–environment interactions are based on a variety of complex psychological processes occurring both at the individual level, as well as at the social group levels, all in the context of our social and environmental ecologies.

Research into the impact of environmental characteristics and situational factors on mental health has been examined in a variety of human living spaces. Environmental factors such as space design, crowding, lighting, indoor air quality and flow, and light all have been demonstrated to have a direct impact on mental health.[32] For example, Holahan[33] observed that rearranging the furniture (e.g. placing the chairs around a table, chairs at a comfortable distance facing each other) promoted social interactions among hospitalized patients, thereby decreasing isolative, passive behaviors. Psychological adjustment was improved by simple amenities such as hallway decorations and weather protections at doorways.[34] The architectural design of the living areas also impacted psychological adjustment and engagement. Patients showed improved mental alertness and social interaction living in small corridors and suites, but no change was observed in the large open sleeping wards (e.g. 15–20 patients in cubicle like space).[35] Evans[32] also found that chronic exposure to noise, crowding, and malodorous pollutants was linked to apathy about recovering and that limited exposure to daylight was correlated with increases in depressive symptoms.

Despite these studies about the importance of environmental factors on mental health in general, much of this information has not been incorporated into the design of prisons or psychiatric facilities. These facilities tend to be underfunded and outdated, in deteriorating states, and buildings are often repurposed for use other than the intended design. A focus on environmental aspects will allow facilities to meet the needs of the wide variety of indistinguishables admitted while also maintaining treatment and security requirements. Indeed, this type of ecological perspective reminds us that it is not just the individual who warrants our focused attention, but also the complex environmental systems in which the individual lives.

Second, there is a need to implement frequent assessment to determine if a person's current level of dangerousness and mental illness requires placement into a facility. Indeed, it is possible that many indistinguishables could show long-term success if they remain in the community. The Eleventh Judicial Circuit Criminal Mental Health Project (CMHP)[36] in Miami-Dade County is one of the most promising examples of coordinated systems solution to decriminalizing mental illness. The Honorable Steve Leifman initiated the CMHP in 2000 to address the high number of untreated and undertreated mentally ill defendants cycling through the courts and jails. Miami-Dade County is uniquely challenging in that it has the highest percentage of residents with serious mental illnesses (nearly three times the national average) but exists within a state system that is ranked 48th in the nation for state funding for community mental health services.[37] The CMHP goes beyond community strategies that attempt to keep mentally ill individuals out of the criminal justice system, by incorporating a comprehensive host of policy and procedural changes that include training law enforcement to recognize signs of mental illness and pre- and post-booking jail diversion programs. In a five-year period, officers within the two largest police departments have responded to approximately 50,000 mental health crisis calls resulting in 9,000 diversions to mental health services and 109 arrests; moreover, the daily census within this jail system dropped from 7,200 to 4,000.[37] As stated in the *New England Journal of Medicine*[37] "the [CMHP] initiative's success is largely attributable to an effort to structure patterns of service delivery and deploy existing resources in ways that are better aligned with the needs of the people coming out of the justice system." In essence, the CMHP has conceptualized a more nuanced solution that transcends the outdated binary model by creating treatment and containment strategies that are contingent upon the defendants' severity of mental illness and level of dangerousness. This model reserves placement in facilities (e.g. jails, prisons, and forensic psychiatric hospitals) for the smaller percentage of individuals that can be best served within them. Programs like the CMHP can increase the chance of indistinguishables receiving the appropriate security and treatment and improving long-term outcomes.

Conclusion

Arguably, there is not just one mental health crisis in America; rather there are multiple mental health crises, one of which involves the criminalization of the mentally ill. The old "mad" versus "bad" dichotomy fails to appreciate the complexity of justice-involved individuals. Innovative programs and policies that address both mental health and dangerousness can result in a greater variety of answers to the remaining question of "how" and "where" to best serve the indistinguishables.

Disclosures

Sean Evans and Shannon Bader have nothing to disclose.

References

1. Chein I. The environment as a determinant of behavior. *J Soc Psychol*. 1954; **39**: 115–121.

2. Dix DL. *On Behalf of the Insane Poor*. Honolulu, Hawaii: University Press of the Pacific; 2001.

3. Rowling JK. *Harry Potter and the Sorcerer's Stone*, 1st edn. New York: A.A. Levine Books; 1998.

4. Penrose LS. Mental disease and crime: outline of a comparative study of European statistics. *Br J Med Psychol*. 1939; **18**: 1–15.

5. Lamb HR. Does deinstitutionalization cause criminalization?: the Penrose hypothesis. *JAMA Psychiatry*. 2015; **72**(2): 105.

6. Large MM, Nielssen O. The Penrose hypothesis in 2004: patient and prisoner numbers are positively correlated in low-and-middle income countries but are unrelated in high-income countries. *Psychol Psychother*. 2009; **82**(Pt 1): 113–119.

7. Kalapos MP. Penrose's law: methodological challenges and call for data. *Int J Law Psychiatry*. 2016; **49**: 1–9.

8. Chaimowitz G. The criminalization of people with mental illness. *Can J Psychiatry*. 2012; **57** (2): 6.

9. Office of the Assistant Secretary for Planning and Evaluation. The psychological impact of incarceration: implications for post-prison adjustment. U.S. Department of Health & Human Services; 2001.

https://aspe.hhs.gov/basic-report/psychological-impact-incarceration-implications-post-prison-adjustment (accessed June 2020).

10. Gramlich J. U.S. incarceration rate is at its lowest in 20 years. Pew Research Center; 2018. www.pewresearch.org/fact-tank/2018/05/02/americas-incarceration-rate-is-at-a-two-decade-low/ (accessed June 2020).

11. Collins WC. *Supermax Prisons and the Constitution: Liability Concerns in the Extended Control Unit.* Ann Arbor, MI: University of Michigan Library; 2004.

12. Riveland C. Prison management trends, 1915–2025. *Crime Justice.* 1999; **26**: 163–203.

13. Grassian S. Psychopathological effects of solitary confinement. *Am J Psychiatry.* 1983; **140**(11): 1450–1454.

14. Kupers TA. Trauma and its sequelae in male prisoners: effects of confinement, overcrowding, and diminished services. *Am J Orthopsychiatry.* 1996; **66**(2): 189–196.

15. Grassian S, Friedman N. Effects of sensory deprivation in psychiatric seclusion and solitary confinement. *Int J Law Psychiatry.* 1986; **8**(1): 49–65.

16. *Madrid v. Gomez,* 889 F. Supp. 1146 (N.D. Cal. 1995).

17. *Jones 'El v. Berge,* 172 F. Supp. 2d 1128 (W.D. Wis. 2001).

18. Bronson J, Berzofsky M. Indicators of mental health problems reported by prisoners and jail inmates, 2011–12. U.S. Department of Justice, Office of Justice Programs, Bureau of Justice Statistics; 2017: 11. www.bjs.gov/content/pub/pdf/imhprpji1112.pdf (accessed June 2020).

19. Broderick C, Azizian A, Kornbluh R, Warburton KD. Prevalence of physical violence in a forensic psychiatric hospital system during 2011–2013: patient assaults, staff assaults, and repeatedly violent patients. In: Warburton KD, Stahl SM, eds. *Violence in Psychiatry.* New York, NY: Cambridge University Press; 2016: 49–63.

20. Convit A, Isay D, Otis D, Volavka J. Characteristics of repeatedly assaultive psychiatric inpatients. *Hosp Community Psychiatry.* 1990; **41**(10): 1112–1115.

21. Cooke DJ, Wozniak E, Johnstone L. Casting light on prison violence in Scotland: evaluating the impact of situational risk factors. *Crim Justice Behav.* 2008; **35**(8): 1065–1078.

22. Swanson JW. Mental disorder, substance abuse, and community violence: an epidemiological approach. In: Monahan J, Steadman HJ, eds. *Violence and Mental Disorder: Developments in Risk Assessment.* Chicago, IL: University of Chicago Press; 1994: 101–136.The John D. and Catherine T. MacArthur

Foundation Series on Mental Health and Development.

23. Swanson JW, Swartz MS, Van Dorn RA, et al A national study of violent behavior in persons with schizophrenia. *Arch Gen Psychiatry.* 2006; **63**(5): 490–499.

24. Clements CB. Crowded prisons: a review of psychological and environmental effects. *Law Hum Behav.* 1979; **3**(3): 217–225.

25. Bader SM, Evans SE. Implementing an ecological approach to violence reduction at a forensic psychiatric hospital: approaches and lessons learned. In: Warburton KD, Stahl SM, eds. *Violence in Psychiatry.* New York, NY: Cambridge University Press; 2016: 263–268.

26. Welsh E, Bader S, Evans SE. Situational variables related to aggression in institutional settings. *Aggress Violent Behav.* 2013; **18**(6): 792–796.

27. Gadon L, Johnstone L, Cooke D. Situational variables and institutional violence: a systematic review of the literature. *Clin Psychol Rev.* 2006; **26**(5): 515–534.

28. Katz P, Kirkland FR. Violence and social structure on mental hospital wards. *Psychiatry Interpers Biol Process.* 1990; **53**(3): 262–277.

29. Lion JR, Pasternak SA. Countertransference reactions to violent patients. *Am J Psychiatry.* 1973; **130**(2): 207–210.

30. Cornfield RB, Fielding SD. Impact of the threatening patient on ward communications. *Am J Psychiatry.* 1980; **137**(5): 616–619.

31. Rossberg JI, Friis S. Staff members' emotional reactions to aggressive and suicidal behavior of inpatients. *Psychiatr Serv.* 2003; **54**(10): 1388–1394.

32. Evans GW. The built environment and mental health. *J Urban Health.* 2003; **80**(4): 536–555.

33. Holahan C. *Environment and Behavior: A Dynamic Perspective.* Berlin, Germany: Springer Science & Business Media; 2012.

34. Timko C. Physical characteristics of residential psychiatric and substance abuse programs: organizational determinants and patient outcomes. *Am J Community Psychol.* 1996; **24**(1): 173–192.

35. Zimring C, Weitzer W, Knight R. Opportunity for control and the designed environment. In: Baum A, Singer J, eds. *Advances in Environmental Psychology.* New Jersey: Erlbaum; 1982; **4**: 171–210.

36. Eleventh Judicial Circuit of Florida. Criminal mental health project. www.jud11.flcourts.org/Criminal-Mental-Health-Project (accessed June 2020).

37. Iglehart JK. Decriminalizing mental illness – the Miami model. *N Engl J Med.* 2016; **374**(18): 1701–1703.

Breaking Down Long-Term Chronic Aggression Within a Forensic Hospital System

Benjamin Rose, Charles Broderick, Darci Delgado, Rebecca Kornbluh, and Stephen M. Stahl

Introduction

Inpatient aggression within psychiatric facilities continues to demand attention. Aggressive acts often cause physical or psychological injury that impact the lives of the patients or staff victims of these incidents. However, it should be noted that the vast majority of psychiatric patients are not aggressive while hospitalized. Studies on inpatient aggression[1-3] showed approximately 25%–35% of inpatients committed acts of aggression. For those inpatients who are aggressive, there is a substantial literature that describes a small subset of "chronically aggressive" patients, who are responsible for the majority of inpatient aggression.[4-11]

Numerous research studies have described clinical characteristics of inpatient psychiatric patients who meet some definition of a chronic aggressor.[4,8,12] While there has not been universal agreement in past studies, several clinical characteristics have been shown to be significant in discriminating between the chronically aggressive and nonaggressive populations, including: cognitive deficits,[4,13,14] suicidal behavior,[12,14] borderline or antisocial personality disorder,[4,15,16] history of substance use,[4] diagnosis of schizophrenia or psychosis,[10,13] hospitalization as a juvenile,[12] and diagnosis of a mood disorder.[4,12]

Given the amount and variety of these clinical characteristics, it is difficult to develop a cohesive theory based on the heterogeneity of the results, and given a finite amount of resources, develop specialty programs that address all of these problems. This informational morass has provided challenges to researchers and clinicians trying to piece together many different clinical features of this population.

Research on the topic of chronic aggression has been clouded by a variety of labels as well as definitions. Studies, that have investigated patients with multiple aggressive acts, have used different terms to describe these patients, such as "chronically aggressive," "repeatedly aggressive," and "chronically violent." While every study reviewed included aggression toward others, there was a lot of variability on the inclusion of aggression toward self, aggression toward property, and verbal aggression. In addition, the primary method of determining if a patient was chronically aggressive has been to set a minimum number of aggressive incidents and a time frame for those incidents to be committed. The number of incidents has ranged from a minimum of 2–20 and the time frame has varied from 5 months to 10 years. This variability creates a problem in clearly defining the group of patients to be studied. A patient committing 20 acts of aggression within 5 months will likely look clinically different from a patient committing 20 aggressive acts within 10 years.

This issue of variability in definitions was highlighted in a study by Krakowsi and Czobor[13] who subdivided a sample of aggressive patients into a "transiently violent" group and a "persistently violent" group. Their findings showed that the transiently violent patients became less psychotic and less violent over a four-week period, whereas the persistently violent did not show any substantial changes in illness or violence. Further investigation showed the persistently violent patients showed more neurological impairment than the transiently violent patients. The positive response to treatment in the transiently violent group highlights the impact that psycho-pharmacological treatment can have for psychosis, but also highlights the relative lack of benefit for persistently violent patients with neurological impairment. Despite the differences in the clinical picture and response to treatment, several studies have lumped these two groups of patients together when conducting research on chronic aggression.

Despite the short four-week duration, Krakowski and Czobor's[13] model, dividing patients into transiently violent and persistently violent groups, provides a useful blueprint for further study. In their model, the transiently aggressive patients were individuals who were aggressive for a period of time but as a result of treatment, time, or other factor, greatly reduced or eliminated their aggressive behavior. The persistently violent patients were those that remained aggressive despite psychopharmacology, therapies, extra resources, reviews by expert clinicians, and other varied interventions. One criticism of their model is the short amount of time that passed before a patient was considered persistently violent. Several psychopharmacological and psychiatric treatments can take months to be effective and so it is unclear if the treatments had worked in the study. In addition, the short duration does not allow researchers to determine if the patient was consistently aggressive.

The aim of the study was to further refine the definition "chronic aggressor" and study patients who had been consistently aggressive over multiple years, labeling this group as, "long-term chronic aggressors." To better understand this group, we then contrasted them with a matched control group to see if we could classify patients into a long-term chronic aggressor group or a nonaggressor group based on the clinical factors that were most related to chronically aggressive patients. More specifically, we aimed to test whether common characteristics of the chronically aggressive patients were present in the long-term chronic aggressive patients.

In an effort to study a long-term chronic aggressor, a more stringent inclusion criterion was used. In this study, we required that a patient have at least 15 incidents of physical aggression, we believed that having a stricter definition would provide a better contrast to the control group. This number is on the high end of what previous studies have required to be considered a chronic aggressor. In addition to the count of aggressive incidents, a consistency factor was implemented, which required a patient to be consistently aggressive five times for three years, for a total of at least 15 aggressive incidents. Only aggressive acts that were physical assaults toward another patient or staff member were counted. Acts such as verbal aggression, aggression toward self, or aggression toward an object or property were not counted in this study.

Method

This study was completed in a state hospital system that comprises five maximum security hospitals and has approximately 6,000 beds. The hospitals are located throughout California and treat patients deemed not guilty by reason of insanity, incompetent to stand trial, mentally disordered offenders, and patients who are civilly committed. Patients have a variety of diagnoses including schizophrenia, schizoaffective disorder, bipolar disorder, major depressive disorder, personality disorders, and cognitive disorders. Approval for this study was obtained through the California Committee for the Protection of Human Subjects.

The study included 30 long-term chronically aggressive hospitalized patients and 30 matched hospitalized controls with zero incidents of aggression within their hospitalization. A long-term chronically aggressive patient was defined as a hospitalized patient who had committed five or more physically aggressive acts each year for three years from January 2011 to December 2015. Physical aggression, within this hospital system, is defined as "hitting, kicking, pushing, or other similar acts directed against another individual to cause potential or actual injury." As mentioned previously, acts of verbal aggression, self-harm, and aggression toward property did not qualify as aggression in this study. A description of the demographic information can be seen in Table 27.1.

A chart review was completed on each individual and information related to aggression, suicidal ideation and behavior, psychiatric diagnosis, psychosocial history, and demographics were recorded. Inter-rater reliability was obtained from the six raters for this study, all who were clinical psychologists or psychiatrists. Kappa coefficients for all of the items exceeded 0.80.

Patient demographic and legal class information were collected from system databases that are routinely used for census tracking. Data on aggressive incidents was collected through a computerized incident management system module of the patient treatment planning database. Within the hospital system, suicidal ideation and behavior are captured in two main areas for each patient. Suicidal ideation and behavior incidents within the hospital are collected from the computerized incident management system. In addition, a thorough lifetime suicidal ideation and behavior history is completed and recorded in a yearly

Table 27.1 Sociodemographic characteristics of the participants

	All patients 2011–2015		Chronic aggressors 2011–2015		X^2 (df = 1)
	n	%	n	%	
Male gender	20,257	85.9	24	80.0	0.86
Diagnosis					
Schizophrenia	17,416	73.9	20	66.6	0.80
Mood disorder	3,935	16.5	7	23.3	1.02
Personality disorder	5,392	22.9	13	43.3	7.11[a]
Cognitive disorder	2,790	11.8	21	70.0	79.34[b]
Ethnicity					
White	9,417	39.9	14	46.6	0.57
Black	6,782	28.8	7	23.3	0.43
Hispanic	5,792	24.6	8	26.6	0.07
Asian	6,79	2.9	1	3.0	0.02
	M	SD	M	SD	
Age	45.01	13.23	51.53	11.29	

[a] $p < 0.05$

[b] $p < 0.01$

suicide risk assessment that is completed by the patient's psychologist. For this study, both sources of information were reviewed for the presence of suicidal ideation or behavior and the presence of suicidal ideation was coded separately from suicidal behavior.

The rest of the variables were obtained from a chart review. Psychiatric diagnosis was recorded from the most recent note written by the treating psychiatrist. A patient was considered to have a cognitive disorder if according to the DSM-5, they had a Neurocognitive Disorder, Intellectual Disability, or Borderline Intellectual Functioning. The psychosocial history was obtained from the treating social worker's notes and demographic information was available in admission assessments.

The aggression databases were queried to obtain lists of patients having five or more aggressive acts for three years from 2011 to 2015. There were a total of 110 patients who met this definition of a chronic aggressor. Due to resource and time limitations, 30 were chosen at random for inclusion in the study. The 30 patients did not significantly differ from the 110 individuals on age ($p = 0.16$), gender ($p = 0.11$), race ($p = 0.90$), or length of stay within the hospital ($p = 0.28$). In order to find a comparison group, 30 patients who had not had any aggressive incidents while

hospitalized within the forensic hospital system were matched to the chronically aggressive group based on variables that have been shown in the literature to be related to aggression: age ±2 years,[17] gender,[18] and length of stay within the hospital.[3,19] It should be noted that patients were not matched on diagnosis. The long-term chronic aggressors and the nonaggressive controls were hospitalized at the same time (with no more than 100 days difference), however, the two groups were chosen from all five hospitals and the matched pairs were not necessarily at the same hospital. Each clinical variable was entered as either present or not present.

SPSS statistical package version 23 was used in completing statistical analyses. To determine if the sample was representative of the hospital system, chi square analyses were used to compare the sample to the population on diagnosis, gender, and ethnicity. Univariate analyses were conducted first to evaluate differences between groups on each variable of interest separately. Variables entered into the model were a history of suicidal behavior, current or previous diagnosis of a personality disorder, current or previous diagnosis of a cognitive disorder, history of psychiatric hospitalization as a juvenile, previous problems with employment, and current or previous diagnosis of a mood disorder. The multivariate analysis was a binary logistic regression, which was chosen because of its ability to use variables to classify cases into a dichotomous dependent variable. Variables were entered in the backwards LR approach to determine the most parsimonious model.

Results

Univariate and stepwise binary logistic regression analyses were run to test the contributions of a presence of history of a cognitive disorder, a history of suicidal behavior, history of hospitalization as a juvenile, presence or history of a mood disorder, presence or history of a personality disorder, and problems with employment in classifying a patient as long-term chronic aggressor or a control group.

The samples of long-term chronic aggressors were randomly selected from all of the long-term chronic aggressors from 2011 to 2015. The age of the sample (M = 51.53 years, SD = 11.29, CI: 47.49–55.57) was not significantly different from the entire sample of long-term chronic aggressors (M = 48.08 years, SD = 11.2), however, the sample of long-term chronic aggressors were statistically older than the hospital population (M = 45.01 years, SD = 13.23).

Univariate Results

Univariate results (Table 27.2) showed that long-term chronically aggressive patients were more likely to have a cognitive disorder than the nonaggressive controls (16.7%), $(x^2[1, N = 60] = 15.43, p < 0.001)$ with 70.0% of the long-term chronic aggressors having a cognitive disorder compared to 16.7% of the controls. In addition, 70.0% of patients had a history of suicidal behavior in the long-term chronically aggressive group compared to 33.3% of controls (66.7%, x^2 [1, N = 60] = 8.08, $p < 0.01$). Psychiatric hospitalization as a juvenile was present in 36.7% of the long-term chronic aggressors and 16.7% of the nonaggressive matched controls. In the univariate analysis, this difference approached significance $(p = 0.08)$.

Multivariate Results

Binary logistic regression was run with a stepwise backwards likelihood ratio entry method. All variables were tested for multicollinearity, with no substantial relationships. With all six variables, the full model correctly classified 80% of the cases. The final reduced model included two variables, Cognitive Disorder $(e^\beta = 10.64, p < 0.001)$ and Suicidal Behavior History $(e^\beta = 4.05, p = 0.03)$ and correctly classified 76.7% of the cases (Table 27.3). The first model and reduced model were compared with the Likelihood Ratio Statistic; there was no statistically significant difference between the full and reduced model. The loss of 3.3% of accuracy in classification was judged to be acceptable. Therefore, the most parsimonious reduced model was used to present these results.

Psychiatric hospitalization as a juvenile, presence of a personality disorder, and the presence of a mood disorder did not make unique contributions to the model and the results are listed in Table 27.3.

Table 27.2 Frequencies and chi square results

	Chronic aggressor n (%)	Control n (%)	x^2 (df = 1)
Diagnosis of personality disorder	13 (43.3)	7 (23.3)	2.70
History of suicidal behavior	21 (70.0)	10 (33.3)	8.08[a]
Cognitive impairment	21 (70.0)	5 (16.7)	15.43[b]
Sporadic employment	26 (86.7)	26 (86.7)	00
Diagnosis of psychosis	20 (66.7)	18 (60.0)	29
History of drug use	22 (73.3)	19 (63.3)	69
Psych hospitalization as juvenile	11 (36.7)	5 (16.7)	3.07

[a] $p < 0.01$
[b] $p < 0.001$

Table 27.3 Binary logistic regression

	Exp(B)	SE	95% CI for Exp(B)		
			p value	Lower	Upper
Cognitive disorder	10.64	66	00[a]	2.90	38.99
Suicidal behavior	4.05	63	03[b]	1.14	14.33

[a] $p < 0.01$
[b] $p < 0.05$

Discussion

Chronically aggressive patients have been a difficult group to study. One reason is the lack of a clear definition of chronic aggression. Definitions have been largely based on meeting a minimum number of aggressive incidents within a time frame, but in previous research the number of incidents and duration of time has varied greatly. In addition, there has been disagreement on whether to include aggression toward self, aggression toward property, or verbal aggression. The lack of a uniform definition has created a mixed clinical profile in the literature that has created problems when researching or developing clinical programs. The result has been a description of chronic aggressors that has varied across clinical, legal, and demographic factors and provided little help to researchers or clinicians aiming to treat these patients more effectively.

This study aimed to rectify the situation by providing a clearer definition of the term "chronic aggressor" and then applying it to patients in our psychiatric hospital system, to better identify targets of treatment. This study adds to the research on the chronically aggressive population by investigating the portion of chronically aggressive patients who have not only met a threshold for the number of incidents, but also met a consistency requirement (number of incidents per year for x amount of years). In addition, the authors also included a nonaggressive control group that was matched for age, gender, and length of stay within the hospital to reduce the effect of known correlates of aggression.

Results of the study identified cognitive disorders as the strongest predictor of the model. This result fits with several previous studies, which also identified cognitive disorders as a key characteristic of the chronic aggressor population.[4,11,13,16] Interestingly, similar to this research project, all of the studies that required 15 or more incidents of aggression found cognitive impairment to be a statistically significant finding.[4,11] Cognitive disorders can come from a variety of etiologies, but ultimately have the same effect of reducing a patient's ability to effectively reason, understand, and function in the world. Cognitive deficits arising from many etiologies are known to be long-term problems, if not lifelong problems. The length and consistency components of our study suggest that these long-term problems play a distinct role in this group of long-term chronic aggressors. Clinically this is important, because while many cognitive disorders have no known cure (e.g. Alzheimer's dementia), cognitive deficits stemming from other disorders have shown to respond to cognitive rehabilitation[20] (e.g. cognitive deficits resulting from severe mental illness).

A history of suicidal behavior was also a statistically significant variable in classifying the long-term chronic aggressors. Previous research has suggested that suicidal ideation or suicidal behavior were related to aggression toward others[4,12] with results that supported the inclusion of a suicidal behavior history variable in a classification model. Interestingly, in Lussier's[4] study, the results suggested that with increasing numbers of aggressive acts, the prevalence of all types of aggressive acts increased, including aggression toward self. The results of the Lussier[4] study, fit with the data from this study, where the presence of suicidal behavior was part of a model that was significantly able to classify between an aggressive and nonaggressive group.

Despite the significance of past suicidal behavior in discriminating between aggressive and nonaggressive groups, a diagnosis of a mood disorder was not significant in univariate or multivariate analyses. This relationship was also seen by Grube[21] who concluded that the exhibition of aggressive behavior is more to do with "disinhibited aggressive potential" and not a specific diagnosis, hypothesizing a neurological basis. Several studies have examined cognitive dysfunction in patients with suicidality and found deficits in executive functioning, attention, memory, and working memory.[22–24]

One interesting finding was that the long-term chronic aggressive patients were significantly older than the hospital population with the average age being 51.53 years. The majority of aggression research suggests that aggressors are much younger, finding a majority of chronic aggressors are in their 20s and 30s.[6,10,12,25,26] One study found that patients with 20 or more aggressive incidents within a seven-month time frame were significantly older, finding a mean age of 60.6. It is interesting to note, that the study by Owen et al.[11] and the current study both required a high number of incidents to be included, 20 and 15 respectively. This difference supports the argument for a subgroup of chronic aggressors that are characteristically different than chronic aggressors as a whole. It is possible that the inclusion requirement of at least three years of aggressive behavior skewed the sample to an older population but the study by Owen et al.[11] had a similar finding with only a seven-month duration.

In addition to a diagnosis of a mood disorder, other variables were investigated and found to not be significant: psychiatric hospitalization as a juvenile, a diagnosis of a personality disorder, and difficulties with employment. One reason for the lack of significance could be due to the inclusion criteria. Acts of aggression toward self, aggression toward property, and verbal aggression were not included as aggressive incidents. Employment problems were equally present within the group, which may suggest that the variable is more an outcome of severe mental illness as opposed to being directly related to aggression.

Conclusion

Based on the data from this study, results of the study showed that long-term chronic aggressors were older, had a cognitive disorder, and had a history of suicidal behavior. We hypothesize that these clinical and demographic variables might all have their roots in cognitive impairment. As people age, cognitive abilities are known to decline, patients with cognitive disorders would have more cognitive impairments by definition, and patients with a history of suicidal behavior have been shown to have deficits in several domains of cognitive functioning. While much is unknown, cognitive deficits appear to play a central role in patients with long-term chronic aggression.

The results of this study showed that presence of a cognitive disorder and a history of a suicidal behavior helped classify patients as either a long-term chronically aggressive patient or a nonaggressive patient. This research lends support to the idea that there are different types of chronic aggressive patients and that long-term chronically aggressive patients may look clinically different from other aggressors, labeled as "chronic" but whose aggressive period was of much shorter duration. Further research may look to replicate these results with a larger sample and prospectively look to determine if age, cognitive disorder, and suicidal behavior history can correctly predict patients who go on to become long-term chronic aggressors.

Clinically, it will be important to screen patients for these problems to identify patients who might be at risk for chronic aggression. A standard psychological intake, review of previous records, speaking with a family member, as well as a formal screening assessment of cognitive abilities could aid in identifying patients who would be at risk for long-term chronic aggression. While this study does not confirm that a cognitive disorder and a history of suicidal behavior

are the clinical factors that cause aggression, it is clinically reasonable to treat conditions that are related to aggression in this population. One promising treatment program for aggression in patients with cognitive deficits is the combination of cognitive remediation and social cognition treatments. Cognitive remediation is the set of treatments designed to improve a person's cognitive abilities and social cognition treatments are designed to improve a person's perceptions and interactions with other people. In a recent systematic review of literature,[27] the authors concluded cognitive remediation and social cognition treatments led to a reduction in aggressive attitudes and physical aggression. In addition to treatments to add, clinicians should carefully weigh the pros and cons of any treatments that could impair cognition. Medications that are known to impair cognition (e.g. anticholinergics and benzodiazepines) could further complicate a person's aggressive behaviors.

This study has several limitations that impact the conclusions. Data were collected retrospectively. We were not able to control for legal commitment and as such, we were comparing patients from one legal commitment to another. Other studies[12] have suggested the need for comparing them separately due to differences in housing and types of treatment available. Cognitive disorders were also combined into one group, which highlighted the clinical feature of cognitive deficits. However, there are a variety of etiologies of cognitive deficits and this study did not distinguish between the different etiologies for cognitive deficits including: traumatic brain injuries, developmental problems, severe mental illness, degenerative neurological conditions, and impoverished environments. Given the nature of the suicidal behavior data, we were not able to distinguish between subtypes of suicidal behavior or report a number of lifetime suicidal behaviors. We expect that having this type of information would improve the ability to understand the data.

Acknowledgments

We would like to thank the many people who were involved in making this study a reality. First, Katherine Warburton who has supported this project and gave us the resources to complete the study. Also, a special thank you to the clinicians who collected the data: George Proctor, Susan Velasquez, Laura Dardashti, Jennifer O'Day, Andrea Bauchowitz, Jonathan Meyer, Michael Cummings, Eric Schwartz, Charles Broderick, Darci Delgado, and Rebecca

Kornbluh. Further, we would like to acknowledge the help of Barbara McDermott and Sean Evans who consulted on key aspects of the study. Also, another thank you to Carl Seele and Angela Stoner, for helping us locate the literature we reviewed. Finally, we would like to thank Stephen Stahl for mentorship in conducting this research.

Disclosures

Benjamin Rose, Psy.D., ABPP, Darci Delgado, Psy.D., Charles Broderick, Ph.D., and Rebecca Kornbluh, M. D. have nothing to disclose. Stephen M. Stahl, M.D., Ph.D., is an Adjunct Professor of Psychiatry at the University of California San Diego, Honorary Visiting Senior Fellow at the University of Cambridge, UK, and Director of Psychopharmacology for California Department of State Hospitals. Over the past 36 months (January 2016–April 2019), Dr. Stahl has served as a consultant to Acadia, Adamas, Alkermes, Allergan, Arbor Pharmaceuticals, AstraZeneca, Avanir, Axovant, Axsome, Biogen, Biomarin, Biopharma, Celgene, Concert, ClearView, DepoMed, Dey, EnVivo, Ferring, Forest, Forum, Genomind, Innovative Science Solutions, Intra-Cellular Therapies, Janssen, Jazz, Lilly, Lundbeck, Merck, Neos, Novartis, Noveida, Orexigen, Otsuka, Pam Labs, Perrigo, Pfizer, Pierre Fabre, Reviva, Servier, Shire, Sprout, Sunovion, Taisho, Takeda, Taliaz, Teva, Tonix, Trius, Vanda, and Vifopharma; He has been a board member to RCT Logic and Genomind; he has served on speakers bureaus for Acadia, Astra Zeneca, Dey Pharma, EnVivo, Eli Lilly, Forum, Genentech, Janssen, Lundbeck, Merck, Otsuka, Pam Labs, Pfizer Israel, Servier, Sunovion, and Takeda, and he has received research and/or grant support from Acadia, Alkermes, Arbor Pharmaceuticals, AssureX, AstraZeneca, Avanir, Axovant, Biogen, Braeburn Pharmaceuticals, Bristol Myer Squibb, Celgene, CeNeRx, Cephalon, Dey, Eli Lilly, EnVivo, Forest, Forum, Genomind, GlaxoSmithKline, Intra-Cellular Therapies, ISSWSH, Janssen, JayMac, Jazz, Lundbeck, Merck, Mylan, Neurocrine, Neuronetics, Novartis, Otsuka, Pam Labs, Pfizer, Reviva, Roche, Sepracor, Servier, Shire, Sprout, Sunovion, TMS NeuroHealth Centers, Takeda, Teva, Tonix, Vanda, Valeant, and Wyeth.

References

1. Broderick C, Azizian A, Kornbluh R, Warburton KD. Prevalence of physical violence in a forensic psychiatric hospital system during 2011–2013: patient assaults, staff assaults, and repeatedly violent patients. In: Warburton KD, Stahl SM, eds. *Violence in Psychiatry*. New York, NY: Cambridge University Press; 2016: 49–63.

2. Daffern M, Mayer MM, Martin T. A preliminary investigation into patterns of aggression in an Australian forensic psychiatric hospital. *J Forens Psychiatry Psychol*. 2003; **14**(1): 67–84.

3. Arango C, Calcedo Barba A, Gonzalez S, Calcedo Ordonez A. Violence in inpatients with schizophrenia: a prospective study. *Schizophr Bull*. 1999; **25**(3): 493–503.

4. Lussier P, Verdun-Jones S, Deslauriers-Varin N, Nicholls T, Brink J. Chronic violent patients in an inpatient psychiatric hospital: prevalence, description, and identification. *Crim Justice Behav*. 2010; **37**(1): 5–28.

5. Daffern M, Howells K, Ogloff J. Interaction between individual characteristic and the function of aggression in forensic psychiatric inpatients. *Psychiatry Psychol Law*. 2007; **14**(1): 17–25.

6. Barlow K, Grenyer B, Ilkiw-Lavalle O. Prevalence and precipitants of aggression in psychiatric inpatient units. *Aust N Z J Psychiatry*. 2000; **34**(6): 967–974.

7. Bjorkly S. A ten-year prospective study of aggression in a special secure unit for dangerous patients. *Scand J Psychol*. 1999; **40**(1): 57–63.

8. Decaire MW, Bedard M, Riendeau J, Forrest R. Incidents in a psychiatric forensic setting: association with patient and staff characteristics. *Can J Nurs Res*. 2006; **38**(3): 69–80.

9. Flannery RB, Jr. Repetitively assaultive psychiatric patients: review of published findings, 1978–2001. *Psychiatr Q*. 2002; **73**(3): 229–237.

10. Cooper SJ, Browne FW, McClean KJ, King DJ. Aggressive behaviour in a psychiatric observation ward. *Acta Psychiatr Scand*. 1983; **68**(5): 386–393.

11. Owen C, Tarantello C, Jones M, Tennant C. Violence and aggression in psychiatric units. *Psychiatr Serv*. 1998; **49**(11): 1452–1457.

12. Bader SM, Evans SE. Predictors of severe and repeated aggression in a maximum-security forensic psychiatric hospital. *Int J Forensic Ment Health*. 2015; **14**(2): 110–119.

13. Krakowski M, Czobor P. Violence in psychiatric patients: the role of psychosis, frontal lobe impairment, and ward turmoil. *Comp Psychiatry*. 1997; **38**(4): 230–236.

14. Krakowski MI, Convit A, Volavka J. Patterns of inpatient assaultiveness: effect of neurological impairment and deviant family environment on response to treatment. *Neuropsychiatry Neuropsychol Behav Neurol*. 1988; **1**(1): 21–29.

15. Langton CM, Hogue TE, Daffern M, Mannion A, Howells K. Personality traits as predictors of inpatient aggression in a high-security forensic psychiatric setting: prospective evaluation of the PCL-R and IPDE dimension ratings. *Int J Offender Ther Comp Criminol.* 2011; **55**(3): 392–415.

16. Kraus JE, Sheitman BB. Characteristics of violent behavior in a large state psychiatric hospital. *Psychiatr Serv.* 2004; **55**(2): 183–185.

17. Gudjonsson G, Rabe-Hesketh S, Wilson C. Violent incidents on a medium secure unit over a 17-year period. *J Forensic Psychiatry.* 1999; **10**(2): 249–263.

18. Staniloiu A, Markowitsch H. Gender differences in violence and aggression – a neurobiological perspective *Procedia.* 2012; **33**: 1032–1036.

19. Barnard GW, Robbins L, Newman G, Carrera F. A study of violence within a forensic treatment facility. *Bull Am Acad Psychiatry Law.* 1984; **12**(4): 339–348.

20. Best MW, Bowie CR. A review of cognitive remediation approaches for schizophrenia: from top-down to bottom-up, brain training to psychotherapy. *Expert Rev Neurother.* 2017; **17**(7): 713–723.

21. Grube M. Which types of aggressive behaviour are associated with suicidal and self-injurious behaviour at the time of admission? *Psychopathology.* 2004; **37** (1): 41–49.

22. Jollant F, Lawrence NL, Olié E, Guillaume S, Courtet P. The suicidal mind and brain: a review of neuropsychological and neuroimaging studies. *World J Biol Psychiatry.* 2011; **12**(5–6): 319–339.

23. Bredemeier K, Miller IW. Executive function and suicidality: a systematic qualitative review. *Clin Psychol Rev.* 2015; **40**: 170–183.

24. Keilp JG, Gorlyn M, Russell M, et al. Neuropsychological function and suicidal behavior: attention control, memory and executive dysfunction in suicide attempt. *Psychol Med.* 2013; **43**(3): 539–551.

25. Hoptman MJ, Yates KF, Patalinjug MB, Wack RC, Convit A. Clinical prediction of assaultive behavior among male psychiatric patients at a maximum-security forensic facility. *Psychiatr Serv.* 1999; **50**(11): 1461–1466.

26. Tardiff K. A survey of five types of dangerous behavior among chronic psychiatric patients. *Bull Am Acad Psychiatry Law.* 1982; **10**(3): 177–182.

27. Darmedru C, Demily C, Franck N. Cognitive remediation and social cognitive training for violence in schizophrenia: a systematic review. *Psychiatry Res.* 2017; **251**: 266–274.

Tipping the Scales of Justice: The Role of Forensic Evaluations in the Criminalization of Mental Illness

Katherine E. McCallum and W. Neil Gowensmith

Introduction

For psychologists or psychiatrists conducting forensic evaluations, a forensic psychological report is a work product – one of many reports they will author over the course of their careers. Many forensic evaluators conduct a large number of evaluations per year; for example, Colorado state evaluators conduct an average of 144 competency to stand trial (CST) evaluations per year.[1] For psychologists or psychiatrists who author a large volume of evaluations, some cases may seem routine. Evaluators may fall into a pattern in which many evaluations appear mundane and typical.

However, for the individual being evaluated, each report holds a tremendous amount of influence. Forensic evaluations cover a wide swath of psycholegal referral questions, and they carry a great deal of influence over the lives of those under evaluation. Although forensic evaluators are not triers of fact, judicial decisions are overwhelmingly correlated to opinions of forensic evaluators;[2] studies have shown that judges follow the opinions of evaluators in 76%–99% of cases.[3–6] These opinions can be far-reaching. For example, evaluations of adjudicative competency or sanity can influence whether a defendant is temporarily detained in a correctional facility, hospital, or released to the community – and they may also ultimately lead to charges being dismissed.[7] Criminal responsibility evaluations can provide the tipping point between acquittal and hospital commitment versus a guilty verdict and imprisonment.[8] Other forensic mental health evaluations may influence whether a parent maintains custody of his/her child, a person is released from a locked facility, a teenager is tried as an adult, a confession is valid, or a plaintiff receives monetary awards. In capital cases, a forensic mental health evaluation can influence whether a defendant is executed.

In addition to the impact on the individual, forensic evaluations have systemic impact. Forensic evaluations that are not conducted within a certain time period can result in a backlog of cases. Many states are currently in the throes of federal lawsuits centered around these delays in evaluation time frames, as defendants with mental illnesses languish in county jails awaiting their evaluations.[9,10] However, when evaluations are conducted too quickly, emerging research shows that forensic opinions are often subject to inaccuracies.[11,12] Further, the quality of reports from state evaluators has been shown to be of mediocre quality in some settings.[13] Reports of poor quality can result in appeals or second opinion requests, compounding the backlog even more. Finally, a great deal of research demonstrates that many evaluators are biased by multiple internal and external factors.[14–24] Biased, unreliable, or low quality forensic mental health evaluations deteriorate the fairness of the justice system overall. Given the important systemic and individual impacts of forensic evaluations, it is critical that they are efficient, valid, reliable, and held to high standards of quality. However, an accumulating body of literature suggests that the efficiency, validity, reliability, and quality of these reports have substantial room for improvement.

Efficiency

Efficiency of conducting forensic evaluations is specifically relevant to CST evaluations, the most frequently ordered mental health evaluations by criminal courts.[25] Courts order an estimated 25,634–51,500 CST evaluations each year nationally, varying from fewer than 50 to approximately 5,000 per year in individual states.[26,27] Numbers of evaluations continue to increase annually. For example, CST evaluations in Wisconsin increased 32.5% from 2010 through 2015,[28] while evaluations in Washington increased 76.3% from 2001 through 2012.[29] Colorado reported a 206% increase in the number of CST evaluations from 2005 to 2014,[30] and Los Angeles County reported a 273% increase from 2010 to

2015.[31] Unsurprisingly, this burgeoning need for CST evaluations has led to long waitlists for evaluations, as states across the nation have struggled to keep pace with the rapid growth of demand. Some states have reported waitlists of more than a year for CST evaluations to be conducted, and several other states are operating under federal or state oversight to ensure that evaluation wait times are reasonable.[10,32] Class action lawsuits in the states of Oregon and Washington successfully lobbied for shorter wait times for CST evaluations and access to competency restoration services.[33,34] Other states are grappling with consent decrees, lawsuits, and legislation on the issue (e.g. Alabama, Colorado, Pennsylvania, Nevada, and California).

Some legislation has resulted in specified time frames for evaluations to be completed. The national average number of days from court order to evaluation report date is 31 days.[32] However, there is considerable variability in these time frames. Oregon and Maryland require CST reports within 7 days, North Carolina has a 10-day time frame for defendants awaiting evaluations in jail, Washington has a 14-daytime limit, and Rhode Island mandates reports within 15 days. Alternatively, several states (Arkansas, Kansas, Missouri, Montana, among others) extend the deadline to 60 days, while 15 states have no statutorily defined time frame at all. Evaluation time frames are currently being adjusted in several states to accommodate the increasing demand for CST evaluations; Colorado's current Consent Decree will decrease the current 28-day time frame for evaluations to 21 days in 2020.[1]

Decreasing these CST evaluation time frames may seem like a good solution to long waitlists for these evaluations. Hiring more evaluators to conduct evaluations more quickly certainly ensures that defendants will be evaluated more quickly. However, emerging research suggests that systems may experience unintended negative consequences if evaluations are conducted *too* quickly.

Most CST evaluators find between 20% and 40% of defendants incompetent to stand trial (IST).[35] However, recent data show that the timing of CST evaluations has a substantial impact on evaluators' opinions. Hawaii data indicate that IST rates were nearly 40% higher in evaluations conducted within seven days of the court order than those conducted beyond seven days.[12] Washington shows a 50% IST rate for CST evaluations conducted within seven days,[34] as does the state of Maryland.[36] This trend seems to be especially true for defendants with psychotic and substance use diagnoses.

Defendants found IST within seven days in the Hawaii sample were more likely to have substance-related and/or psychotic disorders. Additionally, data from a large dataset in Texas show that the rate of IST opinions rose approximately 25% in defendants with a schizophrenia spectrum diagnosis or a substance related disorder when evaluations were completed within 10 days of the court order.[11,37] It seems that quick turnaround time frames for CST evaluations may artificially inflate the numbers of IST opinions in some cases.

Aside from the effects of quick turnaround evaluation on the accuracy of individual competency opinions, these aggressive time frames may also have systemic effects. If courts and attorneys are assured that they will receive CST opinions within 1–15 days, they may in turn request them more often. Paradoxically, shorter time frames for evaluations may incentivize courts and attorneys to order them more frequently – increasing referral numbers, evaluator caseloads, and ultimately defendant wait times. No data are available currently to monitor this possibility; however, Oregon and Washington's recent drastic reductions in evaluation time frames would provide a good naturalistic opportunity to review CST evaluation referral rates, evaluator opinion rates, and systemic effects on wait times.

Quality

The forensic evaluator has considerable influence in how information is included and presented to the court. A quality forensic evaluation is not only defined by good grammar, syntax, and readability, but also the inclusion of critical elements and a well-supported answer to the psycholegal question posed. Poorly written reports could result in a myriad of negative consequences, such as an increasing need for second opinions, compounding the problems noted above. Further, providing the trier of fact with inaccurate or incomplete information risks an unfair trial process.

Several reviews of forensic evaluations have revealed deficits in report quality. Robinson and Acklin found that many critical components, such as historical information, collateral information, or a rationale for the forensic opinion, were not included in 150 CST reports, resulting in an overall "poor" quality rating.[14] A similar review of 150 conditional release reports from Hawaii found that evaluators documented informed consent in only half (52%) of reports and provided a rationale for their opinion of dangerousness in only 34.7% of reports.[13] Skeem et al. found that CST evaluators in

Utah rarely linked the defendant's clinical presentation to the forensic opinion and rarely explained their rationale for arriving at that opinion.[38]

The rising demand for CST evaluations can further threaten the quality of reports by pressuring state systems to widen the pool of qualified evaluators. However, the discipline of the evaluator likely has less influence on report quality than requisite training. Originally, criminal courts only qualified psychiatrists as forensic experts before slowly including psychologists.[39] Despite early concerns about report quality of psychologists, no substantive differences in report quality have consistently been found between disciplines.[40,41] However, both psychiatry and psychology have developed an infrastructure of forensic specialty training through pre- and post-doctoral programs, dedicated subspecialty professional organizations, and high-impact forensic journals.[9] This training and infrastructure is crucial for evaluators to attain minimum quality standards, as forensic evaluations are often complicated, requiring evaluators to consider difficult psychological, legal, and cultural nuances.[15,17,42–44] Simply expanding the pool of eligible evaluator disciplines runs the serious risk of experts offering poorly formulated opinions, unless enough forensic training and infrastructure within that discipline exists.

Reliability

When a psychological evaluation is used in either criminal or civil court, it is expected to be objective and reliable. In admitting either psychiatric or psychological testimony, courts consider factors established by the *Daubert* decision, such as whether it is scientifically valid, whether the "theory or technique can be (and has been) tested," and whether there is a "known potential rate of error."[45] Several scholars have argued psychiatric and psychological testimony do not meet this standard, citing a lack of available base rates, errors in clinical decision-making, and a range of theories too diverse and inconsistent to result in reliable opinions.[23,24] Of course, psychiatric and psychological testimony continued to be present in courtrooms despite these criticisms. In the time since, literature has only accumulated regarding threats to reliability of forensic opinions.

Variability between forensic evaluators is concerningly high. In a sample of 59 evaluators who conducted a total of 4,498 evaluations of legal sanity, 7 evaluators opined the individual was sane in 100% of their evaluations, whereas 3 evaluators opined the individual was sane in 50% of their evaluations.[21] In a sample of 15 evaluators who each completed at least 100 CST evaluations, rates of incompetency findings ranged from 1.7% to 27.9%.[20] Similar discrepancies among evaluators have also been found in the use of forensic assessment instruments. For example, Boccaccini, Turner, and Murrie found that some evaluators assigned consistently higher scores on the PCL-R compared to other evaluators.[46]

This variability may simply be caused by differences between evaluators and the sometimes subjective nature of interpreting statutory language of mental health law. For example, one psychologist may have a higher decision threshold for determining a defendant's "*sufficient* present ability to consult with his lawyer with a *reasonable* degree of rational understanding" (emphasis added).[47] Indeed, Mossman found individual differences in decision thresholds between evaluators in CST evaluations.[48] Though he acknowledged individual differences in feelings and beliefs may contribute to differences in decision thresholds, he also discussed several other influencing variables, such as internal and external expectations and conventions in specific agencies, knowledge of local judicial decision-making trends, or differing understandings of constructs underlying adjudicative competence.

A now well-established threat to reliability is bias of the evaluator toward the side that retained his/her services.[15,17,19] This "adversarial allegiance" effect is present even when evaluators score objective, structured risk assessments designed to mitigate subjective bias.[49] Earlier research has suggested evaluators' opinions are also influenced by the fees they earn.[23,24,50] Additionally, research has found discrepancies in evaluator opinions related to the racial and/or ethnic background of the defendant.[16,18,22] Clearly, these threats to the reliability of forensic opinions must be addressed if evaluations are to reach the highest standards of objectivity and neutrality. The reliability of evaluator opinions is surprisingly low across nearly all psycholegal referral questions,[51] most likely for many of the reasons articulated previously. However, this poor reliability can cause differential and undue harm to certain defendants. Defendants of color, for example, should not be routinely found IST more often than Caucasian defendants; unfortunately, some scholars have shown this to be true in some samples.[16,18] If race or skin color is truly a differential factor for some CST evaluators, then the notion of objective and reliable opinions is clearly tainted. The final forensic opinion (and subsequent judicial adjudication) should not depend on race, skin color, fees, the individual evaluator, or any other idiosyncratic factors. However, if the realities of implicit and explicit bias – as well as other factors related to low reliability across evaluators – are not adequately addressed, then some subpopulations of persons being forensically evaluated may be at risk for injustice.

Validity

The above reliability concerns undoubtedly undermine the validity of forensic evaluations. Unfortunately, research evaluating the accuracy of forensic opinions in the field is substantially lacking because the ground truth is often unknown.[52] Forensic evaluators typically never know if they "got it right" with their opinion, but some research has attempted to measure the accuracy of forensic psychologists. In 2010, Mossman et al. found impressively high accuracy in five forensic evaluators asked to review redacted court reports and provide CST opinions.[53] However, the evaluators provided opinions on a graded scale, rather than a binary one typical for most CST evaluations (competent or not). Though the finding may be encouraging to some, the incredible variability of forensic evaluator opinions summarized above suggests that validity is likely much poorer in the field. Agreement between evaluators intuitively seems to lead to greater accuracy and evidence seems to support this. In Hawaii, when three evaluators evaluated the same defendant for conditional release and unanimously opined release was appropriate, most evaluators "got it right"; about 74% accurately predicted those who would be rehospitalized within three years. Interestingly, agreement of evaluators in their predictions was important. In cases in which three evaluators independently opined in favor of release, only 29.6% of defendants were rehospitalized – compared to a 71.4% rehospitalization rate in cases in which evaluators disagreed as to the person's readiness for release.[54]

Corrective Strategies

Forensic evaluations play an important role in the due process of adjudicating criminal cases with mental health components. Poor forensic standards can unwittingly collude with discriminatory social and judicial practices, such that certain defendants undergoing poor evaluation practices may be more likely to be found competent, sane, dangerous, and so on. It is critical that forensic evaluations provide the court with objective, comprehensive, and accurate information so that the court can utilize the data and opinions in a just manner. Although we have outlined several potential areas in which evaluations can be misused, we now turn to potential mechanisms to mitigate against these threats to evaluation reliability, validity, and quality.

Ensuring High-Quality Evaluations

One possible strategy to improve quality and reliability is training and certification of forensic evaluators.

Approximately half of the states in the US have implemented formal certification processes for psychologists to conduct CST evaluations.[40] In Hawaii, forensic psychologists and psychiatrists who attended a three-day certification training subsequently showed improvement in the quality and reliability of their CST evaluations.[14,55] However, much more research examining the outcomes of these training is needed to truly assess effectiveness.[9] The use of a peer-reviewed evaluation report system can also be used to identify evaluation areas or specific evaluators that need improvement. Although little empirical evidence exists as to the incremental utility of standardized training and peer reviews of reports, it seems safe to assume that high-quality training, and maintenance of high standards among evaluators and their work, will guard against the misuse of forensic evaluations in many contexts.

Evaluation Parameters

The amount of time allotted to complete forensic evaluations appears to matter. Completing evaluations too quickly may lead to inflated rates of incompetent findings among CST evaluations.[11,12,38] However, completing evaluations too slowly can lead to defendants experiencing unconstitutional wait times in jail.[9] To strike a balance, The National Judicial College recommends that CST evaluations be conducted within 15 to 30 days of the initial court order.[56] Although more research is needed to fully assess the optimal time frame of forensic evaluations, the current evidence suggests 15 to 30 may be ideal.[9] In addition to time frames, other conditions of evaluations may affect quality. The ideal testing environment for psychological testing (quiet, uninterrupted time, enough working space, few distractions) is often inaccessible in correctional facilities. Although flexibility is important, evaluators must be willing to require minimally acceptable assessment standards within correctional facilities, lest their evaluation results be potentially tainted.

Even with the ideal evaluation parameters in place, proficient evaluators are paramount in ensuring improved report quality. Creating and maintaining an infrastructure of training and certification of forensic evaluators is a critical step. Additionally, reasonable workloads and competitive salaries will also bolster a workforce of capable evaluators.

Identifying and Mitigating Potential Bias

Employing strategies to identify and mitigate against internal and external evaluation biases is important in ensuring optimal levels of evaluation reliability and validity. Self-monitoring should be a systematic, consistent process for evaluators. However, not all self-monitoring processes are created equal; selecting effective mechanisms is critical. Humans are simply not adept at monitoring their own biases through introspection.[57] Evaluators, like all people, are not only prone to the effects of bias but also to the "bias blind spot" – an insidious phenomenon in which people do not recognize their own biases.[58] Therefore, simply looking in the metaphorical mirror to check one's biases is rarely effective.

Instead, following social psychology's tenets, evaluators should use objective, measurable data to guide the identification and mitigation of biases.[59] For example, evaluators could collect and analyze data from their own evaluations to assess measurable outcomes. Brodsky suggested practitioners can use such a database to measure their own objectivity.[60,61] Some practitioners who have engaged in such self-studies have found surprising and illuminating results.[16,62] Further, if self-monitoring were a standard of practice and data were aggregated across evaluators and settings, we would have far richer information about base rates of opinions in relation to a myriad of potentially significant factors (i.e. geographic locations, relationships to attorneys, fees, workplace environments).

Such an approach can be an especially valuable tool in mitigating the criminalization of mental illness in the forensic evaluation context. If robust data are captured on all forensic evaluations submitted to the court (even, for example, within a state-employed forensic evaluator pool), analyses could illuminate areas of potential discrimination or differentiation.

Certain jurisdictions might be found to refer a high number of spurious cases. Specific evaluators may have unreasonable thresholds for psycholegal criteria. Perhaps defendants from certain races may be found more dangerous than those from other races. Perhaps fees, the referring attorney, or the setting in which evaluations are conducted lead to differential rates of opinions. This sort of data would be tremendously informative in ensuring that systemic biases are identified and addressed in a practical and tangible way, optimizing the reliability and validity of the forensic evaluation process. In doing so, the evaluation process would be less likely to be an unintentional contributor to the criminalization of persons with mental illness.

Conclusions

An unprecedented number of people with mental illness are being funneled to the criminal court in order to access mental health care. Jails and court dockets are increasingly overwhelmed with cases involving mental illness, state hospitals devote far more beds and resources to forensic cases, and people without a criminal commitment are increasingly left waiting for mental health services as forensic cases are prioritized. Each component of the forensic mental health process likely plays a role in maintaining this trend. However, some forensic evaluators appear to operate in a figurative vacuum, assuming that their roles have little impact on the criminalization of people with mental illness; after all, evaluators do not arrest people, raise forensic referral questions, order evaluations, or make any final judicial decisions. However, poorly conducted forensic evaluations can indeed exacerbate the criminalization of persons with mental illness in many ways. Evaluations that suffer from poor reliability, low quality, or evaluator biases can extend criminal commitments unnecessarily, cause delays in the resolution of the case, or posit inaccurate opinions. Research is consistent that evaluation reliability, quality, validity, and accuracy all have room for improvement. In addition, forensic evaluations are inevitably vulnerable to errors and bias, as is all human decision-making. However, when the stakes for individuals and systems are so high, forensic evaluators should always strive for the highest standards. As a field and as individual evaluators, this will involve examining ourselves and our field objectively, ensuring that the standards for our evaluators and our field are as high as possible.

Disclosures

Katherine McCallum and W. Neil Gowensmith report that they have developed an app for mobile phones that allows forensic evaluators to track base rates of forensic opinions. One of the uses of the app is to identify and mitigate against bias. In the current article, the authors encourage practicing forensic evaluators to keep track of their base rates, variables that could affect opinions, and so on. Although the authors do not highlight their app in the current article, and although several options for identifying and mitigating bias were provided, Dr. McCallum and Dr. Gowensmith both state that some readers might equate the recommendation that evaluators monitor their work for bias with the authors' financial interest in the mobile app. To be clear, their ultimate goal is to encourage evaluators to monitor their work reliably and carefully, regardless of methodologies used.

References

1. *Center for Legal Advocacy v. Bicha et al.*, U.S. District Court of Colorado, Case No. 1:2011cv02285. 2011.

2. Redding RE, Murrie DC. Judicial decision making about forensic mental health evidence. In: Goldstein AM, ed. *Forensic Psychology: Emerging Topics and Expanding Roles.* Hoboken, NJ: John Wiley & Sons Inc; 2007: 683–707.

3. Acklin MW, Fuger K, Gowensmith WN. Examiner agreement and judicial consensus in forensic mental health evaluations. *J Forensic Psychol Pract.* 2015; **15**(4): 318–343.

4. Gowensmith WN, Murrie DC, Boccaccini MT. Field reliability of competence to stand trial opinions: how often do evaluators agree, and what do judges decide when evaluators disagree? *Law Hum Behav.* 2012; **36**(2): 130–139.

5. Zapf PA, Hubbard KL, Cooper VG, et al. Have the courts abdicated their responsibility for determination of competency to stand trial to clinicians? *J Forensic Psychol Pract.* 2004; **4**(1): 27–44.

6. Cruise KR, Rogers R. An analysis of competency to stand trial: an integration of case law and clinical knowledge. *Behav Sci Law.* 1998; **16**(1): 35–50.

7. Mowen E. Charges dismissed in crash which claimed family. *Register Herald.* July 7, 2018. www.registerherald.com/news/22514/charges-dismissed-in-crash-which-claimed-family (accessed June 2020).

8. Eaton E. Man who killed Elmendorf police chief found not guilty by reason of insanity. *San Antonio Express News.* July 2, 2018. www.expressnews.com/news/local/article/Man-who-killed-Elemendorf-police-chief-found-not-13044383.php (accessed June 2020).

9. Gowensmith WN. Resolution or resignation: the role of forensic mental health professionals amidst the competency services crisis. *Psychol Public Policy Law.* 2019; **25**(1): 1–14.

10. Locklair B. Due process problems with civil commitment of incompetent defendants: the current round of litigation and the next. Presentation to the American Psychology-Law Society annual conference; 2016, Atlanta, GA.

11. Bryson CN, Boccaccini MT, Gowensmith WN, et al. Does time matter in competency to stand trial evaluations? Presentation to the annual meeting of the American Psychology-Law Society; March 2019, Portland, OR.

12. Gowensmith WN, Metroz H, Bratcher J. The impact of timing on competency to stand trial evaluations. Presentation to the annual meeting of the American Psychology-Law Society; March 2016, Atlanta, GA.

13. Nguyen AH, Acklin MW, Fuger K, et al. Freedom in paradise: quality of conditional release reports submitted to the Hawaii judiciary. *Int J Law Psychiatry.* 2011; **34**(5): 341–348.

14. Robinson R, Acklin MW. Fitness in paradise: quality of forensic reports submitted to the Hawaii judiciary. *Int J Law Psychiatry.* 2010; **33**: 131–137.

15. Boccaccini, MT, Chevalier CS, Murrie DC, et al. Psychopathy – checklist revised use and reporting practices in sexually violent predator evaluations. *Sex Abuse.* 2017; **29**(6): 592–614.

16. Parker G. Come see the bias inherent in the system! *J Am Acad Psychiatry Law.* 2016; **44**(4): 411–414.

17. Chevalier CS, Boccaccini MT, Murrie DC, et al. Static-99R reporting practices in sexually violent predator cases: does norm selection reflect adversarial allegiance? *Law Hum Behav.* 2015; **39**(3): 209–218.

18. McCallum KE, MacLean N, Gowensmith WN. The impact of defendant ethnicity on the psycho-legal opinion of forensic evaluators. *Int J Law Psychiatry.* 2014; **39**: 6–12.

19. Murrie DC, Boccaccini MT, Guarnera LA, et al. Are forensic experts biased by the side that retained them? *Psychol Sci.* 2013; **24**(10): 1889–1897.

20. Murrie DC, Boccaccini M, Zapf PA, et al. Clinician variation in findings of competence to stand trial. *Psychol Public Policy Law.* 2008; **14**: 177–193.

21. Murrie DC, Warren JI. Clinician variation in rates of legal sanity opinions: implications for self-monitoring. *Prof Psychol.* 2005; **36**: 519–524.

22. Hagen MA. *Whores of the Court: the Fraud of Psychiatric Testimony and the Rape of American Justice.* New York, NY, US: Harper Collins Publishers; 1997.

23. Bergeron ML. The use of psychiatric expertise in the forensic context: balm or blunder. *Windsor Yearb Access Justice.* 1994; **14**: 221.

24. Faust D, Ziskin J. The expert witness in psychology and psychiatry. *Science.* 1988; **241**(4861): 31–35.

25. Melton GB, Petrila J, Poythress NG, et al. *Psychological Evaluations for the Courts: A Handbook for Mental Health Professionals and Lawyers, 3rd edn.* New York, NY: The Guilford Press; 2007.

26. Warren JI, Chuahan P, Kois L, et al. Factors influencing 2260 opinions of defendants' restorability to adjudicative competency. *Psychol Public Policy Law.* 2013; **19**: 498–508.

27. Fitch WL. *Assessment #3. Forensic mental health services in the United States: 2014. (Report No. 3, HHSS2834200IT).* Alexandria, VA: National Association of State Mental Health Program Directors; 2014.

28. Wisconsin Department of Health Services. *2015 annual report. (Report No. P-00568).* Madison, WI: Wisconsin Department of Health Services; 2015.

29. Joint Legislative and Audit Review Committee. *State of Washington Final Report: Competency to stand trial, phase II (Report No. 14–1).* Olympia, WA: Joint Legislative and Audit Review Committee; 2014.

30. Colorado Department of Human Services Office of Behavioural Health. Needs analysis: current status, strategic positioning, and future planning. Western Interstate Commission for Higher Education Mental Health Program; April 2015.

31. Sewall A. L.A. County supervisors order report on unexplained surge in mental competency cases. *Los Angeles Times*; March 8, 2016. www.latimes.com/loc al/lanow/la-me-ln-mental-competency-cases-201603 08-story.html (accessed June 2020).

32. Gowensmith WN, Murrie DC, Packer IK. *Report in Response to the Trueblood v. State Washington's Department of Social and Health Services.* Olympia, WA: Office of Attorney General, State of Washington; 2015.

33. *Oregon Advocacy Center v. Mink.* No. 02–35530, 9th Cir.; 2003.

34. *Trueblood v. State of Washington Department of Human and Social Services.* No. 2:2014cv01178, Washington Western District Court; 2015.

35. Pirelli G, Gottdiener WH, Zapf PA. A meta-analytic review of competency to stand trial research. *Psychol Public Policy Law.* 2011; **17**(1): 1–53.

36. Roskes, personal communication, December 12, 2014.

37. Bryson CN, Boccaccini MT, Gowensmith WN, et al. Time matters in competency to stand trial evaluations. Presentation to the American Psychology-Law Society annual meeting; March 2018, Memphis, TN.

38. Skeem JL, Golding SL, Cohn NB, et al. Logic and reliability of evaluations of competence to stand trial. *Law Hum Behav.* 1998; **22**(5): 519–547.

39. Gowensmith WN, Pinals DA, Karas AC. States' standards for training and certifying evaluators of competency to stand trial. *J Forensic Psychol Pract.* 2015; **15**(4): 295–317.

40. Petrella RC, Poythress NG. The quality of forensic evaluations: an interdisciplinary study. *J Consult Clin Psychol.* 1983; **51**(1): 76–85.

41. Poythress NG, Otto RK, Heilbrun K. Pretrial evaluations for criminal courts: contemporary models of service delivery. *J Ment Health Adm.* 1991; **18**: 198–208.

42. Kois L, Pearson J, Chauhan P, et al. Competency to stand trial among female inpatients. *Law Hum Behav*, 2013; **37**(4): 231–240.

43. Mossman D, Noffsinger SG, Ash P, et al. AAPL practice guideline for the forensic psychiatric evaluation of competence to stand trial. *J Am Acad Psychiatry Law.* 2007; **35**: S3–S72.

44. Pinals DA, Tillbrook CE, Mumley DL. Practical application of the MacArthur competence assessment tool – criminal adjudication (MacCAT-CA) in a public sector forensic setting. *J Am Acad Psychiatry Law* 2006; **34**: 179–188.

45. *Daubert v. Merrell Dow Pharmaceuticals, Inc.*, 405 U.S. 597 (1993).

46. Boccaccini MT, Turner D, Murrie DC. Do some evaluators report consistently higher or lower psychopathy scores than others?: findings from a state wide sample of sexually violent predator evaluations. *Psychol Public Policy Law.* 2008; **14**: 262–283.

47. *Dusky v. United States*, 362 U.S. 402 (1960).

48. Mossman D. When forensic examiners disagree: bias, or just inaccuracy? *Psychol Public Policy Law.* 2013; **19** (1): 40–55.

49. Murrie DC, Boccaccini MT, Turner D, et al. Rater (dis)agreement on risk assessment measures in sexually violent predator proceedings: evidence of adversarial allegiance in forensic evaluation? *Psychol Public Policy Law.* 2009; **15**: 19–53.

50. Callahan LA, Silver E. Factors associated with the conditional release of persons acquitted by reason of insanity: a decision tree approach. *Law Hum Behav.* 1998; **22**: 147–163.

51. Gowensmith WN, Murrie DC, Boccaccini MT. Field reliability of competence to stand trial opinions: how often do evaluators agree, and what do judges decide when evaluators disagree? *Law Hum Behav.* 2012; **36** (2): 130–139.

52. Dror IE, Murrie DC. A hierarchy of expert performance applied to forensic psychological assessments. *Psychol Public Policy Law.* 2018; **24**(1): 11–23.

53. Mossman D, Bowen MD, Vanness DJ, et al. Quantifying the accuracy of forensic examiners in the absence of a "gold standard". *Law Hum Behav.* 2010; **34**(5): 402–417.

54. Gowensmith WN, Murrie DC, Boccaccini MT, et al. Field reliability influences field validity: risk assessments of individuals found not guilty by reason of insanity. *Psychol Assess.* 2017; **29**(6): 786–794.

55. Gowensmith WN, Sledd M, Sessarego S. The impact of stringent certification standards on forensic evaluator reliability: further analysis. Paper presented at: The Annual Meeting of the American Psychology-Law Society; March 2015; San Diego, CA.

56. National Judicial College. Mental competencies: best practices model. 2011–2012. www.mentalcompetency. org/pdf/BP-Model.pdf (accessed June 2020).

57. Gowensmith WN, McCallum KE. Mirror, mirror on the wall, who's the least biased of them all?: dangers and potential solutions regarding bias in forensic psychological evaluations. *S Afr J Psychol.* 2019; **49**(2): 165–176.

58. Pronin E, Kugler MB. Valuing thoughts, ignoring behavior: the introspection illusion as a source of the bias blind spot. *J Exp Soc Psychol.* 2007; **43**(4): 565–578.

59. Neal T, Grisso T. The cognitive underpinnings of bias in forensic mental health evaluations. *Psychol Public Policy Law.* 2014; **20**(2): 200–211.

60. Brodsky SL. *Testifying in Court: Guidelines and Maxims for the Expert Witness.* Washington, DC: American Psychological Association; 1991.

61. Brodsky SL. *The Expert Expert Witness.* Washington, DC: American Psychological Association; 1999.

62. Gowensmith WN, McCallum KE, Nadkarni L, et al. Monitoring potential bias within a forensic evaluation agency. Paper presented at: The Annual Meeting of the American Psychology-Law Society; March 2019; Portland, OR.

Competence to Stand Trial and Criminalization: An Overview of the Research

Amanda Beltrani and Patricia A. Zapf

Beginning in the 1960s, a steady decline in the number of inpatient psychiatric beds has occurred across the United States, primarily as a result of stricter civil commitment criteria and a societal movement toward deinstitutionalization. Concomitant with this decrease in psychiatric beds has been a steady increase in the number of mentally ill individuals who are arrested and processed through the criminal justice system as defendants. One consequence of this has been an explosion in the number of defendants who are referred for evaluations of their present mental state – adjudicative competence – and who are subsequently found incompetent and ordered to complete a period of competency restoration. This explosion has resulted in forensic mental health systems that are overwhelmed by the demand for services and that are unable to meet the needs of these defendants in a timely manner. Defendants with mental health concerns are spending an inordinate amount of time incarcerated while waiting for their competency-related services, resulting in what we refer to as criminalization of individuals with mental illness. In many states, lawsuits have been brought by defendants who have had their liberties restricted as a result of lengthy confinements in jail awaiting forensic services. The stress on statewide forensic systems has become so widespread that we have nearly reached the level of a national crisis. Many states and national organizations are currently attempting to study these issues and develop creative strategies for relieving this near-national overburdening of forensic mental health systems.

The purpose of this article is to review the current state of the research on competence to stand trial and to highlight those issues that might be relevant to the issue of criminalization of individuals with mental illness in the United States. Although there is a large and growing literature on issues relevant to adjudicative competence – including its evaluation, the characteristics of competent and incompetent defendants, and restoration services – here, we attempt to focus on those issues that are specifically relevant to the broader issue of criminalization of individuals with mental illness. Space limitations do not permit a comprehensive review, but rather, we present an overview of the competency research as it pertains to criminalization with a focus on recent history and current trends. The interested reader is referred to the other articles in this special issue for more data and detail on related issues, and to other sources.[1–4]

We begin with a brief overview of the competency doctrine and the general procedures used across the United States and then we review the empirical literature on competency to stand trial. We highlight research in three areas – system considerations, evaluation considerations, and treatment considerations – relevant to a complete understanding of the current forensic mental health crisis and for discovering new ways to move forward.

Overview of Competency Doctrine and Procedures

The origins of the competency doctrine can be traced to the Babylonian Talmud and early Judeo-Christian texts along with English common law that emerged at some point prior to the fourteenth century.[5] In English courts of this era, defendants commonly remained mute in lieu of making a plea, which impeded trial proceedings and required English courts to determine whether this muteness was a function of "malice" or "visitation of God."[5] "Mute by visitation of God" encompassed the "deaf and dumb" and expanded to include "lunatics."[6] This distinction provided an opportunity for those suffering from mental illness to avoid the same punishment as those who committed a crime with malicious intent. This was the beginning of the judicial system noting the special needs of the mentally ill in criminal justice proceedings.

Today, a defendant's right to a fair trial is one of the core principles of modern law, which strives to provide all defendants with objective and dignified proceedings (of course, the importance of competence to stand trial in the law is primarily in common law nations and does not extend to many civil law nations). Competency to stand trial (adjudicative competence) is a doctrine of jurisprudence that allows for the postponement of criminal proceedings should a defendant be unable to participate in his or her defense on account of mental disorder or intellectual disability. All defendants are required to maintain a basic level of competence to proceed through the adjudication process; therefore, competency is relevant from arrest or initial detention through sentencing.[7] Adjudicative competence is the most commonly referred forensic evaluation,[8,9] with annual competency evaluation referrals increasing over time.[10,11]

The U.S. standard for trial competence was established in *Dusky v. United States*[12] and all states currently use some variant of the *Dusky* standard, with the exact definition varying by jurisdiction. In *Dusky*, the Supreme Court held:

> It is not enough for the district judge to find that "the defendant is oriented to time and place and has some recollection of events," but that the test must be whether he has sufficient present ability to consult with his lawyer with a reasonable degree of rational understanding – and whether he has a rational as well as factual understanding of the proceedings against him. (p. 402)

Thus, the *Dusky* standard established two prongs for competency: (a) the sufficient present ability to assist counsel with a reasonable degree of rational understanding and (b) the ability to rationally and factually understand the proceedings against him. As the language in *Dusky* is ambiguous, the typical forensic evaluation is left largely unguided by legal statute, with the courts and legislatures giving mental health professionals a large share of the responsibility for defining and evaluating competency, although various states have made attempts to provide delineated statutes to guide the evaluation process. A vast empirical literature on competency evaluation prompted the publication of guidelines[13,14] and best practices[15] to improve competency evaluation procedures.

Modern competency laws vary from state to state; however, most jurisdictions follow similar procedures.

There is a relatively low threshold for ordering a competency evaluation, with all parties to the proceedings responsible for raising the issue of a defendant's competence whenever a *bona fide* doubt exists.[16,17] A written competency evaluation report is typically required for any court-ordered evaluation, with the number of evaluation reports per defendant varying by jurisdiction and ranging between one and three. In most cases, the court readily accepts the opinion of the evaluator (or of the majority of evaluators when three evaluations are conducted, as is the case in Hawaii) and a hearing on the issue becomes unnecessary.[18] In those instances where evaluators are in disagreement about a defendant's competency status, a hearing on the issue is held.

Defendants adjudicated as competent proceed with their cases whereas those found incompetent are ordered to a period of restoration, typically at an inpatient facility but with an increasing number of outpatient restoration programs becoming available in various jurisdictions.[19] Most jurisdictions have time limits for restoration orders and allow for the possibility of extending a restoration order when there is a substantial probability that the defendant will be restored in the foreseeable future. Most defendants (~75%) are restored to competence within a six-month period and returned to court.[20] A smaller proportion take longer than six months but are ultimately restored within a year. And a very small proportion of defendants – primarily those with intellectual disabilities or treatment-resistant psychosis – will not be restored to competence.[21] The current research on competency restoration is superficial, comparing competent and incompetent defendants and identifying characteristics of individuals involved in restoration procedures, not variables that examine incompetent defendants at various stages of restoration.[20]

We now turn to a review of the research on competence to stand trial and highlight issues relevant to the criminalization of individuals with mental illness in the United States.

Empirical Foundations of Competency to Stand Trial

Prior to the 1980s, there was little research on competency to stand trial but the past few decades have witnessed a surge of research, with more than 5,000 publications on this topic since 1980. This vast body of research has explored the characteristics of defendants referred for competency evaluations and those deemed incompetent, the reliability and validity of the evaluation process and of instruments developed for use in competency assessment, predictions regarding the restorability of incompetent defendants, and competency restoration treatment programs.[9] Recently, research has begun to address some of the important system-wide considerations that impact waitlists for evaluations and restoration services.[1–3] We begin by reviewing the empirical literature on competency to stand trial and then highlight various system, evaluation, and treatment considerations important to a complete understanding of the increasing criminalization of individuals with mental illness.

In the United States, between 4% and 8% of all felony defendants are referred for a competency evaluation; however, research indicates that attorneys may have concerns about their clients' competence in as many as 15% of all cases.[22] Of those defendants who are referred for formal evaluation, approximately one in four will be found incompetent, with a meta-analysis of 26,139 defendants indicating a base rate for incompetence of 27.5%.[9]

Symptoms of mental illness, such as the presence of psychosis, play a prominent role in competency determinations.[23] In the past, most evaluators were employed in state psychiatric hospitals and received little formal training in the assessment of competence and matters of law. Therefore, incompetence was equated with psychosis and evaluators rarely considered the specific legal demands of the case.[24] However, empirical research has provided evidence that the presence of psychosis itself is not sufficient for a defendant to be adjudicated incompetent. For example, researchers analyzed data from over 1,000 forensic evaluations conducted over a two-year period and found that only one-half of individuals with a diagnosis of schizophrenia and one-third of those with a diagnosis of intellectual disability were adjudicated incompetent, highlighting that diagnosis alone does not meet the threshold for incompetence.[25] Over the years, researchers sought to identify other variables that are related to competency status.

Comparison studies of competent and incompetent defendants indicate that, relative to competent defendants, incompetent defendants (a) perform poorly on forensic assessment instruments related to legal functional abilities, (b) are more likely to have a psychotic disorder diagnosis, and (c) have psychiatric symptoms that are indicative of severe psychopathology.[23,26,27] Research has consistently demonstrated incompetent defendants to be diagnosed with psychotic disorders at higher rates than their competent counterparts.[28–30] The most robust finding from a meta-analysis of 68 studies published between 1967 and 2008 that compared competent and incompetent defendants was that defendants diagnosed with a psychotic disorder were eight times more likely to be found incompetent than defendants without a psychotic disorder.[9] Furthermore, unemployed defendants were twice as likely to be incompetent than those who were employed and those with a history of psychiatric hospitalization were twice as likely to be incompetent as those without.[9]

Special Populations

Over the last few decades, research has focused on specific vulnerable populations for whom issues of competency are especially important, such as juveniles and individuals diagnosed with intellectual disabilities (formally, mental retardation). More recently, researchers have begun to explore gender and older age in relation to trial competency-related issues.

Individuals with Intellectual Disabilities

In 1990, Bonnie noted that between 2% and 7% of competency evaluation referrals were defendants with intellectual deficits. Adequate representation and proper identification of intellectually disabled defendants in criminal cases were raised as concerns given that previous research had suggested that approximately 15% of incompetent defendants were intellectually disabled.[31] Throughout the 1990s, research reported that about one-half of intellectually disabled defendants were not identified for competency evaluation[32–34] and suggested that these individuals proceed through the criminal justice system without understanding the process or punishments.

Appelbaum[35] provided guidance for identifying individuals with intellectual disabilities in forensic evaluations, highlighting the importance of assessing functional abilities rather than simply relying on IQ score, and underscoring the need for evaluators to consider the tendency for these individuals to be compliant and cooperative and to attempt to conceal their difficulties by pretending to understand.[35] A result of this presentation style is that individuals with intellectual disabilities often do not show signs of poor understanding and/or reasoning. In many cases, this "cloak of competence" gives these individuals the appearance of normalcy in the competency context.[36] Legally, significant impairments then become visible only when the individual also has a severe mental illness or acts in a strange or disruptive manner.[37] Smith and Hudson identified a screening device[38] that could be used to identify intellectually disabled defendants and case studies have provided some guidance for assessing[39,40] and restoring[41] this population to competency.

Bonnie[37] postulated that restoration of incompetent intellectually disabled defendants is highly unlikely and research has since provided empirical support for this, reflecting that most intellectually disabled defendants are not restored to competence.[42] Schouten[43] expressed concern that intellectually disabled defendants may be able to provide correct responses to trial-related questions but not understand their significance. Everington et al.[44] used a simulated research design to examine whether defendants with intellectual disabilities were capable of feigning poor performance on the Competence Assessment for Standing Trial for Defendants with Mental Retardation. Results suggested that, in certain circumstances, intellectually disabled defendants may have the ability to feign poor performance and the authors called for additional research to assess whether these defendants truly understand the repercussions of the outcomes in their actual criminal cases.

Juveniles

Prior to the early 1990s, little was known about juvenile trial competencies. Cowden and McKee[45] conducted the first study, over an eight-year period, to explore the characteristics of juveniles referred for competence evaluations. Findings indicated a positive relationship between age and competence. No significant relationships were found between competency status and sex, race, previous mental health history, and frequency or type of criminal charge. Subsequent research replicated and expanded these findings indicating that, compared to youth not evaluated for trial competence, youth who were deemed incompetent were younger, had special education needs, prior mental health treatment, and histories of being in state custody.[46,47] Other research, however, has not found significant differences between age and performance on a competency assessment measure but the truncated nature of the age range in these samples might explain the lack of significant findings.[48–50]

Ensuring the competency of adolescents has become increasingly important as the juvenile justice system has shifted from a rehabilitative model to a more punishment oriented one and as increasing numbers of adolescents are being either waived or transferred to criminal court.[51] Grisso[52,53] reviewed the developmental literature related to capacities of juveniles to participate in their criminal cases. His review underscores the role that developmental immaturity plays in adolescents' limitations in understanding and appreciating the legal process. Bonnie and Grisso[11] proposed future directions for law and policy related to juvenile adjudicative competence and Katner[54] argued for reforms that would provide greater protection from wrongful adjudication of incompetent youth. Subsequent research has indicated that judges do take developmental maturity into consideration when determining adjudicative competence.[55,56]

Current research suggests that there is greater need to tailor evaluations of adjudicative competence for younger adolescents. Definitions and conceptual guidance for forensic evaluators regarding necessary modifications related to assessing juvenile competence have been outlined in other sources.[57–59]

Gender

Most competency research offers limited rigorous examination of the association between gender and competency outcomes. Riley[60] sought to provide seminal baseline data comparing competent and incompetent female defendants with their male counterparts and, while her results did not show an overall pattern of association between gender and competency adjudication, she argued that research on male-only populations could not be applied equally to female defendants. Crocker et al.[61] used a relatively large sample of female defendants and found support for the notion that women are more likely to be found incompetent relative to males. More recently, Kois et al.[62] explored variables that have historically been associated with competency in samples that are predominately male and found that these associations may not transfer across demographic groups. Pirelli et al.'s[9] meta-analysis found that female defendants were equally as likely to be found incompetent as male defendants. It is noteworthy that this may be due to the small proportion of studies employing females in their samples, since only half of the studies analyzed included females.

Elderly Defendants

Assessing competence in the geriatric population is particularly challenging, primarily as a result of greater deficits in orientation and memory.[63] Approximately one-third of individuals aged 60 years or older who are referred for competency evaluations are deemed incompetent[64] and, compared to younger incompetent defendants, restoration rates for older individuals are much lower.[65] Frierson et al.[66] compared geriatric defendants found incompetent to stand trial with their competent counterparts and found that the most common variables associated with incompetence were older age, presence of dementia, presence of other memory and concentration impairments, and deficits in orientation. Concerns over individual constitutional rights (e.g. *Jackson* time limits) are elevated for competency determinations of elderly defendants as research shows that these defendants are unlikely to benefit from restorative treatment.[65] There is a need for additional research with elderly defendants to further develop our understanding of the implications of age and related impairments on competency evaluation and determination.

We now turn to a discussion of the literature in three areas of relevance to criminalization – system considerations, evaluator considerations, and treatment considerations.

System Considerations

To curtail mass incarceration of persons with mental illness and to support those who would be better served by treatment than punishment, pre-arraignment diversion programs, mental health courts, substance use treatment, and post-incarceration support services have been established in many jurisdictions. However, these alternatives to incarceration are not a panacea as the frequency of competency evaluations and the number of defendants opined incompetent continue to rise. Issues of specific relevance to criminalization of mentally ill defendants include service delivery/system considerations and misuse of the competency evaluation process, each of which are briefly reviewed here.

Service Delivery

LaFortune and Nicholson[67] surveyed judges and attorneys about the competency referral and evaluation process and found that referral for evaluation does not occur for approximately one-third of defendants whose competency is a concern. These researchers and Winick[68] raised concern about the ethical dilemma faced by attorneys when dealing with a client whose competency is in question but the prolonged legal case, involuntary hospitalization involved in the competency process, and the related infringement on the defendant's autonomy may not be seen as being in the best interests of their client.

Various scholars have provided reconceptualizations of competence to stand trial that take into consideration the fiduciary nature of the relationship between defense attorney and defendant. Winick[32] argued that, in some circumstances, it might be in the best interest of the defendant to proceed with a trial even if he or she is incompetent. He postulated that this could take the form of a "provisional trial" where the defense attorney would ensure protection of the defendant, allowing the defendant to proceed with his or her case, with appropriate courtroom behavior. Bonnie[37] proposed two levels of competence – foundational competence to assist counsel and higher-order decisional competence. He argued that defendants found incompetent to assist counsel should be barred from proceeding until they were restored to foundational competence, whereas defendants found decisionally incompetent could proceed by having their defense attorney make decisions on their behalf. Despite the logic presented for these reconceptualizations of competence, provisional trials have not been adopted in any jurisdiction and the decision of the Supreme Court in *Godinez v. Moran*,[69] made clear that decision-making is an important component of a defendant's competence-related abilities.

Throughout the 1980s, various states began making changes to the process by which court-ordered competency evaluations were delivered. Systems evolved from conducting all evaluations at centralized inpatient facilities only to the use of jails and mental health centers as well. Nicholson and Kugler's[26] meta-analysis explored the function of evaluation site (inpatient versus outpatient) on various defendant variables and found that most of the descriptive characteristics that were associated with findings of incompetence did not differ as a result of evaluation setting.

Grisso et al. conducted a national survey to determine the organization of pre-trial forensic evaluation services in the United States.[70] They concluded, "the traditional use of centrally located, inpatient facilities for obtaining pretrial evaluations survives in only a minority of states, having been replaced by other models that employ various types of outpatient approaches" (p. 388). One compelling reason for this shift is cost. Winick[6] estimated that $185 million were spent annually on competency evaluations. By 2012, a conservative estimate of $700 million in annual costs for evaluation and restoration services in the United States was reported.[71]

A more recent national survey was conducted by the National Association of State Mental Health Program Directors and, of the 37 states that responded, only 12 indicated that their state handled competency evaluations solely outside of the psychiatric hospital.[4] Outpatient services varied by state, with various options including jails, outpatient locations, use of community evaluators, and private agencies. The remaining 25 states indicated that some (or most) competency evaluations are conducted at their state psychiatric hospital.[4]

The number of evaluations is growing annually[19] and state reports have documented an increase in the number of forensic patients admitted to state psychiatric inpatient hospitals.[1,2,4] Various states have indicated they are implementing a variety of methods in response to increasing numbers of forensic patients in state hospitals and growing waitlists, including, but not limited to, adding more beds, adapting the admission process, modifying prioritization of waitlists, and developing community- or jail-based programs.[4] Christy et al.[72] noted that defendants in Florida waited an average of 81 days to be admitted to hospital after the court ordered restoration; this research provided the impetus for Florida to reallocate finances to provide additional forensic services.

Few empirical studies have documented the process of the increase in referrals, assessed the scope of the problem, or have identified factors that may be driving it, but these issues are becoming the focus of national attention.[73] Currently, between 10,000 and 18,000 defendants are adjudicated incompetent to stand trial each year and remanded to competency restoration services,[74] with commensurate annual increases as the number of competency evaluations increase. This is an area in need of research and focused attention.

Misuse of Competency Evaluations

As a result of broad deinstitutionalization and legislation changes imposing stricter criteria for involuntary civil commitment, inpatient admissions to psychiatric hospitals declined; however, this was accompanied by a concomitant increase in admissions for forensic services, such as evaluations for competency.[75] Throughout the late 1980s and 1990s various studies explored questions related to whether the competency evaluation process was being used by the courts to obtain inpatient treatment for nondangerous mentally ill individuals.[76–78] Warren et al.[79] examined data from three states and found that defendants charged with public order offenses were more likely to be opined incompetent by forensic evaluators than those charged with more serious offenses. In addition, defendants in Ohio were more likely to be found incompetent than defendants in Michigan and Virginia. These researchers postulated that this difference might be a result of fewer community mental health services in Ohio, leading the courts to use competency referrals as an avenue to obtaining mental health treatment. These data suggest that some portion of inpatient evaluations may be ordered for the primary purpose of securing mental health treatment for the defendant. This "criminalization of the mentally ill" highlights that mental health services are often most accessible through court-ordered services.[80]

The increasing rate of competency referrals and the subsequent increase in incompetent defendants have raised concerns regarding the quality and timeliness of forensic mental health services.[80] Many states are dealing with the challenge of balancing the demands of the legal system, with public safety concerns and limited mental health resources. As of 2015, 37 states had identified specific time requirements for completion of competency evaluations and delineated various settings in which evaluations can be conducted. Gowensmith et al. noted that states with a centralized administration with authority specific to forensic services are in a better position to address delays in competence restoration and inefficiencies in the evaluation and restoration process.[80]

Evaluation Considerations

Several factors regarding the evaluation of competence to stand trial are relevant to a complete understanding of those factors that might play a role in criminalizing individuals with mental illness, including the research on quality of evaluations and reports, evaluator differences, and bias in forensic evaluation. We briefly address each of these here.

Quality of Evaluations and Reports

No published research has examined forensic evaluations but there have been some studies examining the quality of forensic reports, which can, arguably, serve as a proxy for the forensic evaluation. Skeem et al.[81] examined competency evaluation reports in Utah and found that evaluators failed to delineate the rationale or reasoning for their psycholegal opinions and also failed to address some of the specific capacities involved in adjudicative competence. Zapf et al.[18] examined competency evaluation reports in Alabama and found that many evaluators failed to address important, statutorily required, elements. Nicholson and Norwood[82] summarized the research on forensic evaluation reports and testimony and concluded that, "the practice of forensic psychological assessment falls short of its promise" (p. 40).

Several competency assessment tools have been developed to assist in structuring the competency evaluation process.[5,15,83] The benefits of using competence assessment tools include that they provide structure to the evaluation, help to standardize the assessment procedures, improve reliability between evaluators, promote meaningful comparisons across time or between evaluators, facilitate research, improve communication in legal settings, and facilitate deficit-focused restoration efforts.[15,83] Research examining inter-rater reliability for various competency assessment tools indicates higher rates of agreement for overall determinations of competency status, moderate rates of agreement for individual scales, and lower agreement for specific abilities encompassed within each scale.[84–86]

Evaluator Differences

Murrie et al.[87] examined more than 7,000 evaluations, conducted by 60 clinicians, to explore the degree to which individual clinicians varied in terms of their opinions of incompetence. Rates of incompetence opinions varied considerably across evaluators, suggesting that evaluators might differ in terms of how they define, conceptualize, and arrive at opinions regarding incompetence. Although there is greater variability in opinions regarding specific components of competence, there is generally good agreement between evaluators regarding a defendant's overall competency status (i.e. competent or incompetent).[88–90] In a study of competency evaluation reports in Utah where two reports were completed on each of 50 defendants, Skeem et al.[81] found 82% agreement between evaluators regarding overall competency status, but this dropped to an average rate of about 25% when examining agreement between evaluators on whether a particular psycholegal ability was impaired, with agreement on many of the psycholegal abilities examined at less than 10%. In a large field reliability study, Gowensmith et al.[91] examined 216 competency cases in Hawaii, where statute requires three separate evaluations be conducted by independent clinicians for each felony defendant referred for competency evaluation. Results indicated that all three evaluators arrived at the same opinion regarding competence in 71% of cases. Rates of agreement fell to 61% for opinions of competency status for defendants who received restoration services subsequent to being adjudicated incompetent. These results reflect moderate agreement among independent evaluators regarding overarching opinions of competency status but decreasing agreement between evaluators regarding the specific domains and abilities encompassed within competency status. Similarly, these data also indicate that various evaluators may be more or less inclined to opine in a particular direction regarding overall competency status. More research and information is needed regarding the impact of evaluator differences on both the competency evaluation process as well as evaluator decisions and opinions regarding competency status. In addition to evaluator differences, more research on the impact of evaluation context on reliability rates is required.[92]

Bias in Forensic Evaluation

The extent to which bias impacts forensic evaluations is unknown, although consideration of the issue of potential bias and inquiry into ways in which potential bias might be mitigated have become the focus of research and commentary over the past few years.[93–95] Specific issues, such as hindsight bias,[96] and bias awareness[97] have been studied with respect to forensic evaluations. A survey of 1,099 forensic evaluators indicated that most evaluators expressed concern over cognitive bias but held the incorrect view that bias can be reduced by sheer willpower.[98] In addition, evidence for a bias blind spot[99] was found, with evaluators indicating more bias in their peers' judgments than in their own.[98]

Mossman[100] used computer simulation of 20,000 pairs of competency evaluations to test whether bias might account for differences in evaluator opinions regarding competency status. His results indicated that between-examiner disagreements might be attributable to random error rather than examiner biases that imply different thresholds for conceptualizing a defendant's competency status. Murrie et al. have conducted several studies examining the issue of adversarial allegiance – the idea that an evaluator might be more sympathetic to the retaining side – and provided the first empirical support for this allegiance using an experimental research design.[87,101,102]

Although experimental research designs have not been used to address the issue of potential bias in competency evaluations, some research has indicated that certain groups, such as felony defendants and non-White defendants, are more likely to be found incompetent. Further exploration of issues of potential bias are relevant to a complete understanding of criminalization and mental illness.

Treatment Considerations

In 1997, Cooper and Grisso noted that a majority of forensic patients in the United States were receiving competency restoration services but there existed little research on treatment for competency restoration.[34] Two decades later, we remain in dire need of systematic research on competency restoration. Pirelli and Zapf[20] conducted a systematic review of restoration services for 12,781 defendants across 51 studies and found that 81% of individuals were restored to competency, after an average of 175 days. Additional planned analyses could not be conducted because of the limited number of studies using a research design allowing for comparison of defendants at pre-restoration and post-restoration, prompting Pirelli and Zapf to call out the grave state of the competency restoration literature over the last half century.

Although the specific statutes vary by state, restoration services are most typically ordered when treatment is likely to restore competency and no less intrusive alternative exists. In addition, the majority of defendants who are assessed for competency consent to prescribed medication;[103] whereas those who deny their mental illness, or have delusions related to their medications, generally refuse psychotropic treatment.[104] Ladds and Convit noted that most decisions to forcibly medicate defendants are made for clinical reasons rather than legal ones.[104] The United States Supreme Court decision in *Sell v. United States*[105] gave courts legal authority to mandate the involuntary administration of medications to restore competency under certain limited circumstances:

important governmental interests are at stake; the forced medication will *significantly further* those state interests; involuntary medication is *necessary* to further those interests; and administering the medication is *medically appropriate* and will not significantly interfere with the defense or have adverse side effects.

Although psychotropic medication is the most frequent treatment modality utilized for competency restoration, various jurisdictions have established an educational component for competency restoration. Most typically, these educational programs are structured in nature and focus on the goal of providing factual information and decision-making skills to defendants with the goal of restoring the defendant to competence. Siegel and Elwork[106] developed, and empirically tested, a structured psychoeducational program for competence restoration. Scores on a competency assessment instrument were compared for matched groups of incompetent defendants, with one group receiving the psychoeducational competency program and the other serving as a control group. Upon completion of the treatment period, higher ratings of competency were found for the competence restoration group (45%) than for the control group (15%), providing support for the notion that educating incompetent defendants regarding legal aspects specific to trial competence may improve outcomes. Several other researchers have explored educational programs for competency restoration and have provided recommendations for improving the efficacy of competence restoration.[107–109]

The decision of the United States Supreme Court in *Jackson v. Indiana*[110] underscores that incompetent defendants cannot be held indefinitely and, if restoration is unlikely, must either be released or civilly committed. The *Jackson* ruling set the foundation for revisions to state statutes to provide alternatives to commitment as well as limits on the length of commitment.[24] In 1992, Golding[111] speculated that the best predictor of restorability may be a defendant's initial responsiveness to treatment and noted that restoration is unlikely to occur in some cases as a result of the chronic nature of a defendant's psychological or psychiatric issues. Subsequent research sought to gain insight on those defendants who are not likely to be restored to competence. Findings suggested that intellectual disabilities,[42,112,113] and more severe pathology (e.g. schizophrenia spectrum disorder)[114–116] were related to poor restoration outcomes. Hubbard and Zapf[117] explored variables related to clinicians' opinions regarding restorability and found no particular set of variables that produced a high classification rate or that served as reliable predictors of restorability. Warren et al.[116] also explored variables related to restorability and found that defendants considered not restorable were more likely to have intellectual deficits or learning disorders. Mossman et al.[13] also noted that significant cognitive deficits, as well as chronic psychosis, were associated with a low probability of restoration.

Pirelli and Zapf[20] found that when comparing defendants who had been restored to competency with those who had not, non-white defendants and unmarried defendants were less likely to be restored. In addition, defendants with psychotic disorders were two to three times more likely than those without to be incompetent/not restored and defendants who had previously been evaluated for competency were three to five times more likely to be incompetent/not restored than those who had not.

Outpatient Restoration

The high costs and resource demands of treatment for restoration has led some states to examine alternative competency restoration models. In 2003, Miller noted that outpatient restoration treatment was rare, with over 30% of states not legally allowing for such treatment. In 2011, Kapoor reported that 35 states' (70%) statutes allowed for outpatient competency restoration programs, with 16 states having active outpatient programs.[118] Almost half of these 16 states – Florida, Pennsylvania, Virginia, Tennessee, Arizona, Texas, and Louisiana – have attempted jail-based restoration programs, with initial estimates of cost savings from these jail-based programs appearing promising. Yet the lack of mental health staff in jails and the limited number of incompetent defendants a jail has at any given time has caused push-back within several jurisdictions, making jail-based restoration programs difficult to maintain.[118] By 2016, Gowensmith et al. reported that 44 states (86.3%) allowed for outpatient restoration programs and noted that between 2003 and 2016, there was growth in the number of states that allowed for outpatient restoration programs, but that from 2011 to 2016, the number of states that actually utilized such programs remained static at 16.[19] Gowensmith et al. highlighted preliminary but promising results for states using outpatient competency restoration programs.[19] At present, jail-based competency restoration programs require further research to identify the as-of-yet undetermined efficacy and viability of these programs.

Future research on competency restoration is dire to the further development and enhancement of effective competency restoration programs for defendants. Focusing on specific cognitive deficits and symptoms of mental disorder as well as the nexus between these clinical issues/symptoms and the various competency-related abilities and deficits is critical to increasing our understanding of effective interventions for the successful restoration of competency.

Summary and Conclusions

Although there is a large body of research on competence to stand trial, this has primarily focused on the characteristics of defendants referred for competency evaluations and those deemed incompetent, the reliability and validity of the evaluation process and the use of instruments developed for competency assessment, predictions regarding the restorability of incompetent defendants, and competency restoration treatment programs. Larger issues – such as the best methods and procedures for competency restoration and the ways in which the systemic burdens placed on state forensic mental health systems by current standards, statutes, and procedures pertaining to adjudicative competence can be remedied – have not received nearly as much attention. Indeed, Gowensmith[119] argued, "promising policy implications can be rooted in emerging knowledge about the timing of competency evaluations, certification of evaluators, alternatives to inpatient restoration, and changes to evaluations and the associated reports" (p. 1). This brief overview provides a summary of research on competency to stand trial that might be relevant to working through broader issues related to the criminalization of individuals with mental illness. It appears to be time to turn our attention to the wider systemic issues involved in our overburdened forensic systems nationwide in an attempt to understand the contributing factors and how these might be changed to improve service provision and outcomes. The issue of criminalization of individuals with mental illness and how this impacts the competency evaluation and restoration process, as well as the wider systemic demands this places on the state forensic mental health system, are important considerations that are the focus of this special issue.

Disclosure

Amanda Beltrani and Patricia Zapf do not have anything to disclose.

References

1. Pinals DA, Fitch WL, Warburton K. Assessment #10: Forensic patients in state psychiatric hospitals: 1999–2016. /sites/default/files/TACPaper.10.Forensic-Patients-in-State- Hospitals_508C_v2.pdf. August 2017. (Accessed April 1, 2019.)

2. Pinals DA, Fuller DA. Beyond beds: the vital role of a full continuum of care. Treatment Advocacy Centre, National Association of State Mental Health Program Directors; 2017. www.treatmentadvocacycenter.org/storage/documents/beyond-beds.pdf (accessed June 2020).

3. Steadman HJ, Callahan L. Reducing the Pennsylvania incompetency to stand trial restoration waitlist: more than just beds. www.dhs.pa.gov/cs/groups/webcontent/documents/document/c_269519.pdf. December 2017. (Accessed April 1, 2019.)

4. Wik A, Hollen V, Fisher WH. Assessment #9: Forensic patients in state psychiatric hospitals: 1999–2016. Ninth in a series of ten briefs addressing: what is the inpatient bed need if you have a best practice continuum of care? National Association of State Mental Health Program Directors; 2017. www.nri-inc.org/media/1318/tac-paper-9-forensic-patients-in-state-hospitals-final-09-05-2017.pdf (accessed June 2020).

5. Melton GB, Petrila J, Poythress NG, et al. *Psychological Evaluations for the Courts: A Handbook for Mental Health Professionals and Lawyers*, 4th edn. New York, NY: Guilford Press; 2018.

6. Winick BJ. Incompetency to stand trial: developments in the law. In: Monahan J, Steadman HJ, eds. *Mentally Disordered Offenders*. New York, NY: Plenum Press; 1983: 3–38.

7. Murrie DC, Zelle H. Criminal competencies. In: Cutler BL, Zapf PA, eds. *APA Handbook of Forensic Psychology, Vol. 1: Individual and Situational Influences in Criminal and Civil Contexts. APA Handbooks in Psychology*. Washington, DC: American Psychological Association; 2015: 115–157.

8. Morris DR, DeYoung NJ. Psycholegal abilities and restoration of competence to stand trial. *Behav Sci Law*. 2012; **30**(6): 710–728.

9. Pirelli G, Gottdiener WH, Zapf PA. A meta-analytic review of competency to stand trial research. *Psychol Public Policy Law*. 2011; **17**(1): 1–53.

10. Hoge SK, Bonnie RJ, Poythress N, et al. The MacArthur adjudicative competence study: development and validation of a research instrument. *Law Hum Behav*. 1997; **21**(2): 141–179.

11. Bonnie RJ, Grisso T. Adjudicative competence & youthful offenders. In: Grisso T, Schwartz RG, eds. *Youth on Trial: A Developmental Perspective on Juvenile Justice*; Chicago and London: University of Chicago Press; 2000: 73–103. See NCJ-184852.

12. *Dusky v. United States*, 362 U.S. 402 (1960).

13. Mossman D, Noffsinger SG, Ash P, et al. AAPL practice guideline for the forensic psychiatric evaluation of competence to stand trial. *J Am Acad Psychiatry Law*. 2007; **35**(4 Suppl): S3–S72.

14. Wall BW, Ash P, Keram E, Pinals DA, Thompson CH. AAPL practice resource for the forensic psychiatric evaluation of competence to stand trial. *J Am Acad Psychiatry Law*. 2018; **46**(3): 373.

15. Zapf PA, Roesch R. *Evaluation of Competence to Stand Trial*. New York, NY: Oxford University Press; 2009.

16. *Pate v. Robinson*, 383 U.S. 375 (1966).

17. *Drope v. Missouri*, 420 U.S. 162 (1975).

18. Zapf PA, Hubbard KL, Cooper VG, Wheeles MC, Ronan KA. Have the courts abdicated their responsibility for determination of competency to stand trial to clinicians? *J Forensic Psychol Pract*. 2004; **4**(1): 27–44.

19. Gowensmith WN, Frost LE, Speelman DW, Therson DE. Lookin' for beds in all the wrong places: outpatient competency restoration as a promising approach to modern challenges. *Psychol Public Policy Law*. 2016; **22**(3): 293–305.

20. Pirelli G, Zapf PA. A meta-analysis of the competency restoration literature. Paper presented at: 2015 Annual Meeting of the American Psychology-Law Society 2015, San Diego, CA.

21. Zapf PA. *Standardizing Protocols for Treatment to Restore Competency to Stand Trial: Interventions and Clinically Appropriate Time Periods*. Olympia, WA: Washington State Institute for Public Policy; 2013.

22. Hoge SK, Bonnie RJ, Poythress N, Monahan J. Attorney-client decision-making in criminal cases: client competence and participation as perceived by their attorneys. *Behav Sci Law*. 1992; **10**(3): 385–394.

23. Ryba N, Zapf P. The influence of psychiatric symptoms and cognitive abilities on competence-related abilities. *Int J Forensic Ment Health*. 2011; **10**(1): 29–40.

24. Roesch R, Golding SL. *Competency to Stand Trial*. Urbana, IL: University of Illinois Press; 1980.

25. Warren JI, Fitch WL, Dietz PE, Rosenfeld BD. Criminal offense, psychiatric diagnosis, and psycholegal opinion: an analysis of 894 pretrial

referrals. *Bull Am Acad Psychiatry Law*. 1991; **19**(1): 63–69.

26. Nicholson RA, Kugler KE. Competent and incompetent criminal defendants: a quantitative review of comparative research. *Psychol Bull*. 1991; **109**(3): 355–370.

27. Hart SD, Hare RD. Predicting fitness to stand trial: the relative power of demographic, criminal, and clinical variables. *Forensic Rep*. 1992; **5**(1): 53–65.

28. Cooper VG, Zapf PA. Predictor variables in competency to stand trial decisions. *Law Hum Behav*. 2003; **27**(4): 423–436.

29. James DV, Duffield G, Blizard R, Hamilton LW. Fitness to plead: a prospective study of the inter-relationships between expert opinion, legal criteria and specific symptomatology. *Psychol Med*. 2001; **31**(1): 139–150.

30. Viljoen JL, Zapf PA. Fitness to stand trial evaluations: a comparison of referred and non-referred defendants. *Int J Forensic Ment Health*. 2002; **1**(2): 127–138.

31. Miller RD, Germain EJ. Evaluation of competency to stand trial in defendants who do not want to be defended against the crimes charged. *Bull Am Acad Psychiatry Law*. 1987; **15**(4): 371–379.

32. Winick BJ. Reforming incompetency to stand trial and plead guilty: a restated proposal and response to Professor Bonnie. *J Crim Law Criminol*. 1995; **85**(3): 571–624.

33. Smith SA, Broughton SF. Competency to stand trial and criminal responsibility: an analysis in South Carolina. *Ment Retard*. 1994; **32**(4): 281–287.

34. Cooper DK, Grisso T. Five year research update (1991–1995): evaluations for competence to stand trial. *Behav Sci Law*. 1997; **15**(3): 347–364.

35. Appelbaum KL. Assessment of criminal-justice-related competencies in defendants with mental retardation. *J Psychiatry Law*. 1994; **22**(3): 311–327.

36. Edgerton RB. *The Cloak of Competence: Stigma in the Lives of the Mentally Retarded*. Berkeley, CA: University of California Press; 1967.

37. Bonnie RJ. The competence of criminal defendants: a theoretical reformulation. *Behav Sci Law*. 1992; **10**(3): 291–316.

38. Smith SA, Hudson RL. A quick screening test of competency to stand trial for defendants with mental retardation. *Psychol Rep*. 1995; **76**(1): 91–97.

39. Kalbeitzer R, Benedetti R. Assessment of competency to stand trial in individuals with mental retardation. *J Forensic Psychol Pract*. 2009; **9**(3): 237–248.

40. Schlesinger LB. A case study involving competency to stand trial: incompetent defendant, incompetent

41. Stoops R, Hess J, Scott T, et al. Training competency to stand trial in an individual with intellectual disability and behavioral health concerns. *Mental Health Aspects Dev Disabil*. 2007; **10**(2): 47–52.

42. Anderson SD, Hewitt J. The effect of competency restoration training on defendants with mental retardation found not competent to proceed. *Law Hum Behav*. 2002; **26**(3): 343–351.

43. Schouten R. Commentary: training for competence—form or substance? *J Am Acad Psychiatry Law*. 2003; **31**(2): 202–204.

44. Everington C, Notario-Smull H, Horton ML. Can defendants with mental retardation successfully fake their performance on a test of competence to stand trial? *Behav Sci Law*. 2007; **25**(4): 545–560.

45. Cowden VL, McKee GR. Competency to stand trial in juvenile delinquency proceedings – cognitive maturity and the attorney-client relationship. *Univ Louisv J Fam Law*. 1995; **33**: 629–660.

46. Baerger DR, Griffin EF, Lyons JS, Simmons R. Competency to stand trial in preadjudicated and petitioned juvenile defendants. *J Am Acad Psychiatry Law*. 2003; **31**(3): 314–320.

47. Kruh IP, Sullivan L, Ellis M, Lexcen F, Mcclellan J. Juvenile competence to stand trial: a historical and empirical analysis of a juvenile forensic evaluation service. *Int J Forensic Ment Health*. 2006; **5**(2): 109–123.

48. Redlich AD, Silverman M, Steiner H. Pre-adjudicative and adjudicative competence in juveniles and young adults. *Behav Sci Law*. 2003; **21**(3): 393–410.

49. Poythress N, Lexcen FJ, Grisso T, Steinberg L. The competence-related abilities of adolescent defendants in criminal court. *Law Hum Behav*. 2006; **30**(1): 75–92.

50. Schmidt MG, Reppucci ND, Woolard JL. Effectiveness of participation as a defendant: the attorney–juvenile client relationship. *Behav Sci Law*. 2003; **21**(2): 175–198.

51. Salekin RT, Rogers R, Ustad KL. Juvenile waiver to adult criminal courts: prototypes for dangerousness, sophistication-maturity, and amenability to treatment. *Psychol Public Policy Law*. 2001; **7**(2): 381–408.

52. Grisso T. Competence of adolescents as trial defendants. *Psychol Public Policy Law*. 1997; **3**(1): 3–32.

53. Grisso T. What we know about youths' capacities as trial defendants. In: Grisso T, Schwartz RG, eds. *Youth on Trial: A Developmental Perspective on Juvenile Justice*. Chicago, IL: University of Chicago Press; 2000: 139–171.

examiner or "malingering by proxy"? *Psychol Public Policy Law*. 2003; **9**(3–4): 381–399.

54. Katner DR. The mental health paradigm and the MacArthur study: emerging issues challenging the competence of juveniles in delinquency systems. *J Am Acad Psychiatry Law*. 2006; **32**(4): 503–583.

55. Larson K, Grisso T. Transfer and commitment of youth in the United States: law, policy, and forensic practice. In: *APA Handbook of Psychology and Juvenile Justice. APA Handbooks in Psychology Series*. Washington, DC: American Psychological Association; 2016: 445–466.

56. Viljoen JL, Wingrove T, Ryba NL. Adjudicative competence evaluations of juvenile and adult defendants: judges' views regarding essential components of competence reports. *Int J Forensic Ment Health*. 2008; **7**(2): 107–119.

57. Barnum R. Clinical and forensic evaluation of competence to stand trial in juvenile defendants. In: Grisso T, Schwartz RG, eds. *Youth on Trial: A Developmental Perspective on Juvenile Justice*. Chicago, IL: University of Chicago Press; 2000: 193–223. See NCJ-184852.

58. Grisso T. *Forensic Evaluation of Juveniles, 2nd edn*. Sarasota, FL: Professional Resource Press/ Professional Resource Exchange; 2013.

59. Grisso T, Schwartz RG. *Youth on Trial: A Developmental Perspective on Juvenile Justice*. Chicago, IL: University of Chicago Press; 2000.

60. Riley SE. Competency to stand trial adjudication: a comparison of female and male defendants. *J Am Acad Psychiatry Law*. 1998; **26**(2): 223–240.

61. Crocker AG, Favreau OE, Caulet M. Gender and fitness to stand trial: a 5-year review of remands in Québec. *Int J Law Psychiatry*. 2002; **25**(1): 67–84.

62. Kois L, Pearson J, Chauhan P, Goni M, Saraydarian L. Competency to stand trial among female inpatients. *Law Hum Behav*. 2013; **37**(4): 231–240.

63. Frierson RL, Shea SJ, Shea MEC. Competence-to-stand-trial evaluations of geriatric defendants. *J Am Acad Psychiatry Law*. 2002; **30**(2): 252–256.

64. Lewis CF, Fields C, Rainey E. A study of geriatric forensic evaluees: who are the violent elderly? *J Am Acad Psychiatry Law*. 2006; **34**(3): 324–332.

65. Fogel MH, Schiffman W, Mumley D, Tillbrook C, Grisso T. Ten year research update (2001–2010): evaluations for competence to stand trial (adjudicative competence). *Behav Sci Law*. 2013; **31**(2): 165–191.

66. Frierson RL, Shea SJ, Shea MEC. Competence-to-stand-trial evaluations of geriatric defendants. *J Am Acad Psychiatry Law*. 2002; **30**(2): 252–256.

67. LaFortune KA, Nicholson RA. How adequate are Oklahoma's mental health evaluations for determining competency in criminal proceedings?: the bench and the bar respond. *J Psychiatry Law*. 1995; **23**(2): 231–262.

68. Winick BJ. Incompetency to proceed in the criminal process: past, present, and future. In: Sales BD, Shuman DW, eds. *Law, Mental Health, and Mental Disorder*. Belmont, CA: Thomson Brooks/Cole Publishing Co; 1996: 310–340.

69. *Godinez v. Moran*, 509 U.S. 389 (1993).

70. Grisso T, Cocozza JJ, Steadman HJ, Fisher WH, Greer A. The organization of pretrial forensic evaluation services: a national profile. *Law Hum Behav*. 1994; **18**: 377–393.

71. Zapf PA, Roesch R, Pirelli G. Assessing competency to stand trial. In: Weiner IB, Otto RK, eds. *The Handbook of Forensic Psychology, 4th edn*. Hoboken, NJ: John Wiley & Sons Inc; 2014: 281–314.

72. Christy A, Otto R, Finch J, Ringhoff D, Kimonis ER. Factors affecting jail detention of defendants adjudicated incompetent to proceed. *Behav Sci Law*. 2010; **28**(5): 707–716.

73. Callahan L, Dargis M, Ihara E, Irons A. *Foundation Work for Exploring Incompetency to Stand Trial (IST) Evaluations & Competency Restoration for People with Serious Mental Illness (SMI)*. Delmar, NY: Policy Research Associates; 2018.

74. Warren JI, Chauhan P, Kois L, Dibble A, Knighton J. Factors influencing 2,260 opinions of defendants' restorability to adjudicative competency. *Psychol Public Policy Law*. 2013; **19**(4): 498–508.

75. Geller JL, Fisher WH, Kaye NS. Effect of evaluations of competency to stand trial on the state hospital in an era of increased community services. *Hosp Community Psychiatry*. 1991; **42**(8): 818–823.

76. Aubrey M. Characteristics of competency referral defendants and nonreferred criminal defendants. *J Psychiatry Law*. 1988; **16**(2): 233–245.

77. Arvanites TM. A comparison of civil patients and incompetent defendants: pre and post deinstitutionalization. *Bull Am Acad Psychiatry Law*. 1990; **18**(4): 393–403.

78. Steury EH, Choinski M, Steury SR. Incompetency to stand trial and mental health treatment: a case study testing the subversion hypothesis. *Bull Am Acad Psychiatry Law*. 1996; **24**(3): 319–331.

79. Warren JI, Rosenfeld B, Fitch WL, Hawk G. Forensic mental health clinical evaluation: an analysis of interstate and intersystemic differences. *Law Hum Behav*. 1997; **21**(4): 377–390.

80. Gowensmith WN, Murrie DM, Packer IK. *Report in Response to the Trueblood v. State of Washington's Department of Social and Health Services.* Olympia, WA: Office of Attorney General, State of Washington; 2015.

81. Skeem JL, Cohn NB, Berge G, Golding SL. Logic and reliability of evaluations of competence to stand trial. *Law Hum Behav.* 1998; **22**(5): 519–547.

82. Nicholson RA, Norwood S. The quality of forensic psychological assessments, reports, and testimony: acknowledging the gap between promise and practice. *Law Hum Behav.* 2000; **24**(1): 9–44.

83. Grisso T. *Evaluating Competencies: Forensic Assessments and Instruments, 2nd edn.* New York, NY: Kluwer Academic/Plenum Publishers; 2002.

84. Otto RK, Poythress NG, Nicholson RA. Psychometric properties of the MacArthur competence assessment tool – criminal adjudication. *Psychol Assess.* 1998; **10** (4): 435–443.

85. Rogers R, Johansson-Love J. Evaluating competency to stand trial with evidence-based practice. *J Am Acad Psychiatry Law.* 2009; **37**(4): 450–460.

86. Viljoen JL, Roesch R, Zapf PA. Interrater reliability of the fitness interview test across 4 professional groups. *Can J Psychiatry.* 2002; **47**(10): 945–952.

87. Murrie DC, Boccaccini MT, Johnson JT, Janke C. Does interrater (dis)agreement on psychopathy checklist scores in sexually violent predator trials suggest partisan allegiance in forensic evaluations? *Law Hum Behav.* 2008; **32**(4): 352–362.

88. Murrie DC, Boccaccini MT, Zapf PA, Warren JI, Henderson CE. Clinician variation in findings of competence to stand trial. *Psychol Public Policy Law.* 2008; **14**(3): 177–193.

89. Rosenfeld B, Ritchie K. Competence to stand trial: clinician reliability and the role of offense severity. *J Forensic Sci.* 1998; **43**(1): 151–157.

90. Mossman D. Conceptualizing and characterizing accuracy in assessments of competence to stand trial. *J Am Acad Psychiatry Law.* 2008; **36**(3): 340–351.

91. Gowensmith WN, Murrie DC, Boccaccini MT. Field reliability of competence to stand trial opinions: how often do evaluators agree, and what do judges decide when evaluators disagree? *Law Hum Behav.* 2012; **36** (2): 130–139.

92. Guarnera LA, Murrie DC. Field reliability of competency and sanity opinions: a systematic review and meta-analysis. *Psychol Assess.* 2017; **29**(6): 795–818.

93. Dror IE, Murrie DC. A hierarchy of expert performance applied to forensic psychological assessments. *Psychol Public Policy Law.* 2018; **24**(1): 11–23.

94. Neal TMS, Brodsky SL. Forensic psychologists' perceptions of bias and potential correction strategies in forensic mental health evaluations. *Psychol Public Policy Law.* 2016; **22**(1): 58–76.

95. Zapf PA, Dror IE. Understanding and mitigating bias in forensic evaluation: lessons from forensic science. *Int J Forensic Ment Health.* 2017; **16**(3): 227–238.

96. Beltrani A, Reed AL, Zapf PA, Otto RK. Is hindsight really 20/20?: the impact of outcome information on the decision-making process. *Int J Forensic Ment Health.* 2018; **17**(3): 285–296.

97. Zappala M, Reed AL, Beltrani A, Zapf PA, Otto RK. Anything you can do, I can do better: bias awareness in forensic evaluators. *J Forensic Psychol Res Pract.* 2018; **18**(1): 45–56.

98. Zapf PA, Kukucka J, Kassin SM, Dror IE. Cognitive bias in forensic mental health assessment: evaluator beliefs about its nature and scope. *Psychol Public Policy Law.* 2018; **24**(1): 1–10.

99. Pronin E, Lin DY, Ross L. The bias blind spot: perceptions of bias in self versus others. *Pers Soc Psychol Bull.* 2002; **28**(3): 369–381.

100. Mossman D. When forensic examiners disagree: bias, or just inaccuracy? *Psychol Public Policy Law.* 2013; **19**(1): 40–55.

101. Murrie DC, Boccaccini MT, Guarnera LA, Rufino KA. Are forensic experts biased by the side that retained them? *Psychol Sci.* 2013; **24**(10): 1889–1897.

102. Murrie DC, Boccaccini MT, Turner DB, et al. Rater (dis)agreement on risk assessment measures in sexually violent predator proceedings: evidence of adversarial allegiance in forensic evaluation? *Psychol Public Policy Law.* 2009; **15**(1): 19–53.

103. Zapf PA, Roesch R. Future directions in the restoration of competency to stand trial. *Curr Dir Psychol Sci.* 2011; **20**(1): 43–47.

104. Ladds B, Convit A. Involuntary medication of patients who are incompetent to stand trial: a review of empirical studies. *Bull Am Acad Psychiatry Law.* 1994; **22**(4): 519–532.

105. *Sell v. United States,* 282 F. 3d 560 (2003).

106. Siegel AM, Elwork A. Treating incompetence to stand trial. *Law Hum Behav.* 1990; **14**(1): 57–65.

107. Bertman LJ, Thompson JW Jr., Waters WF, et al. Effect of an individualized treatment protocol on restoration of competency in pretrial forensic inpatients. *J Am Acad Psychiatry Law.* 2003; **31**(1): 27–35.

108. Brown DR. A didactic group program for persons found unfit to stand trial. *Hosp Community Psychiatry.* 1992; **43**(7): 732–733.

109. Noffsinger SG. Restoration to competency practice guidelines. *Int J Offender Ther Comp Criminol.* 2001; **45**(3): 356.

110. *Jackson v. Indiana*, 406 U.S. 715 (1972).

111. Golding SL. Studies of incompetent defendants: research and social policy implications. *Forensic Rep.* 1992; **5**(1): 77–83.

112. Salekin K, Olley JG, Hedge K. Offenders with intellectual disability: characteristics, prevalence, and issues in forensic assessment. *J Ment Health Res Intellect Disabil.* 2010; **3**(2): 97–116.

113. Scott CL. Commentary: a road map for research in restoration of competency to stand trial. *J Am Acad Psychiatry Law.* 2003; **31**(1): 36–43.

114. Cochrane RE, Grisso T, Frederick RI. The relationship between criminal charges, diagnoses, and psycholegal opinions among federal pretrial defendants. *Behav Sci Law.* 2001; **19**(4): 565–582.

115. Colwell LH, Gianesini J. Demographic, criminogenic, and psychiatric factors that predict competency restoration. *J Am Acad Psychiatry Law.* 2011; **39**(3): 297–306.

116. Warren JI, Murrie DC, Stejskal W, et al. Opinion formation in evaluating the adjudicative competence and restorability of criminal defendants: a review of 8,000 evaluations. *Behav Sci Law.* 2006; **24**(2): 113–132.

117. Hubbard KL, Zapf PA. The role of demographic, criminal, and psychiatric variables in examiners' predictions of restorability to competency to stand trial. *Int J Forensic Ment Health.* 2003; **2**(2): 145–155.

118. Kapoor R. Commentary: jail-based competency restoration. *J Am Acad Psychiatry Law.* 2011; **39**(3): 311–315.

119. Gowensmith WN. Resolution or resignation: the role of forensic mental health professionals amidst the competency services crisis. *Psychol Public Policy Law.* 2019; **25**(1): 1–14.

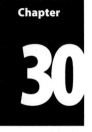

Risk Factors for Recidivism in Individuals Receiving Community Sentences: A Systematic Review and Meta-Analysis

Denis Yukhnenko, Nigel Blackwood, and Seena Fazel

Introduction

Noncustodial sentences are the commonest type of court sanction in many countries.[1–3] Offender management and rehabilitation programs aim to prevent recidivism and the further criminalization of individuals receiving community sentences.[4,5] Although the ultimate goal of these programs is to ensure public safety and to ease the economic burden on justice systems, they assume different rates of repeat criminal behaviors and employ different approaches. The criminogenic needs of individuals (the characteristics of an individual that directly relate to the likelihood of recidivism) are typically broken down into static (nonmodifiable) and dynamic (modifiable) risk factors. Static risk factors are unchanging characteristics of an individual and include gender, age, and prior criminal history. Dynamic risk factors are items that can be influenced or changed during the process of rehabilitation such as employment or substance misuse problems.

Both static and dynamic risk factors are taken into consideration during risk assessment and intervention planning.[6] Static risk factors are strong predictors of future offending behavior, but are, by definition, poor targets for intervention. Moreover, one criticism of many risk assessment approaches is their overreliance on static risk factors and a failure to take time and change into account, although this will need to be linked to effective interventions.[7] Taking into account dynamic factors and their change over time may improve the accuracy of risk assessment.[8] It is also important to study dynamic risk factors for recidivism in community-sentenced populations separately from released prisoner populations. Community sentences are often given to individuals who committed a minor offence, first-time offenders, and other categories considered "low risk." They may also include offenders with better legal representation. Therefore, for individuals serving a community sentence, certain risk factors

may be more or less predictive than in released prisoners, or they may operate through different pathways.

However, many individual studies that examine risk factors for recidivism in community-sentenced populations focus exclusively on static risk factors, typically offenders' demographics and prior contact with justice systems.[3,9,10] This is limited given that, when assessed using standardized diagnostic tools, community-sentenced populations show a higher prevalence of dynamic risk factors such as psychiatric disorders and misuse of illicit substances[11] in comparison to the general population. In addition, prior meta-analyses that have investigated risk factors in community-sentenced populations either examined mixed samples of released prisoners and community-sentenced individuals[12,13] or looked into narrow subpopulations of community-sentenced individuals, for example, sexual offenders[14] or offenders in forensic psychiatric treatment.[15]

In the present study, we examined both static (nonmodifiable) and dynamic (modifiable) risk factors for recidivism in 246,608 individuals receiving community sentences. To the authors' knowledge, this study is the first meta-analysis that examines risk factors for criminal recidivism in a general adult community-sentenced population.

Methods

The systematic review protocol was pre-registered in PROSPERO (CRD42018099606), and PRISMA guidelines[16] were followed (Figure 30.1; Supplement 1).

Search Strategy

Publication search with no time or language restrictions used the following databases: MEDLINE, SAGE, JSTOR, PsycINFO, PsycARTICLE, EMBASE, and Global Health. Search terms consisted of (recidivism OR "re-offending" OR reoffending OR rearrest OR "re-arrest") AND (risk OR predictor OR need) AND (criminogenic OR modifiable OR dynamic) AND ("community service" OR probation OR "community sentence"). We scanned the reference lists of the screened-in articles to identify new studies. In addition, the Google Scholar "cited by" tool was used to identify additional studies. Key investigators with relevant publications were contacted to determine if they had undertaken any new or missed studies.

Study Eligibility and Selection

We included studies of individuals from the general adult (≥18 y.o.) population given community sentences. After the abstracts were screened, 121 full-text articles were assessed for eligibility (Figure 30.1). Individuals released to community supervision after serving a prison sentence (parolees) were excluded.

To be included, a study contained data that enabled estimation of odds ratios (ORs) for at least one risk factor. We excluded studies conducted in narrow subpopulations of individuals given community sentences (e.g. only adolescents, only women, only people with psychiatric disorders), cross-sectional studies, studies of interventions, and validation studies for risk assessment tools. There were no exclusions based on the reported recidivism outcomes, which could include any reoffending, violent and nonviolent reoffending, rearrest, revocation of probation, or technical violations. DY conducted the search and screening of the publications.

Data Extraction

The data extraction process happened in two stages. Standardized forms were used for each stage and several

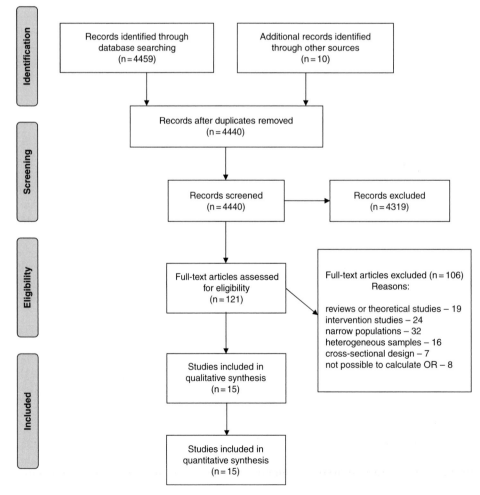

Figure 30.1 PRISMA flow diagram.

variables were pre-specified for later subgroup analysis. First, for each study, we extracted the year of publication, study design, geographical region, coverage (province, state, and country), sample characteristics (number of individuals, selection year, reported outcomes, number of people with reported outcomes, type of follow-up, the length of the follow-up period, gender composition, and mean age), and the list of all risk factors. Second, if at least three studies examined a particular risk factor, the following data were extracted: number of individuals in the exposed and comparison groups, operationalization of risk factor in a particular study, description of comparison group, and source of information (records or risk assessment instrument). Risk factors judged to be similar by their descriptions were collapsed in domains. If a study reported multiple outcomes, the most prevalent outcome for a particular risk factor was extracted to enhance comparability. The most serious outcome was used when the prevalence for two outcomes was the same in a group (in the order of priority: reconviction, probation failure, rearrest, and technical violation). When a study used the same dataset as another study for a given risk factor, the data from the most recent study were extracted.

DY and another researcher (HR) independently performed data extraction. Any disagreements were resolved by discussion with SF.

Several studies that explored data on substance misuse reported it separately for alcohol and drug abuse without providing combined data for any substance misuse. Taking this into account, to avoid duplicating samples, we analyzed individuals with substance abuse problems by three subgroups (problems with alcohol, problems with drugs, and problems with substances in general). In addition, different studies reported risk for ethnicity domain in inconsistent ways. Race and ethnicity might be defined as one or as two separate categories. We used data comparing white and nonwhite individuals, which was the most common way of reporting risk for this domain.

The data were converted to ORs for pooling. If a study reported frequencies or proportions, crude ORs were calculated directly with corresponding 95% confidence intervals. If no such data had been reported, we used other metrics that allowed estimation of ORs. If crude OR estimation was not possible, adjusted ORs were extracted. Reported chi-square values were converted into Cohen's d and, consequently, into log-transformed ORs.[17] All ORs were reported to one decimal place.

Quality assessment was performed using the Newcastle-Ottawa Quality Assessment Scale for cohort studies.[18] This scale evaluates cohort selection, exposure ascertainment, comparability between cohorts, and the quality of outcome measurement. For each item on the scale, the study can be assigned one or two points, with a maximum score of nine points. Any uncertainties about quality rating were resolved by discussion between the authors. Egger's tests were used to assess possible publication bias for each risk factor.

Statistical Analyses

All statistical analyses were done in STATA Version 15 for Windows[19] using *admetan* package.[20] To assess heterogeneity across studies, we used I^2 statistics, which estimates the percentage of variance due to differences between studies. Random effects models were used to provide for more equal weighting between studies. Subgroup analysis was then performed to investigate potential sources of heterogeneity using pre-defined subgroups.

Results

Study Characteristics

We identified 15 studies from 5 countries, which reported data on 246,608 (82% male) individuals from 14 independent samples (Table 30.1). The included studies were published between 1997 and 2018. The majority (11) of the studies were from the USA. Four included papers were reports by governmental agencies,[21,23,30,33] one was a thesis[28] and the rest were published in peer-reviewed journals.

The participants were either representative samples or full cohorts of individuals who received community sentences in a given country or province during a selection period. All included studies utilized a cohort (either prospective or retrospective) design. Rearrest was the most frequently reported outcome (eight studies) and the mean reported follow-up period was 3.5 years (three studies did not provide information on the mean follow-up length). The identified risk factor domains that were examined in three or more studies were gender, income, ethnicity, criminal history, marital status, substance misuse problems, mental health needs, educational problems, employment problems, and association with antisocial peers (Table 30.1). The definitions of exact

Table 30.1 Description of studies included in the meta-analysis

Study	Country	Cohort (selection years, n, % male, mean age)	Outcomes (type and length of follow-up)	Extracted risk factors	NOQAS score
Adams et al.[21]	USA	Individuals sentenced to probation sampled from several counties of Illinois. One individual can be sentenced multiple times (2006, 2770, 82, 31)	Rearrest (during supervision, mean 19.4 months) Revocation (during supervision, mean 19.4 months)	Gender, age, ethnicity, criminal history, marital status, substance abuse, mental health, education, employment, income, and negative peer association	7
Caudy et al.[22]	USA	Individuals sentenced to probation from one urban county of an unnamed southwestern state (2011–2013, 10,642, 76, 34)	Rearrest (fixed end date, mean 1 year)	Gender	7
Department of Justice[23]	UK – N. Ireland	National cohort of individuals receiving noncustodial sentences (2005, 19,047, 85, *33)	Reconviction (starts with a sentence, two years)	Gender and age	7
Grann et al.[24]	Sweden	National cohort of iindividuals receiving noncustodial sentences (1993–2001, 4828, 91, 36)	Reconviction for a violent crime (starts with a sentence + fixed end date, average 4.8 years)	Substance abuse and mental health	7
Harris[25]	USA	A cohort of felony probationers from an unnamed south central state (1993, 3598, 78, 29)	Rearrest, excluding arrests for technical violations (starts with a sentence, three years)	Gender, age, substance abuse, mental health, education, employment, and negative peer association	7
Huebner and Cobbina[26]	USA	Individuals sentenced to probation sampled from several counties of Illinois (2000, 3017, 80, 31) *same dataset as in Olson, 2003	Rearrest (starts with an end of a sentence, four years)	Gender, substance abuse, and employment	7
Humphrey et al.[27]	USA	Individuals sampled from cohort of standard and reparative probationers from Vermont (1998–2000, 4792, 73, 28)	Reconviction (starts with a sentence, five years)	Gender and criminal history	7
Maliek[28]	USA	Individuals sentenced to probation from Texas (2014–2017, 10, 127, 73, 35)	Probation revocation (during supervision, unspecified)	Gender, ethnicity, substance abuse, mental health, education, employment, income, marital status, and negative peer association	7
Minor et al.[29]	USA	Individuals sentenced to probation from Kentucky (1996–1999, 200, 68, median 40)	Probation violation (starts with a sentence, two years)	Gender, ethnicity, criminal history, substance abuse, mental health, education, and employment	8
North Carolina Sentencing & Advisory Commission[30]	USA	Individuals sentenced to probation from N. Carolina (2015, 32,537, 72, 32)	Rearrest (starts with a sentence, two years)	Gender, ethnicity, criminal history, substance abuse, mental health, education, employment, and marital status	7
Olson and Lurigio[31]	USA	Individuals sentenced to probation sampled from several counties of Illinois (1997, 2438, 80, *30)	Rearrest (during supervision, unspecified)	Gender, ethnicity, criminal history, substance abuse, education, and income	7

Table 30.1 (cont.)

Study	Country	Cohort (selection years, n, % male, mean age)	Outcomes (type and length of follow-up)	Extracted risk factors	NOQAS score
Olson et al.[32]	USA	Individuals sentenced to probation from Illinois (2000, 3325, 79, 31) *same dataset as in Huebner, 2007	Rearrest (during supervision, unspecified)	Gender, ethnicity, age, criminal history, substance abuse, education, and income	7
Peillard et al.[33]	Chile	National cohort on individuals receiving noncustodial sentences (2007, 23, 736, 86,≈33)	Rearrest (starts with a sentence, three years)	Gender	7
Sims and Jones[34]	USA	Individuals sentenced to probation from North Carolina (1993, 2850, 83, 87)	Probation failure/ revocation (during supervision, mean 30 months) *cohort is selected based on release date	Gender, ethnicity, age, criminal history, substance abuse, education, employment, income, marital status, and negative peer association	7
Wood et al.[35]	UK – England & Wales	National cohort of individuals from different probation trusts, excluding Tier 1 (low risk) probationers (2009–2010, 125, 718, 24,≈32)	Proven reoffending (start with a sentence, one year for an offence to happen + six months for conviction)	Gender, criminal history, substance abuse, mental health, employment, income, and negative peer association	8

outcomes included in these domains are reported in Appendix 1 in the Supplementary material.

Quality Assessment

Among identified studies, 2 received a score of 8 on the Newcastle-Ottawa Scale, 13 received a score of 7. The commonest identified limitation was missing data for risk factors in a number of individuals or failure to report a nonresponse rate.

Recidivism Risk and Static (Nonmodifiable) Risk Factors

The most commonly reported static risk factor domains were gender, age, ethnicity, criminal history, and educational problems (Table 30.2, Appendix 2 in the Supplementary material).

In the criminal history domain, we included individuals with arrests or convictions that pre-dated an index crime. Having a prior criminal history was strongly associated with recidivism ($k = 9$, $n = 185,491$, pooled OR = 3.0 [CI 95% 1.9, 4.5]; $I^2 = 99\%$). No pre-defined subgroups explained the observed heterogeneity. To determine the association between age and recidivism, we compared adult

individuals younger than 21 years old at the time of their index conviction with older offenders, as this was the most commonly reported age grouping across the studies. Younger age was associated with recidivism ($k = 5$, $n = 160,728$, pooled OR = 1.9 [CI 95% 1.6, 2.3]; $I^2 = 96\%$). Heterogeneity slightly reduced in studies when individuals were followed during their supervision. No other subgroups were relevant for heterogeneity.

Several other static risk factor domains were associated with recidivism. These included educational problems, that is, not having high school diploma or having high educational needs indicated by standardized assessment tools ($k = 9$, $n = 58,342$, pooled OR = 1.6 [CI 95% 1.3, 1.9]; $I^2 = 94\%$), and being male ($k = 13$, $n = 241,481$, pooled OR = 1.4 [CI 95% 1.2, 1.6]; $I^2 = 94\%$). In addition, having nonwhite ethnicity was associated with recidivism (ethnicity domain; $k = 7$, $n = 53,248$, pooled OR = 1.7 [CI 95% 1.3, 2.3]; $I^2 = 97\%$). No subgroups explained heterogeneity in these risk factor domains. Data for the ethnicity domain were reported only by the studies conducted on US samples.

No significant publication bias was identified for any static risk factor (Egger's test results are available upon request).

Table 30.2 Summary of the meta-analysis results (pooled ORs for each identified risk factor domain)

Risk factor domain	Number of studies (k)	Number of individuals (n)	Pooled OR	95% CI	I² (%)
Nonmodifiable					
Gender (male)	13	241,481	1.4	1.2–1.6	94
Age (<21)	5	160,728	1.9	1.6–2.3	96
Ethnicity (nonwhite)	7	53,248	1.7	1.3–2.3	97
Educational problems (not graduating high school or having identified education needs)	9	58,342	1.6	1.3–1.9	94
Criminal history (prior arrest or convictions)	9	185,491	3.0	1.9–4.5	99
Modifiable					
Low income (as specified in jurisdiction)	4	10,302	2.0	1.1–3.4	97
Marital status (single or divorced)	4	40,483	1.6	1.4–1.8	42
Employment problems (unemployed)	8	56,604	1.8	1.3–2.5	98
Substance misuse					
- unspecified	3	47,492	2.3	1.1–4.9	98
- drug misuse	5	13,408	1.7	1.2–2.6	97
- alcohol misuse	3	7953	1.1	1.0–1.2	19
Association with antisocial peers	6	24,175	2.2	1.3–3.7	97
Mental health needs (diagnosed disorder or symptoms that limit functioning)	4	20,049	1.4	1.2–1.6	46

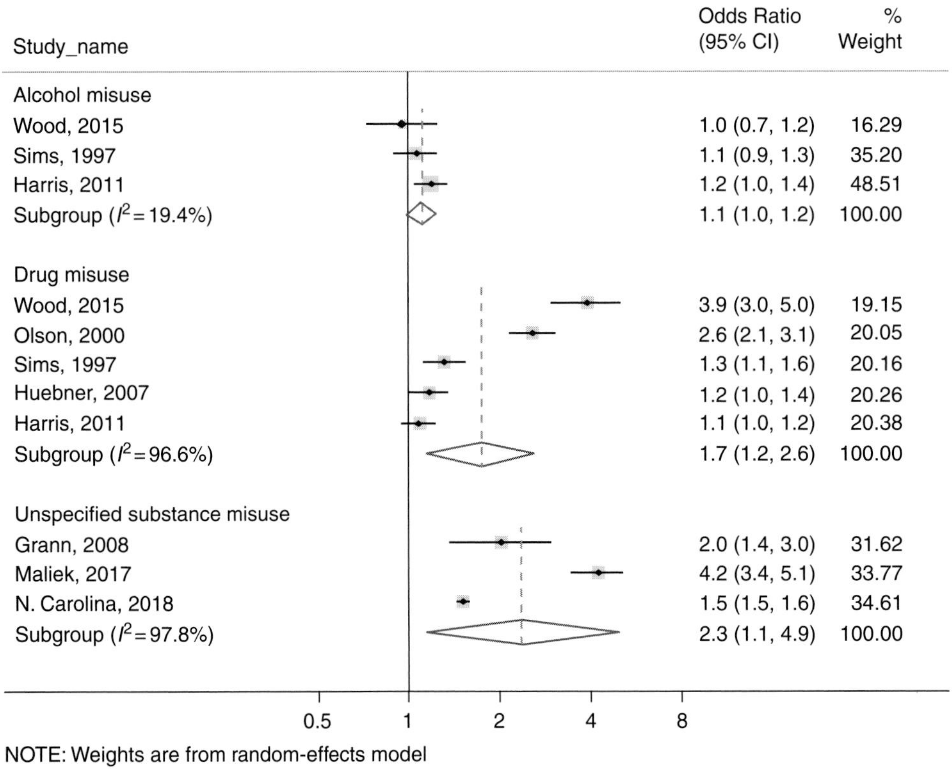

Study_name		Odds Ratio (95% CI)	% Weight
Alcohol misuse			
Wood, 2015		1.0 (0.7, 1.2)	16.29
Sims, 1997		1.1 (0.9, 1.3)	35.20
Harris, 2011		1.2 (1.0, 1.4)	48.51
Subgroup (I² = 19.4%)		1.1 (1.0, 1.2)	100.00
Drug misuse			
Wood, 2015		3.9 (3.0, 5.0)	19.15
Olson, 2000		2.6 (2.1, 3.1)	20.05
Sims, 1997		1.3 (1.1, 1.6)	20.16
Huebner, 2007		1.2 (1.0, 1.4)	20.26
Harris, 2011		1.1 (1.0, 1.2)	20.38
Subgroup (I² = 96.6%)		1.7 (1.2, 2.6)	100.00
Unspecified substance misuse			
Grann, 2008		2.0 (1.4, 3.0)	31.62
Maliek, 2017		4.2 (3.4, 5.1)	33.77
N. Carolina, 2018		1.5 (1.5, 1.6)	34.61
Subgroup (I² = 97.8%)		2.3 (1.1, 4.9)	100.00

NOTE: Weights are from random-effects model

Figure 30.2 ORs for the association between substance misuse and the risk of recidivism in community-sentenced populations by type of misuse.

Recidivism Risk and Dynamic (Modifiable) Risk Factors

The most commonly reported dynamic risk factor domains were substance misuse (Figure 30.2), mental health needs (Figure 30.3), association with antisocial peers (Figure 30.4), employment problems (Figure 30.5), low income (Figure 30.6), and marital status (Figure 30.7).

Substance misuse as a risk factor was reported differently. A standardized diagnosis was only used in one study.[28] Instead, problems with alcohol or

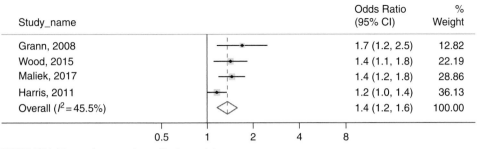

NOTE: Weights are from random-effects model

Figure 30.3 ORs for the association between mental health needs and the risk of recidivism in community-sentenced populations.

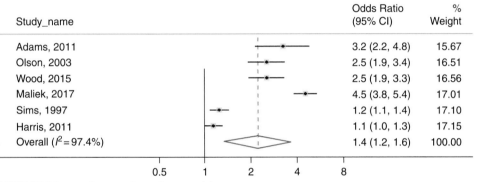

NOTE: Weights are from random-effects model

Figure 30.4 ORs for the association between association with antisocial peers and the risk of recidivism in community-sentenced populations.

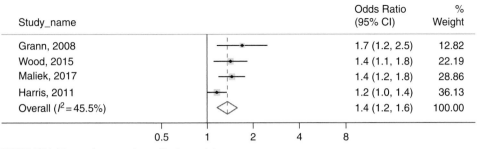

NOTE: Weights are from random-effects model

Figure 30.5 ORs for the association between employment problems and the risk of recidivism in community-sentenced populations.

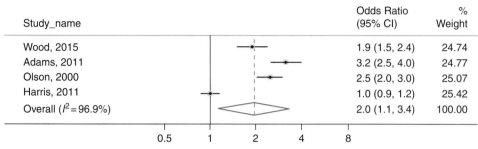

Figure 30.6 ORs for the association between low income and the risk of recidivism in community-sentenced populations.

NOTE: Weights are from random-effects model

Study_name	Odds Ratio (95% CI)	% Weight
Adams, 2011	1.6 (1.3, 2.1)	14.07
Sims, 1997	1.5 (1.3, 1.9)	19.28
Olson, 2008	1.4 (1.1, 1.7)	20.28
N. Carolina, 2018	1.7 (1.6, 1.9)	46.38
Overall ($I^2 = 42.2\%$)	1.6 (1.4, 1.8)	100.00

NOTE: Weights are from random-effects model

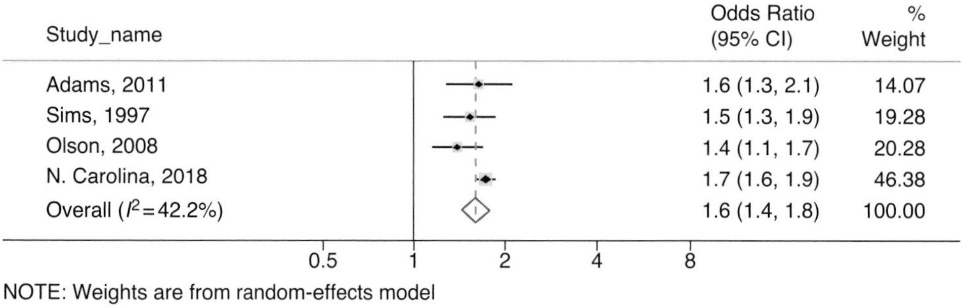

Figure 30.7 ORs for the association between marital status (being single or divorced) and the risk of recidivism in community-sentenced populations.

drugs were typically reported based on interviews and assessments conducted by a probation officer or on record analysis. Recidivism was associated with unspecified substance misuse ($k = 3$, $n = 47,492$, pooled OR = 2.3 [CI 95% 1.1, 4.9]; $I^2 = 98\%$) and drug misuse ($k = 5$, $n = 13,408$, pooled OR = 1.7 [CI 95% 1.2, 2.6]; $I^2 = 97\%$). There was a weak association with alcohol misuse ($k = 3$, $n = 7953$, pooled OR = 1.1 [CI 95% 1.0, 1.2]; $I^2 = 19\%$). The studies that reported a referral to substance misuse treatment programs as a measure of this risk factor were excluded. We considered the referral an unsatisfactory proxy for diagnosis since the referral process is, in many cases, voluntary or may not be a part of a sentence at all, even if an offender has known substance misuse problems. Data from two studies[21,29] were excluded for this reason.

Further subgroup analysis did not identify factors associated with heterogeneity for substance misuse.

Mental health needs (excluding substance misuse) were associated with an increased risk of recidivism ($k =$ 4, $n = 20,049$, pooled OR = 1.4 [CI 95% 1.2, 1.6]; $I^2 = 46\%$). As was the case with substance misuse, medically diagnosed disorders were almost never used as a predictor with the exception of one study.[24] This domain also included presenting with symptoms that limit functioning or having unspecified mental health needs, an assessment of which was often conducted by a probation officer or was not described. Applying a similar rationale to our approach to substance misuse reporting, we excluded data from one study[21] that used a mental health treatment referral as a measure of this risk factor. No pre-identified subgroups explained heterogeneity for mental health needs.

Having antisocial peers was also associated with recidivism ($k = 6$, $n = 24,175$, pooled OR = 2.2 [CI 95% 1.3, 3.7]; $I^2 = 97\%$). This domain included individuals with known gang affiliations, antisocial friends, or lack of prosocial friends. The assessment of this factor was performed mostly by a probation officer or through analysis of records. Heterogeneity was partially explained by lower risk estimates in those below 30 years old compared to 30–35 years old. No other subgroups were associated with lower heterogeneity.

Being unemployed at the time of the conviction was associated with the increased risk of recidivism ($k = 8$, $n = 56,604$, pooled OR = 1.8 [CI 95% 1.3, 2.5]; $I^2 = 98\%$) as well as having low income ($k = 4$, $n = 10,302$, pooled OR = 2.0 [CI 95% 1.1, 3.4]; $I^2 = 97\%$), and being single or divorced (marital status domain; $k = 4$, $n = 40,483$, pooled OR = 1.6 [CI 95% 1.4, 1.8]; $I^2 = 42\%$). No pre-defined subgroups explained heterogeneity for low income, unemployment, or marital status.

No significant publication bias was identified for any dynamic risk factor (Egger's test results are available upon request).

Discussion

This meta-analysis examined the most commonly reported risk factors for recidivism in community-sentenced populations and identified 15 studies involving 246,608 individuals. Three main findings emerge. The first is that dynamic risk factors such as mental health needs, substance misuse, association with antisocial peers, and employment problems increased risk of recidivism in community-sentenced populations. The second is that the strength of these associations was comparable with static risk factors, such as age, gender, and criminal history. The third is that there is a relative dearth of published studies on dynamic risk factors that specifically examine individuals receiving community sentences.

Among static risk factors, younger age and prior criminal history had the strongest association with recidivism. The strength of this association may be considered moderate. Those factors, along with gender, are the common predictors of recidivism in different populations.[36] The frequency of criminal behavior peaks in adolescence and early adulthood, and having a prior criminal history may reflect a lifespan persistent criminal career, which also often begins during adolescence. Educational problems such as not completing high school education may also reflect the early adolescent onset of criminal behavior and be related to persistent problems with social adjustment, which could make the successful reintegration of an offender challenging.

We identified several commonly reported dynamic risk factors that were associated with recidivism in community-sentenced populations, including substance misuse, association with antisocial peers, mental health needs, low income, and problems with employment. The association between substance misuse and recidivism is a common finding in studies on violence and recidivism among released prisoners.[36,37] The association may reflect core endophenotypes for substance misuse such as poor inhibitory control.[38] Drug or alcohol intake may have a disinhibiting effect on an individual thus increasing risk of committing an impulsive crime. Chronic consumption may lead to long-term neurological deficits that are also associated with decreased self-control and increased risk for violence.[39,40] Moreover, drugs may serve as a direct motive for a crime, and illegal possession of drugs may itself be considered a crime. The risk may also depend on the type of drugs used.[41] When alcohol misuse was examined separately, the association was not as strong. Studies in released prisoners have previously shown that diagnosis of alcohol use disorder increased the risk (to the same level as drug use disorder) of reoffending.[42] Most likely, there were not enough identified studies that examined alcohol abuse as a stand-alone risk factor in this meta-analysis. Another possible reason for this finding was the way in which alcohol or drug misuse was measured, typically based on self-report or poorly defined criteria.

Mental health needs were associated with the increased risk of recidivism, which is an important finding. Prior meta-analyses have also found that mental health disorders in general and forensic populations increased the risk of violence.[43,44] However, very few identified studies have investigated the mental health of general community-sentenced populations. Also, using this broad category of mental health needs as a risk factor may not be that practically meaningful for prediction of repeated criminal behavior since different types of disorders may have different associations with recidivism.[24] The existing standardized tools used by probation officers have a "mental health needs/problems" code, but often do not code any specific diagnosis that an individual may have. Using more precise diagnostic categories may be more helpful, although not always possible since this requires professional assessment or access to medical records. Overall, further analysis is required to assess the usefulness of psychiatric diagnoses and their comorbidity in community-sentenced populations.

To determine precise mechanisms of recidivism, it may be informative to examine potential interactions between dynamic and static risk factors, as some factors become more informative for certain subgroups of offenders. For example, Harris[25] compared risk factors among offenders with different criminal career trajectories. Familial problems predicted future rearrest among first-time adult offenders, but they were not a predictor for sentenced offenders with known criminal histories. Many of the factors that may have associations with repeat offending, such as childhood adverse experiences and history of victimization,[45] were examined in the context of general violent behaviour, but not in the context of recidivism studies.

Strengths and Limitations

This is the first meta-analysis, to our knowledge, to investigate risk factors for criminal recidivism in the general population of individuals receiving community sentences. Studies included in the final analysis were of high quality (as assessed by Newcastle-Ottawa Scale) and were conducted using large samples.

The small number of published studies limits the generalizability of the results and leads to several additional limitations. First, it was often not possible to reliably estimate potential sources of heterogeneity, which was high for almost every included risk factor domain. Given the variety of ways in which one risk factor may be defined and measured across different studies, the conclusions should be viewed with caution. Second, it was not possible to separately analyze distal (i.e. prior history of substance abuse/mental health problems) and proximal risk factors (ongoing problems with substance misuse/mental health at the time of the conviction). For this reason, they were combined under their respective domains. Third, we were not able to compare the effects across different outcomes (rearrest, reconviction, technical violation with/without termination of a sentence, and reimprisonment) and different follow-up models (recidivism while serving a sentence versus recidivism after the completion of a sentence). Also, we did not have enough data to compare violent and nonviolent recidivism outcomes.

Another variable that might have contributed to heterogeneity was the difference in sentencing practices among jurisdictions, which our study does not account for. In particular, in jurisdictions where prison sentences are more common, community-sentenced cohorts may be comprised of lower risk individuals when compared to jurisdictions where prison sentences are less common. Differences in sentencing practices result in cohorts with varying compositions that render direct comparisons problematic.

Although there was no identified publication bias, there is still a possibility that some studies may not have provided data for risk factors in cases of nonsignificant findings. Finally, in terms of geographical generalizability, the included studies were limited to Europe and the USA. The US studies were over-represented in the meta-analysis. All studies that examined ethnicity were from the USA, and this risk factor is not generalizable to other countries.

Conclusion and Recommendations

Modifiable risk factors such as mental health needs, substance misuse, association with antisocial peers, low income, employment problems, and marital status were associated with risk of recidivism in individuals receiving community sentences. Further integration of mental health services within criminal justice community supervision agencies requires careful thought and should be based upon the understanding of the treatment needs and recidivism mechanisms of these specific populations. In addition, over-reliance on static (nonmodifiable) risk factors and underplaying of dynamic (modifiable) mental health needs during risk assessment should be avoided as it may lead to less effective rehabilitation practices considering the high prevalence of mental health problems in general community-sentenced populations.

When reporting data for mental health risk factors, diagnostic categories should be provided when the medical records are available, and co-morbidity with substance misuse should be documented. When reporting mental health and substance misuse problems as risk factors, the differences between ongoing problems at the time of a conviction (proximal factors) and problems in the past (distal factors) should be clearly indicated. In addition, researchers and agencies should explore other types of predictors identified in the literature, such as history of maltreatment and victimization, since chronic or ongoing psychological trauma may be an important therapeutic target during rehabilitation. Some of these factors have been extensively studied in other contexts (as predictors of violent behavior and wellbeing), but not within the context of recidivism. Exploring the association of particular symptoms of mental disorders with a plausible connection to recidivism may also be useful. Finally, to make comparisons between studies more meaningful, recidivism data should be reported across different outcomes, including violent and nonviolent recidivism. The use of common reporting guidelines (see Recidivism Reporting Checklist[46]) may facilitate this process.

Acknowledgments

We are grateful to Howard Ryland for assistance with data extraction.

Funding

SF is funded by Wellcome Trust (grant number 202836/ Z/16/Z).

Disclosures

The authors declare that they have nothing to disclose.

Supplementary material

To view supplementary material for this article, please visit https://doi.org/10.1017/S1092852919001056

References

1. Pew Center on the States. *State of Recidivism: The Revolving Door of America's Prisons.* Washington, DC: The Pew Charitable Trusts; 2011.

2. Statistics Denmark. Recidivism. 2018. www.dst.dk/en/ Statistik/emner/levevilkaar/kriminalitet/tilbagefald-til -kriminalitet (accessed June 2020).

3. Ministry of Justice. Proven reoffending statistics: January 2016 to March 2016. 2018. www.gov.uk/gov ernment/statistics/proven-reoffending-statistics- january-2016-to-march-2016 (accessed June 2020).

4. Visher CA, Winterfield L, Coggeshall MB. Ex-offender employment programs and recidivism: a meta-analysis. *J Exp Criminol.* 2005; **1**(3): 295–316.

5. Landenberger NA, Lipsey MW. The positive effects of cognitive behavioral programs for offenders: a meta-analysis of factors associated with effective treatment. *J Exp Criminol.* 2005; **1**(4): 451–476.

6. Bonta J, Andrews DA. Risk-need-responsivity model for offender assessment and rehabilitation. Public Safety Canada; 2007. www.courtinnovation.org/sites/ default/files/RNRModelForOffenderAssessmentAndR ehabilitation.pdf (accessed June 2020).

7. Hanson RK. Long-term recidivism studies show that desistance is the norm. *Crim Justice Behav.* 2018; **45**(9): 1340–1346.

8. Clarke MC, Peterson-Badali M, Skilling TA. The relationship between changes in dynamic risk factors and the predictive validity of risk assessments among youth offenders. *Crim Justice Behav.* 2017; **44**(10): 1340–1355.

9. Central Statistics Office. Probation recidivism 2010 cohort. Central Statistics Office Ireland; 2016. www .cso.ie/en/releasesandpublications/er/pror/probation recidivism2010cohort/ (accessed June 2020).

10. Swedish National Council for Crime Prevention. Recidivism. www.bra.se/bra-in-english/home/crime- and-statistics/crime-statistics/recidivism.html (accessed June 2020).

11. Lurigio AJ, Cho YI, Swartz JA, et al. Standardized assessment of substance-related, other psychiatric, and comorbid disorders among probationers. *Int J Offender Ther Comp Criminol.* 2003; **47**: 630–652.

12. Olver ME, Stockdale KC, Wormith JS.Thirty years of research on the Level of Service scales: a meta-analytic examination of predictive accuracy and sources of variability. *Psychol Assess.* 2014; **26**(1): 156–176.

13. Gendreau P, Little T, Goggin C. A meta-analysis of the predictors of adult offender recidivism: what works? *Criminology.* 1996; **34**: 575–608.

14. Hanson RK, Morton-Bourgon KE. The characteristics of persistent sexual offenders: a meta-analysis of recidivism studies. *J Consult Clin Psychol.* 2005; **73**(6): 1154–1163.

15. Bonta J, Blais J, Wilson HA. A theoretically informed meta-analysis of the risk for general and violent recidivism for mentally disordered offenders. *Aggress Violent Behav.* 2014; **19**(3): 278–287.

16. Shamseer D, Moher D, Clarke M, et al. Preferred reporting items for systematic review and meta-analysis protocols (PRISMA-P) 2015: elaboration and explanation. *Br Med J.* 2015; **350**: g7647.

17. Rosenthal R, DiMatteo MR. Meta-analysis: recent developments in quantitative methods for literature review. *Annu Rev Psychol.* 2001; **52**: 59–82.

18. Wells GA, Shea B, O'Connell D, et al. Quality assessment scales for observational studies. 2004. www.ohri.ca/programs/clinical_epidemiology/oxford .asp (accessed June 2020).

19. StataCorp. *Stata Statistical Software: Release 15.* College Station, TX: StataCorp LLC; 2017.

20. Boston College Department of Economics, Fisher D. ADMETAN: Stata module to provide comprehensive meta-analysis. Statistical Software Components S458561. 2018.

21. Adams S, Bostwick L, Campbell R. *Examining Illinois Probationer Characteristics and Outcomes.* Chicago, IL: Illinois Criminal Justice Information Authority; 2011.

22. Caudy MS, Tillyer MS, Tillyer R. Jail versus probation: a gender-specific test of differential effectiveness and moderators of sanction effects. *Crim Justice Behav.* 2018; **45**(7): 949–968.

23. Department of Justice. *Adult reconviction in Northern Ireland 2005.* Northern Ireland, Belfast: Statistics and Research Branch, Department of Justice; 2011.

24. Grann M, Danesh J, Fazel S. The association between psychiatric diagnosis and violent re-offending in adult offenders in the community. *BMC Psychiatry.* 2008; **8**: 92.

25. Harris P. The first-time adult-onset offender: findings from a community corrections cohort. *Int J Offender Ther Comp Criminol.* 2011; **55**(6): 949–981.

26. Huebner BM, Cobbina J. The effect of drug use, drug treatment participation, and treatment completion on probationer recidivism. *J Drug Issues.* 2007; **37**(3): 619–641.

27. Humphrey JA, Burford G, Dye MH. A longitudinal analysis of reparative probation and recidivism. *Criminal Justice Studies.* 2012; **25**(2): 117–130.

28. Maliek NA. *An Empirical Assessment of the Direct and Indirect Effects of Mental Health Disorders on Probation Outcomes (Thesis).* The University of Texas at San Antonio: ProQuest Dissertations Publishing; 2017: 10617596.

29. Minor KI, Wells JB, Sims C. Recidivism among federal probationers: predicting sentence violations. *Fed Probat.* 2003; **67**(1): 31–33.

30. North Carolina Sentencing & Advisory Commission. Correctional program evaluation: offenders placed on probation or released from prison in Fiscal Year 2015. 2018. www.nccourts.gov/assets/documents/publications/recidivism_2018.pdf?4VQBsstuyz U5dH1Ap7S JQiMe0zTKYU1G (accessed June 2020).

31. Olson DE, Lurigio AJ. Predicting probation outcomes: factors associated with probation rearrest, revocations, and technical violations during supervision. *Justice Res Policy.* 2000; **2**(1): 73–86.

32. Olson DE, Alderden M, Lurigio AJ. Men are from Mars, women are from Venus: but what role does gender play in probationer recidivism? *Justice Res Policy.* 2003; **5**(2): 33–54.

33. Peillard AMM, Correa NM, Cháhuan GW, Lacoa JF. *La Reincidencia en el Sistema Penitenciario Chileno.* Santiago, Chile: Fundacion Paz Ciudadana; 2012.

34. Sims B, Jones M. Predicting success or failure on probation: factors associated with felony probation outcomes. *Crime Delinq.* 1997; **43**(3): 314–327.

35. Wood M, Cattel J, Hales G, et al. *Re-offending by Offenders on Community Orders: Results from the Offender Management Community Cohort Study.* London, England: Ministry of Justice Analytical Series; 2015.

36. Fazel S, Chang Z, Fanshawe T, et al. Prediction of violent reoffending on release from prison: derivation and external validation of a scalable tool. *Lancet Psychiatry.* 2016; **3**(6): 535–543.

37. Stahler GJ, Mennis J, Belenko S, et al. Predicting recidivism for released state prison offenders: examining the influence of individual and neighborhood characteristics and spatial contagion on the likelihood of reincarceration. *Crim Justice Behav.* 2013; **40**(6): 690–711.

38. Ersche KD, Turton AJ, Chamberlain SR, et al. Cognitive dysfunction and anxious-impulsive personality traits are endophenotypes for drug dependence. *Am J Psychiatry.* 2012; **169**(9): 926–936.

39. Arseneault L, Moffit TE, Caspi A. Mental disorders and violence in a total birth cohort: results from the Dunedin study. *Arch Gen Psychiatry.* 2000; **57**(10): 979–986.

40. Sinha R. Chronic stress, drug use, and vulnerability to addiction. *Ann NY Acad Sci.* 2008; **1141**: 105–130.

41. Hendricks PS, Crawford MS, Cropsey KL, et al. The relationships of classic psychedelic use with criminal behavior in the United States adult population. *J Psychopharmacol.* 2018; **32**(1): 37–48.

42. Chang Z, Larsson H, Lichtenstein P, et al. Psychiatric disorders and violent reoffending: a national cohort study of convicted prisoners in Sweden. *Lancet Psychiatry.* 2015; **2**(10): 891–900.

43. Oram S, Trevillion K, Khalifeh H, et al. Systematic review and metaanalysis of psychiatric disorder and the perpetration of partner violence. *Epidemiol Psychiatr Sci.* 2014; **23**(4): 361–376.

44. Fazel S, Gulati G, Linsell L, et al. Schizophrenia and violence: systematic review and meta-analysis. *PLoS Med.* 2009; **6**(8): e1000120.

45. Fitton L, Yu R, Fazel S. Childhood maltreatment and violent outcomes: a systematic review and meta-analysis of prospective studies. *Trauma Violence Abuse.* 2018; epub ahead of print: 1524838018795269. doi:10.1177/1524838018795269.

46. Fazel S, Wolf A, Yukhnenko D. Recidivism reporting checklist. *Open Sci Framework.* 2019. doi:10.17605/OSF.IO/QVTFB.

Developing Policies for Adult Sexual Minorities with Mental Health Needs in Secured Settings

Juan Carlos Arguello

Introduction

Lesbian, Gay, Bisexual, and Transgender (LGBT) people, are more likely to be disproportionally placed in a secured setting.[1] Secured settings such as jails, prisons, and forensic hospitals can be traumatizing, hostile, and dangerous – especially for those who are transgender,[2] which is only compounded when responsive and appropriate policies, procedures, and training are not in place to maintain safety, privacy, and dignity. All LGBT residents, and more importantly those suffering from mental illness, who are in secured environments should be free of discrimination, victimization, and abuse. They should have equal access to safe housing, vocational programs, rehabilitation services, as well as medical and mental health treatments. Many organizations such as National Center for Transgender Equality (NCTE), National Institute of Corrections (NIC), the World Professional Association for Transgender Health (WPATH), and The Joint Commission (TJC) provide guidelines to ensure that LGBT residents are protected. This article provides a general roadmap for developing LGBT policies in secured settings synergizing the recommendations of these organizations with emphasis on policy guidelines for transgender people that are not only standards for good care but also very cost-effective interventions that can help reduce symptoms of mental illness for this population.

Review of Guidelines

LGBT individuals have higher prevalence of mental disorders than heterosexuals and have poorer mental health outcomes.[3] Specifically, higher levels of depression, suicidality, interpersonal trauma, substance use disorders, and general distress have been found for transgender individuals.[4] Recent increased attention of the effects that stigma, discrimination, shame, rejection, and victimization have on LGBT individuals' mental health have been studied.[3] The high prevalence of mental illness in LGBT individuals may be explained by the Minority Stress Model.[5] Minority stress is caused by prejudice, stigma, discrimination, daily hassles, marginality, oppression, hostility, and nonsupportive environments that create unique stressors in LGBT individuals and produces adverse health outcomes, including developing or worsening of mental health disorders. Despite the increased attention to the impact of stigma and discrimination in sexual minority groups, there are few strategies to develop interventions to reduce illness morbidity.[6] Advocacy strategies are recommended to reduce the negative behavioral and environmental experiences by LGBT individuals.[7] Secured settings are hetero- and cisgender-normative environments that, without the appropriate policies to decrease the negative impact of the environment and the attitudes toward LGBT residents, can worsen their mental health. Recommended strategies to decrease minority stress are not only implementable but cost-effective for the facilities.

National Center for Transgender Equality (NCTE)

The NCTE, in 2018, published *Policies to Increase Safety and Respect for Transgender Prisoners: A Guide for Agencies and Advocates* which identified the unique needs of LGBT individuals in secured settings.[8] LGBT individuals endure potential abuse and violence when serving time in these agencies. More specifically, transgender people are 10 times more likely to be sexually assaulted by staff and other residents in state and federal prisons and 40% reported a sexual assault in the previous year.[9] Secured agencies should develop and implement policies that mitigate and reduce these rates of interpersonal violence. The NCTE guide discusses the Prison

Rape Elimination standards that apply to the LGBT population.[10] In 2012, the Prison Rape Elimination Act (PREA) developed standards to protect all inmates including LGBT individuals in federal and state prison.[11] Although, PREA standards are only legally binding in state and federal prisons, adopting these standards in jails and state hospital policies is one substantive step toward the safe provision of services to LGBT residents. The NCTE guide includes how to prevent discrimination, prevent abuse, perform risk assessments, appropriate placement, dignity, respect, privacy, access to health care, and community re-entry.

The NCTE guide recommends that agencies have policies that contain clear nondiscrimination statements. The nondiscrimination statement should bar discrimination and mistreatment based on sex, age, race, national origin, disability, and actual or perceived sexual orientation and gender identity. The policies' nondiscrimination statements should include that LGBT residents will be treated with respect, fairness, and dignity. The policies' nondiscriminatory statements should also contain language that states the agency will have zero tolerance for harassment based on sexual orientation, gender identity, and expression. A simple and low-cost intervention that shows support to LGBT residents is to post nondiscriminatory statements in communal areas.

The NCTE recommends that during the admission or intake process, staff identify vulnerable populations and prevent victimization. Admission or intake policies should contain procedures to identify LGBT individuals, provide for their safety, and establish the appropriate delivery of care. The University of California Los Angeles' Williams Institute website is a helpful resource on how to ask questions about sexual orientation.[12] The Ford Foundation funded a multiyear project at the Williams Institute to identify the best scientific approach to gather data on sexual orientation. Also, PREA standards require assessment and documentation of risk of victimization within days of arrival. It is also an important PREA requirement that the assessments are conducted by staff who are trained in effective and affirmative communication with lesbian, gay, bisexual, transgender, intersex, or gender nonconforming residents in confidential settings. The PREA Resource Center provides training webinars such as "Respectful Communication with LGBTI Offenders" and "Understanding Lesbian, Gay, Bisexual, Transgender, Intersex Inmates, Residents and Detainees" that help staff learn how to interact with LGBT residents with knowledge, respect, and compassion.[13] The period of admission or intake allows time to ask the resident their preferred name and gender pronoun as well as to document this information so that staff are aware of how to address the resident. Policies should also include the resident's preferred staff gender with whom they feel most comfortable when searches are conducted or when staff observe or assist during medical procedures. These simple actions taken by staff during the admission or intake period can prevent stress in LGBT people and can reduce the risk of developing psychological distress. During admission or intake, as with any individual, it is important to assess for the need of mental health services for LGBT. Mental Health questionnaires are often used to identify those individuals that need to be refer to mental health professionals.

Placement or housing assignments of LGBT residents, especially transgender individuals, can be challenging. Policies should include that placement or housing determination will be made through a case-by-case assessment and on an individualized basis. Segregation based solely on their gender or sexual orientation, such as solitary confinement or isolation, is not an appropriate placement for LGBT residents. LGBT individuals are more likely to be placed in solitary confinement than heterosexual residents. The Bureau of Justice Statistics reported that approximately 30% of lesbian, gay, and bisexual prisoners were in restrictive housing in 2011–2012, compared to 18% of heterosexual prisoners, and 22% of lesbian, gay, and bisexual jail inmates had been in segregation compared to 17% of heterosexual jail inmates.[14] PREA standards prohibit individuals at high risk for victimization such as LGBT residents to be placed automatically in involuntary segregated housing, unless there is no other alternative to separate them from likely abusers or for a short period while a placement assessment is completed. Placing LGBT residents who suffer from mental illness in segregation may be detrimental since it may increase their psychiatric symptoms. Some agencies that do not have to comply with PREA standards, such as non-federal jails and prisons, have created LGBT-only housing units. Should these units be available to the organization and utilized, it is important to make residents fully aware that such placement is voluntary and available upon request by the resident. LGBT-only units should have the same privileges, programing, treatment, education, and work opportunities as non-LGBT units. PREA standards also prohibit having a blanket policy to house transgender residents based on their sex assigned at birth or observed anatomy. Every effort should be made to place a LGBT resident in a unit that has residents consistent with their identified gender, unless issues of safety and security prevent such placement.

Many organizations have committees for LGBT residents that assist in placement upon admission into the facility. Some organizations use these committees beyond placement. For example, committees could be involved in determining what property the resident can retain in their possession such as items that supports their identified gender, approving special accommodations such as separate shower times, or authorizing medical treatments such as gender affirming hormone replacement therapy or surgery. It is recommended that the composition of these committees contain medical and mental health professionals who can inform and educate the rest of the committee members on LGBT-specific issues. It is important that these committees advocate for the resident's preferred placement, their access to property related to the gender identity and expression, and their access to the affirmative medical treatment they need.

When developing policies for LGBT residents in secured settings, the NCTE guide emphasizes privacy, dignity, and safety. LGBT patients have the right to privacy. Special attention should be place on policies regarding access to bathrooms, especially for transgender residents, that are consistent with their identified gender. In multiuser bathrooms, privacy can be accomplished with privacy shields or having the resident use it at a different time than other residents. This should be done without limiting the resident's shower time or without isolating them completely from other residents. Having individual toilet stalls with doors and individual showers with curtains are preferred in order to maintain the privacy and dignity of all residents. The CNTE guide recommends that policies should also include the ability of LGBT residents to have access to purchase personal items. These items should not be limited to undergarments but should include items consistent with the person's preferred gender such as clothing, grooming items, cosmetics, and accessories. Some facilities have adopted gender-neutral commissary lists. These commissary lists contain items for all genders. Any resident can purchase any item from the list. Another

recommendation from the CNTE is to allow LGBT residents to have same-sex partner visitations including conjugal visits. LGBT residents should be able to show mutual and consensual displays of affection, such as holding hands and kissing, unless these actions prohibited to all residents in the facility. These additional low-cost efforts, when implemented, can improve the psychological wellbeing of LGBT residents.

Policies should ensure that LGBT patients receive the same access to medical and mental health care as any other resident. Common law cases such as *Sterling v. Borough of Minersville*, *Powell v. Shriver*, *Thomas v. District of Columbia*, and *Moore v. Provo* concluded that the Constitution protects the privacy of highly personal information such as sexual orientation, gender identity, and HIV status. This information shall be kept private by staff unless the LGBT resident discloses this information with others. Special medical treatment considerations in the LGBT community include but are not limited to HIV care and prevention, gender affirming hormone therapy, and gender affirming surgery. Special mental health considerations in the LGBT community include but are not limited to gender dysphoria, trauma-related disorders, anxiety disorders, and depressive disorders. According to the CNTE guide, denying the treatment of these conditions and disorders in institutionalized persons may constitute a violation of the Eighth Amendment. The American Medical Association, American College of Physicians, the American Psychological Association, the American College of Obstetrics and Gynecology, and the World Professional Association for Transgender Health (WPATH) all agree that transition-related treatments are safe, effective, and medically necessary. These treatments are no longer considered cosmetic or experimental. These interventions, including providing gender affirming support by mental health professionals, are the approved treatments for transgender people who are transitioning. The WPATH in their *Standards of Care for The Health of Transsexual*,[15] *Transgender and Gender Nonconforming People* provides guidelines for medical and mental health treatment and includes criteria for gender affirming hormone therapy and gender affirming surgery.

Re-entry planning poses a unique challenge to staff placing LGBT residents back in the community. The same best practices that apply to secured settings should apply to re-entry facilities. PREA standards and fair housing laws that prohibit discrimination against LGBT people should also be applied to community-based facilities (e.g. treatment centers, halfway houses, group houses). Agencies should also ensure that they have contracts with community facilities that adhere to these practices. In addition to appropriate housing, other special considerations for LGBT residents when developing a re-entry or pre-release plans include: ensuring continuity of medical services for LGBT-specific care; helping transgender residents obtain identification documents that reflect their authentic gender identity; and providing LGBT-specific community and online resources.

National Institute of Corrections

The National Institute of Corrections (NIC) in 2015 developed a policy review and development guide, *Lesbian, Gay, Bisexual, Transgender, and Intersex Persons in Custodial Settings.*[16] This guide provides a substantive review of constitutional law that should be considered when developing LGBT affirmative policies. Also, they provide checklists that are based on case law and on PREA standards that apply to LGBT residents. If any of the questions on the checklists are answered "No," the guide recommends addressing that specific issue in policy. NIC contends that the recommended standard is that all policies should be updated to contain all the recommended principles included in the checklists. The NIC's guide also contains appendices containing useful resources for developing policies for LGBT persons.

Another useful aspect to the NIC guide is that it provides examples of case law where institutions have been found to violate the Eighth Amendment, i.e. the right to be free from cruel and unusual punishment. These violations are mostly based on deliberate indifference, or the disregard of the consequences of one's acts or omissions. Agencies were found in violation of the Eighth Amendment when they failed to protect LGBT people from abuse or harassment, used needless segregation, failed to provide medical treatment, failed to protect from unnecessary searches, prohibited same-sex partner visits including conjugal visits, denied marriage to a same-sex partner, prohibited signs of affection between same-sex couples if the same did not apply to heterosexual couples, failed to protect information concerning sexual orientations, failed to protect HIV status, and prohibited possession of nonsexually explicit LGBT materials.

Specifically, regarding transgender inmates diagnosed with gender dysphoria, agencies were found in violation of the Eighth Amendment when they failed to recognize gender dysphoria as a serious medical condition and failed to provide the medically approved treatment for the condition such as gender affirming hormone therapy and gender affirming surgery. Agencies cannot prevent residents diagnosed with gender dysphoria from expressing and adopting the gender consistent with their gender identity since it is considered medical treatment. Treatment for gender dysphoria cannot be denied due to cost or because the agency officials disapprove of the provision of such services. Moreover, according to the NIC guide, agencies cannot use unproven security and safety issues as a reason to deny gender dysphoria treatment.

The Joint Commission

In 2011, The Joint Commission (TJC) published a field guide for *Advancing Effective Communication, Cultural Competence, and Patient- and-Family Centered Care for Lesbian, Gay, Bisexual, and Transgender (LGBT) Community.*[17] The TJC field guide can be useful when developing policies for LGBT residents.

The strategies and recommendations in this field guide are divided into five main areas or domains. These domains are leadership, provision of care, treatment and services, workforce, data collection/use, and community engagement. The following is a brief summary of each domain.

In the leadership domain, TJC recommends integration of LGBT patient needs into the existing and new policies in their accredited facilities. In particular, they recommended that policies contain nondiscriminatory protections for sexual orientation, and gender identity and expression. Policies should provide the patient with the right to identify a support person of their choice in the facility in addition to define family broadly to include different- and same-sex persons related and unrelated to the patients. Policies should have a confidential and reliable method for patients to report discrimination and disrespect. If patients are disrespected, intimidated, harassed, or abused by other patients or staff, a disciplinary process needs to be in place to address these behaviors. Importantly, this domain requires that the facility leadership identifies staff accountable to oversee efforts to provide culturally competent and patient-centered care to LGBT patients and families, as well as establishes a high-level advisory group to monitor supportive efforts, identify gaps, and use information to establish quality improvement activities. The recommendation also includes identifying support staff and physicians with special expertise or experience with LGBT issues.

Regarding the provision of care, treatment, and services domain, TJC recommends the creation and maintenance of a supportive and affirming environment for LGBT patients. Their recommendations include creating a LGBT bill of rights that is posted in high visibility areas of the facility. The common areas, including the visiting rooms, should be welcoming to LGBT patients and their families. It is also recommended that "Safe Zone Area" signs with LGBT-related symbols are posted in these common areas (e.g. rainbow icon). Also recommended is having unisex or single stall bathrooms. The agencies must ensure that visiting policies are fair and nondiscriminatory. The language used by staff with LGBT patients should be inclusive and gender-neutral, and staff should be cautious and avoid bias, stereotypes, and misconceptions about LGBT patients. Staff should also understand and respect the patient's choice to disclose their sexual orientation or keep it private.

The workforce domain ensures that LGBT staff are treated with respect and have equitable treatment and inclusion. Facilities should have policies that protect LGBT staff from abuse, discrimination, bias, and harassment that targets staff members' sexual orientation, or gender identity and expression. Staff working in the facilities should have the same protections as LGBT patients. LGBT staff should be offered health care coverage and benefits equal to any other employee, including coverage of same-sex partners and transgender health. Recruitment and hiring of staff must be inclusive and equitable; human resources departments should provide nondiscrimination policies and statements in writing to new employees.

The data collection and use domain provides examples of what information to gather from all patients to inform facility's policies, program development, quality improvement initiatives, and outreach efforts. These standards around data collection practices assist health care organizations in meeting patient population needs; most importantly, empirical data collection can help health providers to understand their patients and improve the provision of affirmative and competent care. It is recommended that certain data are collected from all patients, including relationship status, sexual orientation, sex,

and gender identity. This information can be collected during the admission and intake process, and patient responses should be voluntary, self-reported, and protected. One important way that health care organizations can improve their patient data collection and better serve their patients is to ensure that electronic medical records have gender identifications beyond the binary of male and female. If the hospital develops a survey, information about sexual orientation and gender should be included. Hospital staff should be trained in how to collect data from all patients, especially those who are LGBT.

Lastly, the TJC recommends that facilities collect feedback from LGBT patients, families, and surrounding LGBT communities to better understand the health needs, identify gaps, and improve areas where deficiencies are found. It is recommended that patient satisfaction surveys include questions on sexual orientation and gender identity. It is important to receive feedback from families on how the facility and staff responded to their needs during the duration of the health care encounter. Also, the facility should engage the surrounding LGBT community and establish outreach partnership efforts that ensure the facility's commitment to provide equitable care to LGBT patients.

Conclusions

This article reviewed existing organizations' guidelines on how to develop policies for LGBT residents in secured settings. They all recommend breaking through institutional barriers and each organization endorsed environmental, behavioral, and social procedures that put emphasis in decreasing stigma, prejudice, discrimination, and harassment. The recommendations increase personal safety and access to medical and mental health services. In addition, they promote dignity, privacy, respect, fairness, and compassion. In the context of the unique inequities experienced by LGBT people, these policy recommendations work to improve mental wellbeing and mitigate or resolve mental health symptoms in LGBT residents, which is cost-effective.

Developing policies for LGBT residents in secured setting is challenging without the guidance of agencies such as The National Center for Transgender Equality, the National Institute of Corrections, the World Professional Association of Transgender Care, and the Joint Commission. Agencies that follow the recommendations of these organizations will have policies that maintain the safety, privacy, and dignity of LGBT residents and promote affirmative environments. Of additional value is that, if these behavioral and environmental interventions are implemented in secured settings, they can positively impact the mental health of LGBT residents.

References

1. Meyer IH, Flores AR, Stemple L, et al. Incarceration rates and traits of sexual minorities in the United States: national inmate survey, 2011–2012. *Am J Public Health*. 2017; **107**(2): 267–273.

2. Center for American Progress, Movement Advancement Project. *Unjust: how the broken criminal justice system fails LGBT people*. Washington, DC 2016.

3. Mereish EH, Poteat VP. A relational model of sexual minority mental and physical health: the negative effects of shame on relationships, loneliness, and health. *J Couns Psychol*. 2015; **62**(3): 425437.

4. Valentine SE, Shipherd JC. A systematic review of social stress and mental health among transgender and gender non-conforming people in the United States. *Clin Psychol Rev*. 2018; **66**: 24–38.

5. Meyer IH. Prejudice, social stress, and mental health in lesbian, gay, and bisexual populations: conceptual issues and research evidence. *Psychol Bull*. 2003; **129** (5): 674–697.

6. Kidd SA, Howison M, Pilling M, et al. Severe mental illness in LGBT populations: a scoping review. *Psychiatr Serv*. 2016; **67**(7): 779–783.

7. Pandya A. Mental health as an advocacy priority in the lesbian, gay, bisexual, and transgender communities. *J Psychiatr Pract*. 2014; **20**(3): 225–227.

8. National Center for Transgender Equality. *Policies to Increase Safety and Respect for Transgender Prisoners: A Guide for Agencies and Advocates*. Washington, DC 2018.

9. Beck AJ, Berzofsky M, Caspar R, et al. *Sexual Victimization in Prisons and Jails Reported By Inmates, 2011–12-Update* (Bureau of Justice Statistics NCJ 241399). Washington, DC 2014.

10. National Center for Transgender Equality. *LGBT People and the Prison Rape Elimination Act*. Washington, DC 2012.

11. United States Department of Justice. Prison Rape Elimination Act (PREA) of 2003 (P.L. 108–79).

12. Badgett MVL, Goldberg N, Conron KJ, Gates GJ. Best practices for asking questions about sexual orientation on surveys. The Williams Institute Sexual Minority Assessment Research Team; 2009. (http://williamsinstitute.law.ucla.edu/wp-content/uploads/SMART-FINAL-Nov-2009.pdf).

13. The National PREA Resource Center. www.preresourcecenter.org (accessed June 2020).

14. Beck AJ. *Use of Restrictive Housing in US Prisons and Jails, 2011–12* (Bureau of Justice Statistics NCJ249209). Washington, DC 2015.

15. Coleman E, Bockting W, Botzer M, et al. Standards of care for the health of transsexual, transgender, and gender-nonconforming people, version 7. *Int J Transgenderism*. 2012; **13**(4): 165–232.

16. Smith BV, Yarussi JM. *Policy Review and Development Guide: Lesbian, Gay, Bisexual, Transgender, and Intersex Persons in Custodial Settings, 2nd edn*. United States Department of Justice, National Institute of Corrections; 2015.

17. The Joint Commission. *Advancing Effective Communication, Cultural Competence, and Patient- and Family-Centered Care for the Lesbian, Gay, Bisexual, and Transgender (LGBT) Community: A Field Guide*. Oak Brook, IL 2011.

An Overview of Jail-Based Competency Restoration

Scott E. Kirkorsky, Mary Gable, and Katherine Warburton

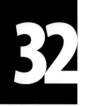

Introduction

Forensic populations in the United States are increasing, driven largely by a rise in individuals determined to be incompetent to stand trial (IST).[1] According to the California Department of State Hospitals' 2017 Annual Report, the most common type of commitment (22% of all commitments) was defendants adjudicated IST.[2] While just five years ago, 343 mentally ill inmates were awaiting placement for competency restoration services, as of 2018, that number has increased to a staggering 819.[3] As defined by the *Dusky v. United States* (1960)[4] standard, a competent defendant must have the capacity to understand the legal proceedings, which includes an understanding of the various participants in the justice process. Defendants must also be able to function within the legal system by consulting with their attorneys. Competency restoration is the process used when an individual charged with a crime is found by a court to be IST. Incompetency to stand trial is generally the result of an active mental illness and/or intellectual disability. A criminal defendant must be restored to competency before the legal process can proceed. State mental hospitals have historically served as the primary source of competency restoration treatment for defendants.

An estimated 60,000 competency evaluations are performed across the United States each year with at least one-fifth of these defendants being adjudicated incompetent.[5] This volume of incompetent defendants occupies a substantial portion of state hospital beds, contributing to an increase in forensic admissions to state hospitals, which increased from 7.6% in 1983 to 36% in 2012.[6] In a 2017 report from the National Association of State Mental Health Program Directors, a 76% increase in forensic patients in state hospitals occurred between 1999 and 2014.[1] (p. 8)

In California, state hospitals maintain about 6,200 beds, and more than 90% of these beds are occupied by individuals from the criminal justice system. Just

a few decades ago, under 50% of patients in state hospitals had come from the criminal justice system. Despite California's recent addition of 700 beds dedicated to competency restoration, still more than 20% of beds occupied by forensic patients are filled with defendants found IST.[2] (p. 3)

Defendants in need of competency restoration services are often held in jail, awaiting admission to a state hospital. The resulting waitlists, which range from days to months, have led to states being held in contempt of court for violating limits placed on how long incompetent defendants can be held in jail. For example, the United States District Court of Washington case of *Trueblood, et al. v. Washington State Department of Health and Human Services et al.*[7] (2015) found that it is a violation of due process for defendants adjudicated incompetent to be held in jail for longer than seven days awaiting competency restoration services. In California, a recent Superior Court order in the case of *Stiavetti, et al. v. Ahlin, et al.*[8] (2016) imposed a 28-day limit to the time a defendant can await competency restoration services, and this trend in litigation can be seen throughout the United States as jails are filling with patients awaiting state hospital admissions.[9] As such, alternatives to state hospitalization for IST patients have been developed, including community-based restoration programs, and jail-based competency (JBCT) restoration programs. JBCT programs provide restoration services in county jails, rather than in psychiatric hospitals. If JBCT treatment is successful, a defendant may bypass a stay at the state hospital, resulting in an expedited resolution of the legal proceedings.

JBCT Programs in the United States

The first JBCT program was piloted in Prince George County, VA in 1997.[10] This program is held at Riverside Regional Jail in a converted unit where 48 cells were adapted into 38 patient rooms and 10 offices for mental health providers. The program is run by Liberty Healthcare (an independent contractor), and, in five years, they have reportedly evaluated and treated "over 1400 inmate-patients and completed 572 formal forensic evaluation reports for the courts."[11]

Over the last two decades, additional states have developed JBCT programs. JBCT programs are now established in Colorado, California, Georgia, Texas, Arizona, Florida, Tennessee, and Louisiana.[10] [(p. 1)] The characteristics of JBCT programs vary significantly in terms of size, selection criteria, physical layout, and availability of mental health services.

JBCT Programs in California

California Penal Code (PC) §1369.1[12] permits the restoration of IST defendants to competency in county jails for a period not to exceed six months. California's[13] JBCT restoration first began in San Bernardino County in 2011 and has expanded to multiple programs across the state with a total of 324 beds.

Total admission for 2018 was 1,289 defendants that were 72% male and 18% female. Average lengths of stays ranged from 57 to 82 days with average days to restore competency ranging from 41 to 66 days. Of the 1,191 defendants discharged from the programs, 748 were evaluated as restored to competency and 10 were evaluated as unlikely to be restored. The remaining 433 defendants were not successfully restored by the JBCT program and were transferred to the state hospital for additional restoration services. The rate of competency restoration of discharged patients from individual California JBCT programs ranges from 52% to 86%.

Selection Criteria

An important consideration when assessing the efficacy of a JBCT program is the spectrum of patients the program is able to treat. Given that these programs are new, guidance in the scientific literature on the selection criteria for JBCT programs is lacking. Using characteristics identified in the literature as predictors of those defendants less likely to be restored may serve as a starting point in developing a set of selection criteria for JBCT programs. In 1992, Carbonell et al. examined 152 hospitalized incompetent defendants and determined that both clinical and demographic variables were poor predictors of restorability.[14] That same year, however, Golding suggested that pre-

morbid functioning, negative symptoms, insidious onset, prior psychiatric history, and a history of response to treatment were the best predictors of restoration of competence.[15] More recently in 2007, Mossman reviewed the records of over 350 defendants hospitalized for competency restoration and found that a lower probability of restoration was associated with older age, misdemeanor charges, and longer stays.[16] In general, older individuals with longstanding, treatment-refractory, severe mental illness or mental retardation as opposed to those with personality and nonpsychotic disorders are less likely to be restored.[17,18]

JBCT programs in California have evolved in terms of the patients that they accept. When the first programs were conceived in 2007 and 2008, the goal was to accept defendants that were expected to rapidly respond to treatment in hopes of quickly and effectively treating this subset of IST defendants. This led to JBCT programs selecting younger defendants that were treatment-naive and resulted in underutilization of available beds. Thus, programs began to accept defendants expected to require an intermediate term of restoration services. These defendants had earlier-onset mental illness and more significant levels of criminal involvement in the form of repeated visits to jail. An estimated 40% of such defendants ultimately went to state hospitals, but over half were successfully treated within the jail setting.

A 2011 study by Colwell and Gianesini.[19] of 71 male defendants ordered to undergo restoration found that those who went more days before medications were initiated were more likely to be found nonrestorable. Recently, JBCT programs began to accept more complicated defendants with multiple incarcerations, longstanding mental illness, co-occurring substance use disorders, psychotic violence, and a history of poor treatment compliance. These defendants often have failed multiple medications or have refractory symptoms. California program administrators expected these defendants to require a longer duration of restoration services, likely necessitating transfer to state hospitals. However, the rationale was that beginning treatment sooner may decrease the length of stay once transferred. Further investigation is needed to determine if treatment in a JBCT program decreases the length of hospitalization for this population.

Certain populations are still difficult to accommodate in California's JBCT programs. For example, defendants with gang affiliations that may limit appropriate housing or their ability to program with peers could be excluded from JBCT. Language barriers may also limit the ability of a JBCT program to accommodate certain defendants. Additionally, individuals with major medical issues that cannot be adequately treated in a jail-based setting, such as those requiring frequent dialysis, can often lack needed accommodations by the JBCT programs. JBCT programs are also frequently unable to provide the necessary level of care to defendants with neurocognitive disorders. However, a brief period of evaluation and treatment in the JBCT setting may allow evaluators to identify these defendants as unlikely to be restored, avoiding an unnecessary attempt to restore competency at the state hospital.

Colorado's Restoring Individuals Safely and Effectively (RISE) program at Arapahoe County Detention Center is an example of a JBCT program that uses specific criteria for identifying appropriate defendants. RISE only accepts defendants that are not an imminent danger to themselves or others; are likely to be restored in 60 days or less; and are medication and treatment compliant. Additionally, candidates must be motivated, medically stable, and able to engage in self-care. Over an approximately 30-month period ending in May of 2016, RISE discharged 221 defendants, restoring 158 (71%) to competence and transferring 43 (19%) to a state hospital facility. RISE's selection criteria are like those used in earlier iterations of California JBCT programs.[20]

Examining the effects of selection criteria on JBCT outcomes requires further study. Evidence-based selection criteria for JBCT program participants may help identify the most efficient use of the various settings where competency restoration services are administered (i.e. inpatient, outpatient, and in county jails). In the absence of selection criteria, JBCT programs may need to adjust their designs to accommodate the most acutely ill patients, who have historically required restoration services in a state hospital.

Medication and Medication Compliance

The issue of involuntarily medicating IST defendants is complex, especially outside of an inpatient psychiatric hospital setting. Most relevant to the issue of involuntarily medicating incompetent defendants is

Sell v. United States (2003).[21] In this case, the Supreme Court of the United States found that medications may be involuntarily administered solely to restore competency when an important state interest is at stake and medication can further that interest by restoring the defendant to competency. Additionally, there can be no less restrictive treatment alternative available. If the *Sell* criteria are met, a Judge may order that a defendant be involuntarily medicated for the purpose of competency restoration. However, even with a *Sell* order in place, the medication must still be administered. The *Sell* criteria need only to be applied when an inmate is not dangerous or gravely disabled. For those inmates that are dangerous or gravely disabled, the Supreme Court of the United States case of *Washington v. Harper* (1990)[22] allows for the involuntary medication of these inmates after administrative review.

In California, "If the defendant is examined by a psychiatrist and the psychiatrist forms an opinion as to whether or not treatment with antipsychotic medication is medically appropriate, the psychiatrist shall inform the court of his or her opinions as to the likely or potential side effects of the medication, the expected efficacy of the medication, possible alternative treatments, and whether it is medically appropriate to administer antipsychotic medication in the county jail," pursuant to PC 1369(a).[23] When identifying those defendants appropriate for involuntary treatment, PC 1370(a)(2)(B)(ii)(II)[24] does not specify that an important state interest be at stake (as is specified in the *Sell* criteria), but does require the defendant be charged with a "[s]erious crime against property or person . . . "

While statutes provide mechanisms for the involuntary administration of medication to JBCT clients, whether involuntary medication is actually administered is facility dependent. In general, medication administration is managed by correctional mental health providers who, as a matter of facility policy, do not involuntarily medicate inmates that are outside of an inpatient psychiatric hospital setting. However, select programs do have dedicated program nurses that administer the medication for JBCT participants.

Fortunately, medication refusals are uncommon in JBCT programs. In California, program administrators estimate that medication compliance is greater than 85%. Voluntary medication administration is emphasized in JBCT programs and various modalities are employed to improve compliance. Defendants are extensively educated on the importance of medication in resolving their symptoms. Additionally, reward systems that incentivize medication compliance may also be permitted. Such incentives can range from access to preferred foods or recreational items to access to additional services or visitation privileges.

While California JBCT programs have not excluded patients that are noncompliant with medications, other states make voluntariness a requirement for admission. For example, Colorado's RISE program lists medication compliance as a selection criterion for participants. In her 2016 National Alliance on Mental Illness (NAMI) presentation, Dr. Galin noted 99% medication compliance for RISE participants.[20] (p. 16)

In 2013, Dr. Patricia Zapf,[25] a national expert in the field of competency restoration, wrote, "The available research and commentary suggests that successful restoration is related to how well the defendant responds to psychotropic medications administered to alleviate symptoms of mental disorders." Attempts to restore most defendants to competency without medications are a futile approach. Thus, if involuntary medications are not consistently administered to JBCT participants, these untreated individuals are at risk of deteriorating and are unlikely to be restored in this setting. At the time of the submission of this manuscript, program-specific data on involuntary medication administration were not available.

Program Staffing

Each California JBCT program has staff that are distinct from that of the jail's psychiatry service. Programs have at least one psychiatrist available to treat JBCT defendants. While participants have daily contact with mental health professionals, psychiatric encounters for medication adjustments generally occur weekly. The amount of time the psychiatrist is available to JBCT defendants varies based on the program size. Emergencies that occur after hours are managed by the jail psychiatrist on call. Jail medical staff manage medical issues.

In addition to psychiatrists, all programs employ psychologists, social workers, and a program director. Ratios of staff to defendants are established upon program inception based on anticipated participants. Recreational therapists and behavioral health technicians may also be employed by larger programs. Social workers run most of the daily programming. Social workers also develop individualized treatment plans

but do not conduct individual therapy. Psychologists perform initial and follow-up assessments and are responsible for submitting progress reports to the court.

Texas uses a similar staffing model, which includes at least one psychiatrist and a multidisciplinary team. Texas' policies for county JBCT programs are outlined in a section of their Administrative Code adopted in August, 2018. Texas emphasizes providing services like those available in an inpatient mental health facility, specifically prescribing similar staffing requirements and hours of restoration services.[26] Additionally, Texas requires the programs to be supported by a "specially trained jailer."[27] Overall, Texas' average ratio of staff to defendants is not to fall below 3.7 to 1.[28]

Colorado's RISE program also makes use of a multidisciplinary team but has added a peer support model approach. Experienced peers help minimize limitations in terms of staff time and materials. Peer support specialists may also enhance the therapeutic milieu by developing trust with defendants participating in the program.

Peers are thought to have a unique appreciation of the circumstances in which other defendants find themselves and can, in theory, provide guidance in overcoming barriers to competence by acting as role models and advocating for other patients. Additionally, Colorado's RISE program makes use of a re-entry specialist who facilitates the return of an individual to the general jail population with the goal of reducing both rates of regression and the need for a second course of competency restoration.[20] (pp. 19–22)

Physical Layout

There are significant differences in the ways that individual JBCT programs house participants. Ideally, defendants undergoing competency restoration are housed separate from the general population. In her 2011 commentary on JBCT restoration, Dr. Kapoor[29] identifies several difficulties inherent to correctional facilities that include: "lock-downs, lack of an officer for transport, 'count' time, shift change, and meals." Dr. Kapoor also notes the potential for incompetent inmates to be victimized by their competent peers. Many of these problems are addressed by separating JBCT program participants from other inmates.

California's JBCT programs are generally housed in a single pod with similar accommodations to those living spaces for the general population. Open cells with yard access are important. Efforts are made to allow defendants to move more freely and attend groups in a more comfortable setting than that of the standard common areas in jail. Large communal areas outside of the cells that are aesthetically discernible from standard jail housing units are ideal. Additionally, an effective JBCT environment is free of loud noises and distractions that are typical of other housing units.

Programs are encouraged to create an environment that feels like a treatment center to enhance the milieu. For example, in some counties, features of the JBCT environment include couches and carpeting. Recruiting custody officers that are amenable to a more relaxed environment and that can have positive interactions with program participants is also desirable. Having access to single cells is critical in order to accommodate more acute or mentally ill participants. If single occupancy cells are not available, unstable defendants may still require their own space, resulting in inefficiencies as one defendant will solely occupy a cell with two beds.

Smaller counties in California have few pre-trial defendants requiring restoration. JBCT programs in these counties are currently being developed, but their design is necessarily different. With one to five total participants at any given time, having a dedicated pod is impractical. Therefore, the milieu environment and peer interaction available to JBCT participants in larger county facilities is limited. Competency restoration specialists schedule visits with these defendants on a regular basis, and psychiatrists are hired for a limited time each week to address medication needs. Given that these smaller county models are in their infancy, the outcomes of these programs and how they will evolve remain uncertain.

Length of Stay

A primary goal of JBCT programs is to more efficiently restore defendants to competency. Rapid competency restoration allows programs to accommodate more defendants and ensures defendants a speedy trial. California program administrators report that historically programs are asked to consider state hospital transfer if a defendant continues to require restoration services after 100 days. As a defendant approaches 100 days, programs evaluate the case closely to determine an appropriate disposition. An emphasis is placed on receiving input from the treatment team to determine the value of additional days of JBCT versus transfer to a state hospital. Recent medication changes and progress may suggest that a transfer is unnecessary. Therefore, it is possible for a defendant to remain in the program for several weeks beyond the 100-day mark. Thus, program administrators do not place hard limits on the duration of JBCT services, empowering individual programs and treatment teams to make decisions on a case-by-case basis.

The average length of stay for California JBCT participants in 2018 was about 69 days. However, the average time to restore patients was only about 52 days. Statewide JBCT administrators identify programs that strictly focus on achieving competency and closely monitor each defendant's progress with routine re-evaluation as characteristics resulting in shorter lengths of stay. Determining what accounts for the period between when defendants are restored to competency and when they are discharged from the JBCT program is an area that requires further investigation.

The average length of stay for California JBCT programs seems consistent with other programs that publish these data. For example, in 2016, Colorado's RISE program reported an average length of stay for restored defendants as 55 days with 76% of defendants restored in less than 60 days and 90% restored in less than 90 days.[20] (p. 16) While average lengths of stay for Texas were not available, their Administrative Code, Rule §416.89, mandates that if a defendant charged with a felony is not restored to competency after 60 days, "the psychiatrist or psychologist must coordinate with provider staff members to link the individual for continued services and supports post discharge from the jail-based competency restoration (JBCR) program to a mental health facility or residential care facility."[30] In a 2010 Request for Information, Louisiana reported that the state maintains a 90-day JBCT program.

Head-to-head studies of competency restoration programs in jails and psychiatric/state hospitals are insufficient to find one environment definitively more efficient than the other. However, in general, JBCT program administrators report an ability to restore defendants to competence as quickly as hospital programs. JBCT programs may allow the restoration process to start sooner and decrease the amount of time IST defendants idle in jail awaiting transfer.

Potential Cost Savings

In their comparison of competency restoration in different treatment environments, Danzer et al.[31] noted that the cost for competency restoration in state hospitals ranged from $300 to $1,000 per day while the cost of competency restoration services in jail ranged from $42 to $222 per day. Although similar efficacy is reported in both treatment environments, because of strict selection criteria in some JBCT programs further comparisons of efficacy are necessary to control for the severity of symptoms, as the most mentally ill IST defendants, and those least likely to be restored, are treated in hospitals. This logical trend may artificially increase the relative efficacy of JBCT programs when compared to hospitals.

Lessons Learned in California

Interviews with program administrators identified the most important take-away lesson is the importance of county government. Trust must be developed. Consistency and follow-through on the part of the JBCT programs are essential. Additionally, many stakeholders may initially oppose JBCT programs. However, opposition may be mitigated by incorporating reputable treatment providers with positive track records in the county that the program will serve.

Conclusion

JBCT is one strategy that states are employing to address the challenges posed by increasing numbers of IST defendants in need of competency restoration services. Potential advantages of JBCT include more rapid access to treatment, decreased costs, and less incentive to malinger.[31] (pp. 7,8) Potential disadvantages include treating IST defendants in a custodial environment, variability in the ability of JBCT program staff to provide involuntary medication despite an involuntary medication order being in place, and, particularly in smaller programs or those with limited staffing, a lack of separation between evaluators and treaters.[30] (p. 311)

Initial outcomes regarding cost savings, efficiency, and efficacy of JBCT programs seem promising, especially in light of the lengthy waitlists for state hospitals due to increasing referrals. However, various questions arise as states consider JBCT programs. Is a JBCT program appropriate for all IST defendants or only those with less-severe mental illness that have a higher probability of rapid restoration? Are jails equipped to treat IST defendants involuntarily, and, if not, should treatment refusal exclude a defendant from participating in a JBCT program? Additional quantitative research is necessary to solidify the role of JBCT services in addressing the increasing burden of IST defendants.

Disclaimer

The findings and conclusions in this article are those of the authors and do not represent the views or opinions of the California Department of State Hospitals or the California Health and Human Services Agency.

Disclosures

Dr. Kirkorsky is a Clinical Assistant Professor in the Department of Psychiatry at The University of Arizona College of Medicine – Phoenix; Dr. Gable is a child and adolescent psychiatrist; Dr. Warburton is the Medical Director of the California Department of State Hospitals. Drs. Kirkorsky, Gable, and Warburton did not receive payment from a third party for any aspect of the submitted work, so there are no conflicts of interest. In addition, Drs. Kirkorsky, Gable, and Warburton have no patents, planned or pending, that are relevant to the submitted work. There are no other relationships or activities that readers could perceive to have influenced, or that give the appearance of potentially influencing, what is written in the submitted work.

References

1. National Association of State Mental Health Program Directors. Assessment #10: forensic patients in state psychiatric hospitals: 1999–2016. 2017. https://nasmhpd.org/sites/default/files/TACPaper.10.Forensic-Patients-in-State-Hospitals_508C_v2.pdf (accessed June 2020).

2. California Department of State Hospitals. 2017 annual report. www.dsh.ca.gov/publications/docs/ADA2017AnnualRept.pdf (accessed June 2020).

3. Weiner J. Breakdown: mental health. 2019. https://calmatters.org/articles/california-mental-health-treatment-in-prisons/ (accessed June 2020).

4. *Dusky v. United States*, 362 U.S. 402 (1960).

5. Wall BW, Ash P, Keram E, Pinals DA, Thompson CR. AAPL Practice resource: evaluation of competence to stand trial. *J Am Acad Psychiatry Law*; 2018. http://jaapl.org/content/jaapl/46/3_Supplement/S4.full.pdf (accessed June 2020).

6. Gowensmith WN, Frost LE, Speelman DW, Therson DE. Lookin' for beds in all the wrong places: outpatient competency restoration as a promising approach to modern challenges. *Psychol Public Policy Law.* 2016; **22**(3): 293–305.

7. *Trueblood, et al. v. Washington State Department of Social and Health Services,* 101 F. Supp. 3d 1010 (W.D. Wash. 2015). https://docs.justia.com/cases/federal/district-courts/washington/wawdce/2:2014cv01178/202545/131 (accessed February 17, 2019).

8. *Stiavetti, et al. v. Ahlin, et al.* Superior Court of California, County of Alameda (2016), Case No. RG15779731, [Tentative] Order Granting In Part Petition for Writ of Mandate (03/15/2019).

9. Warburton K, McDermott BE, Gale A, Stahl. SM. A survey of national trends in psychiatric patients found incompetent to stand trial: reasons for the re-institutionalization of people with serious mental illness in the United States. *CNS Spectr.* 2020; **25**(2): 245–251.

10. Wik A. Alternatives to inpatient competency restoration programs: jail-based competency restoration programs. 2018. www.nri-inc.org/media/1500/jbcr_website-format_oct2018.pdf (accessed June 2020).

11. Jennings JL, Bell JD. The "ROC" model: psychiatric evaluation, stabilization and restoration of competency in a jail setting. 2012. https://doi.org/10.5772/30040 (accessed June 2020).

12. Cal. Pen. Code §1369 (2015).

13. Department of State Hospitals JBCT Metrics Summary for 2018. Received February 8, 2019.

14. Carbonell JL, Heilbrun K, Friedman FL. Predicting who will regain trial competency: initial promise unfulfilled. *Forensic Rep.* 1992; **5**(1): 67–76.

15. Golding SL. Studies of incompetent defendants: research and social policy implications. *Forensic Rep.* 1992; **5**(1): 77–83.

16. Mossman D. Predicting restorability of incompetent criminal defendants. *J Am Acad Psychiatry Law* 2007; **35**(1): 34–43.

17. Morris DR, Parker GF. Jackson's Indiana: state hospital competence restoration in Indiana. *J Am Acad Psychiatry Law.* 2009; **36**(4): 522–534.

18. Morris DR, Deyoung NJ. Long-term competence restoration. *J Am Acad Psychiatry Law.* 2014; **42**(1): 81–90.

19. Colwell LH, Gianesini J. Demographic, criminogenic, and psychiatric factors that predict competency restoration. *J Am Acad Psychiatry Law.* 2011; **39**: 297–306.

20. Galin K, Wallerstein L, Miller R. Restoring Individuals Safely and Effectively (RISE): Colorado's jail-based competency restoration program. Presentation to NAMI national convention; 2016. www.nami.org/getattachment/Get-Involved/NAMI-National-Convention/2015-Convention-Presentation-Slides-and-Resources/A-7-Restoring-Individuals-Safely-and-Effectively-(RISE).pdf (accessed June 2020).

21. *Sell v. United States,* 539 U.S. 166 (2003).

22. *Washington v. Harper,* 494 U.S. 210 (1990).

23. Cal. Pen. Code §1369 (2009).

24. Cal. Pen. Code §1370 (a)(2)(B)(ii)(III) (2018).

25. Zapf P. *Standardizing Protocols for Treatment to Restore Competency to Stand Trial: Interventions and Clinically Appropriate Time Periods (Document No. 13-01-1901).* Olympia, WA: Washington State Institute for Public Policy; 2013.

26. Texas Administrative Code, Title 25, Part 1, Chapter 416, Subchapter C, Rule §416.80. https://texreg.sos.state.tx.us/ (accessed February 18, 2019).

27. Texas Administrative Code, Title 25, Part 1, Chapter 416, Subchapter C, Rule §416.78. https://texreg.sos.state.tx.us/ (accessed February 18, 2019).

28. Texas Health and Human Services. Jail-Based Competency Restoration Pilot Program Third Quarter Report for Fiscal Year 2017. https://hhs.texas.gov/reports/2017/06/jail-based-competency-restoration-pilot-program-third-quarter-report-fiscal-year-2017 (accessed June 2020).

29. Kapoor R. Commentary: jail-based competency restoration. *J Am Acad Psychiatry Law.* 2011; **39**(3): 297–306.

30. Texas Administrative Code, Title 25, Part 1, Chapter 416, Subchapter C, Rule §416.89. https://texreg.sos.state.tx.us/ (accessed February 18, 2019).

31. Danzer GS, Wheeler EMA, Alexander AA, Wasser TD. Competency restoration for adult defendants in different treatment environments. *J Am Acad Psychiatry Law.* 2019; **47**(1): 68–81.

Fixated Threat Assessment Centres: Preventing Harm and Facilitating Care in Public Figure Threat Cases and Those Thought to Be at Risk of Lone-Actor Grievance-Fuelled Violence

Justin Barry-Walsh, David V. James, and Paul E. Mullen

Introduction

Developments in threat assessment, particularly in the area of concerning communications and approaches to public figures, have led to the setting-up in a number of countries of a new style of service for assessing and managing risk to the prominent from the actions of lone individuals. Known as fixated threat assessment centres (FTACs), their central characteristic is that they are jointly staffed by police officers and by psychiatric staff from health services. They are based on the realization that the interests of the prominent in terms of protection overlap with those of the people harassing them in terms of medical care. Research over the last decade has re-established that the majority of those threatening, harassing, or attacking public figures have unmet mental health needs, and that attention to these is often the most effective way of reducing risk, whilst at the same time improving their lot and focusing on treatment, rather than criminalization. The approach has recently been expanded to encompass assessment and intervention in individuals suspected of being radicalized into extreme ideologies and at risk of proceeding to commit terrorist acts.

The presence of psychiatrists in FTACs allows the understanding of motive and mental state which is essential to accurate risk assessment. It also allows health-based interventions to lower or manage risk. The psychiatric involvement here has little to do with the application in courts of the Victorian psychiatric defence of insanity, a legal rather than a medical concept. Nor is it to do with issues of responsibility for an individual's actions which are prominent in some jurisdictions and completely absent in others. Rather, it deals with the reality that mental illness affects people's judgment and behavior, not simply through prominent symptomatology, but through the disinhibition associated with illness, the loss of judgment which comes with social isolation and the absence of a restraining peer group, and the disconnection with social values that often accompanies social decline. Effective interventions will involve compulsory psychiatric treatment in some cases, but in others simple interventions such as connecting the individual with treating services. Networking with statutory agencies such as social work or housing may be highly effective, as may family contact. It is important to note at the outset that the focus of these interventions is prevention of harm. The exercise is not solely concerned with violence, but also with other forms of risk. Concerning communications and approaches may give rise to psychological distress, to fear as to what might happen next, to public embarrassment, to disruption of the ability to perform a public role, and to the use of expensive police resources, some of which prove unnecessary when comprehensive risk assessment is applied.

A key concept in this field is that of fixation. Fixation has been described by Mullen et al. as "an intense preoccupation with an individual, activity, or idea," "an obsessive preoccupation...pursued to an abnormally intense degree."[1] In the public figure context, fixation may be the result of grievances, real or otherwise, of idiosyncratic quests for "justice," of perceived rejection, bizarre amorous attachments or misguided quests for help. Fixation may arise out of mental illness, although this is not always the case. People who engage in stalking behavior and those who become vexatious litigants or querulants commonly are fixated. A striking feature of pathological fixation is the level of psychosocial harm done to the fixated individual as well as the potential for harm both to those closest to the individual and to those who are the object of their fixation. The work of FTACs and similar units in consequence limits harm, not only to prominent people, but to the families and communities from which the fixated individuals come.

The Development of FTACs

In 2003, the British government funded a research project designed to increase the efficiency and effectiveness of the royal and parliamentary protection services.[2] The aim was to improve their ability to evaluate and manage the threat presented by stalkers, threateners, and those who attempted to force their way into the presence of royalty or members of parliament, whether it be with ill or benign intent. For efficiency, read decrease the escalating costs, both of monitoring increasing numbers of potentially problematic people and of providing close protection to an ever-wider circle of royalty and parliamentarians. For effectiveness, read improve methods of recognizing and managing those at high risk of acting to disrupt, or even endanger, the lives of protectees. To give some idea of the magnitude of the problem, the Queen alone, at that time, was the target of the activities of over 2,000 active, problematic individuals.

The commissioning of the research reflected the realization that, in terms of threat towards public figures, although the motivation and modus operandi of terrorist and criminal groups was understood and well-established systems were in place to assess and manage them, there was little understanding of risks posed by disturbed members of the general public who exhibited a pattern of harassment and stalking towards public figures and made repeated attempts to communicate with them or enter their presence. Such individuals did not fit into standard policing methods for assessing and managing threat. Whilst it was recognized terrorist organizations tended to engage in random attacks on mass population targets rather than prominent individuals, isolated loners remained an unknown quantity.

At the outset of the research phase, those of us involved in what was termed the Fixated Research Group believed we would face the classic problem of identifying and prioritizing multiple factors correlated with moving from stalking and threatening to acting in a manner which placed the principals at risk.

In the end, we hoped to generate some kind of predictive algorithm. The researchers were given extraordinary access to the records of the police, protection services, and mental health services. In addition, vast quantities of material generated by the stalkers and threateners were made available. Our initial assumptions about multiple factors and the need for complex algorithms proved mistaken.

As the data accumulated, it became increasingly clear that one factor above all determined both the continuing persistence and intensity of the problem behaviors themselves and the probability of progression to actions which were even more disruptive and on occasion violent. That factor was the presence of untreated mental illness. Most of the persistent stalkers and threateners had serious mental disorders, and virtually all of those attempting to break through the barriers protecting the principals, or making attempted or actual attacks, were psychotic at the time.[3] Severe mental illness was the key both to understanding an individual's motivation and to assessing different forms of risk – the probability of persistence, intensity, and progression to violence. Of course, this is not the same as saying that one has to be mad to target a public figure or that psychotic illness, which is relatively common, could be used as a marker for potential attack. Rather, it affords an avenue for better understanding and assessment of public figure threat cases, as well as opening possibilities for prevention. The treatment of mental illness was revealed as the management method most likely to reduce risk. A predominately criminal justice and security problem became a predominately mental health problem.

The findings of the Fixated Research Group, published in a series of 13 papers in peer-reviewed journals, led to the establishment of the Fixated Threat Assessment Centre (FTAC) in the United Kingdom in 2006 – a model subsequently adopted elsewhere. The unit is located within the Specialist Operations section of the Metropolitan Police, based in London but with a national remit. Its key feature is that it is staffed both by medical personnel from the National Health Service and by police officers, being jointly funded by the Office of Security and Counter-Terrorism at the Home Office and by the Department of Health.

The aims of the approach are twofold: to improve the outcomes for the individuals referred and at the same time to reduce the risk they may pose to the individual they are focused on, or indeed others close to them. The service does not attempt the futile task of attempting to predict who might go on to act in dangerous ways. Rather, it has adopted a population model. It is possible, through looking at the associations of progressing to commit destructive behaviors, to tell which individuals lie in the minority of cases from which problems are likely to come. By intervening in all such cases, it is possible to prevent individuals going on to engage in dangerous actions without knowing which particular individuals would, without intervention, have gone on to do so. An analogy is attention to risk factors in cardiac disease: by identifying those with high cholesterol, obesity, smoking, and so on, it is possible to intervene in a population to reduce the risk of adverse outcomes without knowing exactly which cases, without intervention, would have gone on to suffer them.

A pilot scheme established for 18 months demonstrated the effectiveness of the approach,[4] and led to the unit becoming permanent. The presence of psychiatrists allowed the diagnosis of mental illness and an analysis of its influence on motivation, risk and potential management options. UK FTAC considered referrals of those who made inappropriate approaches or communications to the royal family, senior politicians, and "iconic sites." These referrals led to a process of information gathering by police and mental health professionals and an assessment of the problems each individual might produce. A level of concern was used in describing these,[5] not a level of risk, given that concern levels involve decisions made on limited information in real-time operational situations, as opposed to risk assessment which involves considering large amounts of information at relative leisure. Ways of mitigating or removing concerns were then considered, and a management plan established.[6] This generally involved catalyzing action from statutory services around the country, including police, health services, social services, and even housing. Where mental illness was evident, there was usually liaison with the psychiatric services responsible for the individual's domicile. The role of FTAC was not direct involvement in treatment; rather the emphasis was on the appropriate sharing of information, and the communication of this information in a targeted way to relevant agencies in the part of the country in which the individual lived, with the aim of initiating interventions from other services locally, sometimes on a multiagency basis. In many cases, FTAC arranges a networked community response, which

will involve both the monitoring of cases and practical interventions, with the provision of a support worker. Such practical interventions can be remarkably effective. This reflects the fact that the importance of mental illness to assessing and managing risk concerns not only psychotic symptomatology, but also difficulties in the correct interpretation of events, poor judgment, disinhibition, and social isolation which removes the moderating influence of personal relationships and peer groups.

The range of possible interventions also means that the model can be used in jurisdictions with very different health care arrangements and mental health laws. The UK has advantages in terms of ease of compulsory hospitalization, given the low legal threshold and the existence of the National Health Service. The UK also differs in that responsibility in the mentally ill is only relevant in homicide cases, and hospitalization is routinely used as a final disposal in sentencing at court, with the criteria being the person's health, rather than meeting any insanity criteria. Yet, the model has proved equally useful in countries with quite different systems and in jurisdictions such as Australian states which have a system not dissimilar to the competency/insanity limitations in the USA.

The efficacy of UK FTAC's operations was demonstrated in part by the proportion of referrals in which mental illness was identified. In a study of 100 individuals assessed as being of high or moderate concern by FTAC, 86% were found to be suffering from psychotic illness. Compulsory admission was the outcome in 53% of cases and voluntary admission in 4%, whilst 26.5% were taken on for management by community mental health teams or assertive outreach services.[4] With intervention, 80% of cases had been managed down to a low level of concern by the end of the study period. A more sophisticated assessment of FTAC outcomes used a mirrored design in which individuals were in effect their own controls.[7] The study looked at one- and two-year periods before and after FTAC intervention. It identified highly significant reductions both in the number of individuals engaging in communications and problematic approaches and in the total numbers of incidents of concern.[7] It also saw a reduction in police call-outs, raising the possibility that the exercise might prove cost-neutral.

Reinventing the Wheel

The establishment of the UK FTAC, and the research upon which it was based, can be considered something of a watershed moment in that it brought a focus on mental illness back into threat assessment practice, and it illustrated the overlap between public figure threat assessment and the field of stalking, so enabling insights in terms of motivation, classification, and formalized means of assessing threat to be brought across from stalking research.[8] Threat assessment and management as a construct and a paradigm had seen a resurgence in interest from the 1980s onwards after a century of neglect.[9] This included the development of a threat assessment service in 1986 for Congress in the United States,[10] (which over time increasingly came to resemble the approach taken in the UK FTAC) and the establishment of the LAPD threat management unit in 1990 following the killing of Rebecca Schaeffer by an obsessive fan Robert Bardo in 1990[11,12] and the subsequent introduction of antistalking legislation in California. However, research in the US into harassment, threats, and violence towards public figures had either failed to report findings about mental illness or had failed to interpret them. Dietz and Martell considered threatening and otherwise inappropriate communications to Congress in a lengthy report to the Department of Justice in 1989,[13,14] but did not include their mental illness findings in their subsequent published account.[11] The Exceptional Case Study Project in 1997 conducted for the United States Secret Service further expanded the knowledge base in the United States in this area,[15] but there was a delay in recognizing the significance of mental illness in this population.[16] Its authors looked at 83 cases, of which 45% were assassinations and 54% "near lethal approaches." They found that 61% of the individuals concerned had a history of psychiatric problems, 43% of delusional ideas, and 10% of violent command hallucinations. Nevertheless, the conclusion of the authors was that mental illness was not of particular importance. This is despite the fact that, if one takes the figure for delusional ideas as representing the prevalence of psychosis in the sample and compares it with the point prevalence of psychosis in the general population of around 0.4%,[17] the study cases were 110 times more likely to have a psychotic disorder. Suggestions as to why the mental illness factor was played down are various:[18] it may be that mental illness was thought to be a politically unacceptable form of exculpation, that there was confusion between the (medically meaningless) concept of legal insanity and the presence of psychotic illness, or simply that the

constellation of psychiatric services in the USA was not such that psychiatric care seemed a relevant management option. As regards the legal test of insanity in many Anglo-Saxon jurisdictions, it is relevant to note that its roots lie in criteria set out by the UK's Law Lords in 1843, in the wake of the case of Daniel McNaughton, their specific aim being to demedicalize and recriminalize attacks on public figures by psychotic individuals.

Dietz and Martell,[19] in reconsidering their 1989 findings 21 years later, contended that their omission of their mental illness findings in their published paper was for national security reasons. They then put forward the contention that: "Every instance of an attack on a public figure in the United States for which adequate information has been made publicly available has been the work of a mentally disorder person who issued one or more pre-attack signals in the form of inappropriate letters, visits or statements" (p. 344). This is along the lines of the conclusions of the Fixated Research Group's study of attacks on European politicians[20] which found that death and serious injury were significantly associated with psychosis, the presence of delusions, loner status, and the absence of a political motive. Similar results were obtained in a subsequent and partially overlapping study of violence towards German politicians[21] and also in the Fixated Research Group's study of historical attacks upon the British royal family.[22] However, such conclusions are not new, and it appears characteristic of research in this field that insufficient attention is paid to publications from previous centuries or to those not in the English language. None of the recent US researchers had gone back to the ground-breaking work of Laschi[23] or the 1890 "exceptional case series" by Régis[24] which had described and classified public figure attacks and identified the central role of mental illness.[18] The problem of fixated individuals, it is evident, is common across recent centuries and across different countries within the Western world.

Establishment of FTACs in Other Countries

Interest in the FTAC model led to the formation of the European Network of Public Figure Threat Assessment Agencies, which brought together police and security services from countries within the European Union, as well as further afield, and which functioned as a forum for discussing new developments. An FTAC was then set up in the Netherlands where a study of inappropriate communications and approaches to the Dutch royal family found that 75% were psychotic and a further 11% suffering from mood disorders.[25] Surveys were also conducted of the extent of the problem of harassment and stalking for politicians. In Sweden, a study of members of parliament from the years 1998–2005 found that 74% had been subject to harassment, threats, or violence, and 68% of perpetrators were thought probably to be mentally ill.[26] A survey of regional politicians in Canada found that 30% had suffered harassment, with 87% believing their harassers to be mentally ill.[27]

Next, a survey in the UK of members of the Westminster Parliament found that 81% of respondents were subject to at least one of the intrusive/aggressive behaviors studied.[28] This survey was repeated for the Queensland (Australia) State Parliament in 2011.[29] A similarly high rate (93%) of harassment was identified. The survey was also conducted in Norway[30,31] and in New Zealand.[32] The New Zealand survey benefited from an unusually high response rate (84%) and consistent with the other surveys found that one form of harassment or another was the norm (87% of respondents reporting such behavior) with a distinct increase in the contribution from electronic media compared with the UK (60% reported inappropriate social media contact), likely due to the later date at which the survey was conducted. The effects of such behavior are not trivial, as has been illustrated by James et al.[33] with significant proportions of MPs suffering psychological ill effects. These surveys and the experience of established FTACs also highlighted that it is not the MPs alone who bear the brunt of this behavior, but also their staff, including those in often isolated and vulnerable constituency-based offices.

The Queensland survey led to the establishment of an FTAC in Queensland in 2013 operating under a similar model to the United Kingdom – one with an emphasis on joint work between police and mental health, and a high rate of mental health interventions in those referred.[34] Similarly, in New Zealand, a small pilot service was established in September 2017, with a permanent service following in July 2019. In both these services, referrals are drawn from those who communicate to or intrude upon members of parliament, with a finding of high rate of mental illness amongst the communicators and threateners, again providing an opportunity for intervention and treatment in these individuals.

Within Australia, interest in this approach was accelerated by several high-profile incidents. The inquest into the Lindt cafe siege in New South Wales recommended the establishment of a fixated threat service in that state.[35] The individual at the center of this siege had made abnormal communications to the Queen on several occasions, and the UK FTAC had notified Australian Federal Police of their concerns. In Victoria, the tragic events of January 2017 on Bourke Street in Melbourne where a car was used to attack pedestrians, resulting in the death of six and over 30 wounded, provided further impetus for the establishment of a service in that state. In Australia, FTACs have now been established in New South Wales (2017), Victoria (2018), and Western Australia (2018). In 2016, the Australian Federal Police (AFP) established an FTAC in the Australian capital, Canberra.[36] FTAC capabilities are also evolving in smaller jurisdictions (South Australia, the Australian Capital Territory, Tasmania, and the Northern Territory).

An important finding from the new FTACs is that the cases that they deal with are virtually indistinguishable, regardless of country. This is presumably a reflection of the fact that mental disorders occur with similar frequency across different populations. A consistent finding has been the significant proportion of cases with delusional disorder, a form of psychosis which rarely presents to general mental health services, given that the personality is preserved and it does not lead to disturbance of day-to-day functions in the manner typical of the schizophrenias. Given the association of delusional disorder with querulousness and persistent litigation as well as paranoid and grandiose presentations, this finding is perhaps not surprising. The other group which appears to be consistently over-represented in FTAC samples is autism.

Lone Actors and Grievance-Fuelled Violence

The FTAC approach has obvious parallels with psychiatric diversion schemes at courts and police stations and, like those services, the aim is the prevention of further problem behavior, rather than its criminalization. Court diversion schemes are not new, with services having been set up in Chicago in 1914[37] and Baltimore in 1917,[38] the workings of which are remarkably similar to more recent initiatives developed in the UK in the 1980s and 1990s.[39] Whereas this is a further lesson on the folly of failing to research the lessons of the past, it emphasizes the enduring power of the model adopted by FTAC, which has recently been expanded from the field of public figures threat to that of lone-actor and grievance-fuelled violence, to which this chapter will now turn.

Régis, in his 1890 monograph, divided attackers of the prominent into three types which, restated in the modern idiom, are as follows: first, psychotic cases where the involvement of a prominent person is almost incidental; second, querulants, often suffering from a delusional disorder, pursuing a highly personal and idiosyncratic quest for justice; and a third group which shared a variety of characteristics – underlying mental disorder, a burning grievance fired by perceived maltreatment by society, a world-weariness leading to a suicidal trajectory, a seeking of notoriety in death, sometimes wrapped in religious or political flags. Recent research has found that many of the characteristics of this third group overlap with those of lone actors who engage in acts of violence towards other targets: school/university shooters, workplace killings, rampage killers, and lone-actor terrorism.[40–46] Indeed, the overlap between these various groups is such that they can be considered to form a constellation of behaviors which can be grouped together under the category of "grievance-fuelled violence."[18] Lone terrorists have more in common with fixated individuals and other forms of lone killers than they do with group terrorists. Corner and Gill[47] found that lone actor terrorists are nearly 14 times more likely to have mental health problems than those in terrorist groups, with 40% having a history of diagnosed mental health problems. There is increasing evidence that a proportion of those that engage in this kind of violence may be mentally ill[48,49] and therefore there is a role for mental health professionals.[50] The possible mechanisms through which mental illness may be linked to lone actor terrorism are various.[51] Some mentally disordered people may be susceptible to ideological influences as a result of chronic stress, disenfranchisement, and social isolation.[52] Radical political or religious ideologies may resonate with this group, or tap into their delusional beliefs, so rendering them at risk of indoctrination or radicalization, and more sensitive to the contagion effects of well-publicized lone-actor violence. There may also be fixated persons pursuing some idiosyncratic quest who wrap their cases in the flag of a wider cause in the search for greater

legitimacy. Mental illness may be just one element in the mix that leads to extremist thinking or terrorist activity, rather than the driving force. However, addressing it may be a way of avoiding harmful outcomes in those at risk of progressing to various forms of grievance-fuelled violence. Intervention through the fixated threat model is also supported by research from the threat assessment area that highlights that a number of people that go on to commit these kind of offences are in retrospect found to have engaged in behaviors that flagged their potential (so-called leakage[53,54]).

In the circumstances, it is unsurprising that the FTAC model should expand into these areas in which threat assessment programs incorporating information sharing and multidisciplinary working had become more common.[55–58] The violence represents the end product of a process involving social and psychological forces and effects, with a potentially identifiable and recognizable pathway. In the Netherlands, the National Police Threat Management Team created a multiagency unit for assessing those in danger of radicalization, building on their FTAC model.[59] In London, a collaboration between psychiatric staff from FTAC and antiterrorism police was set up in 2017 to evaluate cases of potential terrorist radicalization. This was under the umbrella of the Prevent program,[60] part of the CONTEST counter-terrorism strategy. Prevent requires statutory agencies to refer to a central point all cases where the radicalization of individuals is suspected. The new development enabled the referral of cases for consideration in terms of mental ill health and risk as part of the overall response. This reflected a development which had already taken place in the Netherlands, following the development of an FTAC-style team in that country. In Australia, the Queensland FTAC expanded its role to incorporate the assessment of cases potentially mentally ill and thought to be at risk of lone-actor violence or grievance-fuelled violence and the Victorian service from inception has incorporated this group.[51] All the Australian FTACs except the Canberra unit have now extended their scope beyond fixation to grievance-fuelled violence in general. With FTAC involvement, counter-terrorism investigations are generally not suspended. But given that mentally ill individuals who have adopted extremist beliefs have fewer inhibitions to violent action, the detailed analysis of their networks and background should not delay critical, risk-mitigating psychiatric intervention. Referral to FTAC may change priorities in the counter-terrorism input. And where mental illness is the predominant factor, there may be no further need for involvement of counter-terrorist measures, with the FTAC services becoming the lead agency in the case. As to research findings from FTACs involved in wider lone-actor cases, only one small series is available in the public domain.[51] Security concerns take time to overcome in the publishing of results in this area.

Further Activities

The UK FTAC has now been running for 13 years. Over time its role has expanded. With the development of expertise, it has become involved in forward security planning for major events, education, training, and research.[6] It coordinated the fixated strand in the security arrangements for the 2012 London Olympics, both in terms of forward-planning and operations on the ground. It fulfilled similar functions for royal weddings and for other major events. Similarly, the Queensland FTAC was involved in security planning and operations for the G20 summit in Brisbane[61] and for the 2018 Commonwealth Games.

A further benefit of research in this area has been the refinement of risk assessment instruments. Such tools involve the use of risk factors, in other words characteristics or behaviors which are significantly associated statistically with the undesired outcome. It proved possible at UK FTAC to combine findings from the literatures on violence, stalking, harassment, and the making of threats with clinical insights and best practice from security agencies and threat assessment centers in the USA and Europe. The work at FTAC over 10 years resulted in the publication of the *Communications Threat Assessment Protocol* (CTAP).[62] This includes a simple one-sided screen for referrers to decide which cases of concerning correspondence should be sent to threat assessment agencies for further action: if any of the list of items on the sheet is scored positive, the case must be referred. Such a screen is of practical importance for, without it, large numbers of inappropriate cases would be referred, so impairing the function of the threat assessment unit, and some cases which should be referred won't have been. A second structured tool within the CTAP allows an initial assessment of concerning communications by a threat assessment unit, allowing triage into different levels of urgency and action. For more detailed threat assessment with more information available, many of the FTACs use an adapted version of the Stalking Risk Profile, which incorporates a section on public figure harassment cases.[63]

Conclusion

The FTAC model emerged as a logical response to rigorous research which demonstrated the importance of mental illness in those who approach and threaten public figures. It involves an innovative approach with police and mental health professionals working together. The primary benefit of the model is the improvement in outcomes for often unrecognized mental illness in individuals whose lives have been blighted and whose condition imperils those around them as well as public figures. It is this that brings such work within the ethical remit of medicine. By focusing on threat assessment and management rather than attempts at prediction, FTACs reduce the potential for further adverse consequences. Since the establishment of the first unit in the United Kingdom, the model has been adopted in a number of jurisdictions and countries, sometimes in modified form. Recent research continues to confirm the value of this approach. An overlap with lone-actor and grievance-fuelled violence has been recognized and this is also an area of growth and development. The emphasis continues to be primarily a public-health one seeking to intervene and improve outcomes for affected individuals at the same time as preventing harm.

Disclosure Information

Justin Barry-Walsh, David V. James, and Paul E. Mullen do not have anything to disclose.

References

1. Mullen PE, James DV, Meloy JR, et al. The fixated and the pursuit of public figures. *J Forens Psychiatry Psychol.* 2009; **20**(1): 33–47.

2. The Fixated Research Group: *Inappropriate communications, approaches, and attacks on the British Royal Family with additional consideration of attacks on politicians.* London: The Home Office; 2006.

3. James DV, Meloy JR, Mullen PE, et al. Abnormal attentions toward the British Royal Family: factors associated with approach and escalation. *J Am Acad Psychiatry Law.* 2010; **38**(3): 329–340.

4. James DV, Kerrigan TR, Forfar R, Farnham FR, Preston LF. The fixated threat assessment centre: preventing harm and facilitating care. *J Forens Psychiatry Psychol.* 2010; **21**(4): 521–536.

5. Scalora MJ, Baumgartner JV, Zimmerman WJ, et al. An epidemiological assessment of problematic contacts to members of congress. *J Forensic Sci.* 2002; **47**(6): 1360–1364.

6. James DV, Farnham FR, Wilson SP. The fixated threat assessment centre. In: Meloy JR, Hoffmann J, eds. *International Handbook of Threat Assessment.* New York: Oxford University Press; 2013: 299.

7. James DV, Farnham FR. Outcome and efficacy of interventions by a public figure threat assessment and management unit: a mirrored study of concerning behaviors and police contacts before and after intervention. *Behav Sci Law.* 2016; **34**(5): 660–680.

8. Mullen PE, Pathé M, Purcell R. *Stalkers and their victims, 2nd edn.* Cambridge, UK: Cambridge University Press; 2009.

9. Farnham FR, Busch KG. Introduction to this issue: international perspectives on the protection of public officials. *Behav Sci Law.* 2016; **34**(5): 597–601.

10. Scalora MJ, Zimmerman WJ, Wells D. Use of threat assessment for the protection of the United States Congress. In: Meloy JR, Sheridan L, Hoffman J, eds. *Stalking, Threatening and Attacking Public Figures: A Psychological and Behavioral Analysis.* New York: Oxford University Press; 2008: 425–434.

11. Pathé M. Stalking public figures: the fixated loner. In: Petherick WSG, Sinnamon G, eds. *The Psychology of Criminal and Antisocial Behavior.* London, San Diego CA, Cambridge MA, Oxford UK: Academic Press; 2017: 295–320.

12. Zona MA, Palarea RE, Lane J. Psyhciatric diagnosis and the offender-victim typology of stalking. In: Meloy JR, ed. *The Psychology of Stalking: Clinical and Forensic Perspectives.* San Diego, CA: Academic Press; 1998: 70–84.

13. Dietz PE, Martell DA. Mentally disordered offenders in pursuit of celebrities and politicians (ICPSR 6007). Inter-university Consortium for Political and Social Research; October 15, 1989.

14. Dietz P, Matthews DB, Martell DA, et al. Threatening and otherwise inappropriate letters to members of the United States Congress. *J Forensic Sci.* 1991; **36**(5): 1445–1468.

15. Fein R, Vossekuil B. Assassination in the United States: an operational study of recent assassins, attackers, and near-lethal approachers. *J Forensic Sci.* 1999; **44**(2): 321–333.

16. James DV. Protecting the prominent?: a research journey with Paul Mullen. *Crim Behav Ment Health.* 2010; **20**(3): 242–250.

17. Kirkbride JB, Errazuriz A, Croudace TJ, et al. Systematic review of the incidence and prevalence of schizophrenia and other psychoses in England. University of Cambridge, IoPatM, Kings College London, Department of Health Policy Research Programme; 2012.

18. James D. *The Fixated, Lone Actors and Grievance Fuelled Violence.* Bangkok, Thailand: Asia Pacific Association of Threat Assessment Professionals; 2015.

19. Dietz P, Martell DA. Commentary: approaching and stalking public figures–a prerequisite to attack. *J Am Acad Psychiatry Law.* 2010; **38**(3): 341–348.

20. James DV, Mullen PE, Meloy JR, et al. The role of mental disorder in attacks on European politicians 1990–2004. *Acta Psychiatr Scand.* 2007; **116**(5): 334–344.

21. Hoffmann J, Meloy JR, Guldimann A, Ermer A. Attacks on German public figures, 1968–2004: warning behaviors, potentially lethal and non-lethal acts, psychiatric status, and motivations. *Behav Sci Law.* 2011; **29**(2): 155–179.

22. James DV, Mullen PE, Pathé MT, et al. Attacks on the British Royal Family: the role of psychotic illness. *J Am Acad Psychiatry Law.* 2008; **36**(1): 59–67.

23. Laschi M LC. Le delit politique. Paper presented at: Actes du Premier Congres International d'Anthropologie Criminelle 1885; Rome.

24. Régis E. *Les Regicides dans L'Histoire et dans le Present: Etude Medico-Psychologique.* Lyon: A. Storck; 1890.

25. van der Meer BB, Bootsma L, Meloy R. Disturbing communications and problematic approaches to the Dutch Royal Family. *J Forens Psychiatry Psychol.* 2012; **23**(5–6): 571–589.

26. Jakten pa makten. *Betankande av Kommitten om hot och vald mot fortroendevalda [The quest for power. Report of the committee on threats and violence against elected officials].* Stockholm: Fritzes; 2006.

27. Adams SJ, Hazelwood TE, Pitre NL, Bedard TE, Landry SD. Harassment of members of parliament and the legislative assemblies in Canada by individuals believed to be mentally disordered. *J Forens Psychiatry Psychol.* 2009; **20**(6): 801–814.

28. James DV, Farnham FR, Sukhwal S, et al. Aggressive/intrusive behaviours, harassment and stalking of members of the United Kingdom parliament: a prevalence study and cross-national comparison. *J Forens Psychiatry Psychol.* 2016; **27**(2): 177–197.

29. Pathé M, Phillips J, Perdacher E, Heffernan E. The harassment of Queensland Members of Parliament: a mental health concern. *Psychiatry Psychol Law.* 2014; **21**: 577–584.

30. Berglund N. Threats on the rise against politicians. *News in English Norway;* 2018.

31. Bjelland HF, BjØrgo T. *Trusler og trusselhendelser mot politikere: En spØrreundersØkelse blant norske stortingsrepresentanter og regjeringsmedlemmer [Threats and threat events against politicians: A survey of Norwegian members of parliament and government officials]*. Oslo: Politihogskolen; 2014.

32. Every-Palmer S, Barry-Walsh J, Pathé M. Harassment, stalking, threats and attacks targeting New Zealand politicians: a mental health issue. *Aust N Z J Psychiatry*. 2015; **49**(7): 634–641.

33. James DV, Sukhwal S, Farnham FR, et al. Harassment and stalking of Members of the United Kingdom Parliament: associations and consequences. *J Forens Psychiatry Psychol*. 2016; **27** (3): 309–330.

34. Pathé MT, Lowry T, Haworth DJ, et al. Assessing and managing the threat posed by fixated persons in Australia. *J Forens Psychiatry Psychol*. 2015; **26**(4): 425–438.

35. Wales SCoNS. *Inquest into the Deaths Arising from the Lindt Cafe Siege: Findings and Recommendations*. Glebe NSW Australia: Department of Justice NSW Government; May 2017.

36. Riddle FJ, Ferriman M, Farmer DG, Baillie KM. Towards a national strategy for managing fixated persons in Australia. *Psychiatry Psychol Law*. 2019; **26** (3): 457–467.

37. Kegel AH. The municipal psychopathic laboratory. *Chicago's Health*. 1930; **24**: 114–120.

38. Rathbone OJ. *Foursquare. The Story of a Fourfold Life*. New York: MacMillan; 1929.

39. James D. Court diversion in perspective. *Aust N Z J Psychiatry*. 2006; **40**: 529–538.

40. Capellan JA. Lone wolf terrorist or deranged shooter?: a study of ideological active shooter events in the United States, 1970–2014. *Stud ConflTerror*. 2015; **38** (6): 395–413.

41. Guldimann A, Brunner R, Schmid H. Habermeyer E. Supporting threat management with forensic expert knowledge: protecting public officials and private individuals. *Behav Sci Law*. 2016; **34**(5): 645–659.

42. Malkki L. School shootings and lone actor terrorism. In: Fredholm M, ed. *Understanding Lone Actor Terrorism: Past Experience, Future Outlook, and Response Strategies*. Abingdon: Routledge; 2016: 182–205.

43. Lankford A. A comparative analysis of suicide terrorists and rampage, workplace, and school shooters in the United States from 1990 to 2010. *Homicide Stud*. 2012; **17**(3): 255–274.

44. McCauley C, Moskalenko S, Van Son B. Characteristics of lone wolf violent offenders: a comparison of assassins and school attackers. *Perspect Terror*. 2013; **7**(1): 4–24.

45. Mullen PE. The autogenic (self-generated) massacre. *Behav Sci Law*. 2004; **22**(3): 311–323.

46. Mullen PE, Pathé M. Assessing and managing threats to commit a massacre. *Aust N Z J Psychiatry*. 2018; **52** (8): 732–736.

47. Corner E, Gill P. A false dichotomy?: mental illness and lone-actor terrorism. *Law Hum Behav*. 2015; **39** (1): 23–34.

48. Gill P, Corner E. There and back again: the study of mental disorder and terrorist involvement. *Am Psychol*. 2017; **72**(3): 231–241.

49. Gill P, Horgan J, Deckert P. Bombing alone: tracing the motivations and antecedent behaviors of lone-actor terrorists. *J Forensic Sci*. 2014; **59**(2): 425–435.

50. James DV, Hurlow J. A 21st century truism. *B J Psych Bull*. 2016; **40**(6): 346.

51. Pathé MT, Haworth DJ, Goodwin T-a, et al. Establishing a joint agency response to the threat of lone-actor grievance-fuelled violence. *J Forens Psychiatry Psychol*. 2017; **29**(1): 37–52.

52. Gill P. *Lone-Actor Terrorists: A Behavioural Analysis*. London: Routledge; 2015.

53. Meloy JR. Approaching and attacking public figures: a contemporary analysis of communications and behavior. *J Threat Assess Manag*. 2014; **1**(4): 243–261.

54. Meloy JR, Hoffman J, James D. The role of warning behaviors in threat assessment: an exploration and suggested typology. *Behav Sci Law*. 2012; **30**(3): 256–279.

55. Coggins MH, Pynchon MR, Dvoskin JA. Integrating research and practice in federal law enforcement: secret service applications of behavioral science expertise to protect the president. *Behav Sci Law*. 1998; **16**(1): 51–70.

56. Cornell D. Threat assessment in college settings. *Change: The Magazine of Higher Learning*. 2010; **42** (1): 8–15.

57. Vossekuil B, Fein RA, Berglund JM. Threat assessment: assessing the risk of targeted violence. *J Threat Assess Manag*. 2015; **2**(3–4): 243–254.

58. Weine S, Eisenman DP, Jackson T, Kinsler J, Polutnik C. Utilizing mental health professionals to help prevent the next attacks. *Int Rev Psychiatry*. 2017; **29**(4): 334–340.

59. B V. Netherlands National Police Threat Management Team. *Annual Conference of the European Network of Public Figure Threat Assessment Agencies*; 2015; London, UK.

60. UK Home Office. Revised prevent duty guidance for England and Wales. London: The Stationery Office; 2015.

61. Pathé M, Haworth DJ, Lowry TJ, et al. A model for managing the mentally ill fixated person at major events. *Aust N Z J Psychiatry*. 2015; **49**(7): 610–615.

62. James D, MacKenzie RD, Farnham F. *Communications Threat Assessment Protocol-25:* *Guidelines for the Initial Assessment of Problematic Communications*. Kent: Theseus LLP; 2014.

63. MacKenzie RD, McEwan TE, Pathé M, et al. *Stalking Risk Profile: Guidelines for the Assessment and Management of Stalkers*. Melbourne, Victoria, Australia: StalkInc and Centre for Forensic Behavioural Science, Monash University; 2009.

Decriminalizing LGBTQ+: Reproducing and Resisting Mental Health Inequities

Tyler M. Argüello

Introduction

Secure settings are, in fact, queer spaces. This is not simply because LGBTQ+ people are found, disproportionately at that, in these settings.[1] ("LGBTQ+" herein refers to people who are lesbian, gay, bisexual, transgender, queer, questioning, Two Spirit, and asexual.) Rather, these spaces are implicitly and explicitly domains for non-normative cultures, behaviors, as well as identities. Often that means various antisocial behaviors, those who have committed crimes, or those who live with severe mental illnesses; or a combination therein. In this review, while those may be operative, the case of those who hold minoritized sexualities and genders will be centralized and examined.[2] It can be that LGBTQ+ people are in secure settings because they have committed crimes and/or live with severe and persistent mental illnesses. However, there are also structural and social forces that contribute to their disproportionate presence in these settings specifically due to existing as a person with a minoritized sexuality or gender, regardless of criminality or mental health. For this review, secure settings mean those locations that are extensions of justice systems; inherently they restrict liberties and rights and they can intersect with mental health and human service systems. These can include jails, prisons, state hospitals, juvenile detention, and immigration detention facilities, among others. Even more, these settings by their very nature of being secure punctuate the lived existences within them through the persistent specter of policing and discipline. The LGBTQ+ individuals, then, who do enter these spaces have a sharply impacted existence by multiple compounding factors, that is, they bring operating oppressive experiences by being a queer person into these settings and those experiences are compounded and even exacerbated by the oppressive nature of such secure settings. The net effect of this, too often, is that the health and mental health of LGBTQ+ people are negatively affected. This does not have to be the case, however.

The purpose of this review is to increase the competence, that is the knowledge and skills, of multidisciplinary practitioners in secure settings to better serve LGBTQ+ clients, albeit to increase equity and justice. In order to achieve this end, this review brings together archives of theoretical, cultural, and empirical research to architect knowledge and skills that are LGBTQ+ affirmative. The review begins with a discussion of critical terminology imperative for understanding and addressing LGBTQ+ existences. Next, the health, mental health, and social inequities that LGBTQ+ people experience are reviewed. From there, the social science paradigm to explain queer disparities, or the minority stress model, is diagrammed. Then, the review moves into more squarely deconstructing how LGBTQ+ people are criminalized and how their health is implicated in that process, moving from pre-detainment experiences, to existing in secure settings, and finally to re-entering the community. In response to this knowledge, applied strategies are offered that are LGBTQ+ affirmative for people and organizations, are promotive of wellbeing, and that are in resistance to criminalizing procedures, pathways, and approaches.

Coming to Terms

Before entering into the nexus of queer inequities, criminalization, and emancipation, it is important to have an understanding of the nature and implications of terms. In this review, "queer" is a preferred term deployed to both signal an umbrella for the ever-amassing collection of identities under the banner of "LGBTQ+" as well as a critical term that signals a persistent disruption and deconstruction of what is normative; often, queer and LGBTQ+ are interchangeable in this review. "Criminalization" is positioned as the often-unconscious process by which sexualities, genders, and other tangible and ideological material become rendered into criminological and forensic terms. "Mental health" is defined in broad terms, following the lead of the World Health Organization's[3] definition that signals it is not simply about the absence of disease or pathology rather it is a function of individuals' attributes in relation with environmental factors.

When it comes to terms around sexuality and gender, binarized and medicalized understandings can predominate. Those are one angle on these terms; a deeper, critical understanding can be helpful to not only broaden awareness, knowledge, self-reflection, and interdisciplinarity – but as well to more effectively work with clients and communities. It is important to keep in mind that this list is necessarily incomplete, unstable, evolving, and generally queer. Table 34.1 provides brief definitions for critical terms when

Table 34.1 Terminology

Term	Definition
LGBTQITSA+	An acronym signifying pointing to ever-evolving identities related to sex/uality, sexual orientation, and gender identity and expression. Often, it stands for: Lesbian, Gay, Bisexual, Transgender, Questioning, Queer, Intersex, Two Spirit, and Asexual. It can be consolidated into labels like "LGBT," "Gay," "LGBTQ+."
Queer	A critical inclusive term for sexualities and genders, as well as better regarded as a verb (versus noun), a strategy, an attitude, or a positionality against the normative.
Biological/Birth Sex	The sex a person is assigned at birth based on visible physiological and anatomical sex characteristics.
Sex/uality	A constellation of biological sex, (chosen) identities, emotional/affectional impulses, sexual attraction/desires, and behaviors with, without, or towards other persons and within one's self.
Sexual Orientation	An individual's physical and sexual attraction toward others.
Sexual Identity	How an individual describes their own sexuality and how it is expressed.
Gender	Refers to the social construction and meaning a given culture associates with a person's attitudes, behaviors, and feelings, and their assigned biological sex.
Gender Identity	A person's sense of being a woman, a man, transgender, cisgender, or other gender identification (e.g. a blend of the aforementioned or beyond those categories).
Gender Expression	The ways a person represents their gender to others, that is, the ways they walk in the world giving life and form to their interior experience of gender, which may or may not be congruent with dominant norms.
Cis or Cisgender	A person whose self-definition (e.g. identity, expressions) is adherent to hegemonic notions of gender – which are also aligned with assigned birth sex.
Trans or Transgender	A person whose self-definition (e.g. identity, expressions) challenges and disrupts traditional binary conceptions and boundaries of gender and sexuality.
Sexism	A system of advantages and oppression that serves to privilege cisgender men, subordinate women (and others), and reinforce normative masculinity.
Biocentrism	The assumption that people whose assigned sex at birth matches their gender identity throughout their lives are more "normal" than those whose assigned sex is incongruent with their gender identity.
Heterosexism	A system of institutional and cultural beliefs, norms, and practices that advantages heterosexuals, and disadvantages those not heterosexual.
Monosexism	A system of institutional and cultural beliefs, norms, and practices that produces the privileged belief that monosexuality (either exclusive heterosexuality and/or homosexuality) is superior to or more legitimate than other identities (e.g. bisexuality).
Heteronormativity	A politics, organized societal system, and social practices that produces and privileges hegemonic heterosexuality.
Homonormativity	A mimic of heteronormativity that does not assume that every person is gay – rather, it assumes that queer people want to be just like heteronormative people.
Mononormativity	Describes the societal expectation that romantic relationships are sexually and emotionally monogamous, as well as points to the organized societal systems that reinforce this.
Cisnormativity	A politics, organized societal system, and social practices that produces and privileges hegemonic cisgenderism.
Coming out, Inviting in, Becoming	The practices, politics, and processes for disclosing or making public one's marginalized sexuality and/or gender.

working with LGBTQ+ people; the following provides more expansive and nuanced definitions.

- *LGBTQITSA+* – A Western-based acronym signifying a mostly stable set of identities related to sex/uality, sexual orientation, and gender identity, and expression. Often, it stands for: Lesbian, Gay, Bisexual, Transgender, Questioning, Queer, Intersex, Two Spirit (TS or 2), and Asexual (and sometimes contentiously Ally). The plus ("+") at the end makes a nod to the fact that there are forever evolving and existing identities along this spectrum of human experiences. For the sake of efficiency, this acronym can be consolidated into labels like "LGBT," "Gay," or "LGBTQ+." Whether represented as an acronym or a single word, this set of labels retains residue of positivistic ways of knowing and essentialized notions of identity. In contemporary times, these labels are often deployed in the promulgation of neoliberal discourse and political economy prioritizing individualism, rights-based social and political agendas, homonormative cultural and economic privileges, and consolidated and sanitized notions of desire and partnering (e.g. "gay marriage" debates). Queer and gay are undoubtedly strange bedmates.

- *Queer* – An umbrella term used by some LGBTQITSA+ people to refer to themselves, often to avoid binary and static conceptions of sex, gender, and sex/uality, among others. Based in critical, feminist, and post-structural perspectives on language, economy, gender, and sex/uality, queer is an antiessentialist, subjectless critique, necessarily indeterminate and referring more to self-identification rather than empirical observation of other peoples' characteristics. It is the suspension and denaturalization of identity as something fixed, natural, and coherent. More appropriately, it can be better understood as a verb (versus noun), a strategy, an attitude, and a position/ality set against the normative.[4–7]

- *Biological/Birth Sex* – The sex a person is assigned at birth based on visible physiological and anatomical sex characteristics; this is most often, and almost exclusively, conferred by a physician and the State, and is conflated with gender (identity).

- *Sex/uality* – A constellation of biological sex, (chosen) identities, emotional/affectional impulses, sexual attraction/desires, and behaviors with, without, or towards other persons and within one's self. Sexuality is a central aspect of being human throughout life, and encompasses (to varying degrees) sex, gender identities and roles, sexual orientation, eroticism, pleasure, intimacy, and reproduction. Sexuality is experienced and expressed in thoughts, fantasies, desires, beliefs, attitudes, values, behaviors, practices, roles, and relationships. While sexuality can include all of these dimensions, not all of them are always experienced or expressed; sexuality is influenced by the interaction of biological, psychological, social, economic, political, cultural, legal, historical, and religious and spiritual factors.[3]

- *Sexual Orientation* – An individual's physical and sexual attraction toward others. This may be to an individual of the same gender (e.g. gay), the opposite gender (e.g. straight), both (e.g. bisexual), asexual, or various others (e.g. pansexual). Sexual orientation may or may not be reflected in someone's outward behaviors or appearance; and, their sexual behaviors may or may not be defined singularly by normative understandings of one's sexual orientation.

- *Sexual Identity* – How an individual describes their own sexuality and how it is expressed. Often, sexual identity interfaces with one's sexual orientation, but not always. For example, a person can have a lesbian orientation and express a heterosexual identity.

- *Gender* – Refers to the social construction and meaning a given culture associates with a person's attitudes, behaviors, and feelings, and their assigned biological sex. Gender-normative or gender-confirming behaviors are those that align with the person's assigned biological sex at birth. Gender nonconformity (or -variant, -creative) occurs when the behaviors, attitudes, and feelings of a person do not align with that person's biological sex and/or gender assigned at birth.

- *Gender Identity* – A person's sense of being a woman, a man, transgender, cisgender, or other gender identification (e.g. a blend of the aforementioned or beyond those categories). Gender identity includes what a person calls themselves (i.e. "preferred gender pronouns") and may or may not be the same as their biological sex.

- *Gender Expression* – The ways a person represents their gender to others, that is, the ways they walk in the world giving life and form to their interior experience of gender, which may or may not be congruent with dominant norms.
- *Cisgender or Cis* – A person whose self-definition (e.g. identity, expressions) is adherent to hegemonic notions of gender – which are also aligned with assigned birth sex.
- *Transgender or Trans* – A person whose self-definition (e.g. identity, expressions) challenges and disrupts traditional binary conceptions and boundaries of gender and sexuality; often times, this self-definition is not aligned with assigned birth sex. Related terms include: gender nonconforming, gender creative, gender variant, genderbending, gender fluid.
- *Sexism* – A system of advantages and oppression that serves to privilege cisgender men, subordinate women (and others), denigrate women-identified values and practices, enforce male dominance and control, and reinforce forms of masculinity that are dehumanizing and damaging to all men. It operates through individual beliefs, practices, institutions, media, and ideas; and is enforced by economic structures, violence, and homo-/trans-/biphobias.
- *Heterosexism* – A system of institutional and cultural beliefs, norms, and practices that advantages heterosexuals. In turn, this system produces prejudice against nonheterosexual people.
- *Biocentrism* – The assumption that people whose assigned sex at birth matches their gender identity throughout their lives are more "real" and/or more "normal" than are those whose assigned sex at birth is incongruent with their gender identity. It is similar to heterosexism but focuses on gender rather than sexual orientation.
- *Monosexism* – A system of institutional and cultural beliefs, norms, and practices that produces the privileged belief that monosexuality (i.e. either exclusive heterosexuality or homosexuality) is superior to or more legitimate than a bisexual or other nonmonosexual orientation (e.g. pansexuality). In turn, this system produces prejudice against bisexual (and other related) people.
- *Heteronormativity* – A politics and everyday practice that produces hegemonic heterosexuality; simply put, the commonsense notion (and

subsequent organized societal systems and social life) that heterosexuality is the only "normal" sexual identity. This belief system assumes that every person is straight – and that their behavior and sexual orientation are in-line with their gender, which is in-line with their genitalia (e.g. penis = male = acts masculine or likes women). Moreover, heteronormativity reproduces not only heterosexuality – but more importantly the expectations, demands, and constraints produced when heterosexuality is taken as normative within a society. Thus, heteronormativity draws on and reproduces discourses of consumption, class/ism, race/ism, ethnicity/ethnocentrism, nation/ality, ability/ableism, privatized intimacy and politics, and domesticity.[8,9]

- *Homonormativity* – A politics that does not contest dominant heteronormative assumptions and institutions, but upholds and sustains them, while promising the possibility of a demobilized gay constituency and a privatized, depoliticized gay culture anchored in domesticity and consumption.[10] This is to say, it is a mimic of heteronormativity that *does not* assume that every person is gay – rather, it assumes that LGBTQ+ people want to be "just like" heteronormative people. Furthermore, it rewards homonormative LGBTQ+ people by bestowing rights, privileges, and access.
- *Mononormativity* – Describes the societal expectation that romantic relationships are sexually and emotionally monogamous. These norms are often reinforced by social and legal institutions, which contribute to dominant narratives about romantic and sexual relationships. Mononormative assumptions are embedded within the words of infidelity and cheating by way of conflating consensual nonmonogamy and *nonconsensual* nonmonogamy (i.e. infidelity), and therefore cannot account for the variety of consensual nonmonogamous relationship experiences.
- *Cisnormativity* – A politics and everyday practice that produces hegemonic cisgenderism; simply put, the commonsense notion (and subsequent organized societal systems and social life) that cisgender is the only "normal" gender identity. This belief system assumes that every person is assigned gender at/before birth – and that their self-identification, behavior, and general presentation in the world everyday are in-line with

this assigned gender, which is in-line with their genitalia. Further, cisnormativity reproduces not only cisgenderism and binarized gender – but more importantly the expectations, demands, and constraints produced when cisgenderism is taken as normative within a society. Thus, cisnormativity draws on and reproduces discourses of consumption, class/ism, race/ism, ethnicity/ethnocentrism, nation/ality, ability/ableism, privatized intimacy and politics, and domesticity.

- *Coming Out/Inviting In/Becoming* – "Coming out" describes voluntarily making public one's sexual orientation and/or gender identity. It has also been broadened to include other pieces of potentially stigmatized personal information. *Inviting in* offers a more critical standpoint and locates agency, choice, and consent within the individual; likewise, *becoming* acknowledges that people are in a continual, lifelong process of coming into their sexuality, gender, and other identities, as well as they are highly contextual. Terms also used that correlate with this action are: "Being out" which means not concealing one's sexual orientation or gender identity, and "Outing," a term used for making public the sexual orientation or gender identity of another who would prefer to keep this information private. Related term: Disclosure.

Health, Mental Health, and Social Inequities

A recent Williams Institute[11] survey estimated that 4.5% of the U.S. population is self-identified LGBT (ranging from 2.7% to 9.8% across the 50 states). Of these LGBT people, 42% are self-identified male and 58% female; 29% are raising children (ranging from 44% to 9% across the states). The majority are white (58%), while 21% are Latino, 12% black, 5% mixed race, 2% Asian, 1% American Indian, and 1% are Native Hawaiian or Pacific Islander. The average age is 37.3 years old, as compared to 47.9 years old for non-LGBT people; within this, 30% of LGBT people are 18 to 24 years old (12% non-LGBT are), and only 7% are over 65 years old (compared to 21% non-LGBT). Just under 10% are unemployed (as compared to 5% heterosexual), with also 15% uninsured (compared to 12%), 27% food insecure (compared to 15%), and 25% have an income less than $24,000 annually

(compared to 18%). And, 41% have completed high school, 30% have completed some college, 17% hold a bachelor's degree, and 13% have post-graduate education (as compared to heterosexuals at 39%, 29%, 18%, and 14% respectively).

What is also known is that LGBTQ+ people bear a disproportionate burden of health, mental health, and social inequities.[12,13] LGBTQ+ individuals have increased risks for obesity, chronic illness (e.g. HIV, diabetes, asthma), mental distress,[14] sexual risk-taking behaviors and unplanned pregnancy,[15] substance use disorder, depression,[16,17] suicide attempts,[17] and smoking.[16] LGBTQ+ people experience higher rates of HIV infection and tobacco, alcohol, and other drug use.[18] They have higher incidence of mental health disorders;[19] it is estimated that the 12-month prevalence for depression for LGB people is at least twice that of heterosexual people, almost twice for anxiety, approximately two to three times for alcohol misuse, and just under three times for other drug misuse. Moreover, research indicates that the interaction of multiple marginalized statuses (e.g. sexual orientation and race) increases the odds of developing mental health challenges,[20] parallel to the fact that rates of mental distress, substance misuse, and disability increase for elderly LGBTQ+ people.[21] However, estimations around LGBTQ+ people and mental illnesses are deceiving.[22] This is in large part due to frequently excluding people known to have a severe and persistent mental illness from studies about sexuality and gender, coupled with the common impulse to regard people living with a mental illness as asexual. As well, there still is a pathologizing of nonheterosexual orientations and nonconforming gender identities. The net result is difficulty in generating representative samples in order to make population-based estimates.

Social stigma, discrimination, and homo- and transphobia against LGBT people negatively affects their quality of life by affecting their employment, income, access to health insurance, and health behavior choices.[23] Social and structural forces may impact LGBTQ+ health and mental health. For example, LGB people living in states with anti-same-sex marriage amendments had significant increases in anxiety and substance disorders compared to LGBT people living in states without these amendments.[24] Also, in states that enacted pro-same-sex marriage laws there were lower levels of psychological distress and reduced medical and mental health care visits.[25] Despite the stereotype that the LGBTQ+ community is predominately affluent, queer people experience poverty at higher rates than their heterosexual and cisgender peers. In particular, LGBT-identified women and men had poverty rates of 21.5% and 20.1% respectively, compared to heterosexual and cisgender women (19.1%) and men (13.4%).[26] Children of same-sex couples are twice as likely to be living in poverty compared to married, different-sex couples, with African American children of gay male parents having the highest poverty rate of 52.3%.[27]

Lesbians have distinct disparities, including higher rates of tobacco use,[28] higher rates of obesity, and lower rates of exercise compared to heterosexual women.[29] They also experience higher rates of anxiety and depression, suicidal ideation, nonsuicidal self-injury related to chronic stress and discrimination, which in turn is related to heavy drinking behaviors.[30,31] They have a heightened risk for reproductive cancers, including breast, ovarian, and endometrial.[32] Elder lesbians are more likely to use tobacco, drink excessively, and suffer from obesity, which are due to overall poor health, cardiovascular disease, and diabetes.[33]

Gay men also experience distinct health and mental health issues, including higher rates of HIV and hepatitis[34] and higher rates of cancers such as anal, prostate, and colon.[35] They are at increased risk for other sexually transmitted infections: gonorrhea, chlamydia, HPV, and syphilis.[34] The ability for gay men to be out about their sexuality and sexual behaviors is essential to receiving comprehensive care. They also experience higher rates of some eating disorders, depression, and anxiety.[36-38] As compared to heterosexual men, gay men are twice as likely to smoke, have higher odds of mental distress and life dissatisfaction, and have more activity limitations due to physical, mental, and emotional problems,[18] as well as less likely to be overweight or obese; still, they are more likely to be vaccinated for flu and have regular HIV tests than heterosexual men.[18] Gay men are more likely to use alcohol and drugs, have higher rates of substance abuse, and are less likely to abstain from use and less likely to continue heavy drinking into later life.[34,39] Gay men are more likely than bisexual or heterosexual men to report discrimination in the past year, especially in healthcare settings, and public spaces such as sidewalks, stores, and restaurants.[40] And, 32% of gay men reported abuse in present or past romantic relationships.[41]

Bisexual people in particular have distinct disparities. Bisexual women are more likely to be uninsured compared to heterosexuals, gays, and lesbians.[42] Bisexual men who have male sexual partners report higher rates of colon cancer and HIV, similar to rates of gay men and other men who have sex with men.[43] Generally, bisexual people experience intimate partner violence, which disproportionately impacts bisexual men and women.[44] As well, biphobia can create barriers to community involvement. Resultantly, bisexual people experience greater social isolation (than their gay/lesbian counterparts).[45] Biphobia may mean that bisexual people do not feel comfortable coming out as bisexual.[46] And, bisexual people are likely to be misidentified as heterosexual or gay/lesbian, depending on the gender of their partner.[47] Some common examples of biphobia include the prejudice that bisexual people cannot be monogamous, are sexually promiscuous, or that they do not have a legitimate identity.

Transgender people endure a myriad of health and mental health inequities.[48] Some (not all) transgender people wish to medically transition (e.g. with hormones or surgeries); not all transgender people have access to or financial means to medically transition in the ways they wish. In this process and generally, transgender people face discrimination, misunderstanding, and at times denial of health care by providers.[49] As well, trans people experience higher rates of suicide attempts and ideation[50] and violence.[51] Rates of depression and anxiety are significantly higher among transgender and gender nonconforming individuals when compared with their cisgender counterparts.[52-54] In the absence of consistent and trans-affirmative care, medical settings can become sites of traumatization for transgender clients. In fact, among transgender individuals accessing health care, 28% were harassed and experienced violence in medical settings, 19% were denied care, and 2% were victims of violence in doctor's offices.[49] These prejudices can lead often to a myth of post-surgical "regret" and therefore a denial of gender-affirming procedures; in fact, estimates are <1–2%.[55-59] Regret is much higher in other medical procedures (e.g. gastric banding); comparatively in the United Kingdom, there is an estimated >65% regret for (nontransgender related) plastic surgery.

In regard to suicide specifically, LGBTQ+ people are at much more risk.[60-62] A meta-analysis of research on LGB mental health showed a twofold excess risk of suicide attempts in the preceding year in men and women, and fourfold excess in risk in gay and bisexual men over a lifetime.[19] There is limited data on suicide completions, deriving mostly from adolescent and young gay males; so far, there is little evidence of increased completions. As for attempts, there are higher rates of attempts compared to heterosexuals worldwide.[63] LGB adolescents are two to seven times more likely to attempt suicide, and they have more lethal means of attempts. The prevalence of suicide attempts in gay or bisexual men is four times that of their heterosexual peers; and, the prevalence for lesbian or bisexual women is twice that of their heterosexual peers. Generally, most attempts tend to occur during adolescence or young adulthood. That said, LGBTQ+ youth who have at least one accepting adult in their life are 40% less likely to report a suicide attempt in the past year.[64] Bisexual people are the most at-risk sexual minority population for poor health outcomes, high-risk health behaviors, and suicidal ideation. Alongside this, transgender people continue to have the highest reported rates of suicide attempts, with 41% of transgender adults reporting a suicide attempt.[49,65,66] Of trans youth, 50% report past suicidal ideation, and 30% report at least one prior suicide attempt. There are increased attempts when trans people have marginal employment (60%) and if they are also of a minority race or ethnicity: black (45%), Latino (44%), and American Indian (56%). Similar to LGB data, most attempts are reported in adolescence and young adulthood. Risk also increases for trans people when they are a sexual minority.

In terms of trauma and interpersonal violence, LGBTQ+ people bear both a disproportionate experience of various assaults and the experience of generally walking in the world feeling completely unsafe, rightfully so. LGBTQ+ people are nearly 2.5 times more likely to experience hate crimes than any other group. Hate-motivated LGBTQ+ homicides increased by 86% in 2017, alongside there being a 400-fold increase in cisgender gay/bi/queer male homicides.[67] LGBTQ+ people of color, youth, gay men, and transgender people are the most likely to suffer injuries and require medical attention as a result of interpersonal violence.[68] In particular, transgender people and LGBTQ+ people of color are most likely to be the victims of anti-queer murders; in the U.S. in 2017, there were 29 reported trans deaths due to fatal

violence, 26 in 2018, and 12 already in 2019 (at the time of writing this review).[69] Often, people resort to violence to "correct" or sensor nonconforming behavior around gender and sexuality.[70] Trans survivors are almost twice as likely to experience physical violence, almost four times more likely to experience discrimination within violent relationships, and 2.5 times more likely to encounter incidents of interpersonal violence in public spaces.[67,71]

For LGBTQ+ people, sexual traumas especially in early life can lead the victim to struggle to separate out the trauma experience from their sexual orientation or gender identity.[72] To link sexual trauma as a cause of sexual orientation or gender identity is a discredited assertion, as is linking pedophilia to an LGBTQ+ orientation. Corrective rape, which is more often experienced by sexual minority women, is abuse caused by someone trying to "fix" the victim's sexual orientation.[72] Young LGBTQ+ people on average experience 3.8 times more sexual abuse, 1.2 times more parental physical abuse, and 1.7 times more assaults at school.[73]

Religious institutions and belief systems have a longstanding difficult relationship with LGBTQ+ communities. Often, religious-based trauma can occur in conjunction with "reparative therapies," which have been denounced by professional organizations.[74] It is estimated that 698,000 LGBT adults (18–59 years old) in the U.S. have received conversion therapy, including 350,000 LGBT adults who received it during their teenage years. Twenty thousand LGBT youth (13–17 years old) will receive conversion therapy from a licensed healthcare professional before they reach 18 in the 41 states that do not ban the practice. Related, 57,000 LGBT youth (13–17 years old) across all states will receive conversion therapy from religious or spiritual advisors before they reach 18. As of this review, conversion therapy is banned in 18 states, one territory, and Washington, D.C., alongside 32 localities most of which are in Florida.[74]

Over the lifespan for LGBTQ+ people, age of coming out is related to the number of victimizations, with the more years a person is publicly out, the more time for the person to be victimized.[75] More generally, traumas can negatively impact an LGBTQ+ person's sense of self and stigmatize their identity. Shame and isolation due to trauma can compound existing negative beliefs and behaviors that the LGBTQ+ person may already face. This said, it can be that coming out can facilitate or hinder healing from traumatic events. Sometimes coming out is empowering and can facilitate increased pride.[76,77] Or, sometimes a person may choose not to come out in fear that their sexuality or gender may be conflated with the trauma.[78]

Minority Stress

Left under the terms of social epidemiology, the forecast for queer people and their wellbeing is dismal. This focus privileges the scientists, psychiatrists, and other medical and mental health professionals alike. Equally, it maintains attention on incidents or event-based oppression, as well persists the focus on the individuals and individualizes the problems.[79] One principal effect of this is the power to define "the problem"; and, queer people have endured this and their problems being defined constantly as "deviant" within medicalized and psychiatric terms. This evacuation of the cultural and the social within the world belies the lived experiences of those who are marginalized and oppressed in society, namely in this instance LGBTQ+ people.

In fact, research and work from the social sciences have developed and applied a model of minority stress that explains the disproportionate rates of illness for LGBTQ+ people.[80] Whereas the original model was developed around lesbian, gay, and bisexual people, its theoretical and practical implications extend to other minoritized and marginalized sexualities and genders as well as experiences of prejudice and oppression.[81–83] Underlying the concept of minority stress are certain assumptions. First, queer people routinely experience stressful events not usually experienced by heterosexuals.[84] Second, stigma and discrimination correlate with poorer health and mental health outcomes.[40] Even perceived discrimination has negative health and mental health outcomes for LGBTQ+ people.[85] And, third, the stressors are unique (i.e. not experienced by nonstigmatized populations), chronic (i.e. related to social and cultural structures), and socially based (i.e. arising from social process, institutions, structures). The minority stress model, then, is used to explain the connections between group-specific processes and negative mental health outcomes among queer people. The application of the framework of minority stress involves three parts: (1) an analysis of minority stress; (2) a consideration of general stress and coping processes; and (3) LGBTQ+-affirmative practice.

In the first part, the analysis of minority stress examines group-specific processes that are distal and proximal. Distal processes are objective prejudice events; these include understanding acute stressful events that have caused significant changes in a person's life as well as regarding the chronic stressful events of everyday discrimination and stigma. In this, it would be effective to become aware of the effects of homo-/bi-/transphobia on the person's development over the life course. Parallel to this, proximal processes involve stigma, internalized negative attitudes, and a concealment of one's sexuality. In the case of stigma, stigmatized individuals have to constantly discern what people think about them, and in turn develop an expectation of stigma and a hypervigilance in interactions with people of the dominant group. This contributes then to an internalization of negative societal attitudes, i.e. internalized homophobia. Resultantly, stigmatized and marginalized people engage in concealment of sexuality as means of protection from a hostile social environment, at persistent threat of their truth becoming public. In addition to these four processes it is important to consider a fifth process of intersectionality. This is to foreground that holding more than one stigmatized identity can exacerbate minority stress, such as a minoritized race, ethnicity, class, or disability. Thus, in attending to people's experiences with minority stress, it is necessary to understand how identities of sexuality and gender intersect with other ones of race and ethnicity, for example.

The next step is to consider general psychological processes of stress and coping. Whereas many minority group members cope with stress through developing and maintaining connections with their communities, there certainly exist individual-level stress and coping that may not be immediately evident. For the fact that queer people experience chronic excess levels of stress, it is important to understand individual-level affected general psychological processes, while also understanding the group-level processes described above. Building off Meyer's[80] minority stress model, Hatzenbeuhler[86] proposed a mediation model linking minority stress with negative mental health outcomes. The general psychological processes encompass affective (i.e. coping abilities and emotion regulation), social (i.e. social supports and interpersonal relationships), and cognitive processes (i.e. maladaptive self-schemas). For example, in the case of concealing one's sexuality, affected psychological responses can include cognitive (e.g. suspiciousness, preoccupation), affective (e.g. shame, guilt, anxiety), behavioral (e.g. social avoidance, impaired relationships), and negative self-evaluation (e.g. identity ambivalence, diminished self-efficacy).[84,87]

The third part in applying a minority stress framework is to engage the person in LGBTQ+-affirmative work. Instead of being a singular evidence-based clinical intervention or method (such as cognitive behavior therapy or Dialectical Behavioral Therapy [DBT]), work involves overlaying or imbuing the methods used and the clinical relationship at-large with positivity, validation, multilevel attention and action, and overall affirmation for LGBTQ+ people, their sexuality, gender, and their lived experiences as intersectional people.[84,88–92] In a way, this affirmative care enhances existing methods or models being deployed by the practitioner; to that end, however, a crucial element to this work is the reflexivity of the practitioner and their willingness and ability to interrogate their own biases and prejudices.

This affirmative work necessarily begins with analyzing the information gathered from the first two steps above, and then formulating the person's case from an explicit LGBTQ+-affirmative standpoint, that is, making sense of "what is going on" or "what the problem is" given the person's experiences of living in this world over their lifetime as a queer person. Such a case formulation accounts for chronic stress, persistent prejudices, coping abilities, traumatic events, as well as a positive regard for the development of sexuality and gender over time. This formulation then links the person into a treatment plan that addresses the problems at hand as well as engages the person in an action plan to affirm their identities. This work involves continual attention to the quality of the therapeutic alliance, cultural competence, strengths of the person, and accounting for the presenting issues within a social context. It involves taking active steps to address or intervene with histories and current experiences of stigma, issues around disclosure, coping and social skills, as well as attending to presenting issues around the person's intersecting identities. Finally, there needs to be attention and action around connecting into or with community resources, building affirmative interpersonal relationships, and other potentially indicated more macro-oriented action like taking part in community organizing efforts. This is one important implication of

understanding LGBTQ+ health and mental health inequities within a minority stress framework: given the multilevel experience of chronic stress, persistent discrimination, and overall oppression experienced by queer people, the attendant interventions to redress negative affects must be multilevel as well, not singularly intra- or interpersonal.

How LGBTQ+ Risk and Inequities are Criminalized

Compounding chronic, harmful minority stress, LGBTQ+ people and their health, mental health, and social inequities have been and are still today criminalized in a variety of ways. At baseline, while LGBTQ+ people are a small minority in the context of the entire U.S. population, the incarceration rate of LGB people versus all U.S. adults is 1,882 versus 612 per 100,000 people.[93] For transgender people in particular, per a national survey, 2% of trans respondents reported having been incarcerated in the past year, a rate more than twice the general population (0.87%);[94] this rate increased accounting for trans people of color and low-income respondents. In general, it is estimated that one in six trans people – and one in two trans black people – has been to prison.[95] When taking into account age, LGB young people represent 12% to 20% of those youth in juvenile detention, with 85% of all incarcerated LGB youth being people of color.[94] Male sexual minorities are 6.2% of jail populations and 9.3% of prisons; while female sexual minorities are 35.7% and 42.1% respectively. The status of being a sexual minority is correlated with negative outcomes in correctional settings, in that, sexual minorities are more likely to receive prison terms over 20 years, more likely to have spent time in solitary confinement or disciplinary segregation, and more likely to be sexually victimized while incarcerated.[93] And, in all, 29.3% of gay and bisexual men have experienced serious psychological distress (as compared to 13.6% straight men), and 24.7% of lesbian and bisexual women have as well (compared to 18.8% straight women).

While these rates and overall inequities for queer people are both alarming and distressing, to say the least, LGBTQ+ people and their identities are not inherently criminogenic. In fact, queer people are *de facto* of acute interest to society in so far as their self-identifications around gender and sexuality challenge, disrupt, or reinforce heteronormative ideologies and structures. This is to say that bodies, ways of life, and survival strategies that *do not* conform to or manifest heteronormativity become subject to both social and formal policing as well as technologies of discipline, corrections, detention, and punishment.[96] This criminalization has occurred through various ways and by various societal systems over time based on the ways in which LGBTQ+ people have been regarded. Historically and contemporaneously, queer people have been subjected to the medicalization of homosexuality (e.g. deviants, infectious, aberrations), the psychiatrization of their mental health (e.g. sick, objects of interventions, insane, pathological sexual interests), and the pathologization of queer socializing and ways of life (e.g. immoral, dangerous, degenerates). There are well-known archives interrogating these experiences and histories.[97–102] The intention here is not to replicate those works, rather to diagram how these processes that promote criminalization continue to occur by structures and societal systems and in the everyday lives of LGBTQ+ people across the U.S. Below, this criminalization is diagrammed from pre-detainment experiences, through detainment and experiences being in the system, and then through re-entry into the community.

Before entering into the diagram of criminalization, it is imperative to understand that LGBTQ+ people become criminalized through their experience of holding multiple identities. Queer people are not singularly their sexuality or gender, rather they hold multiple identities that intersect; and, from an intersectional perspective,[103] the lived experience of minority stress, oppression, and inequities is a function of how these multiple identities are targeted and/or allowed by social structures and systems. For example, a person is not queer or black, rather they are queer *and* black *and* other identities around class, ethnicity, gender, age, and beyond. What is important about using an intersectional analysis is that the more intersecting identities that are operating in people's lives, the more compounding are the injustices and inequities. While all queer people are criminalized in various ways, that experience of criminalization is only intensified by additional experiences of racism, ethnocentrism, sexism, classism, ageism, and beyond.[96] This is starkly exemplified by the U.S. criminal justice system – a system that is over-represented by black people, people of color, immigrants, people living with mental illness and/or addiction, and low-income people. When squared

with sexuality and gender in particular, as is discussed in the whole of this review, those LGBTQ+ people who are further disproportionately over-represented and captured into the system are young queer people and people of color, trans and gender nonconforming people, and those of low income and homeless.[1,2]

Prior to Detainment

Before entering the system, LGBTQ+ people face a number of factors that increase the chance of their life trajectory interfacing with law enforcement and ending up in detention: discrimination and stigma, discriminatory enforcement of laws, and negative policing strategies.[96,104] First, queer people are subjected to discrimination and stigma from early ages and over the life course; minority stress aptly diagrams this experience. Young LGBTQ+ people face family rejection, abuse, neglect, bullying, harassment, and behavioral problems, which can lead to being thrown out of the home, choosing to run away, dropping out of school, or being placed (or ending up) in the child welfare system.[105] For too many, this can lead to experiencing homelessness and barriers to academic success. Generally, for young and older queer people, chronic exposure to discriminatory experiences and policies contribute to difficulties in earning living wages, securing stable housing, meeting basic needs, and accessing medical and mental health care. This puts all queer people, regardless of age, at risk of homelessness as well as turning to survival economies that, in turn, increases encounters with law enforcement. Worsening this situation is that the safety net, or continuum of social services, that should be available to protect and care for vulnerable people like LGBTQ+ people is chronically underfunded.

In terms of discriminatory enforcement of laws, LGBTQ+ continue to face a legal system that effectively targets them and their perceived or real behavior. Regardless of advances in treatment for and prevention of HIV, 82% of LGBTQ+ people live in a state that has HIV-specific criminal law or broader criminal laws related to perceived or potential exposure or transmission of HIV; even more, 15% of queer people live in a state that does not have an HIV-specific law but where general criminal law has been used to prosecute people living with HIV.[106] In one survey in California, 99% of those charged under HIV-criminalization statutes were convicted and 91% were sentenced to prison or jail; similarly, approximately two-thirds of these people were black or Latino.[96] Alongside these laws, LGBTQ+ people have been subjected to antisodomy laws that have regulated consensual sex between adults.[1,96] In 2003, the U.S. Supreme Court (in *Lawrence v. Texas*) ruled that states could not legislate private, consensual behavior between adults. Whereas that ruling should prohibit queer people being targeted, in fact, at least 10 states still have antisodomy laws on the books and gay and bisexual men, in particular, continue to be targeted by police where they congregate or have sexual contact.

Young queer people are additionally targeted by laws regulating sex between minors, by which they are held to account for consensual behavior that their straight peers are not and ultimately must too-often register as sex offenders and receive harsher punishments.[96] Related, the current U.S. drug policy has resulted in disproportionately impacting urban communities, people of color, and those living in poverty. Many of these people are also LGBTQ+, as research does show that queer people are more likely to abuse substances, including those that are illegal.

Finally, queer people are subject to harmful policing strategies. Commonly nowadays, local law enforcement agencies have concentrated on quality-of-life and zero-tolerance policing strategies; that is, focusing on minor crimes like littering or not paying public transit fares as well as criminalizing public behaviors like loitering, making too much noise, or public drinking.[1,96] Queer people get caught up in these strategies often due to the broad discretion of officers, for example, young queer people being subject to arrest for congregating outside an LGBT center or engaging in survival sex. Similarly, transgender people in particular, but LGB people more broadly, are targeted by police due to the perception of transgressing gender norms or profiled as being more disorderly. This extends to police also aggressively enforcing antiprostitution statutes. Queer people engage in survival sex and sex work due to a number of reasons, including family rejection, discrimination, poverty, and homelessness.[1,96,104] More than 79% of trans people have reported interactions with the police, and trans people of color trading sex are more than twice as likely to be arrested (as opposed to white counterparts).[107] Too often, officers use wide discretion to stop LGBTQ+ people for suspicion of prostitution due to carrying condoms, and when they do charge them they can add additional charges. In a larger frame, queer people are also subject disproportionately to search-and-frisk strategies for any perceived suspicious behavior in public.

When queer people experience hate crimes and other interpersonal violence, they are met with discrimination and more violence by police. In one study, 20% of hate crimes were due to sexual orientation and 0.5% due to gender; and, while 54% of survivors reported the crimes, only 6% were later classified as a hate crime.[108] Moreover, when queer people report hate crimes, they can experience more physical violence by police. Trans people are 6.1 times more likely to experience physical violence, and 5.8 times more likely to experience harassment, threats, bullying, and vandalism. Queer and HIV-affected people of color are 2.4 times more likely to experience physical violence, and younger queer and HIV-affected people are 2.2 times more likely. In all, LGBTQ+ people also face abuse and brutality by law enforcement including negative sexual, verbal, and physical contact.[96]

Detainment and Being in the System

Once queer people are caught up in the legal system, they face another set of criminalizing experiences. As queer people enter into legal proceedings, they must contend with inadequate access to counsel, discrimination by judges, prosecutors, and court staff, as well as discrimination by juries.[1,2,96,104] This can play out by queer people having improper or no representation. They can experience less pre-trial release, discrimination during proceedings like the use of a gay "panic" defense or being perceived as having character defects, and receiving harsher sentences. Also, LGBTQ+ people can be discriminated against by not being placed on a jury singularly for their perceived or real gender or sexual orientation, or juries may enact anti-LGBTQ+ biases despite being directed to disregard such information.

After these experiences throughout trial and sentencing, LGBTQ+ people face unfair and inhumane treatment in jails, prisons, and detention facilities.[1,96,104,105] Commonly, this abject treatment manifests as improper placements, harassment and sexual assault by staff and inmates, inadequate access to health care, unmet basic needs and services, and a lack of recourse. Still today, there is little federal oversight of detention facilities; yet, in 2003, the federal government enacted the Prison Rape Elimination Act (PREA) to reduce and eliminate sexual assault by both inmates and staff. Significantly, PREA identifies LGBTQ+ people as a vulnerable population and gives guidance for how such inmates should be treated and protected.[96] In terms of placements, too often LGBTQ+ people are placed in segregated units or solitary confinement. One U.S. Bureau of Justice report showed 28% of nonheterosexual inmates were in solitary confinement in prison over the past year (versus 18% heterosexual) and 22% in jail (versus 17%); overall, 85% of LGBTQ+ inmates have ever been in solitary, which has negative mental health effects including increased self-harm and suicidality.[96,109] Despite PREA directing facilities to provide placement responsive to gender, trans people are still placed almost exclusively by the sex recorded on their birth certificate.

While being in a facility, queer people face harassment and sexual assault by staff and inmates. This manifests as unnecessary searches and strip searches, harsh treatment, and punishment like withholding food. Even more, this occurs as sexual assault.[96] Young LGBTQ+ people are at particular risk, with one in five reporting sexual victimization by another inmate or facility staff. Generally, for queer adults, 24.1% of trans and 12.2% nonheterosexual inmates report sexual assault, as opposed to 1.2% heterosexual and 2% of all inmates.[110–112] Consequently, this can negatively affect the person's mental health and potential for recidivism. Related, LGBTQ+ inmates can have inadequate health care due to lack of funding for such services or their own resources to pay for them, to a lack of competent health care providers, and to an increased need for mental health care. In addition, there can be limited HIV testing and poor access to transgender-related care. LGBTQ+ inmates face their basic needs being left largely unmet, as well. This occurs through a lack of outright respect, a lack of supportive or adjunct services like GED programs, or restricted family visitations. Underscoring these disparities, queer inmates have little recourse against violence, cruel punishment, or denial of basic rights. Despite the act, inmates cannot sue other inmates or staff under PREA.[1,2,96] More generally, inmates have limited access to legal support while incarcerated, and if they do, they face the discriminatory issues and stigma again in those legal settings as noted above.

Re-Entry into the Community

Once LGBTQ+ people have served their time and completed their sentence, they face a host of issues after detention that produce risk for recidivism and further experience of criminalization. At-large, LGBTQ+ people face a lack of competency within prison-based re-entry programs, such as lack of respect and appreciation for the multiple levels of discrimination around accessing housing or jobs.[96,104,105] As

well, trans inmates can have extreme difficulty in obtaining documents reflective of their authentic gender. Before release, LGBTQ+ inmates are at increased risk for being detained indefinitely through civil commitment procedures, secondary sex-related crimes, as noted earlier, for which queer people are targeted by police and laws disproportionately. Upon probation and parole, there is a lack of queer competency, which can manifest as lack of sensitivity for the difficulties in obtaining work or needing to travel beyond proscribed limits to access competent health care. For those housed in re-entry programs like halfway houses, they can face harassment, discrimination, and violence within the facility. This is only intensified for those in religiously affiliated programs.

As an LGBTQ+ person is working the process of re-entry, they can face numerous challenges.[96] These include difficulty finding housing and employment, inadequate health care after release, being ineligible for public assistance, mis- or overuse of sex offender registries, barriers to education, severed or denied parenting rights, challenges reconnecting with family, difficulty obtaining name changes, and loss of political participation. Re-entry is challenging for any person post-incarceration; however, these difficulties layered with additional LGBTQ+ discrimination and prejudice make the path more treacherous for queer people's health, mental health, and recidivism.

Strategies for LGBTQ+ Wellbeing: Decriminalizing Safe(r) Spaces and Operationalizing Affirmation

The wellbeing of LGBTQ+ people is a function of the person in environment, drawing on the expansive framework of the World Health Organization regarding health and mental health.[3] Central to this calculus is an appreciation for the maneuvers of chronic minority stress as well as the haphazard incitement to treat bodies, sexualities, and genders as criminogenic when they exceed the confines of heteronormative conceptions and practices. The known inequities that continue to be borne by queer people, while both troubling *and* preventable, do offer an instructive opportunity to consider how intentional work can be done in order to resist, redress, and repair those inequities. The multilevel nature of the chronic stress both targeting and experienced by LGBTQ+ people points to the fact that the interventions professionals deploy necessarily must be multilevel and multifaceted. In this section on applied practices, it is obvious that an exhaustive list is not provided for all the ways in which institutions and practitioners could operationalize culturally responsive and affirmative practices with LGBTQ+ communities. Rather, these multilevel strategies offered here are ones readily applicable to the work in correctional, forensic, and other detention facilities, as well as to the clients who may be seen in the community at risk for detention or who hold that history therein. And, these practices are ones that can be enacted by individuals, teams, organizations, and institutions. They include provider competence, affirmative case work, indicated interventions, and progressive policies.

Provider Competence

It can be common nowadays to hear practitioners talk about having or holding some variant of cultural competence. Unfortunately, this is not a static archive or experience nor is it an intellectual endeavor satisfied by one continuing education course. At baseline, cultural competence is a direct function of building relationships and trust with clients, consciously developing knowledge, and deploying interventions and assessments that are dynamic and consistent with the worldview of clients. Even more, it involves actively engaging with one's self and one's own culture and experience. It is an ongoing process. And, it appreciates the vulnerabilities and strengths of clients and communities, as well as the experiences of power, privilege, and oppression for both the clients and the practitioner. And, this process does involve an interrogation by the practitioner of their own biases, prejudices, and behaviors.

This is an apt issue for practitioners to take seriously when working with LGBTQ+ people. In considering minority stress, the queer person's experience of chronic stress is only compounded by the fact that almost every healthcare provider is not receiving adequate education and training to provide culturally competent care to LGBTQ+ people.[113] In a survey, only 41% of LGBTQ+ patients believed their providers had sufficient knowledge about queer issues.[114] When providers were surveyed, over three-quarters of nurses reported they never received any LGBT-oriented training, and almost 80% of their employers acknowledged providing no education on the topic.[115] This is consistent in medicine, social work, and mental health.[116–120] And, without baseline education or other mandatory training, providers are largely left up to their own

experience, prejudices, stigmas, and choice to adhere to their profession's ethical standards. It is not uncommon that people in general – which includes providers – can have a spectrum of reactions to and engagement with the disclosure of a minority gender or sexual orientation by their clients.[104] These typical reactions include pity (i.e. believing heterosexuality is preferred and pitying others who are not), dismissal (i.e. outright denying the client's identities), romanticizing (i.e. relegating clients to being "special" populations), sensationalizing or objectifying (i.e. viewing clients as parts or less than human), fetishizing (i.e. focusing only on aspects of gender or sexuality), tolerance (i.e. putting parameters down as in one's sexual orientation is just a phase to grow out of), disgust (i.e. rejection and demoralizing), acceptance (i.e. having to accept the client but in light of their gender or sexuality as problems), and liberal (i.e. generally friendly yet have not engaged in self-reflection about one's own biases and privilege).

These reactions can direct providers toward various behavior that may or may not be promotive of wellbeing. Along the spectrum of possibilities, providers could actively participate in prejudiced or phobic actions, deny the stress and discrimination experienced by queer people, or recognize there are inequities and harms but take no action. As well, they may educate themselves, educate others, support or advocate for queer people, and even initiate or prevent change in organizations and institutions. Again, while these possibilities do generally exist for any provider, it is known that it is less common for LGBTQ+ clients to encounter providers on the end of the spectrum toward education, advocacy, and promoting organizational change. In fact, heterosexist attitudes among practitioners can reduce their empathy for LGBTQ+ people and even harm them.[121] Like the general population, healthcare providers can and do have subtle (though sometimes active) phobias and practices toward LGBTQ+ people that are left unexamined and therefore appear in their practice. These prejudices coupled with low knowledge and self-awareness create poor service delivery, misdiagnosis, pathologizing, and deprecation. In turn, a queer client's experience of this sort of nonaffirmative practice can result in dissatisfaction with services, avoiding care, or omitting critical information during it.

To this point, it is important for practitioners to engage with an ongoing exploration of their own understanding and biases related to sexuality and gender identities, as self-awareness is a crucial part of effective practice. In addition, practitioners should adhere to their profession's ethics and best practice standards; endemic to current-day standards, conversion therapy is never indicated for LGBTQ+ people.[122–129] Equally important is for organizations, agencies, and institutions to identify and provide adequate trainings for all staff. This would necessarily include an assessment of policies and practices, identifying those not LGBTQ+-affirming and taking action to transform them into more inclusive and affirming ones.

LGBTQ+-Affirmative Case Work

Holding education about or having competence with LGBTQ+ communities and common issues does not equate to the intentional action of conducting queer-affirmative work with individuals, groups, organizations, or institutions. Continuing the discussion on this topic began above, affirmative work (see Figure 34.1) starts at baseline with an explicit validation of and appreciation for the wide spectrum of LGBTQ+ identities and expressions therein. And, sexualities

and gender identities and expressions are not incidental demographic variables to check off assessment boxes, rather they are figured at the center of the client's life experience as well as considered a central part of how they are coping and behaving in detention facilities. Building off an understanding of minority stress and a model for stress and coping,[130–133] an affirmative approach is a three-part process that can be overlaid onto whatever intervention or modality a team or individual practitioner commonly uses.[88,134] The first part is to adequately assess the client's experience of queer stress, accounting for histories with stigmas, phobias (external and internal), chronic stress (both individual and community level), and disclosure and concealment of identities. The second part is to assess for coping, understanding abilities and skills for emotion regulation, social and interpersonal functioning, cognitive schemas, and sexual and intimate relationships. This area also tends to qualities of resilience that the clients hold in these areas and beyond. The third part is to formulate the case within a queer-affirmative perspective parallel to the clinical modality or tradition that the practitioner uses. For example, a DBT-oriented practitioner

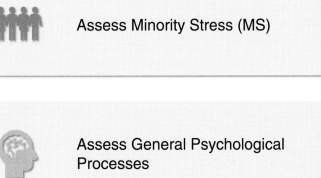

Assess Minority Stress (MS)

Exposure to prejudice events
Operating stigmas
Internalized homophobia
Sexuality, gender concealment

Assess General Psychological Processes

Coping/emotional regulation, social/interpersonal functioning, cognitive schemas, relationships
Resilience; develop MS analysis on psychological functioning and health risking behaviors
Formulate case with clinical methods and MS analysis

Design Queer-Affirmative Approach, Treatment

Attend to therapeutic alliance
Address stigma, disclosure, coping, social skills, intersectionalities
Develop positive self-identity, connections with community
Multilevel interventions

Figure 34.1 LGBTQ+-affirmative case work.

formulates the case within a tradition of behaviorism as well as one that is queer-affirmative. To this end, alongside the traditional interventions conducted with the client, queer-affirmative action is taken. This would include consistent attention to the therapeutic alliance, cultural competence, strengths, and a person-in-environment understanding of mental health. As well, the interventions offered tend to issues of stigma, disclosure, stress and coping, and intersectional identities. This is all in service of cultivating wellbeing, a positive sense of self, and increased connections with communities. Finally, the work is multi-level, when possible, as chronic minority stress is multilevel; therefore, interventions need to appropriately and adequately address forces that impinge on or facilitate the client's mental health.

It can be illusive in practice to see blatant examples of queer-affirmative work; or, practitioners may side-step such an approach to formulating and intervening with cases due to a variety of reasons, one of which may be lack of training and education. Nonetheless, queer-affirmative work can operationalize in an endless number of ways as, ultimately, it is contextually oriented to the setting, population, client, and team of providers.[88] This is when consultation, supervision, as well as thorough and ongoing conversations with clients can be helpful. For example, it can be helpful for organizations to have an LGBTQ+ client advocate on care teams when staffing clients, or to appointment one or more lead clinicians who are obligated to ensure that the advocacy and care for LGBTQ+ clients is responsive and affirmative.

One decided place to start is considering the lines of inquiry utilized in intake paperwork, onboarding clients into new systems, and clinical assessment interviews and initial encounters. A persistent problem and effect of heteronormative and cisnormative systems and institutions is the encouragement toward an uncritical usage of identity categories, an insistence on minority sexualities and genders as deviant or problematic, as well as an individual focus at the expense of an appreciation for client's experiences interacting with prejudiced systems. Equally, providers may have the best intentions to serve LGBTQ+ clients, but they can at times focus too much or too little on the client's sexuality or gender identity, either overassociating or undercorrelating it with health and mental health issues.[104] Accordingly, a queer-affirmative approach would encourage a conversation with clients about how they square their sexuality and gender with the

situation or problems at hand.[135] This can be achieved through more narrative-oriented lines of inquiry; for example: *How do you describe or think about your sexuality and/or gender to yourself? Is your sexuality or gender important to how you see yourself; if so, in what ways? Are there any other important areas of your identity? Have you had concerns about your sexuality or gender? How does your sexuality or gender figure into your health and mental health?* From there, it is important for clinicians and staff to consider how is this information documented, recorded, and then used to inform treatment and care.

Indicated Interventions: Language

Co-extensive with an affirmative approach as well as increasing provider competence, a series of interventions are indicated that are multilevel focused. The first of which is an attention to the language and communication around sexualities and gender used throughout organizations and institutions, and this occurs in a number of aspects. First, a persistent problem with effectively serving LGBTQ+ communities is the dearth of data about them; either it is not collected, or it is inaccurately collected.[13] Whereas it is helpful to use some standardized categories for sexualities and genders, it is equally helpful to have more dynamic or open-ended response categories throughout the intake, assessment, and termination processes.[104] Second, in auditing the affirmative and inclusive climate of any organization or institution, it is helpful to assess for how inclusive as well as neutral language is in clinical, administrative, and interpersonal communication. For example, in the case of transgender clients, this would include utilizing preferred gender pronouns, ensuring use of authentic (versus "dead") names, creating opportunities for clients to notify about changes to self-identification, and holding colleagues and systems accountable for misuse of pronouns. In this instance, it is known that using preferred gender pronouns and authentic names alone is linked to a reduction in negative mood and suicidality.[136] Other ways to enact more neutral and inclusive language is to address clients and colleagues with the title "Mx." ("mix") instead of Mr. or Ms., or generally to use they/them/theirs pronouns and passive forms of writing, or to defer to more inclusive nouns such as "partner" versus wife or husband. More broadly and third, it is equally helpful to allow for clients to have opportunities over time and relationships with various staff and clinicians to self-identify, but moreover within fluid frameworks, regarding sexuality and gender along a spectrum. This kind of logic resists the tendency to regard sexuality and gender within binaries, which often cannot accommodate the lived experiences, let alone self-identification practices of clients. Fourth, it is important to account for how representation exists across an organization's built environment that reflects inclusivity, affirmation, validation, as well as accountability. Professional associations continue to give much direction about how this can manifest.[122–129]

Indicated Interventions: PrEP

In the U.S., HIV continues to disproportionately affect gay and bisexual men, men who have sex with men, transgender women, and people of color.[137] When doing affirmative work with LGBTQ+ people, assessment and dialogues must include attention to sexual health – in particular HIV prevention and care. This can be part of an initial assessment or incorporated increasingly into the routine interactions with clients.[104] Technologies for HIV prevention have evolved; HIV testing and condom use are no longer the only or primary ones. Since 2012, the CDC has published guidelines for Pre-exposure Prophylaxis, or PrEP.[138,139] This is a single daily dose of one antiretroviral medication, which can reduce transmission risk by more than 90%. It is indicated for populations at increased risk, and who adhere to a daily pill regimen along with routine testing and monitoring. And whereas PrEP has been a substantial advance in HIV prevention technologies, its awareness and use lags. A number of the primary barriers to PrEP getting to those most at risk include the fact that only one in three prescribing providers knows about PrEP, parallel to the problems of homophobia, stigma, and discrimination. It is important to know that any provider with prescriptive authority can prescribe PrEP.[138–140]

Indicated Interventions: Trauma-Informed Care

As discussed previously, LGBTQ+ people are disproportionately at risk for and experience victimization, violence, and trauma. Whether or not an organization or institution provides treatments for traumatic stress, they can organize their culture and programming within a trauma-informed approach.[141] Similar to a queer-affirmative approach, this is one that is overlaid onto existing policies, protocols, and interventions commonly used in organizations already. In that,

there are a number of core tenants to a trauma-informed approach. First, the organization's culture and work recognize the impacts of violence and victimization for LGBTQ+ people. Second, recovery is a central goal of treatment, which includes an attention to empowerment, choice, having voice, and control when possible. In this, the therapeutic alliance is one of a relational collaboration and it avoids retraumatization. Third, the framing and understanding of trauma for queer people is diagrammed in a way to acknowledge how individual experiences are connected to larger macro forces as well as that marginalized communities have experienced historical traumas over time. Fourth, as interventions are deployed, attention is given to the intersectional identities of clients such that they can see their culture and experience represented and reflected in the work. Finally, a trauma-informed approach actively acknowledges and seeks out opportunities to understand and validate the resilience and post-traumatic growth that often can occur after or because of traumatic experiences.[142]

Progressive Policies

Organizations and institutions have various capacities to enact policy change that can be responsive to decriminalizing the understanding of and practices around LGBTQ+ health and mental health. Mounting best practice recommendations and progressive guidance has been offered to these ends; however, the deployment of such knowledge and applied practice can too often be left to political will, the negative effects of prejudices and stigmas as discussed previously, or the financial health of organizations.[94,96,104,105,117,118,122,129,143] Nonetheless, offered here are four policy recommendations that target some of the central ideological mechanisms that contribute to the continued criminalization of LGBTQ+ people and their mental health:[96]

- *Modernize HIV criminalization laws.* States should repeal laws that criminalize the transmission of HIV and other diseases. In considering revisions to current laws, lawmakers and advocates should take into consideration unique or additional burdens these laws place on individuals living with HIV/AIDS, and the extent to which existing laws do not take into account the most recent science around prevention, transmission of, and care for HIV.
- *End criminalization of consensual sex.* State and local law enforcement should not criminalize

consensual sex between adults. They should ensure that laws policing sex are not discriminatorily enforced against LGBT people, in particular reduce and cease entrapment scenarios targeting gay, bisexual, and men who have sex with men. States should pass legislation ensuring access to condoms without fear that their possession or presence will be used as evidence to justify stops, arrest, or prosecution for any sex work or lewd conduct-related offense.

- *Increase data collection about LGBTQ+ people's experiences with law enforcement.* Governments, academics, and advocates should strengthen data collection about the experiences of LGBTQ+ individuals with law enforcement through anonymous and other surveys that protect participants. The Bureau of Justice Statistics should add questions concerning sexual harassment of and misconduct toward LGBTQ+ community members by law enforcement. The Centers for Disease Control should add similar questions to the National Intimate Partner and Sexual Violence Survey. And, community-based organizations such as the National Center for Transgender Equality should be fortified in their work on work like the U.S. Transgender Survey.

- *Enact PREA requirements for placement of LGBTQ + people.* Detention facilities should enforce PREA regulations for placement of LGBTQ+ people. In this, queer people should be consulted about their needs and safety concerns in determining the most appropriate housing assignments. In particular, transgender individuals should be housed based on their authentic gender identity, rather than anatomical sex or the sex on their birth certificate. LGBTQ+ individuals should not be placed in solitary confinement based solely on their sexual orientation and/or gender identity.

Conclusion

Ironically, all the while that dominate and heteronormative cultural practices, ideologies, and systems construct and reinforce secure settings, these secure spaces are queer. They are replete with non-normative behaviors and existences, some of which are queer people. The presence of LGBTQ+ people make these spaces something more than what they were originally developed for, that is, discipline, correction, punishment,

(social) policing, or rehabilitation, and more. Queer people confound these spaces, as their presence within them starkly represents that society deems minoritized sexualities and genders as abject problems. That said, LGBTQ+ identities continue to expand, transform, gain visibility, challenge language, and receive attention and advocacy. In that attention and analysis, it is increasingly clear that queer people have always been and continue to be criminalized *de facto* because of their sexuality, gender identity, and/or gender expression – regardless of putative criminal behavior. The stigma, disparate treatment, and policing around this are only compounded when accounting for their other intersecting statuses and identities of mental health, class, race, ethnicity, documentation, and ability, among others.

The effects of this approach are numerous. The multilevel efforts, historically and currently, to sanction, police, detain, and intervene upon LGBTQ+ people for their very existences, in effect, has diverted much attention clinically, socio-politically, and in research from the basic criminality of LGBTQ+ people *apart* from their sexuality and gender. This is to say that the persistent efforts to criminalize queer people has done the work to obscure a more accurate understanding of LGBTQ+ offenders, victims, and the relationships therein.[105] Another effect has been to reduce attention to the chronic minority stress, disproportionate health and mental health inequities, substantial experiences of victimization and historical traumas, as well as social inequities too often left invisible. Accordingly, systems and interventions have been less focused on recovery, rehabilitation, and prevention; instead, they have been reinforcing that queer people are understood as generally expendable[144] in U.S. society, let alone other parts of the world. Effectively, then, whereas systems may have the preeminent intention to be helpful and rehabilitative, this distressing picture of LGBTQ+ people is one that exacerbates mental health symptoms, contributes to (self-)harm, and fosters problematic relationships with substances, all the while disrupting the relationship between LGBTQ+ people and society.[105]

Again, this does not have to be the case. The approach by secure systems and practitioners therein can be different; LGBTQ+ people deserve it to be so. Ultimately, it should be clear that providers need not be LGBTQ+-identified to provide culturally competent and affirmative services that are responsive to the needs and issues of the queer people they serve.[145]

As discussed in this review, that process can begin with attending to language practices, interrogating biases in oneself and the systems under which one works, and challenging normative ideologies, policies, and practices. As well, in a larger effort to decriminalize LGBTQ+ people and their mental health prior to entering the system, there are various moments to target during their stay in a secure setting and while working the process of re-entry into the community. And as the chronic stresses and strains on queer people are multilevel, the effective responses to redress and repair inequities must be multilevel, beginning with a LGBTQ+-affirmative formulation. There is certainly work to be done.

Disclosures

Conflicts of interest: Tyler Argüello has nothing to disclose.

References

1. Mogul JL, Ritchie AJ, Whitlock K. *Queer (In)Justice: The Criminalization of LGBT in the United States.* Boston, MA: Beacon Press; 2011.

2. Stanley E, Smith N, eds. *Captive Genders: Trans Embodiment and the Prison Industrial Complex.* Oakland, CA: AK Press; 2011.

3. World Health Organization. Mental health action plan: 2013–2020. 2013. www.who.int/mental_health/publications/action_plan/en/ (accessed June 2020).

4. Jagose A. *Queer Theory: An Introduction.* New York, NY: New York University Press; 1996.

5. Sullivan N. *A Critical Introduction to Queer Theory.* New York, NY: New York University Press; 2003.

6. Warner M. *Publics and Counterpublics.* Brooklyn, NY: Zone Books; 2002.

7. Eng DL, Halberstam J, Muñoz JE. Introduction: what's queer about queer studies now? *Social Text 84–85.* 2005; **23**(3–4): 1–17.

8. Rubin GS. Thinking sex: notes for a radical theory of the politics of sexuality. In Parker R, Aggleton P, eds. *Culture, Society and Sexuality: A Reader.* New York, NY: UCL Press; 1999: 143178.

9. Warner M. Fear of a queer planet. *Social Text 29.* 1991: 3–17.

10. Duggan L. (2004). *The Twilight of Inequality?: Neoliberalism, Cultural Politics, and the Attack on Democracy.* Boston: Beacon Press; 2014.

11. Williams Institute. LGBT demographic data interactive. 2019. https://williamsinstitute .law.ucla.edu/visualization/lgbt-stats/?topic=LGBT# density (accessed June 2020).

12. Institute of Medicine. *The Health of Lesbian, Gay, Bisexual, and Transgender People: Building a Foundation for Better Understanding.* Washington, DC: National Academies Press; 2011.

13. US Department of Health and Human Services. Healthy people 2020: lesbian, gay, bisexual, and transgender health. Office of Disease Prevention and Health Promotion; 2010. www .healthypeople.gov/2020/topics-objectives/topic/les bian-gay-bisexual-and-transgender-health (accessed June 2020).

14. Conron KJ, Mimiaga MJ, Landers SJ. A population-based study of sexual orientation identity and gender differences in adult health. *Am J Public Health.* 2010; **100**: 1953–1960.

15. Saewyc EM, Poon CS, Homma Y, et al. Stigma management?: the links between enacted stigma and teen pregnancy trends among gay, lesbian, and bisexual students in British Columbia. *Can J Hum Sex.* 2008; **17**: 123–139.

16. Heiden-Rootes KM, Salas J, Scherrer JF, et al. Comparison of medical diagnoses among same-sex and opposite-sex-partnered patients. *J Am Board Fam Med.* 2016; **29**(6): 688–693.

17. Ryan C, Huebner D, Diaz RM, et al. Family rejection as a predictor of negative health outcomes in white and Latino lesbian, gay, and bisexual young adults. *Pediatrics.* 2009; **123**: 346–352.

18. Blosnich JR, Farmer GW, Lee JG, et al. Health inequalities among sexual minority adults: evidence from ten US states, 2010. *Am J Prev Med.* 2014; **46**: 337–349.

19. King M, Semlyn J, Killaspy H, et al. *A Systematic Review of Research on Counselling and Psychotherapy for Lesbian, Gay, Bisexual, and Transgender People.* London, UK: British Association for Counselling and Psychotherapy; 2007.

20. Bostwick WB, Boyd CJ, Hughes TL, et al. Discrimination and mental health among lesbian, gay, and bisexual adults in the United States. *Am J Orthopsychiatry.* 2014; **84**(1): 35–45.

21. Fredrikson-Goldsen KI, Kim H-J, Emlet CA, et al. The aging and health report: disparities and resilience among lesbian, gay, bisexual and transgender older adults. SAGE (Services & Advocacy for GLBT Elders); 2011. https://issuu .com/lgbtagingcenter/docs/full-report-final-11-16-1 1 (accessed June 2020).

22. Kidd S, Howison M, Pilling M, et al. Severe mental illness among LGBT populations: a scoping review. *Psychiatr Serv.* 2016; **67**(7): 779–783.

23. Centers for Disease Control and Prevention. Stigma and discrimination. 2019. www.cdc.gov/msmhealth/stigma-and-discrimination.htm (accessed June 2020).

24. Hatzenbuehler ML, McLaughlin KA, Keyes KM, et al. The impact of institutional discrimination on psychiatric disorders in lesbian, gay, and bisexual populations: a prospective study. *Am J Public Health.* 2010; **100**(3): 452–459.

25. Russ TC, Stamatakis E, Hamer M, et al. Association between psychological distress and mortality: individual participant pooled analysis of 10 prospective cohort studies. *Br Med J.* 2012; **345**: e4933.

26. Gates GJ, Newport F. Special report: 3.4% of U.S. Adults Identify as LGBT. Gallup; 2012. www.gallup.com/poll/158066/special-report-adults-identify-lgbt-aspx (accessed June 2020).

27. Badgett MV, Durso LE, Sheneebaum A. *New Patterns of Poverty in the Lesbian, Gay, and Bisexual Community.* Los Angeles: The Williams Institute; 2013.

28. Nyitray A, Corran R, Altman K, Chikani V, Negrón EV. Tobacco use and interventions among Arizona lesbian, gay, bisexual and transgender people. Arizona Department of Health Services and Wingspan; 2006. www.lgbthealthlink.org/Report-Cards/Arizona/2016 (accessed June 2020).

29. Brittain DR, Baillargeon T, McElroy M, et al. Barriers to moderate physical activity in adult lesbians. *Women Health.* 2006; **43**(1): 75–92.

30. Blosnich J, Andersen J. Thursday's child: the role of adverse childhood experiences in explaining mental health disparities among lesbian, gay, and bisexual US adults. *Soc Psychiatry Psychiatr Epidemiol.* 2015; **50**(2): 335–338.

31. Poteat T. Top 10 things lesbians should discuss with their healthcare provider. Gay and Lesbian Medical Association; 2012. www.glma.org/index.cfm?fuseaction=Page.viewPage&pageID=691 (accessed June 2020).

32. Zaritsky E, Dibble SL. Risk factors for reproductive and breast cancers among older lesbians. *J Women's Health.* 2010; **19**(1): 125–131.

33. Fredriksen-Goldsen KI, Kim H-J, Barkan SE, et al. Health disparities among lesbian, gay, and bisexual older adults: Results from a population-based study. *Am J Public Health.* 2013; **103**(10): 1802–1809.

34. Centers for Disease Control and Prevention. HIV and gay and bisexual men. 2019. www.cdc.gov/hiv/group/msm/index.html (accessed June 2020).

35. World Health Organization. Hepatitis: Q&A. www.who.int/health-topics/hepatitis#tab=tab_1 (accessed June 2020).

36. Carper TL, Negy C, Tantleff-Dunn S. Relations among media influence, body image, eating concerns, and sexual orientation in men: a preliminary investigation. *Body Image.* 2010; **7**(4): 301–309.

37. Mosher WD, Chandra A, Jones J. Sexual behavior and selected health measures: men and women 15–44 years of age, United States, 2002. *Adv Data.* 2005; **15**(362): 1–55.

38. Wichstrom L. Sexual orientation as a risk factor for bulimic symptoms. *Int J Eat Disord.* 2006; **39**: 448–453.

39. Ostrow DG, Stall, R. Alcohol, tobacco, and drug use among gay and bisexual men. In Wolitski RJ, Stall R, Valdiserri RO, eds. *Unequal Opportunity: Health Disparities Affecting Gay and Bisexual Men in the United States.* New York: Oxford University Press; 2008: 121–158.

40. Bostwick WB, Boyd CJ, Hughes TL, et al. Dimensions of sexual orientation and the prevalence of mood and anxiety disorders in the United States. *Am J Public Health.* 2010; **100**(3): 468–475.

41. Houston E, McKirnan DJ. Intimate partner abuse among gay and bisexual men: risk correlates and health outcomes. *J Urban Health.* 2007; **84**(5): 681–690.

42. Diamant AL, Wold C, Spritzer K, et al. Health behaviors, health status, and access to and use of health care: a population-based study of lesbian, bisexual, and heterosexual women. *Arch Fam Med.* 2000; **9**(10): 1043–1051.

43. Winn RJ. *Ten things bisexuals should discuss with their healthcare provider.* Gay and Lesbian Medical Association; 2012.

44. VanKim NA, Padilla JL. *New Mexico's Progress in Collecting Lesbian, Gay, Bisexual, and Transgender Health Data and its Implications for Addressing Health Disparities.* Albuquerque, NM: New Mexico Department of Health, Chronic Disease Prevention and Control Bureau; 2010.

45. Balsam KF, Mohr JJ. Adaptation to sexual orientation stigma: a comparison of bisexual and lesbian/gay adults. *J Couns Psychol.* 2007; **54**(3): 306–319.

46. Scherrer KS. Clinical practice with bisexual identified individuals. *Clin Social Work J.* 2013; **41**(3): 238–248.

47. Bradford M. The bisexual experience: living in a dichotomous culture. *J Bisexuality.* 2004; **4**(1–2): 7–23.

48. Landers S, Gilsanz P. The health of lesbian, gay, bisexual, and transgender (LGBT) persons in Massachusetts. Massachusetts Department of Public Health; 2009. www.mass.gov/eohhs/docs/dph/com

missioner/lgbt-health-report.pdf (accessed June 2020).

49. Grant JM, Mottet LA, Tanis J, et al. Injustice at every turn: a look at Black respondents in the National Transgender Discrimination Survey. National Center for Transgender Equality and National Gay and Lesbian Task Force; 2011. www.thetaskforce.org/wp-content/uploads/2019/04/Injustice-at-Every-Turn-2009.pdf (accessed June 2020).

50. Grossman AH, D'Augelli AR. Transgender youth and life-threatening behaviors. *Suicide Life-Threat Behav.* 2007; **37**(5): 527–537.

51. Stotzer RL. Violence against transgender people: a review of United States data. *Aggress Violent Behav.* 2009; **14**(3): 170–179.

52. Budge SL, Adelson JL, Howard KA. Anxiety and depression in transgender individuals: the role of transition status, loss, social support, and coping. *J Consult Clin Psychol.* 2013; **81**(3): 545–557.

53. Nemoto T, Bodeker B, Iwamoto M. Social support, exposure to violence, and transphobia: correlates of depression among male-to female transgender women with a history of sex work. *Am J Public Health.* 2011; **101**: 1980–1988.

54. Nuttbrock L, Hwahng S, Bockting W, et al. Psychiatric impact of gender-related abuse across the life course of male-to-female transgender persons. *J Sex Res.* 2010; **47**: 12–23.

55. Cohen-Kettenis PT, Pfäfflin F. *Transgenderism and Intersexuality in Childhood and Adolescence: Making Choices.* Thousand Oaks, CA: SAGE; 2003.

56. Kuiper AJ, Cohen-Kettenis PT. Gender role reversal among postoperative transsexuals. *Int J Transgenderism.* 1998; **2**(3).

57. Pfäfflin F, Junge A. *Sex Reassignment. Thirty Years of International Follow-Up Studies after Sex Reassignment Surgery: A Comprehensive Review, 1961–1991* (Translated by Jacobson RB, Meier AB). Kissing, Germany: Symposium Publishing; 1998.

58. Smith YL, Van Goozen SH, Kuiper AJ, et al. Sex reassignment: outcomes and predictors of treatment for adolescent and adult transsexuals. *Psychol Med.* 2005; **35**(1): 89–99.

59. Dhejne C, Oberg K, Arver S, et al. An analysis of all applications for sex reassignment surgery in Sweden, 1960–2010: prevalence, incidence, and regrets. *Arch Sex Behav.* 2014; **43**(8): 1535–1545.

60. Cochran SD, Mays VM, Sullivan JG. Prevalence of mental disorders, psychological distress, and mental health services use among lesbian, gay, and bisexual adults in the United States. *J Consult Clin Psychol.* 2003; **71**(1): 53–61.

61. Haas AP. Suicide and suicide risk in lesbian, gay, bisexual, and transgender populations: review and recommendations. *J Homosex.* 2011; **58**(1): 10–51.

62. Kertzner RM, Meyer IH, Frost DM, et al. Social and psychological well-being in lesbians, gay men, and bisexuals: the effects of race, gender, age, and sexual identity. *Am J Orthopsychiatry.* 2009; **79**(4): 500–510.

63. Mathy RM. Suicidality and sexual orientation in five continents: Asia, Australia, Europe, North America, and South America. *Int J Sex Gender Stud.* 2002; 7(2/3): 215–225.

64. The Trevor Project. National survey on LGBTQ mental health. 2019. www.thetrevorproject.org/survey-2019/ (accessed June 2020).

65. Moody C, Smith NG. Suicide protective factors among trans adults. *Arch Sex Behav.* 2013; **42**(5): 739–752.

66. Olson J, Schrager SM, Belzer M, et al. Baseline physiologic and psychosocial characteristics of transgender youth seeking care for gender dysphoria. *J Adolesc Health.* 2015; **57**(4): 374–380.

67. Waters E, Yacka-Bible S. A crisis of hate: a mid year report on lesbian, gay, bisexual transgender and queer hate violence homicides. National Coalition of Anti-Violence Programs; 2017. http://avp.org/wp-content/uploads/2017/08/NCAVP-A-Crisis-of-Hate-Final.pdf (accessed June 2020).

68. Rothman EF, Exner D, Baughman AL. The prevalence of sexual assault against people who identify as gay, lesbian, or bisexual in the United States: a systematic review. *Trauma Violence Abuse.* 2011; **12**(2): 55–66.

69. Human Rights Campaign. Violence against the transgender community in 2019. 2019. www.hrc.org/resources/violence-against-the-transgender-community-in-2019 (accessed June 2020).

70. Zou C, Andersen JP, Blosnich JR. The association between bullying and physical health among gay, lesbian, and bisexual individuals. *J Am Psychiatr Nurses Assoc.* 2013; **19**(6): 356365.

71. Gandy-Guedes M, Havig K, Natale AP, et al. Trauma impacts on LGBTQ people: implications for lifespan development. In Dentato M, ed. *Social Work Practice with the LGBTQ Community: The Intersection of History, Health, Mental Health, and Policy Factors.* New York, NY: Oxford University Press; 2018: 118–136.

72. Walker MD, Hernandez AM, Davey M. Childhood sexual abuse and adult sexual identity formation: intersection of gender, race, and sexual orientation. *Am J Fam Ther.* 2012; **40**(5): 385–398.

73. Friedman MS, Marshal MP, Guadamuz TE, et al. A meta-analysis of disparities in childhood sexual abuse, parental physical abuse, and peer victimization among sexual minority and sexual nonminority

individuals. *Am J Public Health*. 2011; **101**(8): 1481–1494.

74. Movement Advancement Project. Conversion "therapy" laws. 2019. www.lgbtmap.org/equality-maps/conversion_therapy (accessed June 2020).

75. D'Augelli A. Lesbian and bisexual female youths aged 14 to 21: developmental challenges and victimization experiences. *J Lesbian Stud*. 2003; **7**(4): 9–29.

76. Balsam KF. Traumatic victimization in the lives of lesbian and bisexual women. *J Lesbian Stud*. 2002; **7**(1): 1–14.

77. Balsam KF. Trauma, stress, and resilience among sexual minority women: rising like the phoenix. *J Lesbian Stud*. 2003; **7**(4): 1–8.

78. Salmon KA. *Sex Abuse?: Just as Long as You're Not Gay: An Exploratory Study with Queer Adults on Childhood Sexual Victimization (Master's thesis)*. Northampton, MA: Smith College; 2014.

79. Das G. Mostly normal: American psychiatric taxonomy, sexuality, and neoliberal mechanisms of exclusion. *Sex Res Soc Policy*. 2016; **13**: 390–401.

80. Meyer IH. Prejudice, social stress, and mental health in lesbian, gay, and bisexual populations: conceptual issues and research evidence. *Psychol Bull*. 2003; **129**: 674–697.

81. Cyrus K. Multiple minorities as multiply marginalized: applying the minority stress theory to LGBTQ people of color. *J Gay Lesbian Ment Health*. 2017; **21**(3): 194–202.

82. Moradi B, Wiseman MC, DeBlaere C, et al. LGB of color and white individuals' perceptions of heterosexist stigma, internalized homophobia, and outness: comparisons of levels and links. *Couns Psychol*. 2010; **38**(3): 397–424.

83. Parra LA, Benibgui M, Helm J, et al. Minority stress predicts depression in lesbian, gay, and bisexual emerging adults via elevated diurnal cortisol. *Emerg Adulthood*. 2016; **4**(5): 365–372.

84. Alessi EJ, Hartman E. Incorporating minority stress theory into clinical practice with sexual-minority populations. In: Dentato MP, ed. *Social Work Practice with the LGBTQ Community: The Intersection of History, Health, Mental Health, and Policy Factors*. New York, NY: Oxford University Press; 2018: 249–265.

85. Holley LC, Mendoza NS, Del-Colle MM, et al. Heterosexism, racism, and mental illness discrimination: experiences of people with mental health conditions and their families. *J Gay Lesbian Soc Serv*. 2016; **28**(2): 93–116.

86. Hatzenbuehler ML. How does sexual minority stigma "get under the skin"?: a psychological mediation framework. *Psychol Bull*. 2009; **135**(5): 707–730.

87. Pachankis JE. The psychological implications of concealing a stigma: a cognitive-affective-behavioral model. *Psychol Bull*. 2007; **133**: 328–345.

88. Argüello TM, ed. *Queer Social Work: Cases for LGBTQ+ Affirmative Practice*. New York, NY: Columbia University Press; 2019.

89. Davies D. Towards a model of gay affirmative therapy. In Davies D, Neal C, eds. *Pink Therapy: A Guide for Counsellors and Therapists Working with Lesbian, Gay, and Bisexual Clients*. Buckingham, England: Open University Press; 1996: 24–40.

90. Herek GM. The psychology of sexual prejudice. *Curr Dir Psychol Sci*. 2000; **9**(1): 19–22.

91. King M, Semlyen J, Tai SS, et al. A systematic review of mental disorder, suicide, and deliberate self harm in lesbian, gay, and bisexual people. *BCM Psychiatry*. 2008; **18**(8): 70.

92. Tozer EE, McClanahan MK. Treating the purple menace: ethical considerations of conversion therapy and affirmative alternatives. *Couns Psychol*. 1999; **27**: 722–742.

93. SAMHSA. Sexual minority representation in US jails and prisons. 2019. www.samhsa.gov/gains-center (accessed June 2020).

94. National Center for Transgender Equality. LGBTQ people behind bars: a guide to understanding the issues facing transgender prisoners and their legal rights. 2018. https://transequality.org/transpeople behindbars (accessed June 2020).

95. Lambda Legal. Transgender incarcerated people in crisis. 2019. www.lambdalegal.org/know-your-rights/article/trans-incarcerated-people (accessed June 2020).

96. Movement Advancement Project, Center for American Progress. Unjust: how the broken criminal justice system fails LGBT people. 2016. www.lgbtmap.org/file/lgbt-criminal-justice.pdf (accessed June 2020).

97. Grzanka PR, Miles JR. The problem with the phrase "intersecting identities": LGBT affirmative therapy, intersectionality, and neoliberalism. *Sex Res Soc Policy*. 2016; **13**: 371–389.

98. Foucault M. *The History of Sexuality, Vol. 1: An Introduction* (Translated by R. Hurley). New York: Vintage Books; 1978/1990.

99. Chauncey G. *Gay New York: Gender, Urban Culture, and the Making of the Gay Male World, 1890–1940*. New York, NY: Harper Collins; 1994.

100. Bland L, Doan L, eds. *Sexology Uncensored: The Documents of Sexual Science*. Cambridge, UK: Polity Press; 1998.

101. Irvine JM. *Disorders of Desire: Sexuality and Gender in Modern American Sexology, 2nd edn.* Philadelphia, PA: Temple University Press; 2005.

102. Terry J. *An American Obsession: Science, Medicine, and Homosexuality in Modern Society.* Chicago: University of Chicago Press; 1999.

103. Crenshaw K. Mapping the margins: intersectionality, identity politics, and violence against women of color. *Stanford Law Rev.* 1991; **43**: 1241–1299.

104. O'Brien RP, Walker PM, Poteet SL, McAllister-Wallner A, Taylor M. Mapping the road to equity: the annual state of LGBTQ communities, 2018. #Out4MentalHealth Project; 2018. https://califor nialgbtqhealth.org/wp-content/uploads/2018/12/O4 MH-Mapping-the-Road-to-Equity.pdf (accessed June 2020).

105. Woods JB. LGBT identity and crime. *Calif L Rev.* 2017; **105**: 667–732.

106. Hasenbush A, Miyashita A, Wilson BDM. *HIV Criminalization in California: Penal Implications for People Living with HIV/AIDS.* Los Angeles, CA: The Williams Institute; 2015.

107. Fitzgerald E, Espeth S, Hickey D, et al. Meaningful work: transgender experiences in the sex trade. Best Practices Policy Project, Red Umbrella Project, National Center for Transgender Equality; 2015. www.bestpracticespolicy.org/wp-content/uploads/2 015/12/Meaningful-Work-Full-Report.pdf (accessed June 2020).

108. Ahmed O, Jindasurat C. Lesbian, gay, bisexual, transgender, queer, and HIV-affected hate violence in 2014. National Coalition of Anti-Violence Programs; 2015. https://avp.org/wp-content/upload s/2017/04/2014_HV_Report-Final.pdf (accessed June 2020).

109. Kaba F, Lewis A, Glowa-Kollisch S, et al. Solitary confinement and risk of self-harm among jail inmates. *Am J Public Health.* 2014; **104**(3): 442–447.

110. Beck AJ, Harrison PM, Guerino P. Sexual victimization in juvenile facilities reported by youth, 2008–09. US Department of Justice Bureau of Justice Statistics; 2010. www.bjs.gov/content/pub/pdf/svjfr y09.pdf (accessed June 2020).

111. Jenness V. Transgender inmates in California's prisons: an empirical study of a vulnerable population. Presentation to The California Department of Corrections and Rehabilitation wardens' meeting; April 8, 2009. http://ucicor rections.seweb.uci.edu/files/2013/06/Transgende r-Inmates-in-CAs-Prisons-An-Empirical-Study-of-a-Vulnerable-Population.pdf (accessed June 2020).

112. Beck AJ, Berzofsky M, Caspar R, et al. Sexual victimization in prisons and jails reported by inmates, 2011–12. US Department of Justice Bureau of Justice Statistics; 2013. www.bjs.gov/content/pub/pdf/svpjri1112.pdf (accessed June 2020).

113. Schweiger-Whalen L, Noe S, Lynch S, et al. Converging cultures: partnering in affirmative and inclusive health care for members of the lesbian, gay, bisexual, and transgender community. *J Am Psychiatr Nurses Assoc.* 2019; **25**(6): 453–466 doi.org/10.1177/1078390318820127.

114. McCann E, Sharek D. Survey of lesbian, gay, bisexual, and transgender people's experiences of mental health services in Ireland. *Int J Ment Health Nurs.* 2014; **23**(2): 118–127.

115. Carabez R, Pellegrini M, Mankovitz A, et al. "Never in all my years…": nurses' education about LGBT health. *J Prof Nurs.* 2015; **31**: 323–329.

116. Obedin-Maliver J, Goldsmith ES, Stewart L, et al. Lesbian, gay, bisexual, and transgender-related content in undergraduate medical education. *J Am Med Assoc.* 2011; **306**(9): 971–977.

117. Sequeira GM, Chakraborti C, Panunti BA. Integrating lesbian, gay, bisexual, and transgender (LGBT) content into undergraduate medical school curricula: a qualitative study. *Ochsner J.* 2012; **12**(4): 379–382.

118. White W, Brenman S, Paradis E, et al. Lesbian, gay, bisexual, and transgender patient care: medical students' preparedness and comfort. *Teach Learn Med.* 2015; **27**(3): 254–263.

119. Bell SA, Bern-Klug M, Kramer KW, et al. Most nursing home social service directors lack training in working with lesbian, gay, and bisexual residents. *Soc Work Health Care.* 2010; **49**(9): 814–831.

120. Willging CE, Salvador M, Kano M. Unequal treatment: mental health care for sexual and gender minority groups in a rural state. *Psychiatr Serv.* 2006; **57**(6): 867–870.

121. Love MM, Smith AE, Lyall SE, et al. Exploring the relationship between gay affirmative practice and empathy among mental health professionals. *J Multicultural Couns Develop.* 2015; **43**(2): 83–96.

122. American Medical Association. LGBTQ population care. 2019. www.ama-assn.org/delivering-care/creat ing-lgbtq-friendly-practice (accessed June 2020).

123. American Psychological Association. APA LGBT resources and publications. 2019. www.apa.org/pi/l gbt/resources (accessed June 2020).

124. American Psychological Association. Guidelines for psychological practice with transgender and gender nonconforming people. *Am Psychol.* 2015; **70**(9): 832–864.

125. National Association of Social Workers (NASW). Lesbian, gay, bisexual & transgender (LGBT). www .socialworkers.org/Practice/LGBT (accessed June 2020).

126. Craig SL, Alessi EJ, Fisher-Borne M, et al. *Guidelines for Affirmative Social Work Education: Enhancing the Climate for LGBQQ Students, Staff, and Faculty in Social Work Education.* Alexandria, VA: Council on Social Work Education; 2016.

127. Austin A, Craig SL, Alessi EJ, et al. *Guidelines for Transgender and Gender Nonconforming (TGNC) Affirmative Education: Enhancing the Climate for TGNC Students, Staff and Faculty in Social Work Education.* Alexandria, VA: Council on Social Work Education; 2016.

128. American Nurses Association Ethics Advisory Board. *Position statement: nursing advocacy for LGBTQ+ populations.* Silver Spring, MD: ANA; 2018.

129. Lim FA, Brown DV, Jones H. Lesbian, gay, bisexual, and transgender health: fundamentals for nursing education. *J Nurs Educ.* 2013; **52**(4): 198–203.

130. Alessi EJ. A framework for incorporating minority stress theory into treatment with sexual minority clients. *J Gay Lesbian Ment Health.* 2014; **18**(1): 47–66.

131. Craig SL, Austin A, Alessi E. Gay affirmative cognitive behavioral therapy for sexual minority youth: clinical adaptations and approaches. *Clin Soc Work J.* 2013; **41**(3): 258–266.

132. Crisp C, McCave EL. Gay affirmative practice: a model for social work practice with gay, lesbian, and bisexual youth. *Child Adolesc Soc Work J.* 2007; **24**(4): 403–421.

133. Pachankis JE. Uncovering clinical principles and techniques to address minority stress, mental health, and related health risks among gay and bisexual men. *Clin Psychol: Sci Pract.* 2014; **21**(4): 313–330.

134. Argüello, TM. HIV stress exchange: HIV trauma, intergenerational stress, and queer men. Presentation to the 13th International Conference on Interdisciplinary Social Studies; 2018. Granada, Spain.

135. Semp D. Questioning heteronormativity: using queer theory to inform research and practice within public mental health services. *Psychol Sex.* 2011; **2**(1): 69–86.

136. Russell ST, Pollitt AM, Li G, et al. Chosen name use is linked to reduced depressive symptoms, suicidal ideation, and suicidal behavior among transgender youth. *J Adolesc Health.* 2018; **63**(4): 503–505.

137. Centers for Disease Control and Prevention. HIV. www.cdc.gov/hiv/default.html (accessed June 2020).

138. Centers for Disease Control and Prevention. PrEP. www.cdc.gov/hiv/basics/prep.html (accessed June 2020).

139. Centers for Disease Control and Prevention. Daily pill can prevent HIV: reaching people who could benefit from PrEP. www.cdc.gov/vitalsigns/hivprep/ (accessed June 2020).

140. pleasePrEPme.org. Helping people access pre-exposure prophylaxis. www.pleaseprepme.org/pre pnavigatormanual (accessed June 2020).

141. Substance Abuse and Mental Health Services Administration. *SAMHSA's Concept of Trauma and Guidance for a Trauma-Informed Approach.* Rockville, MD: Substance Abuse and Mental Health Services Administration; 2014.

142. Helgeson VS, Reynolds KA, Tomich PL. A meta-analytic review of benefit finding and growth. *J Consult Clin Psychol.* 2006; **74**(5): 797–816.

143. World Professional Association for Transgender Health. Standards of care for the health of transsexual, transgender, and gender nonconforming people. https://wpath.org/publica tions/soc (accessed June 2020).

144. Lamble S. Queer necropolitics and the expanding carceral state: interrogating sexual investments in punishment. *Law Critique.* 2013; **24**: 229–253.

145. Klein E. Using social support for LGBTQ clients with mental illness to be out of the closet, in treatment, and in the community. *J Gay Lesbian Soc Serv.* 2017; **29**(3): 221–232.

Building a Therapeutic Relationship Between Probation Officers and Probationers with Serious Mental Illnesses

Matthew W. Epperson, Leon Sawh, and Sophia P. Sarantakos

Introduction

Addressing Mental Health in an Era of Smart Decarceration

For the first time in nearly four decades, the incarcerated population in the United States has begun to level off and decline, suggesting that mass incarceration has reached a tipping point.[1] Additionally, there is growing empirical evidence that incarceration does not meet its stated goals of increasing public safety and rehabilitating individuals; in most cases, incarceration does just the opposite.[2] Incarceration is also not applied evenly, as people of color and people with behavioral health disorders are grossly over-represented in jails and prisons.[3–5] In recent years, criminal justice systems across the country have begun to develop new decarceration policies and practices in attempts to reduce the overuse of incarceration.[6] However, decarceration efforts will be most successful if they intentionally target and reverse disparities, an approach termed "smart decarceration."[7]

This article presents a smart decarceration approach to addressing mental health disparities in the criminal justice system, with a particular focus on probation. First, we discuss the role of probation within the criminal justice system and the complex needs of probationers with serious mental illnesses (SMI). We then describe the multistage collaborative development of an intervention that focuses on building a therapeutic relationship between probation officers and probationers with SMI in order to better address their unique and complex needs. We present findings on intervention content as a result of a stakeholder-engaged process, as well as acceptability and feasibility findings through qualitative interviews and observations with probation officers and probationers with SMI.

Probation as a Key Site for Intervention

There are nearly seven million people under the control of the U.S. criminal justice system and more than half of these individuals are on probation, making probation the largest segment of the criminal justice system.[8] Probation entails a "community supervision" sentence, often in lieu of incarceration, with specific court-ordered conditions such as abstinence from substances, avoiding additional criminal activity, and engaging in rehabilitative supports. People on probation are at a critical juncture, either successfully completing the terms of probation and exiting the criminal justice system or violating the terms of their supervision and falling deeper into the system via incarceration.

For decades, a persistent over-representation of people with mental illnesses has been documented in the criminal justice system.[4,5] As a result, probation departments across the United States supervise approximately half a million probationers with SMI, which includes schizophrenia spectrum, bipolar spectrum, and major depressive disorders.[9] As highlighted in the Sequential Intercept Model,[10] a framework that details opportunities for intervening with justice-involved persons with SMI, service provision is needed across continuous points of contact in the criminal justice system. Key tasks of those who work throughout the system include identifying justice-involved persons with SMI and providing them with linkages to mental health treatment, counseling, and psychiatric care, as well as other needed wraparound services such as family, housing, and employment supports. Despite probation being an optimal site for intervention, there is limited research that has fully developed the capacity of probation to meet the multifaceted legal and treatment needs of justice-involved persons with SMI.[11,12]

Addressing the complex needs of persons with SMI presents unique challenges to probation departments. When persons with SMI are sentenced to probation, the symptoms of their disorders often hinder the individual's ability to successfully comply with the terms of their probation, further exacerbating the difficulties associated with successful community tenure.[13] Compared with those without mental illnesses, probationers with SMI have a greater likelihood of violating their probation and are at higher risk of reincarceration.[14] Probationers with SMI are also more likely to have a co-occurring substance use disorder than those without SMI,[15] resulting in a greater need for integrated treatment services for both types of disorders.[16] Meeting the treatment needs of probationers with SMI while simultaneously assessing and intervening on criminogenic risk factors have become tandem goals for probation departments.[17,18]

Due to the influx of individuals with SMI in probation departments, specialized mental health probation caseloads have grown considerably over the last 25 years. Consisting of probation officers who have been trained in supervising probationers with SMI, specialized mental health probation is one of the most prevalent criminal justice/mental health collaborative models, next to mental health courts, and has been designed to more effectively meet the needs of probationers with SMI. In specialized mental health probation units, probation officers are tasked with serving dual law enforcement and case management types of functions. For example, specialized probation officers receive mental health training, work to establish relationships with local mental health treatment and wraparound service providers, and utilize problem-solving approaches (e.g. case management, counseling techniques) to better link probationers with SMI to needed services.[18]

Research on the positive effects of specialized probation on reducing criminal justice involvement for probationers with SMI has grown in recent years. In a longitudinal study designed to test whether use of specialized mental health caseloads resulted in better public safety outcomes than standard probation programming, those probationers assigned to specialized probation were less likely to be rearrested for any crime than probationers in the standard group, with this effect lasting for up to five years after program enrollment.[19] Another study found a greater decrease in jail days for people on specialized probation compared with probationers with SMI on standard probation, although there was also an increase in probation violations.[20] In

a study comparing specialized and standard probation approaches, specialized mental health probation officers were able to establish higher quality relationships with probationers, participate more directly in probationer treatment, utilize positive compliance strategies, and report fewer violations than the standard probation group.[21] Most recently, Skeem et al. found that use of specialized mental health caseloads was more cost-effective than standard probation in supervising probationers with SMI due to savings associated with reduced recidivism and behavioral health care costs.[22]

Importance of the Therapeutic Relationship

A positive working relationship between professional and client is a key ingredient in effective delivery of human services.[23] This working relationship is achieved through a shared understanding of goals, clear assignment of therapeutic tasks, and development of a bond between worker and client.[24] Studies across a range of therapeutic services have identified essential therapist characteristics that positively influence the working relationship, including attributes such as warmth, empathy, and trustworthiness and techniques such as exploration, reflection, and conveying support.[25] Thus, the therapeutic relationship (also referred to as working relationship or working alliance) is a strong predictor of clinical outcomes, particularly for people with mental health and substance use disorders.[26]

Growing evidence demonstrates that the importance of building a therapeutic relationship is also critical within criminal justice settings such as probation, and this is particularly true of programs that work with clients with SMI.[27] Studies examining the effectiveness of specialized programming for justice-involved persons with SMI consistently agree that sole reliance on surveillance and punishment is ineffective at improving mental health and preventing further criminal justice involvement.[28] Working with probationers with SMI complicates the work of the probation officer to include roles such as advocate, helper, and confidant, and conflict between these support-oriented and law enforcement roles can hamper the effective work of probation officers.[29,30] In order to successfully navigate these roles, officers must build a positive therapeutic relationship with their clients in order to address sensitive issues such as mental health symptoms and specific treatment needs.[31,32]

Although limited in scope, several empirical studies have shown that a positive probation officer/client therapeutic relationship is related to several desired outcomes, including reduced substance use,[33] response to treatment for spousal abuse,[34] and reduced criminal recidivism, including lessened time spent in jail.[35–37] Although most research on the therapeutic relationship in community supervision settings has been conducted with the general probation and/or parole population, some work has explored this relationship specifically among justice-involved persons with SMI, identifying key characteristics of a positive therapeutic relationship such as caring, fairness, trust, and support.[23,28,29] Moreover, successful engagement of justice-involved persons with SMI is related to an increased sense of procedural justice (or fairness) and lower perceptions of coercion, both of which are indicators of higher participation in mental health treatment and criminal justice programming.[40,41]

In a study conducted by members of the study team,[43] qualitative interviews with 21 probation officers were conducted to better understand how officers in a specialized mental health probation unit, mental health court, and standard probation program utilize different supervision approaches and balance the perceived dual roles of law enforcement and rehabilitation when working with SMI probationers. As part of the same study, researchers analyzed data from a sample of 98 probationers with SMI who completed the Dual-Role Relationship Inventory – Revised (DRI-R),[35] as well as qualitative interviews in which probationers discussed their experiences with probation officers while on specialized and standard probation. The DRI-R was developed to assess the quality of relationships between justice-involved individuals and the professionals who supervise them, and the developers state that the instrument is best validated for probation and parole settings.[35] After controlling for significant covariates, probationers in mental health court rated the quality of their relationships with their probation officers higher than probationers in specialized mental health probation or standard probation groups.[23] However, officers who were assigned to supervise mental health caseloads were perceived by the probationers under their supervision as more caring, trustworthy, supportive, and less authoritarian than those probationers assigned to standard probation. The authors conclude that being treated with genuine care, fairness, and support is therapeutic and can be transformative for probationers with SMI. The challenge, however, is the operationalization of these ideas into regular day-to-day practices within probation programs.[23] Some existing probation officer training programs address core correctional practices including limited content on relationship quality, but these approaches have not been adapted for probationers with SMI.[44,45]

Although these studies demonstrate that the quality of the relationship between officer and client is a critical ingredient in achieving better mental health and criminal justice outcomes, no evidence-based interventions have been developed to target this relationship among probationers with SMI. The purpose of this study was to engage in a collaborative process to develop a probation officer-led intervention that aims to enhance the therapeutic relationship between officers and probationers with SMI. We discuss a systematic process of engagement with a range of stakeholders to identify core intervention components, and assess their acceptability and feasibility in a real-world probation setting. Within this approach, the building of a therapeutic relationship is conceptualized as a foundational element on which additional intervention components can be delivered to facilitate service engagement and reduce criminal justice involvement for people with SMI on probation.

Methods

BIPSE Intervention Development Process

This section focuses on the iterative process undertaken by our team to develop and refine an intervention, named *Brief Intervention to Promote Service Engagement (BIPSE)*, designed specifically to assist probation officers who work with people on probation with SMI. We took a "design for implementation" approach to the development of this intervention, in which we sought to engage key stakeholders in an iterative planning process, in order to accelerate the intervention's implementation in a real-world probation setting.[46] The process began by convening collaborative stakeholder meetings with staff from the proposed implementation site – a specialized mental health probation unit within a large Midwestern U.S. adult probation department. Stakeholder meetings were comprised of probation officers and unit supervisors, community-based mental health treatment providers, individuals with SMI who were previously on probation, and representatives from local and regional advocacy groups. Three stakeholder meetings were held over the course of six months, with an average of 15 stakeholders attending each meeting. Each stakeholder meeting focused on generating priority areas for intervention through a process of facilitated discussion, consensus-building, and articulation of follow-up action steps. Between stakeholder meetings, members of the research team conducted literature and intervention reviews to identify content and approaches that aligned with topics prioritized by the stakeholder group. We also held additional consultation meetings with probation staff and supervisors in order to gain a better sense of the unit's practices and procedures.

The stakeholder meetings helped to elicit probation officer priorities, tasks, and roles, and also elucidated personal and treatment needs of persons with SMI on probation. Several consistent themes emerged from these meetings, most of which focused on enhancing the probation process to help probationers with SMI connect to needed services in order to achieve greater stability and avoid unnecessary punishment. These conversations often came back to the central issue of the relational dynamics between probation officer and client, and the foundational importance of clients being able to trust and engage with their probation officer in order to discuss issues of mental health, substance use, relationships, and other personal needs. This theme resonated with earlier research our team had done with probationers with SMI, who emphasized the interconnection of trust, support, and caring as powerful components of a relationship with their probation officer that facilitated motivation and engagement in services.[23] Furthermore, stakeholder meetings addressed logistical issues such as existing training and stated needs of officers, examination of current probation protocols and required paperwork, and officer acceptability of intervention concepts.[47]

Next, members of the research team observed 15 scheduled sessions with mental health unit probation officers and their clients with SMI in order to better understand the context and environment in which probation supervision meetings take place. Observations of probation officer/client interactions yielded important information, which further assisted the research team in identifying components to incorporate into the BIPSE intervention. Many scheduled sessions were not completed because of client no-shows, and completed sessions were often quite brief, with few concrete activities to structure the sessions beyond monitoring compliance of court-ordered probation conditions. Individual officers did exhibit behaviors to facilitate connection with their clients, but these strategies seemed to be limited to personal style and conversational approaches, and they were not embedded in routine probation processes. Following this first round of observations, the research team reviewed the existing research literature to identify interventions and approaches being used with the probation population. Interventions from other disciplines were also reviewed (e.g. medicine, social work) to see whether it might be possible to adapt them for use within the mental health probation setting.

Collectively, the stakeholder meetings, our observations of probation officer/client interactions, and our review of the existing intervention literature led to the articulation of three key intervention components that were critical to the probation process for people with SMI: (1) engagement; (2) shared decision-making; and (3) strategic case management. The first two components, engagement and shared decision-making, were conceptualized as foundational components to establish a strong therapeutic relationship on which strategic case management approaches could be built (in this article, we will focus on these two relational components). Within these components, the research team developed and/or modified a variety of tools and activities that could be used by probation officers to develop and strengthen the therapeutic relationship (Figure 35.1).

Assessing BIPSE Components

To vet the acceptability and feasibility of the BIPSE intervention materials, we conducted a three-stage process within the specialized mental health probation unit. First, we facilitated a two-hour workshop in which we presented the materials to three probation officers who were randomly selected from the available mental health unit team. These probation officers were given a BIPSE intervention binder containing an overview of the intervention and draft activities/tools for use with their clients. Some examples of activities include a cost/benefit worksheet, goal-setting exercises, introduction to use of the teach-back method, and development of an overview of probation roles and expectations. During the workshop, we facilitated

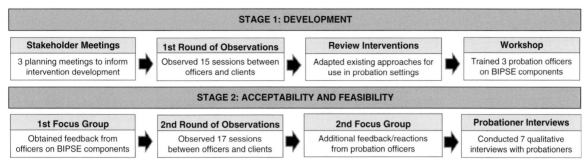

Figure 35.1 Brief Intervention to Promote Service Engagement: development process.

role play scenarios in which officers practiced various activities.

Following this workshop, we held two focus groups with these three officers – one immediately following the workshop and the other approximately three months later. In the interim, officers were asked to try out some or all of the activities with their clients as they seemed relevant and applicable. Second, during that same three-month period, we observed 17 sessions between these three probation officers and their clients to assess whether and how any of the activities in the workshop were being used. Third, we conducted seven interviews with probationers assigned to these three probation officers to better understand how officers interact with their clients and assist them in adhering to the terms of their probation, getting linked to treatment and other needed wraparound supports, achieve their goals, and the extent to which the components of engagement and shared decision-making facilitated these processes.

Focus groups and individual probationer interviews were audio recorded and transcribed verbatim. For observations of sessions between probation officers and clients, field notes were written at the conclusion of each meeting. The focus group and interview transcripts and observation notes were analyzed for thematic content related to the development of a therapeutic relationship within the context of a specialized mental health probation unit.

Results

The iterative and stakeholder-engaged BIPSE development process led to the articulation of two key intervention components that target the development of a therapeutic relationship between probation officer and client: (1) engagement and (2) shared

decision-making. Within the BIPSE intervention, these two components are viewed as a necessary foundation on which strategic case management services can be delivered to address mental health needs, criminal risks, and attending to the multiple support and compliance-monitoring functions that are required when supervising probationers with SMI. In this section, we describe the two relational BIPSE components of engagement and shared decision-making, as well as findings from focus groups, observations and interviews on the feasibility and acceptability of activities and processes related to each component. We also present findings on the re-examination of probation officer roles in the context of building a therapeutic relationship with clients.

BIPSE Component: Engagement

Engagement as a Core Relational Practice

Probation settings are characterized by an overarching climate of power differentials and compliance-monitoring in which the enforcing of probationers' adherence to court conditions typically relies on punitive sanctions and, in cases of repeated noncompliance, unsuccessful termination from probation and incarceration.[48] Successful engagement of probationers with SMI is the first and core focus area of BIPSE, serving as a foundation for other intervention components. Through our previous review of relevant literatures and interventions, we have identified several promising characteristics that informed engagement-focused intervention activities. First, intentional engagement should begin with the probation officers' very first encounter with a probationer, and the first several months of probation supervision are a key period for continued engagement activities. Initial engagement activities we included in BIPSE involve an initial phone check-in prior to the first probation meeting,[49] discussion of probationer life goals and incorporation of some of these goals into the probation relationship and treatment planning,[50] and use of key motivational interviewing techniques such as affirmation and reflective listening.[51]

Opportunities for Engagement

In our workshop of BIPSE components with probation officers, we defined engagement as, "Effort made by the officer to connect with and develop a relationship with a client in such a way that encourages and maintains the client's active interest and participation in completing probation successfully." Elements of engagement that were discussed as being most salient were building rapport, demonstrating respect, seeking feedback, focusing on immediate concerns, and clarifying the process of probation. Probation officers noted that effective engagement was a critical component of their work in supervising probationers with SMI. As one officer stated: "It's important that they are not only engaged in what is asked of them on probation but engaged in their treatment, because it's a very collaborative effort between the treatment providers and us to get them through probation successfully." Several probationers also reflected in their interviews that attempts by their probation officer to engage and connect with them were appreciated and effective, as illustrated by this quote from a probationer who had previously been on probation in another unit: "It's completely different. It's like coming here, I'm not afraid. I'm not fearful, like, oh am I going to be in trouble if I go there and see them? I'm kind of like, excited to come here, it's like a little therapy session."

One element of engagement that was deemed highly acceptable by officers and probationers was the task of clarifying the process and expectations of probation. Probationers expressed that they were not always aware of all the terms and requirements of specialized mental health probation and thought that it would be helpful to have more communication around these requirements and how probation officers could support them. Officers also acknowledged that existing intake materials were somewhat confusing for their clients with SMI, and that providing clear and understandable expectations could be a key task in early probation engagement. In response to the presentation of the teach-back method, an approach commonly used in healthcare settings to ensure that information was communicated effectively,[52] one

probation officer noted how this approach could facilitate engagement and relationship-building: "I also see the usefulness of the teach-back method. Especially how on the back end, you can do like a review with the client, make sure that they understand what's expected of them. I think that it promotes their engagement in probation as well as in whatever task is being set before them. I think it promotes the relationship between the client and the officer as well."

BIPSE Component: Shared Decision-Making

Shared decision-making is well established as a critical element for persons with SMI to actively and meaningfully participate in their treatment to achieve better outcomes.[53–55] For many probationers with SMI, probation serves as the gateway for linkage to needed mental health treatment and other wraparound supports. Thus, it is critical for probationers with SMI to share decision-making opportunities with their probation officer in the context of their probation supervision. However, power differentials present barriers to probationers having a more active role in their treatment, and officers are frequently unable to scale back their own power to facilitate greater involvement by probationers.[43] A core focus area of BIPSE involves helping officers to identify and utilize opportunities for probationers with SMI to make collaborative decisions regarding their treatment plans.

Facilitating Shared Decision-Making

In the BIPSE workshop, we stressed that it is important for probation officers to clearly explain the dynamics of probation, the various roles and functions officers must take on, and the responsibilities and expectations of probationers. Establishing open communication between officer and client is critical to creating an environment in which probationers with SMI feel empowered to express their preferences. Therefore, probation officers must be trained to identify key opportunities where probationers can be invited to discuss options and weigh-in on decisions.[56] BIPSE incorporates several structured activities for probation officers through which they can facilitate shared decision-making with their SMI clients about issues such as treatment referrals, timing and location of probation appointments, articulation of goals and objectives, and building of problem-solving skills. During initial BIPSE development, we incorporated elements of shared decision-making to facilitate greater participation by

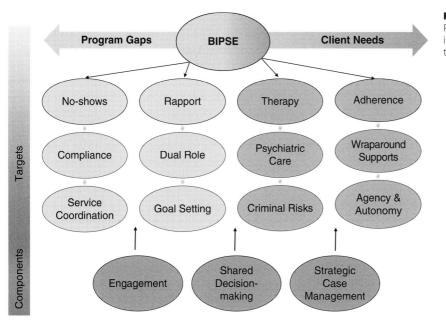

Figure 35.2 Brief Intervention to Promote Service Engagement: intervention components and targets.

probationers in probation activities, increased choice-making, reduced perceived coercion, and increased perceptions of procedural justice, as each of these mechanisms has been shown to be related to greater service engagement (Figure 35.2).[41,53,57]

Probation officers and probationers alike endorsed the acceptability of the BIPSE intervention component of shared decision-making. As one officer stated regarding their work with probationers with SMI, "If they are having input on the decision of maybe where to do treatment or what type of treatment program they want to enter, they are more likely to engage in and complete it successfully. It kind of helps them come to a more prosocial way of thinking through working with them and making better decisions." Beyond treatment-focused decisions, the goal-setting BIPSE component, in which probation and nonprobation-related goals are elicited from the client, generated an opportunity for probation officers to learn about their client's goals and priorities and how to form a shared approach to achieving them. Reflecting on this as a positive experience with their probation officer, one probationer stated, "Yeah, they try to help you figure out what your goals are … she [officer] pretty much wants to know my goals."

During our observations of officer and probationer meetings, one officer elected to utilize the BIPSE cost/benefit worksheet to discuss an issue of probationer noncompliance. In response to a probationer testing positive for drug use, the probation officer employed the worksheet to elicit from the probationer their perceptions of the negative and positive aspects of using drugs. Through the completion of the worksheet, the probationer revealed that using drugs helped them to escape feelings of loneliness, as they have a deep desire to be in an intimate relationship. Learning this new information, the probation officer was able to validate the probationer's feelings and acknowledge their personal goal. As opposed to using a punitive-based approach, the officer's use of the cost/benefit worksheet facilitated a collaborative discussion on how to avoid future drug use in which the probationer was an active participant. The officer later reflected on this interaction and how it helped navigate role conflict, stating, "That could have been a challenging confrontation, but instead I felt like we were working on the problem together."

Re-examining Probation Officer Roles

During the focus group immediately following the BIPSE workshop, probation officers expressed that they would be willing to try using some of the tools we provided in their day-to-day practice. However, officers pointed out that they already informally used aspects of several of these relational strategies. Officers also liked the way in which certain tools were designed and could envision using them with their clients as these tools provided a way for them to incorporate input from their clients into the session. Officers acknowledged that they often struggled with connecting with their clients, stating that many clients were unable or unwilling to open up to them. What became clear through our observations of probation meetings was that officers may occasionally employ relational strategies with their clients, but these attempts were somewhat haphazard and not connected to clear relational targets or probation processes. Additionally, officers may find it difficult to develop a therapeutic relationship in the midst of navigating tasks such as supervision, monitoring, and providing services and supports. Through our workshopping of intervention activities and providing feedback after observations, officers began to appreciate the importance of more intentionally incorporating relationship-building strategies into their regular practice, and utilizing BIPSE activities to structure and track their efforts. In this way, officers expressed a desire to build a more formalized skill set on therapeutic relationship-building with their clients.

Many of the feasibility concerns expressed by officers demonstrated limited attention to the multiple roles that probation officers embody. Although discussed in previous research as dual roles of care and control,[35] most of the structured processes and procedures that probation officers are expected to employ support the law enforcement or surveillance role. For example, we suggested that probation officers attempt to contact their new clients by phone prior to their first intake session. Although officers agreed that this could be an effective early engagement strategy, they also noted that intakes are often scheduled at the last minute, and calling ahead of time would likely be infeasible. Additionally, officers noted that a cost-benefit component was included in their existing risk assessment case planning paperwork. However, officers' use of this cost-benefit activity seemed to be more focused on criminogenic risk reduction, and not on cultivation of a therapeutic alliance. Our observations of probation sessions confirmed that most of the officers' activities were driven by required paperwork and case supervision tasks, and the bulk of these tasks were not directly related to therapeutic relationship-building.

Discussion

Probation officers that work with clients with SMI essentially occupy two complex and sometimes conflicting roles: a law enforcement role as an officer of the court, and a supportive role to identify treatment needs and coordinate care. This article details a process of intervention development to help officers develop a therapeutic relationship with probationers with SMI while fulfilling these two roles. Through a multistaged "design for implementation" approach, relational elements were identified as core components of effective intervention for probationers with SMI. Focusing on the therapeutic relationship between probation officer and client is supported by research that demonstrates that, particularly for probationers with SMI, the quality of the relationship is predictive of increased treatment engagement and reduced recidivism.[21,22] Despite this evidence, no interventions currently exist that focus on the enhancement of the therapeutic relationship between probationers with SMI and their officers. As part of an overall intervention approach, key BIPSE relational components of engagement and shared decision-making are conceptualized as building the foundation of a therapeutic relationship, on which other intervention components can be built to facilitate use of mental health services and reduce criminogenic risk.

The process of the BIPSE intervention development yielded many important findings that can inform enhancement of the therapeutic relationship between probation officers and probationers with SMI. As emphasized in stakeholder meetings and in interviews with probationers, power imbalances between officer and client are a clear barrier to the development of rapport and the establishment of a collaborative working alliance. Additionally, lack of clear communication around individual and shared roles and responsibilities can result in probationers with SMI disengaging from meaningful involvement in probation supervision and related services in the community. The BIPSE component of engagement helps to overcome these barriers by establishing early and supportive methods of communication and relationship-building that demonstrate supportive officer roles and respond to immediate concerns of the probationer. By incorporating targeted elements of active listening and respect, officers can counteract perceptions of being overly punitive and harsh, replacing them with approaches that represent fairness and caring. In this way, BIPSE could serve to help officers navigate the multiple roles and identities that they must take on when supervising clients with SMI.

Shared decision-making as a core BIPSE element demonstrates promise in creating a working alliance between probationer and officer in which collaboration toward agreed-upon goals can emerge. Identifying opportunities for shared decision-making requires officers to re-examine their roles and the limitations of their own power within the therapeutic relationship. Through our workshopping of BIPSE components and focus groups with probation officers, we were able to collaboratively identify initial opportunities for a shared process between officer and client. One such example is in cases of noncompliance, wherein officers can explore the underlying issues that their clients are experiencing, and jointly develop a response that is both meaningful and supportive. This process does not require officers to cede their power, but rather to reframe the demonstration of power in order to form mutual agreement on goals and tasks with clients.

The activities related to BIPSE components of engagement and shared decision-making were viewed favorably by both probation officers and clients. However, officers suggested that they were already engaging in therapeutic relationship-building by demonstrating empathy and respect to their clients. Although a personal disposition of respect and empathy is certainly conducive to better relationship quality, we found that officers tended to rely upon common probation structures and routine practices, often to the detriment of enhancing their relationships with clients. By focusing on key relational targets and concrete associated activities, BIPSE attempts to structure and enhance relationship-building approaches by probation officers that had previously been haphazard or unplanned.

The importance of active involvement from a range of stakeholders in the BIPSE "design for implementation" development process cannot be overstated. Through our collaboration with probation officers, current and former probationers with SMI, community treatment providers, and advocates, we were able to develop a shared understanding of the challenges of providing effective probation supervision to clients with SMI. Providing opportunities for probation officers to practice BIPSE activities, and eliciting feedback from probationers resulted in meaningful input on the intervention. As a result, the BIPSE components that have been developed serve to expand the scope and role of probation officers while also acknowledging the real-world constraints of supervising large caseloads with limited resources.

Our findings related to BIPSE development and refinement support the promise of additional research on the intervention. Existing activities related to engagement and shared decision-making should be further refined and tailored to fit within common probation practices, and approaches must be identified to efficiently document the delivery of intervention activities and connect them to probation officer expectations and procedures. These processes will lead to the development of a BIPSE treatment manual, which will include a more full development of the strategic case management component. Ultimately, BIPSE will be pilot tested to assess preliminary effects on hypothesized intervention targets of the therapeutic relationship, client motivation, participation in services, and perceived coercion and procedural justice. These targets will then be assessed against short-term outcomes of probation attendance, adherence, and completion, as well as longer-term outcomes of sustained mental health service engagement, mental health stability, and reduced recidivism.

Conclusion

The therapeutic relationship between probation officer and client is a critical component to programmatic success for people with SMI on probation. This study demonstrates that meaningful criminal justice-based interventions to enhance the therapeutic relationship can be built in ways that are both acceptable to officers and probationers, and feasible to implement in specialized probation practices. If interventions such as BIPSE prove to be effective, additional evidence-based interventions can be built upon this foundation of the therapeutic relationship to achieve positive mental health and criminal justice outcomes for probationers with SMI.

Acknowledgments

We would like to acknowledge the members of our stakeholder panel, people currently and formerly on probation, and probation officers for their collaborative work on this project. Additionally, we acknowledge research assistants Jesse Self, Emily Claypool, and Kathryn Frances who assisted with stakeholder meetings, focus groups, and interviews.

Funding

This work was supported by the National Institute of Mental Health (grant #K01MH103446).

Disclosure

Matthew W. Epperson, Leon Sawh, and Sophia P. Sarantakos do not have any disclosures.

References

1. Epperson MW, Pettus-Davis C. *Smart Decarceration: Achieving Criminal Justice Transformation in the 21st Century.* New York, NY: Oxford University Press; 2017.

2. Travis J, Western B, Redburn S. *The Growth of Incarceration in the United States: Exploring Causes and Consequences.* Washington, DC: National Academies Press; 2014.

3. Mauer M. Addressing racial disparities in incarceration. *Prison J.* 2011; **91**(3): 87S-101S.

4. Steadman H, Osher F, Robbins P, Case B, Samuels S. Prevalence of serious mental illness among jail inmates. *Psychiatr Serv.* 2009; **60** (6): 761–765.

5. Fazel S, Danesh J. Serious mental disorder in 23,000 prisoners: a systematic review of 62 surveys. *Lancet.* 2002; **359**: 545–550.

6. Doob AN, Webster CM. Creating the will to change: the challenges of decarceration in the United States. *Criminol Pub Policy.* 2014; **13**:(4).

7. Epperson M, Pettus-Davis C. Smart decarceration: guiding concepts for an era of criminal justice transformation. In: Epperson M, Pettus- Davis C, eds. *Smart Decarceration: Achieving Criminal Justice Transformation in the 21st Century.* New York, NY: Oxford University Press; 2017.

8. Kaeble D, Glaze LE, Tsoutis A, Minton TD. Correctional Populations in the United States, 2014. Bureau of Justice Statistics; 2015. www.bjs.gov/index .cfm?ty=pbdetail&iid=5519 (accessed June 2020).

9. Skeem J, Emke-Francis P, Eno Louden J. Probation, mental health, and mandated treatment: a national survey. *Crim Justice Behav.* 2006; **33**(2): 158–184.

10. Munetz MR, Griffin PA. Use of the sequential intercept model as an approach to decriminalization of people with serious mental illness. *Psychiatr Serv.* 2006; **57**: 544–549.

11. Epperson M, Wolff N, Morgan R, et al. Envisioning the next generation of behavioral health and criminal justice interventions. *Int J Law Psychiatry.* 2014; **37** (5): 427–438.

12. Wolff N, Frueh B, Huening J, et al. Practice informs the next generation of behavioral health and criminal justice interventions. *Int J Law Psychiatry.* 2013; **36**: 1–10.

13. Council of State Governments. Criminal Justice/ Mental Health Consensus Project Report. 2002. www .ncjrs.gov/pdffiles1/nij/grants/197103.pdf (accessed June 2020).

14. Louden JE, Skeem JL, Camp J, Christensen E. Supervising probationers with mental disorder: how do agencies respond to violations? *Crim Justice Behav.* 2008; **35**(7): 832.

15. Lurigio A, Cho Y, Swartz J, et al. Standardized assessment of substance-related, other psychiatric, and comorbid disorders among probationers. *Int J Offender Ther Comp Criminol.* 2003; **47**(6): 630.

16. Solomon P, Draine J, Marcus SC. Predicting incarceration of clients of a psychiatric probation and parole service. *Psychiatr Serv.* 2002; **53**(1): 50.

17. Morgan RD, Flora DB, Droner DG, et al. Treating offenders with mental illness: a research synthesis. *Law Hum Behav.* 2011; **36**(1): 37.

18. Babchuk LC, Lurigio AJ, Canada KE, Epperson MW. Responding to probationers with mental illnesses. *Feder Prob.* 2012; **76**(2): 41–48.

19. Skeem J, Manchak S, Montoya L. Comparing public safety outcomes for traditional probation vs specialty mental health probation. *JAMA Psychiatry.* 2017; **74** (9): 942–948.

20. Wolff N, Epperson M, Shi J, et al. Mental health specialized probation caseloads: are they effective? *Int J Law Psychiatry.* 2014; **37**: 464–472.

21. Manchak S, Skeem J, Kennealy P, Louden J. High-fidelity specialty mental health probation improves officer practices, treatment access, and rule compliance. *Law Hum Behav.* 2014; **38**(5): 450–461.

22. Skeem J, Montoya L, Manchak S. Comparing costs of traditional and specialty probation for people with serious mental illness. *Psychiatr Serv.* 2018; **69**(8): 896–902.

23. Epperson M, Thompson J, Lurigio A, Kim S. Unpacking the relationship between probationers with serious mental illnesses and probation staff. *J Offender Rehabil.* 2017; **56**(3): 188–216.

24. Bordin E. The generalizability of the psychoanalytic concept of the working alliance. *Psychother Theory Res Pract.* 1979; **16**(3): 252.

25. Ackerman S, Hilsenroth M. A review of therapist characteristics and techniques positively impacting the therapeutic alliance. *Clin Psychol Rev.* 2003; **23**(1): 1–33.

26. Martin DJ, Garske JP, Davis MK. Relation of the therapeutic alliance with outcome and other variables: a meta-analytic review. *J Consult Clin Psychol.* 2000; **68**(3): 438.

27. Canada K, Epperson M. The client-caseworker relationship and its association with outcomes among

mental health court participants. *Community Ment Health J*. 2014; **50**: 968–973.

28. Lamberti J. Preventing criminal recidivism through mental health and criminal justice collaboration. *Psychiatr Serv*. 2016; **67**(11): 1206–1212.

29. Clear TR, Latessa EJ. Probation officers' roles in intensive supervision: surveillance versus treatment. *Justice Q*. 1993; **10**(3): 441–462.

30. West AD, Seiter RP. Social worker or cop?: measuring the supervision styles of probation & parole officers in Kentucky and Missouri. *J Crime Justice*. 2004; **27**(2): 27–57.

31. Seiter RP, West AD. Supervision styles in probation and parole: an analysis of activities. *J Offend Rehabil*. 2003; **38**(2): 57–75.

32. Skeem J, Eno Louden J. Toward evidence-based practice for probationers and parolees mandated to mental health treatment. *Psychiatr Serv*. 2006; **57**(3): 333.

33. Blasko BL, Friedmann PD, Rhodes AG, Taxman FS. The parolee-parole officer relationship as a mediator of criminal justice outcomes. *Crim Justice Behav*. 2015; **42**: 722–740.

34. Brown P, O'leary K. Therapeutic alliance: predicting continuance and success in group treatment for spouse abuse. *J Consult Clin Psychol*. 2000; **68**(2): 340.

35. Skeem J, Eno Louden J, Polaschek D, Camp J. Assessing relationship quality in mandated community treatment: blending care with control. *Psychol Assess*. 2007; **19**(4): 397–410.

36. Taft C, Murphy C, King D, Musser P, DeDeyn J. Process and treatment adherence factors in group cognitive-behavioral therapy for partner violent men. *J Consult Clin Psychol*. 2003; **71**(4): 812.

37. Walters G. Working alliance between substance abusing offenders and their parole officers and counselors: its impact on outcome and role as a mediator. *J Crime Justice*. 2016; **39**(3): 421–437.

38. Latessa E, Lemke R, Makarios M, Smith P. The creation and validation of the Ohio Risk Assessment System (ORAS). *Feder Probat*. 2010; **74**: 16.

39. Kennealy P, Skeem J, Manchak S, Eno Louden J. Firm, fair, and caring officer-offender relationships protect against supervision failure. *Law Hum Behav*. 2012; **36**(6): 496–505.

40. Canada K, Watson A. "Cause everybody likes to be treated good": perceptions of procedural justice among mental health court participants. *Am Behav Sci*. 2013; **57**(2): 209–230.

41. Watson A, Angell B. Applying procedural justice theory to law enforcement's response to persons with mental illness. *Psychiatr Serv*. 2007; **58**(6): 787–793.

42. Blasko B, Taxman F. Are supervision practices procedurally fair?: development and predictive utility of a procedural justice measure for use in community corrections settings. *Crim Justice Behav*. 2018; **45**(3): 402–420.

43. Epperson M, Canada K, Thompson J, Lurigio A. Walking the line: specialized and standard probation officer perspectives on supervising probationers with serious mental illnesses. *Int J Law Psychiatry*. 2014; **37**: 473–483.

44. Robinson C, Lowenkamp C, Holsinger A, et al. A random study of Staff Training Aimed at Reducing Re-arrest (STARR): using core correctional practices in probation interactions. *J Crime Justice*. 2012; **35**(2): 167–188.

45. Smith P, Schweitzer M, Labrecque R, Latessa E. Improving probation officers' supervision skills: an evaluation of the EPICS model. *J Crime Justice*. 2012; **35**(2): 189–199.

46. Epperson M, Sawh L. Developing an intervention for probationers with SMI: a "design for implementation" approach. 24th Mental Health Services Research Conference; 2018., National Institute of Mental Health, Bethesda, MD.

47. Epperson M, Sawh L. Implementation-focused development of an intervention targeting probationers with serious mental illnesses. 11th Annual Conference on the Science of Dissemination and Implementation in Health; 2018. Washington, DC.

48. Epperson M, Sarantakos S, Thompson J, Self J. Tactical compliance versus self-transformation: adaptive responses of probationers with serious mental illnesses [under review].

49. McKay M, Hibbert R, Hoagwood K, et al. Integrating evidence-based engagement interventions into "real world" child mental health settings. *Brief Treat Crisis Interven*. 2004; **4**(2): 177.

50. Ward T, Brown M. The good lives model and conceptual issues in offender rehabilitation. *Psychol Crime Law*. 2004; **10**(3): 243–257.

51. Walters S, Clark M, Gingerich R, Meltzer M. *Motivating offenders to change: a guide for Probation and Parole*. Washington, DC: US Department of Justice, National Institute of Corrections; 2007.

52. Dinh TTH, Bonner A, Clark R, Ramsbotham J, Hines S. The effectiveness of the teach-back method on adherence and self-management in health education for people with chronic disease: a systematic review. *JBI Datab Syst Rev Implement Rep*. 2016; **14**(1): 210–247.

53. Joosten E, DeFuentes-Merillas L, De Weert G, et al. Systematic review of the effects of shared decision-making on patient satisfaction, treatment

adherence and health status. *Psychother Psychosom.* 2008; **77**(4): 219–226.

54. Deegan P, Drake R. Shared decision making and medication management in the recovery process. *Psychiatr Serv.* 2006; **57**(11): 1636–1639.

55. Adams J, Drake R, Wolford G. Shared decision-making preferences of people with severe mental illness. *Psychiatr Serv.* 2007; **58**(9): 1219–1221.

56. Elwyn G, Frosch D, Thomson R, et al. Shared decision making: a model for clinical practice. *J Gen Intern Med.* 2012; **27**(10): 1361–1367.

57. Munetz MR, Ritter C, Teller JL, Bonfine N. Mental health court and assisted outpatient treatment: perceived coercion, procedural justice, and program impact. *Psychiatric Serv.* 2014; **65**(3): 352–358.

Length of Stay for Inpatient Incompetent to Stand Trial (IST) Patients: Importance of Clinical and Demographic Variables

Charles Broderick, Allen Azizian, and Katherine Warburton

Introduction

State psychiatric hospitals face increasing referrals for the evaluation and restoration of individuals whose mental health symptoms render them incompetent to stand trial (IST).[1] As referrals can overwhelm capacity for admission, state hospitals at times are unable to admit IST patients in a timely fashion. The resulting use of "waitlists" has the undesirable consequence of forcing symptomatic individuals to endure long waits (while jailed) for admission to a psychiatric hospital. These long wait times have been determined to be unconstitutional, resulting in litigation against the responsible state mental health authorities.[2] Unfortunately, available options to expedite hospital admission of these IST patients can have significant clinical and economic consequences. Simply admitting patients without sufficient treatment resources risks overcrowding, while building increased hospital capacity is time-consuming, costly, and contrary to the drive for community treatment for mental illness.

Another solution is to examine patient factors leading to a longer length of stay, with the goal to increase treatment efficiency. This in turn would reduce length of stay and increase overall availability of state hospital beds without the need to build additional capacity. Our study examined patient variables impacting length of stay, with the goals of identifying factors related to patient length of stay as well as identifying targets of treatment that could result in more efficient treatment delivery for IST patients.

The topic of competency restoration has a large literature base, but few studies have directly focused on the specific topic of hospital length of stay for IST patients. Previous research into the topic of pre-trial competency has generally studied three broad areas: (i) factors regarding which arrestees are found incompetent,[3] (ii) factors to identify who can and cannot be restored to competency,[4–6] and (iii) length

of hospitalization, or time to restoration after being found incompetent.[7–13] However, most studies purporting to have investigated length of stay instead actually examined percentage of patients remaining hospitalized at predetermined time intervals (e.g. patients restored to competency within six months, those restored within one year, etc.) or differences in time hospitalized between those found restorable compared to those found not restorable[7,8,12] rather than actual hospital length of stay.[9–11,13]

Research on the topic of length of stay has been marked by a lack of utilization of clinical variables. The studies mentioned above that investigated length of stay typically examined demographic variables (e.g. age, sex, ethnicity, marital status) and perhaps a single clinical variable, such as diagnosis. Clinical factors that could describe hospital course and response to treatment have not been investigated as thoroughly. Our study sought to extend current research by investigating additional clinical variables likely to impact length of stay in IST patients. Specifically, we were interested in what the variable "number of violent acts while hospitalized" could reveal about hospital length of stay in IST patients, as our hospital's annual reports on patient violence have informally documented a relationship between violence and increased length of stay.[14] We were also interested in how such a clinical variable compared (in terms of relative importance) to the other variables typically studied (such as the demographic variables) in a model used to describe length of stay in these patients. Our hypothesis was that individual patient clinical factors would be more important than demographic factors in a statistical model of patient length of stay.

Methods

This study was reviewed and approved by the California Health and Human Services Agency Committee for the Protection of Human Subjects (CPHS), the IRB with oversight over all research with human subjects in the California Department of State Hospitals (DSH).

Description of Setting

The California DSH operates five different state hospitals across the state, with current populations ranging from 600 to 1,500 patients at each facility. All facilities except the designated Sexually Violent Predator (SVP) hospital treat IST patients. Typical housing is a dorm-style room with unit sizes ranging from 35 to 70 patients. All units for IST patients are single-sex.

Subjects

The study subjects consisted of adult patients (age 18 and greater) admitted under the IST statutes (California Penal Code sections 1367–1376) between January 1, 2010 and June 30, 2018 and included n = 3,748 females and n = 16,292 males with a mean age of 38.4 years (range = 18.0–89.2; SD = 12.6). The total number of patients admitted was 20,041, however a single patient was discharged to an outside hospital on their day of admission and so was not included. Thus, the number of subjects included in the study was N = 20,040 (see Table 36.1 for a full description of subject demographics). Starting point for each patient in the study was their admission date on or after January 1, 2010 through to June 30, 2018. Each patient was tracked until their discharge date or December 31, 2018 (whichever occurred first) to ensure sufficient follow-up time was allowed to record any violent behavior. Patients not discharged by December 31, 2018 were treated as right-censored. Length of stay ranged from 1 day to 1,247 days, with a median of 105 and a mean of 157.4 days (interquartile range 58–189). As the median and interquartile range indicate, most patients were treated and discharged rapidly; only 9.3% of patients were hospitalized for longer than 365 days.

Study Variables

Variables were chosen based on previous research which showed a relation to length of stay, as well clinical expertise in what could reliably differentiate shorter-stay patients from longer-stay patients. As mentioned previously, the annual reports of violence in our hospital system have noted (informally) a link between the number of violent acts by a patient and length of stay; in this study we wished to investigate this formally.[14]

In the current study, the clinical variables of: (i) diagnosis, (ii) number of violent acts, (iii) level of functioning at admission, and (iv) history of previous California DSH hospitalization (potentially a sign of long-term illness chronicity) were included, as these were clinical variables available for all patients. While diagnosis had been studied before, to the best of our knowledge violent acts had not been studied, and the other clinical variables have rarely been included in studies such as this.

To judge the importance of clinical variables in such a model, we also included demographic variables typically included in previous investigations of this topic, such as: (v) age at admission, (vi) treating hospital, (vii) ethnicity, and (viii) sex. In this manner, we could examine how consistent our study was with past studies, as well as compare the importance of clinical variables to demographic variables in modeling patient length of stay.

Data Collection

Patient demographic and legal class information were collected from system databases routinely used for census tracking. Data on violent incidents were collected through the computerized incident management module of the patient treatment planning database.

Diagnosis and level of functioning were collected from the computerized patient treatment planning system.

Regarding diagnosis, for discharged patients the formal discharge diagnosis (DSM-IV-TR or DSM-5)[15,16] given by the treating psychiatrist and team was used, as this would be the most accurate diagnosis. For censored (i.e. not discharged) patients in the study, the most recent treatment team diagnosis was used. Since patients commonly had multiple diagnoses, only the primary diagnosis was used. Over 280 different primary diagnoses were collapsed according to the DSM-5 category or chapter title, and the following eight overarching categories were used: (i) any bipolar diagnosis, (ii) any schizophrenia diagnosis, (iii) any schizoaffective diagnosis, (iv) any other psychotic disorder not schizophrenia or schizoaffective, (v) any neurocognitive or neurodevelopmental disorder, (vi) any mood disorder, (vii) any malingering diagnosis, and finally (viii) an "other" category which included all diagnoses used which did not fall into any previously mentioned category. The number of patients in each category can be seen in Table 36.2.

Table 36.1 Summary of subject demographics by ethnicity

Ethnicity	Number		Age at study start		
			Mean	SD	Range
Overall study	Total	20,040	38.4	12.6	18.0–89.2
	Female	3,748	39.4	11.9	18.0–84.2
	Male	16,292	38.2	12.8	18.1–89.2
African-American	Total	5,998	38.3	12.4	18.1–84.2
	Female	1,185	39.1	11.9	18.9–84.2
	Male	4,813	38.2	12.5	18.1–81.8
Asian	Total	628	40.6	12.7	18.6–89.2
	Female	118	43.5	11.6	21.6–75.0
	Male	510	39.9	12.9	18.6–89.2
Hispanic	Total	5,554	34.7	11.6	18.0–88.3
	Female	859	35.5	10.9	18.0–75.8
	Male	4,695	34.5	11.7	18.1–88.3
Native American	Total	133	37.2	11.4	19.0–67.8
	Female	29	38.9	8.68	20.3–56.1
	Male	104	36.7	12.0	19.0–67.8
Other/Unknown	Total	252	36.3	12.0	18.8–79.9
	Female	24	39.0	12.9	20.8–79.9
	Male	228	36.0	11.9	18.8–75.3
Pacific Islander	Total	323	37.7	12.6	18.4–77.9
	Female	65	39.8	13.6	20.6–77.9
	Male	258	37.2	12.3	18.4–74.7
White	Total	6,981	41.4	12.8	18.2–89.1
	Female	1,468	41.6	11.9	18.8–81.2
	Male	5,513	41.4	13.0	18.2–89.1

Violence during the study was defined as physical assaults directed against either another patient or a staff member, as defined in the California DSH policies (see our earlier article for a full description).[17] Analogous codes and definitions also exist for verbal aggression and property damage, but were not used in this study as we examined only physical violence. A total count of physically violent acts where the patient was determined to be the aggressor was obtained and was studied as the variable of interest. Out of the 20,040 patients in this study, 5,240 (26.1%) had one or more violent acts during their hospitalization (full range for the study population was 0–90), with 2,618 (13.1%) having two or more violent acts.

Level of functioning at admission was collected from the patient admission diagnosis, which included the admission GAF score. While not formally a part of DSM-5, admission GAF scores were still determined by DSH psychiatrists as it served as a quick and standardized method of describing a patient's level of functioning when admitted.[18] The remaining variables (treating hospital, age at admission, previous DSH hospitalization, ethnicity, and sex) were all obtained from the databases used for census tracking and population reports.

Statistical Analyses

Data preparation and analyses were performed with R version 3.5.1.[19] Data files were provided by the centralized data management office of the California DSH for all patients who were in residence or admitted to the hospitals during the periods 2010–2018; from these were extracted the records of all patients resident or admitted to a hospital between January 1, 2010 and June 30, 2018 inclusive and the IST patients were determined based on their legal code at admission. Data files were also provided for all the records of violent acts by patients, which were again further refined to extract just the acts in which physical contact was made or attempted, recorded during the period between January 1, 2010 and December 31, 2018 inclusive.

We first carried out a univariate descriptive analysis of variables potentially related to hospital length of stay using Kaplan–Meier analyses, to evaluate statistical significance of each variable individually. We then conducted a multivariate survival regression utilizing a Weibull parametric survival model to obtain direct quantification of improvement of survival time based on the variables of interest, as compared to the reference level for each variable.[20] A Weibull parametric survival model was chosen because this would facilitate comparisons of length of stay, as well as other distinct advantages over other models.[21] Since the demographic data showed differences in the average age across ethnicities, and we had hypothesized that age would also be related to length of stay, we included the interaction between ethnicity and age at admission in the model as a variable to control for this. Lastly, we evaluated the variables in the model to delineate which variables were most important, as these could potentially be priorities to target in treatments.

Results

Full demographic data are available in Table 36.1, as well as a detailed breakdown by ethnicity. Of the 20,040 study subjects, the primary diagnosis was missing for 83 and admission GAF score was missing for 867 subjects. Inspection of the missing admission GAF scores showed that the missing data were evenly distributed across all years, with no discernible pattern. No data were missing for any patients on the remainder of the variables (age at admission, violence, hospital, ethnicity, sex, or previous admission).

Univariate analyses were conducted on all subjects with the data available for that variable. Multivariate analyses could only be conducted on subjects with complete data for all variables. Since the patients with missing data comprised only 4.7% of the total and complete data was available for 19,091 patients, we decided to drop the cases with missing data from the multivariate analysis, rather than impute missing data.

Each variable was first examined in a univariate analysis. Table 36.2 provides the results of the univariate analyses conducted on each variable, using Kaplan–Meier statistics, showing the median length of stay in days for each variable. For categorical variables, the Kaplan–Meier analyses were carried out by stratifying the levels of the categorical variables; for continuous variables, the variable was divided into blocks and the resulting blocks became the stratification levels (e.g. age at admission was divided into blocks comprised of those aged 18–19, 20–29, 30–39, etc.).

Evaluation of the multivariate model characteristics showed adequate validity of the Weibull distribution for the data when compared to both (a) the quantile-quantile probability plot of observed versus theoretical values, and (b) comparison of Weibull residuals to Kaplan–Meier residuals.[20] The results of the multivariate analysis are shown in Table 36.3, which presents the maximum likelihood estimates of the Weibull model parameters (the β-coefficients) and the exponentiated coefficients (the column labeled "e^{β}").

Clinicians will most likely be interested in the exponentiated coefficients. In the Weibull model exponentiated coefficients are traditionally called "accelerated failure time" statistics, which in this context are better described as "accelerated time to event" statistics (the "event" in this case being discharge). Exponentiated coefficients less than 1 are indicative of a shorter length of stay relative to the reference group (or for continuous variables, indicative of increasing acceleration to discharge, as the value decreases from 1). Exponentiated coefficients greater than 1 indicate a longer length of stay relative to the reference group (for continuous variables, exponentiated coefficients greater than 1 indicate increasing time to discharge, the higher the value). As an example, Table 36.3 shows that a diagnosis of bipolar disorder has an exponentiated coefficient value of 0.558 (95% CI 0.536–0.581), indicating an "accelerated time to discharge" (i.e. decreased length of stay) by a factor of 0.558 when compared to the reference level diagnosis of schizophrenia.

Using these coefficients in the model, one can calculate the projected length of stay for categories of patients. Extending the example mentioned in the previous paragraph, using a prototypic patient with reference or median values (for example, a diagnosis of schizophrenia, median age = 36.01, no violent acts,

Table 36.2 Summary of univariate Kaplan–Meier Analyses for hospital length of stay (LOS), in days

Variable	N	Median LOS	Lower 95% CI	Upper 95% CI
Primary diagnosis	83 obs missing			
Bipolar	2,023	77	76	78
Malingering	772	49	49	53
Neurocognitive	445	194	171	217
Other	1,625	64	62	70
Personality	201	50	44	56
Psychosis (other)	1,824	77	73	77
Schizoaffective	3,716	119	113	121
Schizophrenia	9,351	126	124	129
Age at admission	No missing obs			
18–19	343	81	76	93
20–29	5,944	92	91	97
30–39	5,620	98	92	99
40–49	3,981	105	104	110
50–59	3,105	126	119	131
60–69	939	147	140	164
70+	198	203	187	246
Total violent acts	No missing obs			
0 (none)	14,800	92	91	93
1	2,622	119	117	126
2	1,093	145	136	155
3–4	829	161	148	175
5–9	492	202	189	218
10+	204	316	273	382
Hospital	No missing obs			
Hospital A	3,225	106	105	112
Hospital B	4,014	127	125	129
70 or higher	50	42	35	63
Ethnicity	No missing obs			
African-American	5,998	98	93	99
Asian	628	133	120	147
Hispanic	5,554	105	104	109
Native American	133	111	92	146
Other/Unknown	252	111	98	131
Pacific Islander	323	126	112	140
White	7,152	105	101	106
Sex	No missing obs			
Female	3,748	91	88	97
Male	16,292	106	105	108
Previous admission	No missing obs			
No	12,805	97	93	98
Yes	7,235	119	115	120

Table 36.3 Summary of multivariate parametric survival model statistics

Variable	β	S.E.	Wald Z	Pr(>|Z|)	exp(β)	95% CI
(Intercept)	4.7856	0.0418	114.51	< 0.0001		
Primary diagnosis						
Bipolar	−0.5834	0.0206	−28.28	<0.0001	0.558	0.536–0.581
Malingering	−0.7970	0.0308	−25.90	<0.0001	0.451	0.424–0.479
Neurocognitive	0.0288	0.0418	0.69	0.4897	1.029	0.948–1.117
Other	−0.5215	0.0227	−23.00	<0.0001	0.594	0.568–0.621
Personality	−0.8203	0.0599	−13.69	<0.0001	0.440	0.392–0.495
Psychosis (other)	−0.4846	0.0213	−22.79	<0.0001	0.616	0.591–0.642
Schizophrenia	0				1	
Schizoaffective	−0.1390	0.0162	−8.60	<0.0001	0.870	0.843–0.898
Age at admission	0.0162	0.0008	20.99	<0.0001	1.016	1.015–1.018
Total violent acts	0.0947	0.0037	25.44	<0.0001	1.099	1.091–1.107
Treating hospital						
Hospital A	0.0193	0.0173	1.11	0.2799	1.019	0.985–1.055
Hospital B	0.1012	0.0168	6.02	<0.0001	1.107	1.071–1.144
Hospital C	0.2468	0.0159	15.57	<0.0001	1.280	1.241–1.322
Hospital D	0				1	
Admission GAF score	−0.0084	0.0007	−12.66	<0.0001	0.992	0.990–0.993
Ethnicity						
African-American	0.0310	0.0477	0.65	0.5148	1.032	0.940–1.133
Asian	0.0587	0.1187	0.49	0.6210	1.060	0.840–1.338
Hispanic	0.1012	0.0477	2.12	0.0340	1.106	1.008–1.215
Native American	0.7782	0.2663	2.92	0.0035	2.178	1.292–3.670
Other/Unknown	−0.0750	0.1794	−0.42	0.6760	0.9278	0.6528–1.319
Pacific Islander	0.1119	0.1431	0.78	0.4343	1.118	0.845–1.481
White	0				1	
Sex						
Female	−0.1035	0.0156	−6.64	<0.0001	0.902	0.875–0.930
Male	0				1	
Previous admission						
No	0				1	
Yes	0.0373	0.0128	2.91	0.0036	1.038	1.012–1.064
Interaction terms						
Age at admission * African-American	−0.0016	0.0011	−1.43	0.1516	0.9984	0.996–1.001
Age at admission * Asian	0.0053	0.0028	1.88	0.0596	1.005	0.999–1.011
Age at admission * Hispanic	0.0001	0.0012	0.08	0.9351	1.000	0.998–1.002
Age at admission * Native American	−0.0218	0.0070	−3.12	0.0018	0.978	0.965–0.992
Age at admission * Other/Unknown	0.0058	0.0047	1.22	0.2237	1.006	0.996–1.015
Age at admission * Pacific Islander	0.0023	0.0036	0.63	0.5309	1.002	0.995–1.009
Age at admission * * White	0				1	

Table 36.4 Summary of variable importance in the multivariate model

Variable	X^2-Df	Deviance	Df	Deviance / Df	BIC
Primary diagnosis	1896.31	2014.08	7	287.73	1945.08
Age at admission	1057.52	745.02	1	745.02	735.16
Total violent acts	646.10	1051.94	1	1051.94	1042.08
Treating hospital	256.37	283.07	3	94.36	253.51
Admission GAF score	159.40	157.53	1	157.53	98.39
Ethnicity	147.02	149.15	6	24.86	139.29
Sex	43.12	46.84	1	46.84	36.99
Age at admission * ethnicity	12.86	17.58	6	2.93	−41.49
Previous admission	7.46	8.5	1	8.5	−1.36

treating hospital D, admission GAF score median = 31, white, male, with no previous admission), one can compute a median length of stay of 123.94 days. By altering the diagnosis to bipolar but keeping all other variables constant, the calculated median length of stay is 69.16 days. As can be seen, dividing these numbers and rounding yields 0.558, showing that the time to discharge for the example bipolar patient was "accelerated," and that the length of stay differed proportionally by the exponentiated coefficient for bipolar disorder, when compared to the reference diagnosis of schizophrenia.

Summarizing the multivariate results presented in Table 36.3, all diagnoses had a significantly shorter length of stay than the reference diagnosis (schizophrenia) with the exception of neurocognitive disorders (which also included neurodevelopmental disorders). Age at admission had the effect of increasing the length of stay as age increased, e^β= 1.016 (95% CI 1.015–1.018). Violent acts had the effect of increasing length of stay as the number of violent acts increased, e^β = 1.099 (95% CI 1.091–1.107). The findings for the variable treating hospital were mixed as two hospitals had a statistically significant longer length of stay than the reference hospital (which had the most admissions); the remaining hospital also had a longer length of stay but the result was not statistically significant. Level of functioning at admission (as measured by the admission GAF score) was also significant with an exponentiated coefficient of = 0.992 (95% CI 0.990–0.993), indicating that patients with a higher level of functioning had a shorter length of stay. Regarding ethnicity, due to differences in the median age across groups, an interaction term was included in the model to control

for these differences. Compared to the reference group (whites), both Hispanics = 1.106 (95% CI 1.008–1.215) and Native Americans = 2.178 (95% CI 1.292–3.670) had a longer length of stay. Compared to males (the reference group), females had a shorter length of stay with e^β= 0.902 (95% CI 0.875–0.930). Having a previous admission increased the length of stay e^β= 1.038 (95% CI 1.012–1.064) compared to not having had a previous admission.

To better aid clinicians in identifying target variables for treatment prioritization, we evaluated each variable for its importance in the model. We first used the traditional method of computing the proportion of explainable log-likelihood for each variable (the chi-square statistic minus its degrees of freedom) for assessing the partial effect of each variable in the model.[20] Using these results to guide order of entry, each variable was then entered into the model one step at a time and we computed: (a) the deviance for each variable, (b) the deviance penalized by degrees of freedom, and (c) the Bayesian information criteria (BIC), for each variable.[22]

As can be seen in Table 36.4, these various methods consistently found that: (1) diagnosis, (2) number of violent acts, and (3) age at admission were the most important variables in the model. The other variables (treating hospital, level of functioning at admission, ethnicity, sex, previous admission), while statistically significant, were not as influential in the model as these three variables.

Discussion

This study examined the significance and relation of clinical and demographic variables to hospital length of stay for patients involuntarily committed to

California state psychiatric hospitals under the state's IST statutes. In addition to finding significant differences in length of stay for the clinical and demographic variables studied, our study found that the most important variables in the model for determining length of stay were diagnosis, number of violent acts, and age at admission. These findings highlight that variables describing a patient's clinical status and response to treatment were important in the model determining length of stay, more so than demographic variables typically used in many previous studies. Clinicians, policymakers, and researchers looking at this topic should be actively seeking ways to include more patient clinical variables in their studies to better inform treatment and policy decisions.

Regarding diagnosis, our study found that patients diagnosed with schizophrenia (the largest single patient group) had statistically significant longer lengths of stay at the hospital than all other diagnoses, with the exception of those diagnosed with a neurocognitive disorder. While our study cannot definitively answer "why" diagnoses had different lengths of stay, the finding that patients diagnosed with schizophrenia or a neurocognitive disorder had longer lengths of stay than other diagnoses raises several issues. A concern with treating psychosis or neurocognitive disorders is the issue of patients not benefitting from treatment, or "treatment resistance," which is typically described as affecting up to 30% of patients with a psychotic mental disorder.[23] While the length of stay for study subjects overall was relatively short (median length of stay overall was 105 days, interquartile range 58–189 days), the rate of patients hospitalized longer than a year was 9.3% for all diagnoses, 22.5% for patients with a neurocognitive disorder, and 12.4% for those with a primary diagnosis of schizophrenia.

Recent research examining treatment resistance in schizophrenia has pointed out several factors, including issues of cognitive functioning or cognitive disability in schizophrenia.[23,24] A study which conducted long-term follow-up of schizophrenia patients showed that those with the poorest response to treatment typically had higher rates of negative symptoms and worse cognitive functioning at baseline.[25] Likewise, another study recently found that measures of cognitive functioning accurately predicted treatment response to antipsychotic medication, even when there were no differences in measures of psychopathology between treatment responders and nonreponders.[24]

Given the relation between poor treatment response and cognitive functioning, it is worth noting that cognitive impairment of some form is considered a hallmark of schizophrenia.[26–28] Generally, in our hospitals, we have found most patients actively psychotic are stabilized with the use of antipsychotic medication early in their hospital stay. However, treatments to restore trial competency are not just pharmacological but are also didactic and involve procedures that can be cognitively challenging.[8,29] For example, competency restoration activities such as a "mock trial" entail role-playing, behavioral rehearsal, and abstract reasoning about case factors as well as anticipating arguments from the prosecution and weighing alternative ideas, such as chance of success for various alternatives. A factor in longer length of stay for patients diagnosed with schizophrenia and neurocognitive disorders could be cognitive issues which impact their ability to learn relevant facts and apply this learning to their case in a manner that demonstrates to a treatment team enough understanding and progress to be returned to court as restored to competency.

While it could be argued that the same cognitive deficits are also found in other serious mental illness disorders (such as bipolar disorder) recent research focused on this question has found that cognitive deficits in those diagnosed with bipolar disorder are much less severe, and if present have the greatest impact during acute episodes and not while under treatment.[30,31] Also, in patients diagnosed with bipolar disorder, severity of the cognitive impairment is directly related to the severity of the psychotic symptoms.[32] This may explain why relative to those diagnosed with schizophrenia, the patients diagnosed with bipolar disorders had a much shorter length of stay, while those diagnosed with schizoaffective disorder had a length of stay more consistent with the patients diagnosed with schizophrenia.

Regarding violence while hospitalized, to the best of our knowledge, ours was the first study to examine patient violence as a factor in length of stay in IST patients. In our study, patient violence while hospitalized was both statistically significant in the model and was also one of the most important variables influencing length of stay. This was consistent with our belief that clinical variables reflective of a patient's current level of psychopathology or response to treatment are more informative about their length of stay than demographic variables. This was also consistent with our clinical experience, in which we have noted a pattern to violence, response to treatment, and subsequent length of stay.[14]

We should note that not all patients in the study were violent. Although all study subjects were involuntarily hospitalized while facing felony charges and considered "dangerous" due to this, only 26.1% were violent during their hospital stay. However, our analyses (both univariate and multivariate) showed that if a patient was violent during their hospitalization, this behavior was meaningful and had a significant impact on extending their length of stay.

Consistent with the other studies that directly investigated length of stay, this study showed that younger patients typically had a shorter length of stay than older patients. Again, while our study cannot directly point to "why" this is, it could be possible that age acted as a proxy variable for the long-term effects of life-long chronic mental illness, i.e. older patients have had the disease longer and are more likely to be impacted by the debilitating disease effects on domains such as cognition and learning, in addition to medical problems associated with other factors (e.g. cardiovascular disease, metabolic syndrome, etc.).[33] Thus, it is possible the impact of age on length of stay could be due to the interplay between serious mental illness and its longer-term debilitating effects on health and cognition over the course of the patient's life.

The finding that treating hospital had a statistically significant impact on length of stay is also consistent with previous research.[12,13] In our study, the hospital that treated the most forensic patients had the shortest median length of stay. This is consistent with the finding by Morris and Parker, who found that the state hospital dedicated to treating forensic patients had the shortest length of stay, when compared to the other hospitals which did not specialize in treating these forensic patients.[12] This finding emphasizes that hospitals not well-practiced in specialized programs required for IST treatment could likely have longer lengths of stay.[1]

Our finding that level of functioning at admission, while statistically significant, was not as important as other variables is understandable in that most patients actively psychotic can be stabilized relatively quickly with medication. However, treatment for restoration of competency, as discussed earlier, is extensive beyond just psychiatric stabilization. Treatment for competency restoration also involves didactic teaching and cognitively challenging tasks addressed at having the patient anticipate and prepare for hypothetical circumstances in court as well as anticipating ways to mitigate challenges and engage resources (such as cooperating with their attorney) for a better court outcome. We should note, however, the measure used (admission GAF score) has known limitations and potentially a more focused measure of functioning could have been more informative.[18]

Demographic variables such as ethnicity and sex, while statistically significant, were not as important statistically as the clinical variables discussed above. Of concern was the finding that Native-American patients overall had a significantly longer length of stay. Due to the small number in the study (compared to other ethnic groups), there was large variation in individual patient length of stay, which limits conclusions. However, this finding merits future study. Likewise, previous admission was statistically significant, yet not as important as the other variables examined.

Clinicians often ask, "Which variable is most important?" to receive guidance on treatment prioritization. Variable importance is a complicated topic (especially in terms of "clinical" versus "statistical" importance). However, there are several methods of evaluating variables for their importance in an analysis. While the differing methods yielded slight differences, all the currently accepted methods of determining variable importance consistently placed diagnosis, violence while hospitalized, and age at admission in the top three most important variables. Our results add to, and are consistent with another study, which studied a smaller subset of variables consisting largely of demographic (but not clinical) variables.[13,34] This emphasizes the importance of utilizing clinical variables when studying clinical outcomes, such as length of stay.

The present study is not without its limitations. With the size of the staff involved, lack of inter-rater reliability checks among the diagnosing psychiatrists is a limitation, but a reality that exists in clinical settings. The use of a system-specific special incident tracking tool for violence limits comparability with other studies. However, the fact that the violence reporting form was integrated into regular nursing duties likely was advantageous, as it meant that the nursing staff did not view completing the form as an extra duty and enabled the collection of data for a far longer period of time than in previous studies. This also likely reduced under-reporting. The fact that the prevalence of violence in our study was at levels comparable to other studies, or even higher than some other studies, provides assurance that violent incidents were routinely reported and were not systematically overlooked. The collapsing of the patient's diagnoses into overarching DSM-IV-TR or DSM-5 diagnostic categories undoubtedly led to a loss of specificity. However, given the fact that there were over 280 different primary Axis I diagnoses, few options existed for us to present diagnostic data in a concise, meaningful way.

Conclusions

Our study found significance between length of stay and the clinical and demographic variables studied. Our analysis indicated that the most important variables in the model were: (1) diagnosis, (2) number of physically violent acts, and (3) age at admission. These findings point to the need for implementing treatments aimed at mitigating these factors. The fact that patients diagnosed with schizophrenia or neurocognitive disorders spent significantly longer time hospitalized compared to other diagnostic groups shows that assessment and treatment of learning and cognitive abilities should be highlighted early in admission. These patients may need smaller groups and more focused interventions addressed at their cognitive strengths, rather than traditional treatment interventions. Age at admission may be an important factor as it can impact various aspects of a patient's functioning and health, such as increasing health issues in older patients, long-term effects of co-morbid medical issues commonly found in the seriously mentally ill (e.g. cardiovascular disease, diabetes), as well as cognitive issues seen in older patients with serious mental illness.

The finding that violence by a patient while hospitalized significantly increased length of stay points to the need to assess patients for violence risk factors early in their hospital stay, and to conduct routine violence risk assessments throughout the duration of their stay. Violence should also be considered a clinical target for both psychopharmacological and psychosocial treatment. While the issue of violence by the mentally ill in the general population may be controversial, the issue of violence in patients recently jailed for serious crimes and involuntarily hospitalized for competency restoration should be a treatment priority routinely addressed in this population.

Funding

This research received no specific grant from any funding agency, commercial, or not-for-profit sectors.

Disclosures

Dr. Broderick has nothing to disclose.

Dr. Azizian has nothing to disclose.

Dr. Warburton has nothing to disclose.

References

1. National Association of State Mental Health Program Directors. Assessment #10: Forensic Patients in State Psychiatric Hospitals: 1999–2016. 2017. https://nasmhpd.org/sites/default/files/TACPaper.10.Forensic-Patients-in-State-Hospitals_508C_v2.pdf (accessed June 2020).

2. Bellisle M. After paying $83 million in fines, Washington settles jail mental-health lawsuit. *Seattle Times*. December 12, 2018.

3. Pirelli G, Gottdiener WH, Zapf PA. A meta-analytic review of competency to stand trial research. *Psychol Public Policy Law*. 2011; **17**(1): 1–53.

4. Gay JG, Vitacco MJ, Ragatz L. Mental health symptoms predict competency to stand trial and competency restoration success. *Legal Criminol Psychol*. 2017; **22**(2): 288–301.

5. Morris DR, DeYoung NJ. Long-term competence restoration. *J Am Acad Psychiatry Law*. 2014; **42**(1): 81–90.

6. Morris DR, Parker GF. Effects of advanced age and dementia on restoration of competence to stand trial. *Int J Law Psychiatry*. 2009; **32**(3): 156–160.

7. Grossi LM, Green D, Schneider M, et al. Personality, psychiatric, and cognitive predictors of length of time for competency to stand trial restoration. *Int J Forensic Ment Health*. 2018; **17**(2): 167–180.

8. Colwell LH, Gianesini J. Demographic, criminogenic, and psychiatric factors that predict competency restoration. *J Am Acad Psychiatry Law*. 2011; **39**(3): 297–306.

9. Toofanian Ross P, Padula CB, Nitch SR, et al. Cognition and competency restoration: using the RBANS to predict length of stay for patients deemed incompetent to stand trial. *Clin Neuropsychol*. 2015; **29**(1): 150–165.

10. Nicholson RA, Barnard GW, Robbins L, et al. Predicting treatment outcome for incompetent defendants. *Bull Am Acad Psychiatry Law*. 1994; **22**(3): 367–377.

11. Mossman D. Predicting restorability of incompetent criminal defendants. *J Am Acad Psychiatry Law*. 2007; **35**(1): 34–43.

12. Morris DR, Parker GF. Jackson's Indiana: state hospital competence restoration in Indiana. *J Am Acad Psychiatry Law.* 2008; **36**(4): 522–534.

13. Renner M, Newark C, Bartos BJ, McCleary R, Scurich N. Length of stay for 25,791 California patients found incompetent to stand trial. *J Forens Legal Med.* 2017; **51**: 22–26.

14. Department of State Hospitals. Violence Report DSH 2010–2017. 2019. https://web.archive.org/web/20190 729220318/https://www.dsh.ca.gov/Publications/Rep orts_and_Data/docs/Violence_Report_DSH_2010–2 017.pdf (accessed January 2020).

15. American Psychiatric Association. *Diagnostic and Statistical Manual of Mental Disorders, 4th edn. Text Revision (DSM-IV-TR®).* Washington, DC: American Psychiatric Association Publishing; 2000.

16. American Psychiatric Association. *Diagnostic and Statistical Manual of Mental Disorders, 5th edn. (DSM-5®).* Washington, DC: American Psychiatric Association Publishing; 2013.

17. Broderick C, Azizian A, Kornbluh R, et al. Prevalence of physical violence in a forensic psychiatric hospital system during 2011–2013: patient assaults, staff assaults, and repeatedly violent patients. *CNS Spectr.* 2015; **20**(3): 319–330.

18. Monrad AIH. Global Assessment of Functioning (GAF) properties and frontier of current knowledge. *Ann Gen Psychiatry.* 2010; **9**(1): 20.

19. R Core Team. R: a language and environment for statistical computing. R Foundation for Statistical Computing; 2018. www.r-project.org/about.html (accessed June 2020).

20. Harrell FE. *Regression Modeling Strategies: With Applications to Linear Models, Logistic and Ordinal Regression, and Survival Analysis.* New York and Switzerland: Springer International Publishing; 2015.

21. Carroll KJ. On the use and utility of the Weibull model in the analysis of survival data. *Controlled Clin Trials.* 2003; **24**(6): 682–701.

22. Hilbe JM. *Logistic Regression Models.* Boca Raton, FL: CRC Press; 2009.

23. Kinon BJ. The group of Treatment-Resistant Schizophrenias: heterogeneity in Treatment-Resistant Schizophrenia (TRS). *Front Psychiatry.* 2018; **9**(9): 757.

24. Bak N, Ebdrup BH, Oranje B, et al. Two subgroups of antipsychotic-naive, first-episode schizophrenia patients identified with a Gaussian mixture model on cognition and electrophysiology. *Transl Psychiatry.* 2017; **7**(4): e1087.

25. Chang WC, Ho RWH, Tang JYM, et al. Early-stage negative symptom trajectories and relationships with 13-year outcomes in first-episode nonaffective psychosis. *Schizophr Bull.* 2019; **45**(3): 610–619.

26. Elvevag B, Goldberg TE. Cognitive impairment in schizophrenia is the core of the disorder. *Crit Rev Neurobiol.* 2000; **14**(1): 1–21.

27. Green MF. Cognitive impairment and functional outcome in schizophrenia and bipolar disorder. *J Clin Psychiatry.* 2006; **67**(9): 3–8; discussion 36–42.

28. MacCabe JH. Population-based cohort studies on premorbid cognitive function in schizophrenia. *Epidemiol Rev.* 2008; **30**: 77–83.

29. Schwalbe E, Medalia A. Cognitive dysfunction and competency restoration: using cognitive remediation to help restore the unrestorable. *J Am Acad Psychiatry Law.* 2007; **35**(4): 518–525.

30. Palmer BW, Loughran CI, Meeks TW. Cognitive impairment among older adults with late-life schizophrenia or bipolar disorder. *Continuum (Minneap Minn).* 2010; **16**(2): 135–152.

31. Reichenberg A, Weiser M, Rabinowitz J, et al. A population-based cohort study of premorbid intellectual, language, and behavioral functioning in patients with schizophrenia, schizoaffective disorder, and nonpsychotic bipolar disorder. *Am J Psychiatry.* 2002; **159**(12): 2027–2035.

32. Lewandowski KE, Whitton AE, Pizzagalli DA, et al. Reward learning, neurocognition, social cognition, and symptomatology in psychosis. *Front Psychiatry.* 2016; **7**: 100.

33. Fagiolini A, Goracci A. The effects of undertreated chronic medical illnesses in patients with severe mental disorders. *J Clin Psychiatry.* 2009; **70**(3): 22–29.

34. Scurich N. Personal communication requesting clarification of table dated November 14, 2017. ed.

Severe Mentally Ill Patients: Our Global Migrants

Neuroethical Issues in Psychiatry and Pharmacology Today. A Brief Manifesto Toward the World Symposium 2021

Alberto Carrara

The overarching aim of this editorial is to present a dream: a World Symposium in the eternal city of Rome in which prominent psychiatric experts, neuroethicists, and lawyers dialogue on severe mentally ill patients as our global migrants. The aim is to foster an inclusive and fruitful interdisciplinary conversation and draw up practical proposals in order to protect and promote the dignity of human persons afflicted by severe mental disorders.

Clausen and Levy define neuroethics as a real, systematic, and informed reflection on and interpretation of neuroscience and related sciences of the mind (psychology in all its many forms, psychiatry, artificial intelligence, and so on), in order to understand its implications for human self-understanding and the perils and prospects of its applications. Neuroethics has developed as a response to the increasing power and pervasiveness of the sciences of the brain and the mind.[1]

According to the World Health Organization (WHO), good mental health is related to mental and psychological wellbeing. It is amply documented but little is known that mental disorders affect one in four people around the globe. Moreover, we are still facing the complex and social issue of abolishing the stigma of mental illnesses. Mental dysfunctions rooted in the nervous system's disorders are still not considered on the same level as cardiovascular disease, cancer, kidney disease, and other illnesses. Although public knowledge about neurosystemic mental diseases is usually seen as valuable, knowledge about severe mental illness (SMI) is often disregarded. As a consequence, many persons suffering from severe mental disorders still avoid asking for help, and they may not receive appropriate therapeutic and social support also due to the community's lack of awareness.[2] Out of a world population of 7.7 billion, 2% suffer from an SMI. Depression affects about 264 million people (2.7% males; 4.1% females); anxiety disorders strike around 284 million individuals (2.8% males; 4.7% females); bipolar disorder amounts to 46 million; whereas eating disorders and schizophrenia affect around 16 million and 20 million, respectively (https://ourworldindata.org/mental-health).

To give a sense of the scale of the problem, the contemporary global migration crisis involves roughly the same amount of individuals.

The subject of psychiatry is not a brain, a dysfunctional piece of neural tissue, but human patients, whom can be compared to our society's eternal migrants who have never had a home. In addition, there is the correlated tragedy of suicide: one person dies every 40 seconds. Every suicide has long-lasting effects on the people left behind.

In Pope Francis' Message for the 105th World Day of Migrants and Refugees 2019 (September 29, 2019), he repeatedly highlights the fact that the contemporary migration burden is not just about migrants, but instead is about evil, terrorism, violent conflicts, all-out wars that continue to tear humanity apart. Injustices and discrimination follow one upon the other, economic and social imbalances on a local or global scale, individualism, utilitarian mentality, indifference, and so forth. At the end, and above all, it is the poorest of the poor and the most disadvantaged who pay the price.

How can we fail to recognize a very close analogy, or even, an identification between our SMI patients and today's migrants? They are all extremely vulnerable people seeking help.

In order to promote mental wellbeing, to prevent severe mental disorders, and to protect human rights and the care of people affected by those painful conditions, herein, we propose *a global call for action* focused on a gathering in Rome of experts in the field of medicine, psychiatry, pharmacology, and neuroethics, as well as law, and others. The aim is to foster an inclusive and fruitful interdisciplinary dialogue and present proposals able to protect and promote the dignity of the human person afflicted by severe mental disorders. Our speakers could organize their topics around Pope Francis' four key verbs – *"welcome, protect, promote, integrate"* – concerning the nature, treatment, ethical issues, and policies related to SMI. Our "guiding star" of reflection is the protection and promotion of all SMI patients as human persons. They are also members of our Common Home: our real existential peripheries, which we need to attend with specific and effective proposals.[3]

Designed by Stephen M. Stahl, Donatella Marazziti, Armando Piccinni, and myself, the First World Symposium 2021 on "Severe Mentally Ill Patients: Our Global Migrants. Ethical, Legal, and Social Issues in Psychiatry and Pharmacology Today" will take place in Rome at the European University of Rome (via degli Aldobrandeschi, 190). Numerous institutions are involved, among which I want to mention and thank the Pontifical Academy for Life in the person of its President, Bishop Vincenzo Paglia.

Each day, experts in medicine and neuroethics will discuss the main questions related to SMI migrants. For example, is there free will when you are psychotic? Does incompetence entail loss of free will? What is the meaning of life if you suffer from schizophrenia? Why has this illness been shunned by humanity over the centuries? Can religious faiths help find the right options? What does SMI teach us about ourselves?

During the symposium, Pope Francis himself will speak on the relevance of ethical reflections in psychiatry.

Disclosure

Alberto Carrara has nothing to disclose.

References

1. Clausen J, Levy N. *Handbook of Neuroethics.* Dordrecht, Netherlands: Springer; 2015.

2. Mannarini S, Rossi A. Assessing mental illness stigma: A complex issue. *Front Psychol.* 2019; **9**: 2722. doi:10.3389/fpsyg.2018.02722.

3. Pope Francis. *Encyclical Letter Laudato si'.* Rome, Italy: Ignatius Press; 2015.

Index